Integrated Behavioral Healt

MW00803279

degree from the point of view that they still are not really aware of what is going on inside of them. Full responsibility for their actions does not come until there is full awareness, although the responsibility to be courteous, considerate, compassionate, and kind is *always* there, whether they are aware or not.

If someone had been able to observe the beginning of the whole issue in childhood, and if that someone had been able to help the person in question understand the inner workings of the fear that then created the unconscious defense mechanism, then that person might have never come to be an adult with all these issues that have such a pervasively toxic influence on many of his/her relationships, as well as on the well-being of his own heart.

Some Causes of Emotional Unavailability & Neediness

As I imagine you realize, this is not a precise science. Even the DSM-5 (The Diagnostic and Statistical Manual of Mental Disorders, a widely-distributed classification and diagnostic tool published by the American Psychiatric Association) is under continual scrutiny and wide-spread criticism because there is little agreement about how to diagnose disorders that for some might appear to be measurable, and for others less so. Those of us who work with the human mind, heart, and soul observe certain behaviors and draw conclusions. We then attempt to understand if those behaviors may be due to factors that took place in childhood, or to later trauma, or, perhaps, to chemical imbalances in the brain and body, or other causes.

A vitally important element that is most often not taken into account, not understood, and may even be studiously ignored is the soul (also called non-local consciousness). Such ignoring may have a very deleterious effect on our well-being, and of course on helping those who seek people such as myself out with the hope of finding solutions to their pain.

Attachment Issues

The attachment bond that is so crucially important to early childhood development, and that depends on someone being available to the child from birth onward, in a lovingly continuous, caring, responsible, and dependable fashion, for this attachment bond to be healthy, has been written about at length in countless clinical and lay books. Particularly the first two years of life lie within the timeframe that concerns us with regards to the manner in which the later emotional development might be affected negatively.

What happens when that bond is not healthy, or, at least not as healthy as it could be, is a major reason why professionals that work in my field are able to have clients. This is at the base of one of the greatest issues people have in their emotional and relational life. Poor attachment bonds create all manner of difficulties in trusting and relating to others - whoever those others may be - and they create those problems due in part to the difficulty the individual has not only in expressing emotionally, but also in accepting, understanding, and empathizing with emotional expression from others. Furthermore, lacking healthy attachment bonds also leads to a lack of self-love and poor boundaries, to name only a few of the added difficulties such individuals face.

It's not difficult to understand the origin of this problem. Another matter is solving it. As small children we give our hearts easily and willingly. The first people we give them to are almost always our parents, or whoever it is that spends most of their time taking care of us. But it is in the confines of this early relationship that we can find the seed of the adult relationship problem.

Am I saying it is the fault of our parents? Not necessarily. It might simply be the mistaken perception of the child that believes subconsciously and subliminally that love is painful. In this chapter we will examine several cases where what the child perceived was abandonment, when in fact, it was not. And even if it were the fault of our parents, we would then need to examine (with compassion) how they themselves grew up, and what happened to *their* hearts at that early stage of *their* lives at the hands of their own parents, and so forth.

Early childhood attachment is a theory espoused by developmental psychologists John Bowlby and Mary Ainsworth that basically states that depending on the degree of safety and security a child feels due to its relationship with its primary caretaker in the early years of life (and this of course depends largely on the self-awareness that the same caretaker has, the sense of inner security that caretaker has, and the relationship that caretaker has with his or her *own* emotions, as well as how much of an *adult* the parent/caretaker is, and that is not necessarily a question of chronological age, as well as whether he has learned how to love himself), there will be a greater or lesser degree of comfort in close relationships in later life.

The relationship with our primary caregiver in childhood, that is, the main person or persons who are in charge of taking care of us, is largely responsible for how our attachment bonds are formed. By means of an experiment in which children are brought to an office or lab – a place where the children have not been before - and then briefly separated from their parents, developmental psychologists have concluded that there are four main types of attachment that impact our psycho-emotional health, our adult relationships, the manner in which we love, or do not love ourselves, and of course, our concept of ourselves. These are:

- **Secure Attachment**
  These children explore happily while the parent is still in the room, they get upset when he leaves and are comforted when he returns. They also know they can

count on the parent for comfort when they are upset because of the way the parent normally responds to the child. If a stranger comforts them while they are upset, they respond well, but clearly prefer the parent. This parent responds well and lovingly to the child at all times.

- **Avoidant Attachment**
  These children explore, but not in connection with the parent. When the parent leaves, they are not upset, nor are they happy when the parent returns and if the parent picks them up they turn away, and show little reaction. If a stranger tries to connect with them they react in a similar – avoidant - fashion. The kind of parent these children have does not react in loving and helpful ways to the distressed child, and further, has shown the child that he prefers the child not to cry and furthermore, that *independence* from – and not *need* for - the parent is a desirable trait.

- **Ambivalent / Resistant Attachment**
  These children distrust strangers, become very upset when the parent leaves but cannot be consoled when the parent returns. There may be low maternal availability in the home or the parent may be inconsistent between appropriate and neglectful behavior. In other words, the child lacks consistent loving reactions from the parent and hence does not know what to expect, which in turn causes him to not know how to react.

- **Disorganized Attachment**
  These children have a lack of clear attachment type. When the parent returns to the room, the child may freeze or rock itself. The parent may be frightened or frightening, may be withdrawn, intrusive or abusive. Because the child feels both comforted and frightened

by the parent, it becomes confused and disorganized in its attachment.

If the attachment bond we formed with our parents was not secure, there is a reasonably high chance that we experience some – or much - difficulty in loving the self. This will negatively impact our adult relationships as well, until we seek conscious awareness and understanding. (For more about his topic, see Chapter 14).

You can well begin to imagine how a child - who is now an adult - with any but the secure attachment type enumerated above might behave in a relationship such as a marriage, or otherwise committed live-in situation. There could be a continual push-pull situation. One day this partner loves you and seeks out your company, and may even surprise you with needy, dependent, or obsessive, possessive, and controlling behavior; another day he/she may be cool, even cold, rejecting, indifferent, and distant. You never quite know where you stand with such a partner. Clearly poor attachment in childhood ties in very closely with emotional unavailability and neediness.

The less securely attached a child was in his early life, the more he will balk at close emotional ties, or the more he may seek to establish ties (all the while filled with yearning) that often quickly devolve into neediness, or the more he will be at great odds with those ties, even if he/she opens his heart to them. The work of the therapist is to find ways during sessions to offer a new road (in the safety of the therapist's office: that safe, sacred and holy place that Jung called the *temenos*) to that security that was missing in early life in the relationship with the primary caretaker. This of course implies that eventually the client will be able to find that safety and security within, and once it is placed there, it can no longer be threatened by emotions in the same way it is continually being threatened as long as the client is seeking safety and security through the relationship with *another* as opposed to with the self.

If you become aware of pulling in your emotions on more than one occasion; if you become aware of feelings of discomfort when you begin to get too emotionally close to someone, or he/she demands greater emotional closeness from you, and you find such a request unreasonable, then the fact that you are becoming *aware* of this is telling you something about yourself.

I remember an instance of a female client who was in a relationship with a married man. He seemed to always hold her at arm's length, and her pain at this distance from him was often at the forefront of our sessions. Nevertheless, when he left her for another woman, although he stayed with his wife, my client eventually found another man - who was *also* married. This clearly demonstrated our principle of insecure attachment leading to dis-ease, or lack of *ease* in close relationships. She was far more comfortable with a man who was not truly available for her than she would have been with one who made emotional demands on her. In some fashion by living like this she did not need to solve her underlying issue because her very way of life allowed her to live within the safe confines of her emotional comfort zone.

And so we return once more to the manner in which you distance yourself from your emotions. You may find yourself uncomfortable around your own emotions. You are probably also uncomfortable around the emotions of others. You may notice that you find it easy to display emotions when you watch a movie or see something sad on the news because in both instances the people involved (movie actors or hungry children in a sub-Saharan country) have nothing personal to do with you. Are you recognizing bits of yourself?

Distant or Cold Parents

While a parent who is cold and distant might contribute to the underlying factors for poor or unhealthy attachment bonds, in fact, this may occasionally not be the case. In my files, I have instances of parents who appear to have been reasonably adequate in those early bonding years, and yet due to any number of later circumstances became more distant and cold, perhaps even disapproving in the next (still crucial) part of someone's early childhood. Some of those circumstances may be due to: hardships suffered by the parent during war, death of the spouse, death of another child in the family, an unexpected turn for the worse financially causing greater stress, or more work, or both, and hence less quality time for the child, all of which of course, in the case of a truly adult and mature parent, would not cause such cold and distant behavior, but in the case that applies to most of us before we become conscious and aware individuals, such behavior is not necessarily surprising.

Surprising or not, the child that is now subject to the coldness, or outright rejection, or perhaps lack of interest, and the caring that greater interest would imply, may suffer in ways that will impinge on his/her future adult relationships. Wariness, a lack of trust, a fear of giving the heart to the potential partner, and many other similar issues may cloud the relationship horizon for people with this background.

Missing Parents

Occasionally children miss out on having a parent due to death or illness, and even a certain weakness of character on the part of the parent may signify that in some fashion the parent is not there for the child in ways that make the child feel secure and loved (see more about this in Chapter 6). While this is not the same as not bonding when the child is still a baby and small infant, it may nevertheless also lead to a lack of true connection with the parent, which in turn may lead to difficulties in the child's adult relationships. Other ways in which parents may count as missing, is when continual work is put ahead of the family - our society calls it workaholism - or even when a social or spiritual life is put ahead of the family.

Adoption

Adoption is a very special issue within this section of attachment issues. When adoption takes place immediately or nearly almost immediately at birth, the potential for adult relationship issues based on attachment and bonding problems is greatly decreased. If, however, adoption takes place later, perhaps after spending some time with the birth mother, then living a period of time in a foster home or orphanage, and only then does the actual adoption occur - even when all of this takes place in the first 24 months of life, it may nevertheless create numerous bonding concerns. When adoption takes place later in the child's life, assuming no real bonding took place prior to age two, the potential for adult relationship issues increases even more dramatically.

This by no means signifies that the individual so affected will not be able to help himself (or find outside help). What may, however, not occur at all, or - at best - take time to occur, is the recognition that despite having had loving adoptive parents, the issues that were left unresolved from a very early age, were probably not assuaged on the basis of that love. In and of itself, wonderful though such adoptive parental love and care may be, it is often simply not enough.

Hence you can see the pressing need for information. Information about your own early years; about the meaning of attachment and bonding; about the recognition of danger signals - often in your body (see more in Chapter 7), such as a twisting in the gut, or a tightening in the region of the heart - that can alert you to the fact that what is in fact going on probably has less to do with the person with whom you are interacting at that moment, and more to do with the fact that that specific person is possibly just a good 'hook' for something that is connected to your childhood as indicated by the signals you are receiving. Hence it becomes clear that the emotional and physical symptoms that are being felt have so much more to do with unresolved attachment issues than with the other person. This kind of information can go a long way towards helping you begin to resolve a great deal, in particular, if you have the desire and intention to do so.

Partners of such people will often spend a good deal of effort and time trying to understand exactly what is going on in the person who is emotionally unavailable and/or needy, and due to this understanding (via information), may try to share it with the partner. Often that leads nowhere, simply because the partner is not yet ready (and may never be) to tackle his/her own problems that arose from the early years of life.

So exactly what happens with adoption? Many elements can influence the development of the adopted child. Here are some with which we can begin our exploration:

- Was the child given up for adoption because he/she was not wanted? (It's difficult to know the answer to this, but the child and adult that was once adopted, may always wish he had the answer).
- Was the child born to a young mother, who might have liked to keep him/her, but due to her age, incomplete education, or financial instability, decided to give him up for adoption?
- Was the child taken from the mother for some legal reason (abuse, neglect, mental instability, substance abuse, criminal activity, etc.)? This will vary from country to country, and what may apply in one, will not necessarily apply in another, it also depends whether this individual was adopted in 1950 or in 2011, as much has changed regarding adoption and parental rights, etc., on a global basis).

- Was the child left on the steps of a cloister, police station, church, or orphanage?
- Are there any records at all of the birth parents and their own provenance, age, professions, etc.? (Sometimes there are not, which may make everything even more complicated for the child's development).
- There is a word used frequently in adoption literature. It is *relinquishment* and the word's very definition and connotations are something the adopted child grapples - often in vain - to come to terms with because it refers to what parents who give up a child do: they *relinquish their baby.* They let it go. This - clearly - is not always easily assimilated, even by the best-adapted adoptees.
- Change issues - such as moving to another home or city, changing schools or friends, or divorce of the adopted parents - are frequently accompanied by much greater stress, anxiety, turmoil, and even trauma for an adopted child, than they are for other children because on some level it brings back what already happened - great change - albeit in other forms.

The next element to consider is the awareness of the adoptive parents. Some - but not nearly all - learn as much as they can about adoption and its potential effect on their child. Others - perhaps the majority - fall into the generalized belief as mentioned earlier, that love is the answer. And certainly, without a doubt, love is a great part of the answer, but it is - unfortunately - not the entire answer. As said, the more information the parents have about all of the above factors, and the more information the growing adopted child, adolescent, and young adult has about how whatever it was that happened - or didn't happen - around his or her early bonding could potentially create later emotional difficulties for the adoptee, in particular with regards to relationships, the better. As already stated, it is *precisely* in this arena that the adopted individual can benefit enormously by recognizing (thanks to information of the kind supplied here and in many other sources, or via a counselor or therapist) his/her own signals that *allow him to know* when something is occurring that triggers a potential fight-or-flight response due to stress, fear, anxiety, or any number of other emotions.

As we will see further on, a similar fight or flight signal and trigger, either emotional, or physical, or both, occurs with others who were not necessarily adopted, but whose early bonding scenarios were challenged. Also see Chapter 14.

Separation / Abandonment

There may be a separation from the parents in the very early life of the child for any number of reasons. Even if such a separation is only temporary, it may leave an indelible mark.

A nine-month-old baby was left at a hospital during war-time Belgium. The mother lived in a remote village and had to return there in order to work, and hence was only rarely able to come to visit her baby. It was nearly impossible to obtain travel permits, and even when she could, money was scarce. Due to the illness the child had, he had to stay at the hospital for eleven months. We can only speculate what happened on psychological and emotional levels by virtue of this individual's later life trajectory, as actual memories of such a young age are hard (although not impossible) to come by. We assume the early bonding process was interrupted. Not only interrupted, but broken somehow, as the 9-month-old baby's interpretation of this - obviously not a conscious interpretation - would have been to equate feelings of loss, pain, and abandonment, and the subconscious connection of that loss and pain to love.

Somehow the psyche might have 'decided' that love was a very dangerous thing indeed, and that when love arose, it would signal - in those subconscious ways learned as a baby - even when the individual was already well into adulthood, that danger lurked, and that hence it might be best to withdraw emotionally. Remember that this is all fear-based, and that the fear is connected to the pain the baby experienced - we might say on a visceral level - when the mother's presence was no longer there. Pain was felt, and when anything occurs to cause that particular pain to arise, albeit subconsciously, fear also appears, and there you have the defense mechanism designed to *escape* these feelings showing its face.

Another example from my case files was quite similar, except that in this case the boy was already eight or nine when the separation that was perceived as abandonment took place. Due to motor problems involving a lengthy stay at a specialized rehabilitation center in his native Switzerland, during which time the child felt deprived of his mother's presence and love, the result was great difficulty in committing emotionally in his later adult life. I might add, that this person's mother, in addition to not being able to be there for her son in the manner just described, was also a slightly cool woman. Not unkind. Not unloving, but not demonstrative; not very physically affectionate, in a way her son might have wished. And so he had to do without such clear affection on several levels. Over the course of our sessions, he told me that subsequently, as an adult, whenever a woman grew close to him, he tended to move away from her. He felt suffocated and needed by the woman in ways he was not prepared to give back to her.

It's at this particular point that it has to be clearly understood that this is *not* (at least generally) an individual who is incapable of giving, or of being emotionally committed, but one whose defense mechanisms grew to become very strong, and thus there is fear not only of the emotion expressed by the partner because it is love, which is something that has a history of having hurt this person in the past, but there is also a fear of being vulnerable, because that state - being vulnerable - means that you're open to being hurt. A vicious circle, you might say. But *not*, as said, due to callousness or other character faults (at least generally) on the part of the one who pulls away, is cool, rejecting, uncommitted, or emotionally unavailable.

Having said that, it does not make it any easier, of course, for the partner who wishes greater closeness, but that is a topic we'll deal with in greater detail in Chapters 12, 13, and 14.

Another Type of Separation or Abandonment

There is a variation on this theme of *apparent* abandonment by the parent/s, and that is when the biological parent, in particular the mother, leaves the child with someone for the early months or perhaps even years of the child's life.

This can happen for a variety of reasons. In the first half of the twentieth century, when bearing an illegitimate child was generally still frowned upon, such children that were not given up for adoption, were occasionally 'farmed out' to a convenient relative until the biological mother was in a better position to be able to care for the child herself.

One such client lived with an older sister of her mother's from birth to nearly the age of two. As we have already seen, those are crucially important bonding months and years. She even came to call this aunt 'mommy' (whether this happened automatically and was then tacitly 'allowed' by the aunt, or exactly how it came about, was not something my client knew). In the meantime her biological mother had met a caring and understanding man who not only wished to marry her, but also wished to adopt her little daughter. The city they chose to settle in was in a distant location, many hours from the city in which the aunt lived. As far as my client was able to piece the story together when she was older and discovered what had happened, her biological mother arrived one day (remember, this was at a time when mobiles, email, faxes did not yet exist, and even just regular old-fashioned landline telephones were not the norm in the most typical of households) to tell her older sister that she was now ready to take charge of her little daughter. She then packed her up and drove away with her new husband.

Imagine - if you can - what such deprivation of her beloved 'mommy' must have occasioned to my client. Imagine even more, that her mother in all likelihood had not the slightest inkling about the immense trauma she had just provoked in her little daughter, trauma that would haunt her daughter for the great majority of her life, showing up in little-understood resentment of her mother (who on her side, felt she had a naughty, recalcitrant, and unlikeable little girl on her hands), living in great emotional dependence (neediness) on her adoptive father, who regrettably died in an automobile accident when she was only 21, leaving her with another gaping wound she only poorly understood, and finally, showing up in both emotional unavailability as well as neediness in her future adult relationships, further mirrored to some degree, even with her own children.

Another older client from a similar period in the early 20th century was born illegitimately to a young woman about to set off on a career in law, and who in fact, when she realized she was pregnant, was just in the early part of her studies. Again, for similar reasons as in the case above, she sent her little baby off to a foster home until she had completed those studies, and become engaged to be married to her future husband, who again was happy to adopt the little girl, now four or five years old. Despite the new marriage and theoretically ideal conditions for the child, the mother nevertheless, once again farmed her little daughter off to an older relative for another few years, then brought her back home, and ultimately sent her off to boarding school.

The fact that the little girl lived some very good years with this relative is nevertheless not as important in understanding her inner world, as is the fact that when she was once again summoned to her rather cold mother, she was again *bereft*. She had - in her young life - already lost her earliest love connections, and had learned a very hard lesson indeed: loving another brought pain; loving another was *not* safe; loving another had to be guarded against. Clearly, none of this was thought out in an adult way. Rather, it was subconscious; visceral, and took place entirely on the feeling and physical level. She erected defense mechanisms in order to not feel such pain again, and even as an older adult when she came to see me the first time, was still not truly aware of what was going on. She was very obviously not in contact with her own emotions, and despite a greater than average knowledge of the psyche, she appeared quite divorced from her own.

And in one final example of this nature we fast forward into the second half of the 20th century, into the life of a man who had been born into a loving and close-knit family in the 60's. He remained only briefly with his parents, who had immigrated to the United States, in order to build a better life for themselves and their family. They soon realized that in order to create this new life, which required long and arduous hours of dedication, their first-born infant baby would not receive the care he needed and so with heavy hearts, decided to take him back to their family in Guatemala. There he remained for those all-important first two years of his life, until his parents were more settled in the United States and were therefore in a position to be able to fly back home and get their little boy. You already know what this means. Despite their great love for their child, he nevertheless experienced and perceived being ripped away from all those who filled his heart and gave him security. He experienced the pain of abandonment, because although he was not abandoned - neither by his parents when they first took him back to Guatemala, nor by his grandparents when his parents came to take him back to the United States - he nevertheless perceived it as such on that very deep, visceral, and primordial level. And as such - bearing in mind no one in his world was aware of the psychological and emotional ramifications of all of this - he internalized a certain fear of the pain of abandonment by an object of love. This contributed to his fear of commitment, and hence a certain emotional unavailability and simultaneously to his deep yearning for love, and his neediness. It contributed to what some authors call the *push-pull* effect in adult relationships, and it also contributed to his poor boundaries.

This is the case because even if part of you is emotionally unavailable, the yearning and needy part of you that so hopes for and wants and *needs* love, will often do or *allow* whatever it takes in order to maintain that love. Once reassured and feeling secure again, the cooler, emotionally unavailable part of you may rear its head - perhaps in retaliation, or perhaps simply in order to uphold the status quo that assures that power or control of the relationship remains in your hands, because ultimately that power gives you the greatest measure of security. As long as you have it, you need not allow any kind of vulnerability into your life.

It is interesting to note that in all three of these examples, when the child returned to the biological mother or parents, another child was either already on the way, or had already been born, and career and other work-related issues were also taking up the parents' time, and thus usurped, we might say, the final opportunity for these individuals to receive the undivided attention from the biological mother - at least for a time in what was left of their childhood - in order to potentially lessen, perhaps even ameliorate some of the psycho-emotional trauma they were undergoing.

Sadly, and it must by now be clear to you that this is simply how it is, these specific parents I've described here, as well as so many other parents in these and similar situations over the centuries, were and are simply *not aware* of what their behavior - often well-intentioned and caring - had wrought in their children. Nor were/are they aware of any of the psychological and emotional approaches and psychological tools that they could have provided and brought to the table in order to help their child come to a better resolution of the trauma he/she had undergone. In most instances it becomes a lose-lose situation for the child until someone - often the child himself, albeit well into adulthood - realizes that help and understanding are required in order to heal the wounds and to be able to move on from them.

Further Childhood Dilemmas That May Cause Attachment Issues:

- **Mother/Father with a succession of lovers**

Another instance is a kind of abandonment that is not on the physical level as much as it is on the psycho-emotional one. A parent who is divorced or single, and of course occasionally even one who is married, and who has sexual relationships with a succession of lovers, may create a great deal of turmoil for the child, especially if it concerns the parent of the opposite gender.

This is not directly related to jealousy, oedipal or Electra complexes, or anything like that, as much as to the child being able to observe what I am going to call the *flightiness* or lack of steadfast loyalty of the parent on the emotional level, due to the parent's relatively frequent and easy exchanging of these partners. The mother may be perceived (even if the child is not yet familiar with the terminology, because the observation of these events often begins to occur when the child is still very young) to be a kind of butterfly and the father a Don Juan, or 'player'.

Two reactions may occur: the child may decide (subconsciously, viscerally) that with whatever ease he/she has observed the parent abandon each lover, it may soon be applied to him/herself, i.e., to the child and one thing any child fears more than most other things, is, of course, abandonment - both physical and emotional. The second possible reaction is that the child decides (subconsciously, viscerally) that *love causes pain*. Either way - and indeed, the child may take both variants onboard - the child now has the beginnings of a fear of love entrenched in his psycho-emotional make-up because of the pain he/she has observed love to cause.

Trust is also involved, because it is *his/her* beloved parent (often the parent of the opposite gender) who is inflicting such pain on the other person, as observed by the child, and yet because it is the beloved parent doing this, the child literally begins to doubt and worry about the trustworthiness regarding his or her own self of this parent who is capable of these acts.

You might be questioning how it is possible that a small child could observe all of this, and of course more than actually observing it, as most of it is, as said, *not* conscious, it is a question of the child taking it in on a more visceral level, even if it's from a distance.

The explanation of how this occurs is often ridiculously simple: the child may be playing in the next room while the parent is telling the current partner that the relationship is over. It may simply be a telephone conversation that the child overhears. Or the child may have been taken to the park, or a beach, or a playground, and while there, the parent and the current partner of choice have a meeting or telephone conversation that the child witnesses in this subconscious fashion. The child may also be present as the parent tells a friend of the *dénouement* of the relationship with the latest partner, and thus gets a blow-by-blow account of all it entailed. Of course, he/she may also be witness to much greater emotional drama, if he happens to be physically present when the parent tells a partner that he/she is no longer wanted and the partner has an emotional melt-down.

The result, as said, may be twofold. One is the belief that *love causes pain*. To a greater or lesser degree, this is what the child has assimilated, and now begin the attachment issues that may lead the psyche and heart of this child down that stone and boulder-strewn path of neediness and emotional unavailability in his/her adult relationships. The second potential result may entail a lack of trust in the opposite gender; a feeling of deep visceral anxiety regarding the steadfastness and trustworthiness of their expressed love.

- **Mother or Father mistreats the other parent (in the child's perception)**

When one parent mistreats the other, particularly if the mistreated parent is of the same gender as the child, another variation on the theme occurs, giving rise to potentially poor attachment as well.

Generally the kind of mistreatment referred to here is not domestic abuse, but emotional pain. If the child observes the parent of his own gender reacting in pain to something the other parent has said, particularly if it concerns marital - or even simply *emotional* - infidelity, and particularly if the parent who throws it in the face of the other partner (because in this type of situation the *offending* parent can be cruel in this manner) does not appear to be very repentant, or even seem to care, the child may pick up cues about the *pain that love may cause*. These cues, just as others that have been discussed in this chapter, are subliminal. They may create a physical reaction or they may create a dynamic of psychological and emotional fear that is not conscious (for more about physical and emotional reactions in emotional unavailability and neediness, see Chapter 7). Eventually, as the child grows up, these evolve into a pattern and become intertwined with a subconscious defense mechanism, in order to protect the child against that physical reaction, or against that fear, *every time* the individual - who is now an adult - experiences either of these. (For more about adult reactions to emotions and physical sensations and triggers from childhood, see Chapter 14, as these lie at the crux of both the problem, as well as its resolution).

And of course because the defense mechanism referred to above is subconscious, it tends to occur automatically, with no adult cognition and understanding involved in the manner in which the mechanism manifests when the triggers - be they emotional, or physical, or both - arise, no matter what the age of the individual. Without this *adult* understanding and cognition - which is what this book offers the reader - the resolution of these issues is almost impossible, although, as you will see, the cognition is not enough.

- **Abuse by Someone the Child Loves**

This modality of early conditions that may lead to attachment issues is perhaps one of the most well-known and understood by the layman. If a child trusts and loves an adult, or an older person who is somehow involved in the child's care, and that person at some point physically, sexually, emotionally, and/or psychologically abuses the child, the message may again be some modality of *love causes pain* and *I can't trust those I love*.

There are so many varieties of this particular phenomenon that it has crept into popular literature and film, starting at the black end of the continuum with serial killers and psychopaths who were devastatingly abused by a parent or caretaker, and whose dreadful pain and yearning in infancy and childhood for loving care eventually led them down such a path, to the other end of the continuum where you often find the most needy, in some fashion the most helpless, but who may also become the most plaintive and manipulative, leaning on their family and friends for ever greater caretaking under the guise of their endless need due to having been such a victim of their parent or caretaker in childhood.

And I'd like to add in passing that such neediness is often related to emotional vampirism (see Chapter 4) on the part of the abused person, very poor boundaries, and of course, a lamentably absent regard and love for the self.

****

Note - as stated earlier - that it is interesting to observe the relatively high frequency with which adult individuals who have learned some of the above subconscious lessons and are still currently manifesting them in their relationship lives, and hence often demonstrate great difficulty expressing emotions with their loved ones, nevertheless habitually appear to have none of these difficulties with friends, animals, or the children of other people. They may also be very easily drawn to tears and emotion when they see a certain kind of film. Yet let their spouse come to them with pain about something they (the emotionally unavailable person) have provoked, and they may maintain an aloof poker face, as though they had not the slightest of connections with their own emotions or those of the partner. And indeed, to a degree this is true due to the wall surrounding their emotions that the defense mechanisms they erected in childhood have created.

Chapter 4

Patterns

Most of us start out our relationship lives by reliving a pattern we've brought in from childhood. This is not our fault. It just is. But it is our responsibility to become aware of it, although again, at the beginning we are not aware of it, and that also simply is not our fault. It just is.

It's essentially when the patterns start repeating themselves, that it becomes our responsibility to be conscious enough to become aware of them, as opposed to blaming our partner or our bad luck.

But why do we often start our relationship lives that way? What happened in our childhood that caused us to fall into a pattern of some kind? Shall we just blame our parents? The answer to that is a rotund no. Even if we could prove that our parents were not good parents, there is simply no point in blaming them. It solves nothing.

Furthermore, by the time many of us realize that we have a given pattern, and that it might be related to some element of our early upbringing and emotional closeness or lack thereof, we are already in our 30's and 40's or more, and often our parents are no longer around.

More than casting our eye about in order to find someone to blame, compassion is the word we need to keep on the front burner when we undergo such realizations. Generally speaking our parents clearly became the way they did due to their own upbringing. It's so much more important to focus on the fact that now, thanks to having become aware of the pattern, we can actually do something about it. And by so doing, we can move beyond it, to another kind of relationship that need not consist of the blindness or the compulsions or obsessions which made up the gist of our earlier relationships.

So back to our question of why our relationship lives often begin that way: by living out a pattern. Imagine having an emotionally unavailable parent that the child desperately tries to draw into its circle of love. What happens when the child realizes this is impossible? There are numerous possible outcomes. One potential scenario is that the child believes it is unlovable. Or perhaps it believes it is not loved due to its own fault, for not doing this or that or the other thing right. It may begin to believe that love is not safe because it hurts.

Or imagine a parent who continually criticizes the child, never once giving the child the satisfaction of hearing words such as: *I am so proud of you ... you did such a good job*. The child therefore simply is never given the possibility to feel that he/she is good enough. Imagine the devastation this creates in the way that child begins to love itself, or better said, imagine how nearly impossible it will be for such a child to begin to love itself, or in any way truly and deeply feel good about itself.

Furthermore, this child may develop into an over-achiever, where he only feels good about himself when he hears the accolades or receives the honor after reaching a goal. Rarely do these individuals enjoy the journey. And to add insult to injury, once the goal has been achieved, they feel compelled to seek another goal or achievement, in order to reap yet more accolades, honor, or recognition, because that tends to be the only way they are able to feel good about themselves.

Or imagine having a parent who uses the child's love to manipulate the child emotionally: making it feel guilty or bad or inadequate in some way. This again works against the child's best interests and precludes a healthy love for the self, a strong belief in the self, and the necessary acceptance of the self in order to lead a productive life. The consequences of such destruction wrought on the fragile childhood psyche can only be fully appreciated decades into the future through the many issues that arise for such an individual throughout his/her adult life.

Or imagine the parent who shows the child that someone *or something* else (the other parent, a new partner, another sibling, a profession or any kind of an activity, perhaps a sport, or even shopping, a spiritual ideal, or a 'mission') is always more important in the parent's life than the child itself.

Or imagine the parent who in some fashion abandons the child, whether emotionally, physically, financially, or in other ways. This not only leaves scars, but also sets the child up for relationships that somehow re-enact some of these abandonment scenarios.

And *that*, in a nutshell, is precisely the reason why we have patterns: on subconscious levels we choose partners with whom we are able to re-enact our childhood scenarios. Why, you ask, would we want to do this? I don't believe we *want* to do it - at least not consciously - but our psyche (some might say it's the soul) somehow knows that this is a process that can lead to healing whatever was wounded in childhood, although of course what heals us is *not* the repetition of a pattern, but the *recognition* of the pattern and the cleansing of the part of the self that got us there - as adults - in the first place. And that recognition, as said, does not generally happen until we have gone through the pain and frustration of a failing or failed relationship, as well as - most of the time - several such relationships.

So we may subconsciously pick partners that will do to us what our parents did, or what the parent with whom we had the difficulty did. Obviously this does not happen during the honeymoon phase of the relationship, or we would *never* get into the relationship in the first place. We generally first 'cement' our relationships with a marriage certificate, or the joint purchase of a home, or a baby, before we get into the painful part. Some authors believe this cementing occurs (again subconsciously) so that we are unable to easily leave the relationship. Therefore - because we are obliged, at least in the beginning, to stay in the relationship - we have a chance of trying to understand what is happening - by initially remaining there - although unfortunately for many of us, that does not always happen, and most particularly, it does not always happen the first time around.

And just to reiterate, *please* do not make the mistake of trying to figure out why your parents were like this; why they did this to you; why they were not more loving, more caring, kinder, more approving and accepting of you. Remember also, they had their own set of parents who were probably not as ideal as they could have been, and so on, for as far back generationally as you care to go. So *why* this all happened is not nearly as important as understanding that simply by realizing it happened and that it has colored your adult relationships (not only your love relationships, but your friendships as well), *you now stand on the threshold of changing it, or changing yourself, and in*

the process of so doing, gaining immeasurable freedom.
Further, if you change yourself, you offer your children new
horizons which can be instrumental in putting an end to the
cycle of psycho-emotional pain.

So having seen now how some of these patterns
arise in our personalities, let's examine a few very specific
types of relationship patterns that we fall into. And just to
reiterate a point already made earlier in this book, and that
I've always considered of prime importance for
understanding the dynamics of our relationships, Carl
Gustav Jung, who along with Sigmund Freud was one of the
most renowned figures in the early annals of
psychoanalysis, said that it is precisely the infinite
intelligence of the psyche (in its quest toward individuation,
growth, and wholeness) that leads us to become attracted
to certain individuals. In our emotional lives this also leads
us to be attracted - as we have seen - to those people who
have attained (or stagnated at) the *same* level of emotional
maturity as we have.

These individuals, as indicated above, will enable us
to re-enact our childhood parental dynamics and scenarios
that will more often than not - if we are paying attention -
lead us to feel physical sensations in our body and feel
emotions that are strangely *familiar* to us. And of course the
reason they are familiar is because we have felt them all
before, when we were small.

That, by the way, is also the reason why our
reactions in those situations are often the reactions of a
child. *Not* because we are childish, but because this part of
us has never grown or matured emotionally and
psychologically; it remained arrested at that stage of
development. But it *can mature* and - the more conscious
and aware we become - *it will* indeed do so). This attraction
to certain individuals that then leads to a relationship, may
then - eventually - due to the later frustration and possible
pain these individuals may bring to our lives (and we to
theirs) ultimately offer us the opportunity to come to

understanding and growth. This always leads to greater inner freedom.

Finally, you may wonder why so many patterns are described, if this book focuses on emotional unavailability and neediness. *Your* road to the consequences of this double-sided coin may have been quite different from that of another person's road there. By reading about numerous patterns you will more readily begin to understand more clearly how your own pattern emerged. In Chapter 5 you will find an exercise designed to show you how to discover your own patterns.

PATTERNS:

Take Care of Me (Let Me Take Care of You!), AKA Poor Boundaries & Co-Dependence

It seems that as long as we remain unaware and unconscious in our lives, there is always a price to pay in our relationships. A woman may fall into the figurative lap of a man who offers to take care of her on some level (and it need not necessarily be financial, as the components of the caring could be emotional or psychological, perhaps academic, professional or even social). If she lies back, releasing a great sigh of relief, and allows him to do so, she almost always immediately relinquishes a part of her autonomy. It seems to be part of the *deal*, or simply the way the process works - subconsciously - for both partners.

In relinquishing part of her autonomy, she sets herself up to have her boundaries overstepped on some level. Perhaps the partner demands that in return she be there for him at all times, which precludes having a career of her own. Or he may demand she follow in his chosen field of academics or law or business, but in *his* footsteps, and not in those of her own making. This may lead to resentment and bitterness which may eventually erode the relationship, and/or the health of both partners. But it has its roots in the early relationship each of these partners had with their parents. One being cared for, acquiescing in some fashion, but paying a cruel price due to a fundamental lack of independence, and the other feeling he is only truly loved and needed if his "way" of thinking or behaving is adhered to, and if not, it is considered an act of high treason and proof of a lack in the way he is loved.

Or perhaps - this is another sample case - one of the partners recognizes a potential addiction problem in the other at an early stage in the relationship and decides that they will 'cure' that person. They just *know* they will be able to do so, and furthermore, they also just know that once the other partner sees how truly wonderful they are - the way the one who wants to cure the other *sees* them - then they will be able to begin to live out the magnificence of their life and purpose. (All of this is possible, by the way, just not likely ... at least not before these individuals begin to recognize that they are repeating a pattern). So here we have co-dependence rearing its ugly head, as well as, just like the previous example, boundaries being overstepped, especially once the addicted person lets loose on their substance of choice.

And remember: if *your* boundaries are being crossed by your *partner*, it is *not* first and foremost your partner's fault, although they do carry responsibility for their own behavior and lack of awareness. However, it is *your* responsibility to ensure that your own boundaries are healthy. And as long as you are enabling someone in a co-dependent relationship (by covering up the tracks - perhaps so that no one in your social circle notices - of a drinking or substance-abusing partner, for example, instead of setting some firm consequences if they do not clean up their act and then following through on those consequences), you are certainly not setting up healthy boundaries for yourself. This will affect your health, your state of mind, and last, but not least, the health of the relationship. And if this is your first partnership of this type, you may not yet have recognized the pattern, and may be thinking: *why do I have such bad luck in choosing my partners?*

But here, once again, you are reliving some element of your past. Perhaps one of your parents was an addict of some kind, even if *only* workaholic, shopaholic, or bulimic. And perhaps you learned early on to cover up their tracks so that no one would notice. The die is cast. And until you recognize it in your relationship patterns, you will continue to revisit this dynamic in your relationships, even though at the beginning of each relationship you are so very convinced that *this time it is truly different.*

And remember: the reason we (subconsciously) seek the repetition of a dynamic is *not* to feel what we felt as helpless or unloved or manipulated children, but to *resolve* those unresolved issues that linger from our childhood.

If - in the above enumerated examples that deal with poor boundaries - you now recognize that you tend to choose individuals who will step on your boundaries, and if you now consciously work on creating healthy boundaries, you will begin to attract another kind of individual into your life - or said in other words - you will begin to be attracted to another kind of person, and hence, your future relationships, while they will in all probability have another - new - kind of issue to work on, will nevertheless have progressed beyond *this* particular issue, freeing you up enormously on those inner levels that are so important to well-being and inner harmony.

Poor Boundaries & Emotional or Energetic Vampires

Most of us have been conditioned to regard vampires as the very substance of our most dreaded nightmares - the absolute epitome of horror. And yet many of us lead lives with more than just a nodding acquaintance with one or more emotional and energetic vampires.

Perhaps the most daunting aspect of this – *if we wish to do something about it* - is that a good number of people with this type of personality often *appear* to be anything but emotional or energetic vampires. They *appear* to be kind, generous, considerate, and hospitable. And certainly, in many ways – at least on the surface – that is exactly what they are. So why do you feel so awful when you are with them? Weakened, drained, exhausted, sapped. Your energy is gone. Your vitality is gone. Your good mood is gone. You've been sucked dry in the truest sense of the word.

Remember, emotional unavailability and neediness - if not always, then certainly with great frequency - go hand-in-hand with poor boundaries. Hence, the more you understand them, how they arise, and your role in allowing them into your life, the more you will be able to create healthier ones, and therefore this rather lengthy description about emotional vampires and how they almost always form part and parcel of poor boundaries that follows. Please also note that they often arise in childhood, before adult cognition sets in, and the most efficient way of starting the process of eradicating them, is to understand their early provenance.

Here's how to recognize when you're in the presence of one of these people, and please note that it's helpful to use your feelings as a gauge. Do you feel a tightening in your gut? A restriction in your chest? A queasiness? An uneasiness? These body sensations, as well as what follows, which is taken from the way we feel, gives you a hint that you might be in the presence of an emotional or energetic vampire. *Remember: the way your body feels when you spend time with someone, as well as your emotions always indicates something that is going on that you would do well to investigate. It may not always mean you are faced with a person of the type I have been describing, but it certainly warrants some careful consideration.*

- Guilty (we feel guilty as we ask ourselves how we can possibly be feeling some of the things we are feeling, if this person is being *so good* to us *or so helpful and hospitable.*)
- Drained and sapped
- Tired and weak
- Unenthusiastic (or if we were enthusiastic earlier in the day, after some time in their presence, our enthusiasm is gone)
- Pushed and pulled in directions you don't want to go (ever heard of subliminal manipulation?)
- You may even feel befuddled, less clear in your head, as if you had been mildly drugged

Who are they? They can be anywhere and everywhere. Or not. What I mean is this: if you have someone like this in your life, that person, or those persons, could be in any sector of your life. Very close to you. Or more distanced. But if they are emotional or energetic vampires, you will know it because of the way you feel when you are with them for more than a few moments.

Let's examine some typical scenarios:

The "nothing you do or say is ever valued" vampire

This type is never happy for you if something good happens. Or, rather than showing happiness when you tell them about something good, or something you are proud of, they find a reason to put it down, or to show you how it could go wrong, or why it will never work. If, after many of these situations, you finally say something about it, there is a good chance that they may defend themselves by telling you: *well someone has to be realistic.* If you mention that they never seem to be happy for you when something goes well, they may seem puzzled and ask: *but what do you mean? Of course I'm happy for you.* If you don't catch on, you won't see the connection between your low feelings after being with them, and their lack of joy about your good news. Or you may find yourself striving to do something really spectacular, just to get a favorable reaction from them. In some fashion your well-being depends on them. And when it does not come, the circle repeats itself, with your vitality and enthusiasm going lower and lower each subsequent time.

The "I know it better than you do" vampire

This vampire is not a vampire because they actually *do* know something better than you do. I mean when they talk about those areas where they truly have expertise, you do not feel drained or empty. What happens here is something different. You tell them about something. You are enthusiastic. It could be something you did, or experienced or heard about or read. And immediately they have some kind of one-up-man-ship. It could be that they heard about it long before you. They were doing this when you were still a baby. Or they know all about feeling that way (if you had been describing feelings), but now they are well launched into their own description of their experience of this type of thing. Whatever it is, they have been there, done that, or know about it. You begin to feel flattened, drained, sucked dry whenever you speak to them.

The "victim" vampire

This one can actually be putting on a very brave face, interlaced however, with much possible sighing, and a soft, suffering - but brave - voice. Here there has been - in the eyes of the vampire - a great injustice done to the to him, perhaps it is the family that has let the person down, perhaps it was a spouse, or friends, occasionally this vampire may *even blame him or herself* for some events, but nevertheless, *because they view themselves as victim*, albeit brave and all-suffering, *you* are put into the untenable role of someone who is expected to *help* this person, generally at the expense of your own well-being. Your help may come in the guise of marathon talk sessions, ideas, something you physically *do* for the other to help them get stronger or better, but whatever it is, *it drains you*. And of course, if you stop accepting the role of helper, builder-upper of strength (the other's), you feel *guilty* for being such a bad friend (or relative, or partner).

The "monologue" vampire who never lets you get a word in edgewise

This one isn't just talking endlessly about what is not going well in his/her life; the endless talking can also be about potentially interesting subjects, but there is simply no interest whatsoever in what you might have to say about it. So the monologue goes on and on. And since this particular vampire has never done anything to offend you, you feel you would be rude or discourteous by complaining. And so you continue to listen as your life blood (your energy) drains out of you. This can go on for decades if you allow it (or if you choose to continue to engage in the *dance*).

The "I just want to be like you and do everything you do" vampire

This one suffocates you by their desire to emulate you to the nth degree. They may begin by dressing like you, going to the same tailor or designer, using your salon, picking up your discards when you no longer date someone (or after you've divorced someone). Later they may actually try to date them even when you are still with someone. They want to go everywhere you go, participate in all your activities, they may decide to sign up at your gym or your yoga class, they may show up unbidden at restaurants when you are dining out with other friends. But basically, because *all* they are really doing is trying to be like you – which we often take as something complimentary – you may not notice how much you are being suffocated until it has reached a point of strong frustration. And then, if you want to keep your head over water, you may need to totally ostracize them from your life.

The "please take care of me" vampire

This one is another type of *victim* vampire, but comes dressed in new clothing. This vampire comes right out and says he/she needs your help, needs you to take on responsibility for some portion of *their* existence. *And for some reason*, you fall right into the role. It could be because at the beginning it makes you feel good, or strong, or valuable. Or perhaps they admire you as go about whatever it is that you do for them. But eventually it suffocates you, because you are now in the strait-jacket of *having to be responsible for the other*. And to remove the strait-jacket, to stop being suffocated, you may need to take drastic measures, never an easy step. To begin with, it will probably make you feel highly guilty to refuse to continue in the role. But if you *do continue* in the role, you may feel, apart from suffocated, very resentful, low in energy and enthusiasm, *because life just is no longer very good.* How can it be, if your life blood runs through their veins? Don't forget, that in some fashion, vampires are parasites.

The "I can't live without you" vampire

This is a cousin of the *please take care of me* vampire, i.e., another type of *victim* vampire, but this one is bigger and stronger. This one may even get the kids to help reel you back into the fold in order to re-establish the status quo. This one may have been feeding off you for an entire marriage. Or as your sibling an entire lifetime. Or your parent, or even your child. You *know* that you feel drained and empty, perhaps even *hopeless* in their presence (hopeless because you just don't know how to stop it). So finally you take the big step and give them an ultimatum – or, even more drastic - remove them from your life. *Now they use strategic tactics to undermine your recently-found strength*. They pull at your heart-strings by sending you the children (possibly adult children) to let you know how they are not able to live without you. Or they send you your parent (in the case of a sibling) to pass on the same message. The result? You feel so guilty, so terrible about your own *selfish* behavior (for wanting to be out of their presence), you feel so responsible for their well-being, that you may capitulate. *Don't. It's your life that is at stake.* You are responsible for *you*. They are responsible for *themselves*. They need to learn how to exist without feeding off you, and it is not your role to teach them how.

The "I need to know everything about your life" vampire

This one really suffocates as well, but here the suffocation has nothing to do with imitating you or behaving like a victim who *needs* you to be responsible for them or who can't live without you. Here we're talking about someone whom you have become used to giving blow-by-blow accounts of the details of your life. You may be friends and talk on the phone every day and all the fine points are gone over in minute detail. Or you may be colleagues with a similar scenario. At the beginning it just happened. If someone asked you how it came about, you might say that you aren't really certain. It felt good, and it was lovely to be able to share with someone in such intimate fashion. At some point however, it started to become an obligation - perhaps a moral obligation. You felt guilty if you didn't share all. You sometimes began holding some bits back, noticed it, and then felt resentful if the other pried, or prodded you into saying more. In time, you started feeling drained as you recounted your daily life to the vampire. But by now – at least on the surface – you are so close, that it seems to make no sense that you want out, or that you have any negative feelings, so guilt builds up on more guilt. *And you feel more drained.*

Note: This listing is not meant to be definitive. There are many, many other versions of emotional and energetic vampires. Some, who appear in the workplace as your superiors, have not even been touched upon here, and they can make life a living hell. Others can appear in your bedroom. That will eventually also turn into a living nightmare.

How can we understand what it means? There is high degree of manipulation in the art of being a vampire – manipulation directed at you in order that you will offer your neck (and your life blood) willingly.

In the early stages of the relationship, you may have a feeling of being worthy, of having value, but when you begin to feel drained and robbed of energy, *you know that those feelings were merely part of the unresolved issues in you that need work.* The vampire:

- Does not have to take care of the self
- Does not have to work on being responsible for the self
- Feels alive by draining others
- Feels powerful by draining others

There is also something very needy about the vampire – why else would they be draining you of your life blood? However, this kind of neediness is exceedingly dangerous and toxic for you, if you decide to "help" them with it. Where they are needy, *they are dysfunctional.* And that is totally their own responsibility. That doesn't mean you couldn't be a supporting friend or partner, should they decide to do something about it. But as long as they *expect* to get their *blood* from you, and you comply, *you are both highly dysfunctional.*

In order to deal with this, you might try talking openly. Maybe you can salvage the relationship, although I don't think it's very likely because in order for this to happen, the other person will have had to do some *growing* of their own, and more often than not growth takes place at different time in individuals' lives. Try explaining. If none of that works, keep as much distance as you can, both physically and emotionally. Examine everything that is being said and done, and remember that whatever it is that is being said and done has *nothing* to do with you, and *everything* to do with the other person. Consciously *choose* to hear it and observe it, but to *not* let it affect you the way it has up to now. Leave the presence of the other person as soon as you can. But in some cases you may need to walk away - perhaps in a definitive way - by ending the relationship.

Having emotional and energetic vampires in your life eventually teaches you about boundaries, about the fact that you have poor boundaries, about the fact that you have now (as you truly become aware of this in your life) developed a real *allergy* to this, to people who do not respect you. In either calling them *to order*, or in *ridding your life* of them, you become much more aware and conscious about yourself. Due to this you are now in a position to move to an entirely new level in your life because of this new awareness and your conscious decision not to let individuals of this type continue to be an influence in your life.

This *reorganization* of your inner self and the subsequent move to an entirely new level is immensely important. It means you become responsible for your *entire self*, not just for your physical well-being, for example. By so doing, you ensure that your environment – in this case the type of individuals that people your world – is healthy for you. Another magnificent step to inner freedom.

Victim-Savior

This next relationship pattern is rather easy to understand, although less so when you are immersed in the middle of living out the scenario. If you are one of those very benevolent and generous individuals who spends a good portion of their time helping and giving to others, we speak well of you. We admire you. We believe you are a person to emulate. And perhaps you are. But perhaps not.

When you help others and give to others, there are a number of potential scenarios. Imagine a mentor, who furthers his protégé's knowledge about their mutually chosen field of endeavor. The protégé may eventually outrun or surpass his mentor, and in so doing, obviously becomes autonomous at the very least, and possibly may find his mentor is no longer necessary. At this point some mentors become very angry and feel betrayed, while others *feel gratified*.

Or imagine helping someone who is new in town - showing them around, introducing them to all your friends, helping them find a place to live and then a job. And then, maybe some time down the road when they are a bit more established, you discover that they have organized a party and invited most of those people you introduced them to, *but not you*. At this point you may become very angry and feel betrayed, or you may feel very sad. Either way, clearly this is not the way someone we admire for how generous they are in the help they give others, should feel.

Let's take the examples a bit closer into the love relationship arena. You meet someone who is not making ends meet. You believe they've had a rough deal in life so far. You take them under your wing. In the process, you fall in love. You cherish this person (and I've seen this example in both genders, i.e., sometimes the person who had a rough deal is the woman, and sometimes it is the man). You take care of them in all senses of the word. You pay for furthering their education, you pay for a better wardrobe (also in part so that you can feel good about them when you are seen together), and eventually you get married. You want to make your partner feel equal to you in all things, so you open a joint bank account, and when you buy a house, you put half in your partner's name. You have some children, and so of course your partner doesn't really ever have time to pursue a career, if she is the wife, and if it's the husband who had the rough life prior to meeting you, clearly you are the one who continues working directly after giving birth, and your husband may stay home with the baby. You can see where this is going. At some point your partner either makes more and more demands while giving less and less, and you begin to see you have been used, and want to break away from the relationship yourself, or your partner announces out of the blue that he/she wants a divorce and before you know it, you are served papers that show that you are going to be taken to the cleaners and that your children will - in all likelihood - be wrested from you. You are in shock. You feel enormous rage and outrage. You feel betrayed. And you feel deep sadness. Not at all the way someone who started out being kind, generous and helpful should wind up feeling, right?

But let's examine what happened in the examples I've offered where the 'generous' person wound up feeling angry and betrayed. Could we say that he 'saved' the other person from having to do something on his own? Could it be that he saved the other person from standing on his own two feet? Or could it be that he did it, not because he was so generous and helpful (at least not in the first instance), but that he did it because of *how good it makes him feel* to have another be so grateful to him? Or to admire him for his skills, abilities, or social contacts, or for his ease at accomplishing things?

Let's take that one step further: while it is true that at the beginning the gratitude and even admiration the other person shows you is authentic, it is also true that after a time it may pall. Perhaps they now wish to strike out on their own but feel stymied by your need to be needed in this particular way. Or perhaps they become resentful of your 'power' over them. That could be financial, social, academic, professional, and so on. Either way, they are no longer happy to be with you, and definitely not with your demands, unspoken or otherwise, to be kept up on a pedestal. And so the savior, who has rescued the victim, is abandoned, shunned or otherwise cast off.

But where did this relationship pattern come from? As a child you may have unwittingly and unwillingly been cast into the savior role: a role that should never be foisted on anyone, least of all an unsuspecting and helpless child. You might be the little boy who became mommy's 'little helper' and whom she admired so much, as long as you did exactly what she expected of you. You felt the brunt of her disapproval when you were not there for her in the way she expected, and because it was never resolved (most probably because you never truly understood the dynamics of the role that had been thrust on you by an adult who herself refused to be an adult and expected you to take that on), you have (your *psyche* has) the need - albeit subconscious - to relive this particular drama until you are given that love, admiration and approval that you craved as a child.

Evidently when you repeat this as an adult, it typically ends badly, and therefore you are literally forced to seek another solution. And that *lies within you* and not in the other person's approval, love, and admiration of you. But you won't understand that until you have undergone the process and begun to work it out.

The other way this pattern can work is that you are the victim. You were always saved as a child by your parent or parents. When you got into scrapes, or when you broke the neighbor's window with your baseball, or shoplifted adult magazines from the store, and were found out, your parent covered for you. Or paid someone off. Or made excuses for you. Or you bullied someone at school and your parent 'fixed' it. Or maybe you couldn't get into college, but your parent had a friend on the board and you scraped by with your not-so-outstanding grades and got in thanks to that. Whatever happened, you learned to rely on another to get you through. And now this other - perhaps your wife or husband - has had enough of you not pulling your weight. And so they leave you. And you find yourself another savior or rescuer. And after a time it happens again. And you are beginning to glimpse the possibility that there may be a pattern. Because of course what you need to learn is to find the wherewithal in *you* to resolve your problems, as opposed to getting another to do it for you.

Please Love Me & Never Leave Me (*Don't* Suffocate Me): The Paradox of Neediness & Emotional Unavailability

In this pattern dynamic - which is the central theme of this book - we find couples that come together because they *depend* on each other, although at first glance one is the dependent partner and the other is the *independent* partner. Yet, after careful examination, we come to the conclusion that they both depend on each other very deeply for very similar reasons: they represent - as we have seen and are discussing throughout this book - two sides of a single coin.

The more obviously dependent partner is clearly needy, mostly in the emotional sense, although it may also be in other ways. Emotional neediness basically means that the partner believes he or she is unable to live without the love of the apparently more independent partner. It means he believes that he is not sufficient for his own well-being. It means he has not learned to love himself. It means - and this is the most important aspect of it - he/she will do almost *anything* at all in order to ensure the maintenance of the love of the partner that is considered so necessary for his/her well-being.

An external need, in others words, when we depend on something *external* to ourselves for our well-being, frequently carries within it the seeds of failure. In the case of a relationship, it may often be the cause of power plays between the two people, the less *needy* one being the one to dominate the relationship, and the *needier* one to resentfully accept this dominance due to his or her need for the other partner.

Power plays are not the only manifestation of relationships mired in mutual need. Another frequent expression is obsession or possessiveness, or a need to control. And you can imagine – if you haven't been there – the kind of resentment and negative feelings that this can generate on the part of both people. Akin to any substance addiction, obsession or possessiveness or the need to control can take people to hellish places in their hearts and minds that few of us would wish to visit. I have created an entire workshop on this topic, because although this type of addiction is often masked by a veneer of sophistication, it occurs more frequently than most people suspect, and makes the existence of those that suffer from it a living nightmare.

So why do we become needy in relationships? Of the roughly 40% men and 60% women that come to my private practice, many would initially answer that 'needing' your love partner is how it should be. But why should love imply a feeling that almost always develops into something negative, and at best, makes those who feel it that they could not live without the beloved, thus 'proving' in their minds, that this is really love? Is that really what love is all about?

Wouldn't it make more sense to assume that love means freedom rather than independence? What does needing our partner tell us?

Let's start with the falling in love part. What are we actually falling in love with? Stated simply, we fall in love with those bits and pieces of *ourselves* that we have not yet recognized, but that we find (via projection) in the partner. Is she tender and understanding? Is he funny and the center of the party? Is she strong and enterprising? Is he confident, with a great sense of integrity? All of those qualities may well be part of your partner's character, but the fact that you fell in love with those specific traits, tells you that they are actually part of your own character *as well*.

Since you do not yet manifest those qualities, because you have not yet recognized them in yourself, you need your partner to be able to 'be in touch with' that part of you. That is what 'hooks' you on your partner. Your partner's presence in your life gives you contact to those parts of you that you have not yet developed, making you feel that your partner is absolutely indispensable to your well-being.

So then, when something happens to the relationship, or your partner leaves, or threatens to leave, is when the strong feelings of need arise. This is the time when you should realize that these strong feelings of need are a vast red flag letting you know something is going on inside of you *that only you can do something about*. If you ignore it, or translate it into *"I was deeply wounded by my partner"*, or *"my partner did not return my feelings when I most needed him/her, so I guess that means I always choose the wrong people"*, or *"next time I will choose better, so that this kind of thing never happens to me again"*, then instead of resolving your inner dilemma, you will merely perpetuate it by maintaining the status quo inside of you, falling in love with yet another person that puts you in touch with bits of you that you have not yet recognized in yourself, and thus setting yourself up to be 'needy'.

The other side of the coin in this particular relationship pattern is emotional unavailability which can be devastating to everyone touched by it. People often mistakenly understand it as a ploy on the part of the emotionally unavailable person to *use* others, or to *get without giving*, and while it is true that some of that may happen at times, it is also true that it consistently undermines the existence of the one who suffers from it, and consequently wraps its painful tentacles around those who are in the life of that person.

As we have seen, it's a subject fraught with pain and difficulty, potentially more so for the person on the receiving end of an emotionally unavailable partner or parent or friend, but also on the side of the individual who "plays" out the role of the emotionally unavailable person, as they too, can suffer tremendously from it.

Looking For Daddy (or Mommy)

This one can work in several ways. You might not have had *enough* of your opposite gender parent as a child. Or you might have had too much, in the sense of being over-protected, over-loved, and over-spoiled. Either way, it was dysfunctional, and you will seek - subconsciously - to correct the dysfunction by repeating the pattern with your adult partners. As long as they play the role you were accustomed as a child, nothing changes. But if they should leave you, or if you, by any chance, decide that not being loved properly (in the case where you are repeating the pattern of a missing, absent of rejecting father or mother, for example) is not good, and hence *you*, yourself, are in fact the one who leaves, you will initially crave another relationship that allows you to work out the pattern, you will assume you have chosen badly, or had bad luck in your choice of partner. Nevertheless, as already stated repeatedly in this chapter, once you recognize that there is a pattern (after several such failed relationships), you may begin to take note and proactively seek to change your psyche. (For a more detailed discussion about this pattern see Chapter 6).

****

There are numerous other patterns in relationships, variations on those already described here, as well as different ones. However, the purpose of this chapter is not to exhaust the possibilities, but merely to point out that this - the patterns - is a phase in our relationship lives that occurs more often than not, and that the sooner we can recognize our particular pattern and understand its purpose in our lives, the sooner we will be able to move beyond it, and attract another kind of relationship into our lives.

Chapter 5

Discovering Your Patterns

One of the ways of discovering your patterns is by doing a very simple exercise, that then - once you've completed it - nevertheless will require a good deal of courageous self-reflection.

Take a sheet of paper for every important romantic or love relationship in your life. This may include even the time you were utterly infatuated with the boy/girl next door when you were still in your early teens, depending on the depth of your feelings, your yearning, or your despair about the situation. Here is how you do it:

1. On separate sheets of paper write the name of the person, the year or years it took place, as well as your

and their age during the time the relationship lasted (even if it only existed in your head).

2.   Next write down how you met.

3.   For each relationship, now list everything that initially attracted you to that person. *Not* their physical attributes, as much as something about them as a person, some inner quality: their joy, the capacity to stand up for others, their seriousness, their intellectual capacity, their inner strength, their sense of humor, etc.

4.   Now contemplate the demise of the relationship: Who ended it: you, or your partner?

5.   What caused it to end? Were there specific events that led to that point? Or did it have more to do with how you *now* perceived the other, as opposed to how you used to see them earlier?

6.   Or do you remember your partner saying much the same to you, to justify why he/she was ending it: that he/she believed that *you* had changed and were no longer the person you had made yourself out to be at the beginning?

7.   Make a few notes (some brief bullet points will do) about how you felt when it was over: relieved, devastated, enraged, sad, resentful, in agonizing emotional and perhaps even physical pain, etc.

8.   Assuming you've now done this for *each* of those relationships, the next part has to do with you discovering what *connects* all these people that formed part of your life and heart over a period of time. This may require some deeper thinking because at first glance you may continue to believe that they were all

very different. And of course, on some level they were: older, younger, bigger, smaller, successful, less successful, but on another level - and this is the level that interests us for the purposes of this exercise - they *affected* you in similar ways. What were those ways?

9. Did you wind up feeling you had married your father? Your mother? Or someone who always criticized you and never approved of anything you did? Someone who wanted you all to him/herself and got jealous if you spent time with your friends or on your hobbies? Someone who tried to isolate you from the life you had before meeting this person? Or perhaps you felt that the more time you spent together, the more this person became cool, aloof, and perhaps even cold. Or no longer wanted to have sex. Or refused to be physically affectionate. Or was incapable of saying loving words. Or giving a compliment. Or perhaps they were so demanding, so jealous, so needy, that you thought you might suffocate.

10. I imagine you get the drift. Your job now is to discover in what ways the different individuals who have populated your relationship life to this point, were, in fact, quite similar, *especially* in how they affected you.

11. This is of crucial importance, because it is a strong indicator of one of your prime relationship patterns - probably born in the depths of your earliest childhood in relationship to one or both of your parents, and that you have been grappling with since you were a child, and most particularly since you first fell in love.

12. It explains in quite clear and exact fashion why you continually attract 'this' type of person into your love life. If you will read the chapter on relationships, you will see that our relationships are jewels in our life that

serve to help us grow. And of course the way they help us grow is by causing us to overcome our patterns by resolving - *in ourselves* - that which was left unsolved when we were children due to incomplete parenting. Note: we almost *all* had incomplete parenting, as did our parents have incomplete parenting, as did theirs (our grandparents), and so on. Until the world changes what it teaches us at school, and until the world decides that the conscious inner quest including self-love and self-responsibility is *at least* as important as outer success in life, we can assume that parents will continue to muddle through as best they can, and unfortunately, often that 'best' is not nearly good enough.

13. At this point, if you are being honest and courageous in your process of self-reflection, you will recognize that the 'things' you are blaming on, or accusing your past partners of, are, in fact, matters that tie in to your own issues. Was your partner cold? *Perhaps you are too needy and hence attract cold partners.* Was your partner too suffocating? *Perhaps you are too emotionally unavailable and hence attract needy people to your life.* Was your partner too critical? *Perhaps you have a total lack of self-love and self-esteem.* Was your partner too over-bearing, inconsiderate, etc.? *Perhaps your boundaries are not healthy and need to be shored up.* Do you see how it always comes back to you? It may very well be true that your partner needs to do some extensive work on his/her own issues, it may even be that your partner is/was an absolute jerk, but *that is completely beside the point for our concerns here.* All you need to worry about is how to resolve your *own* issues. That is all you are responsible for, in order that your life may improve; thereby improving the very quality of all your hours and days and your inner well-being.

14. So it's crucial that you understand - and I reiterate - that these people who have come into your life, and who are now, by virtue of your analysis of your relationships, showing you one or more patterns, *are the key to solving your issue.* They themselves have nothing to do with it. You might even still be in a relationship with the last of these. The resolving lies in your own hands, but it lies there now, thanks to what you discovered about yourself due to these relationships.

15. What you now do in order to resolve the issue will allow you to move to another level in your development. And what you now do will comprise most of the following:

    a. being conscious and aware

    b. being mindful in such a way that you remain present, as opposed to wandering off to the past or future in your thoughts

    c. taking full responsibility for all you think, feel, say, do, and how you react

    d. knowing you always have a choice

    e. beginning to love yourself by *always* fully taking care of the state of your inner energetic frequency, your inner well-being, as well as your balance, equilibrium, or inner state of peace (how to bring about change and improvement in all these points and more is fully addressed in Chapters 13 and 14).

16. At this point you will begin to pull the projection from *out* there in to yourself. Why? Because what you projected *out there* when you were falling in love - some of those specific qualities that endeared the other to you so much - now begin to form part of your own personality, character, and psyche. *The reason you projected them out there was because you had not yet recognized them as forming part of yourself in a nascent*

*state. That was the reason why you had to 'love them'
out there in the guise of the other person. That was why
you 'needed' that other person's presence so much, and
why you felt so unbelievably good when you were with
him/her. It allowed you - in this roundabout fashion - to
connect with yourself. It allowed you - in other words -
to be able to love yourself.* So of course, when the other
no longer behaves the way you *need* them to, in order
to get that feeling, or when the other leaves, you are
bereft in ways that may leave you reeling. Until loving
the self is not learned along with learning how to walk,
we will always be faced with this dilemma (also see my
book *The Power of Your Heart: Loving the Self*).

17. A final thought about this process of discovering your
    patterns and learning what to do with the information
    you have acquired, is that you now have the
    opportunity - should you *not* be in a relationship at this
    time - to *observe* yourself consciously in any new
    relationship that you may begin. You will see in a much
    more transparent fashion what your typical triggers are,
    and where - in the process of beginning a relationship
    with another - you begin to make movies in your head
    regarding that other person. And of course, if you've
    done your home work as in point 15, you will now be
    conscious and aware enough to both change that inner
    dialogue about the other in your head, as well as to
    have already supplied yourself with self-love in such a
    way, that although you obviously wish to include love in
    the gamut of possibilities of your life, you will *never*
    again allow your *need* for love to dictate anything at all.
    Why? Because you will be fulfilling your own need for it,
    and hence, when you come to the table, you won't
    need it. You won't become a dependent half of a
    dysfunctional relationship. Rather, you will open the
    door to a totally different kind of love where neither of
    you is dependent on the other, because you both

complement each other. You might also benefit from re-reading pages 5 and 6 in the Foreword, as you may now derive a new meaning from those paragraphs.

Chapter 6

Fatherless Women & Motherless Men

The lack of the opposite gender parent in a child's life can have numerous significant ramifications as we shall see in this chapter. The parent may have died physically, or is 'dead' because he/she is absent from the child's life in a meaningful way, not only due to abandonment or divorce, but also due to simply not caring for the child in those necessary ways during the early developmental stages of our lives that help us grow into healthy adults. If the biological parent is gone and an adoptive parent (or new partner of the remaining parent) has taken on the role of the missing biological parent, then the adoptive parent's lack of caring - should that be the case - is just as toxic to the child's healthy development as the biological parent's lack of caring would have been.

Note that what we are examining here is *not* poor bonding or attachment, which we have already discussed in Chapter 3, and which typically occurs in very early infancy and childhood, but an absence - perceived or real - of one of the parents by the child.

Absence due to death may occasionally even be easier to deal with both psychologically and emotionally, than the *other* absence in which the parent is very much alive but missing from the child's life in that meaningful way.

The problems that bring adult clients to my office in the instance of having had a supportive opposite-gender parent are very different from those that occur for individuals whose parent did not give them a sense of security, protection, love, caring, and last, but most certainly not least, of caring about them and the content of their lives.

This lack of interest and caring about them and the content of their lives implies that *getting* those feelings of being loved and being protected always entails a struggle of sorts. It is *never* something they are automatically assured of having simply because they happen to be the child of that parent. That struggle, in turn, implies a chronic underlying anxiety related to love. As you can see, these individuals are already on the road to feeling - almost always subconsciously - that they need to protect themselves somehow; to erect some sort of defense mechanism in the arena of love.

Clearly then, the condition in early life of motherlessness and fatherlessness frequently depends not on the death of the parent, but on the fact that the parent of the opposite gender is not there for the child in the optimal and ideal way that is necessary for emotional, psychological, spiritual, and in some cases, even physical development to take place in a healthy fashion. Therefore, due to this lack of parenting which may often occur even when the parent is doing their best, dysfunctionality in the personality of the growing boy or girl evolves. The reason it often occurs, even when the parents are doing their level best, is due to what I call the *non-adult, non-self-reflective, and uninformed parent syndrome* which is touched on several times throughout this book, but most particularly in Chapter 14. Remember, as we have already seen, when individuals who are themselves the product of this "parent syndrome", and then *also* become parents, it will require much awareness, re-thinking, and re-educating in order for them to evolve into a healthier role model for their own children.

Adult Women Raised Without a Father

Little girls who live without a father do so not only due to death, abandonment, or divorce, but also due to physically present fathers but who are emotionally absent, or ill over a lengthy period of time in some way (clinical depression, terminal disease, etc.), or because the father is a workaholic, or because in some fashion the father is a disappointment to the daughter, as might be the case when the father is weak or ineffectual. Such differing types of absence in the girl's life may have major consequences of varying kinds, since an ideally healthy emotional and socio-psychological developmental trajectory in the early years of life *does* require some type of positive paternal role model.

Optimally, a little girl needs to see herself reflected in the love she sees for herself in her father's eyes. This is how she develops self confidence and self esteem. This is how she develops a healthy familiarity with what a positive expression of love feels like. This is how she develops an appreciation for her own looks and her own body. This is how she develops what Jungians would call her "animus", her counter-sexual self; her masculine self, which will help her be proactive, productive, and creative in the outer world as she grows into adulthood.

If, however, the little girl does *not* have such a relationship with the father, if she sees rejection or emotional coldness or withdrawal in him, or if he simply is not available at all, her sense of self will be tainted, her self confidence warped or non-existent, her portrait of a loving relationship may be distorted or dysfunctional, and she may find herself, no matter how pretty, vivacious, lovable, funny, or intelligent, lacking in appeal.

Clearly, self confidence and self esteem can be forged through one's own endeavors during the life course, even if a father has not been present, but the path to success in such endeavors, and the *reasons* for which they are even attempted, tend to be quite different in the adult woman who was raised with a positive relationship to her father, as opposed to the one who was not. The former may excel simply because she believes in herself, while the latter *needs* to excel in order to catch a glimpse of approval and recognition in the eyes of those who give her a message of approval, honor, or prestige. The value of such a belief in oneself, easily acquired by the woman with a positive relationship to her father, is immeasurable in the adult life. Conversely, the lack of it in many of the countless women who were raised without a positive father image may cause the life course to be fraught with difficulties.

Perhaps the arena in which the most painful process of learning how to deal with the early lack of a father is played out is in that of relationships. If a girl has not been assured of her value as a woman by that early relationship with the father, she finds it difficult to relate to men precisely because she may often unconsciously seek to find that recognition in the eyes of the beloved and this may lead her down an early path of promiscuity which in turn makes her feel she is "bad", but on she marches, relentlessly visiting bed after bed, locking in a fierce embrace with man after man, in the hope that *this* one or *that* one, or the *next* one will finally give her that which she never had as a child – validation of herself for herself.

Other women may choose another route, falling in love with an older man and thus marrying "daddy". At this point many different scenarios may ensue. If the man is at all psychologically aware (something often, but not always lacking in older men who like younger girls), he may have a vague inkling of what is going on. Therefore, once she starts – within the secure confines of the relationship or marriage – the process of growth, which will inevitably lead her to separate from her husband in some ways that are emotionally and psychologically necessary in order for her become her own woman, he will not blanch in fear at this process, and allow her the necessary space and freedom to do so. In that case, the marriage will in all likelihood thrive and continue to grow. If, however, the man is not aware, and sees her search for growth as a threat to the superiority he felt upon marrying a young, and as yet undeveloped woman, he will attempt to stifle her, to manipulate her psychologically by making her believe she is worthless, silly, or, and this appears to be a perennial favorite, that she "needs professional help in order to calm down and behave like she used to before".

Another possible scenario is that of avoiding relationships totally, or *of avoiding the engagement of one's emotions.* Examples here abound: the maiden aunt, who dedicates her life to her nieces and nephews, or who becomes a teacher and dedicates her life to her career; the nun, who dedicates her life to God, or the prostitute, who, although she may engage her body, rarely engages her emotions. Another example is that of the eternal seductress, who needs to remain in control by seducing the man and never actually involving her own feelings. A slightly more difficult to recognize version of the same scenario is played out by the woman who consistently has relationships with married men who never leave their respective wives for her. On an unconscious level this suits her just fine because it gives her the perfect excuse never to have to commit herself totally.

The core of the matter is, of course, that the self-confidence and recognition so avidly sought must be found within oneself rather than in the outer world – at least initially - in order to be of lasting and true value. The world of emotions that is avoided out of fear or because one never really learned what love is, must first be found in oneself (i.e., it is necessary to love the self *before* one loves another). The task of accomplishing this, requires that the individual become aware of him or herself (by observing the self, the *self-talk*, and all emotions that occur, good or bad, since all of these serve to give clues about the true self), and that *absolute honesty* about oneself be employed in this endeavor. Let the reader be warned: this process is not a simple weekend project; it must be ongoing throughout life; it must become second nature, but it *will* pave the road to finding inner self-confidence and love for oneself, which will in turn lead to eliminating the need for finding these things in another. This is one of the roads to inner freedom that psychological knowledge offers.

Case Studies

The clinical case studies that follow are not exhaustive as there are many more types of fatherless women and motherless men than those discussed here, but this will give you an idea of some of the backgrounds of people whose childhoods missed out on having an intact and healthy relationship with the parent of the opposite gender, even when that parent was trying his or her best.

Obviously as we've already seen throughout this book, one of the problems is that the parents often have many unresolved issues from their own childhood, and if they don't have the benefit of information such as this, then of course, these parents may not even *know* that their way of behaving is dysfunctional, and are most certainly *not* consciously working on changing their behavior, thought patterns, and manner of reacting.

Remember also, as you read these case studies, that what is being depicted by the light strokes of the brush each description offers is merely an outline of the beginning of the pattern that then comes to trouble the individual later on in life.

Clinical case studies of the background and pattern of fatherless women

"Liz": "The Caretaker"

- This girl frequently has an alcoholic father, or a father who is addicted to either another substance, or some kind of addictive behavior such as gambling, over-working, etc.

- She loves him very much and by caring for him in any way a little girl can, such as fetching him his slippers when he comes home, or getting him a soft pillow, she ensures her importance in his life.

- She also quickly becomes aware of the fact that there are days where it is best not to speak to him, or to only speak in certain ways, or to only use a certain tone of voice.

- As she grows older, making sure no one sees his addiction, by hiding his bottles, or covering up for him when he slurs his words, or in any other way manifests his addictive behavior or its consequences, she continues her role of importance in his life, and lives in this caretaking role.

- The pattern here tends to be that she takes on responsibility for what is not - and never should have been - hers to be responsible for - she becomes the caretaker of others' problems.

- She blossoms; she feels good, when she does this, either because she feels that her father, and later others will be grateful to her when she takes care of them and solves their problems for them, or because this way she feels needed, or because she believes that this is the way to be loved by another.
- This will evidently affect her behavior in her adult relationships.

"Michelle": "Daddy's little girl - as long as you adore me - another kind of betrayal and rejection"

- This girl's father comes in several versions.
- In one version he appears and reappears in the girl's life because he no longer lives with the mother, but his interaction with the daughter is not stable, so she can never count on him in those ways that are necessary for her healthy psychological and emotional development.
- In another version he actually lives with the family, but his presence is somehow not stable, either because he travels a great deal, or spends much time working, or socializing with business associates, and thus does not participate in family events, causing a similar kind of absence for his little girl.
- Furthermore, this daddy either sexually abuses his daughter, or is somehow inappropriate in the way he behaves with her - possibly because there are sexual innuendos in how he treats her.
- Due to this behavior from the time she is very little, she comes to believe it is normal which means her sexual boundaries as an adult woman will be skewed.
- The father also tends to be emotionally immature, and is incapable of showing his little daughter warmth and acceptance, except insofar as it coincides with his own needs, in which case they are given priority over hers, and this creates even greater insecurity in her.

- She may strongly dislike her mother because she feels that her mother comes between herself and her beloved father.
- She may feel guilty towards her mother.
- The pattern here tends to be that the daughter always feels insecure about her father's love for her, about her "lovability", and about – as she grows older – her desirability as a woman.
- She probably feels strongly rejected or abandoned whenever her father is not present, or when he is anything but warm and accepting of her, which is something that obviously only happens - if at all - on the rarest of occasions. It is as though his love and acceptance always come at a price.
- Later on, sex may be fraught with dysfunctionality for her, either due to herself or the partners she attracts into her life who may be somewhat dysfunctional in the matter, or a combination of both.
- This will evidently affect her behavior in her adult relationships a great deal

"Robin": "Daddy never saw her - as though she never existed."

- This father never knew he had a little girl.
- It was almost as though she never existed.
- When he looked at her, she felt he was looking through transparent glass, and not at her.
- He rarely speaks directly to her, or if he does, he generally ignores what she says, or he gives little or no importance to her wants, likes and dislikes.
- He may become aware of the fact that she is sexually precocious at a young age, and she may know that he knows, and yet he fails to react in any fashion.
- The pattern here tends to be that she feels that her wishes, her thoughts, her wants, likes, and dislikes are of no importance and value, almost that she has no

right to them, and will therefore discount her own worth.

- She probably finds it very difficult to give herself any kind of recognition and she will find it difficult to appreciate any of her gifts.
- She may often apologize for herself.
- She may be artificially gay and give the appearance of being vivacious and full of life, or intellectually very bright, in order to grab daddy's attention, but when she is alone she wonders where all her gaiety or intelligence went.
- This will evidently affect her behavior in her adult relationships a great deal.

"Janine": "Blind love and betrayal of the girl through the mother"

- This daddy is adored by his daughter.
- Her adoration is blind – as it frequently is in the case of a dysfunctional relationship between father and daughter.
- She observes how her mother suffers through her father's affairs, but no one ever discusses it.
- There is an enormous elephant in the home while she is growing up, but it feels as though she is the only one who sees the elephant.
- Somehow she sees her mother as weak.
- Therefore her father must be excused for behaving as he does; for having affairs, because if the mother is weak, or clinging, or cries a lot, or is cold to him, then there must be a good reason for daddy to look for other women.
- Sometimes daddy even produces little half-brothers and half-sisters for her, and although she sees mummy's pain, she somehow accepts them in order to be able to continue loving daddy.

- She is determined not to ever be like the mother and so becomes extremely capable and as she grows older, she becomes a virtual expert in always taking care of any problems that arise.
- Frequently mommy does not behave like a mother, either because she is too much of a child herself, or too weak, or too cold, or too emotionally immature. She tends to be quite manipulative.
- This daughter takes the place of her mother in many ways, even though the mother is not dead or otherwise not available to the household - she is just either weak, or sick and frail, or occasionally she may be occupied with her career.
- The pattern here tends to be that she has great difficulty in seeing anything good about having been born a female because of what she sees happening to her mother.
- Nevertheless, since she must search for daddy in her adult relationships, she does have to be feminine, and may – despite her extreme capability and intelligence – take an inferior role or even a powerless role to the men in her life. In many ways, she is broken, just like her mother, because of her fear of the pain daddy provoked in mommy that could come to visit her in her own relationships.
- This will evidently affect her behavior in her adult relationships a great deal.

"Marilyn": "Love is pain; pain is love"

- This daddy is truly abusive.
- He may sexually abuse his daughter.
- He may also physically abuse her.
- And he may emotionally and psychologically abuse her
- What leaves the greatest marks on her, however, is the sexual and physical abuse.

- She may self-mutilate, become addictive, develop eating disorders, and most likely will search for a father substitute as an adult, because her daddy was not a real daddy. (Note: not all people who manifest such behaviors have been abused by a parent).
- Until she begins resolving the issues, however, the substitute daddy may also turn abusive.
- The pattern here tends to be that her life is felt to be in total chaos, that she has no control over what happens to her, and that she has no sense whatsoever of her value.
- This will evidently affect her behavior in her adult relationships a great deal.

"Maya": "You are so precious and wonderful, *only* I know how to love you"

- This daddy offers life to his little girl on a silver tray.
- Nothing is too good for his little girl.
- He spoils her endlessly and gives her not only whatever she wants, but anything he thinks she should have.
- He typically attempts to mold her in the image of the perfect woman that he has in his mind.
- (This father does not generally abuse or behave sexually inappropriately with his little girl in any way).
- He continually tells her how precious she is and how much he loves her.
- He tells her that no one will ever love her like he does.
- He tells her that no one will ever take care of her the way he does.
- He tells her that the world is full of predatory men.
- He creates a golden cage for her.
- The *pattern* here tends to be that she grows up believing she is entitled to having all her wishes fulfilled, and that all men will behave with her the way her father does.

- She never has a chance to experience disappointment.
- She never has to be patient to wait to receive something or to achieve something because (depending on his financial means and social connections) daddy always makes sure she gets it immediately, whether it is a doll, or a pony, a BMW, or being admitted to Harvard, Yale, or Oxford.
- This will evidently affect her behavior in her adult relationships a great deal.

Adult Men Raised Without a Mother

As we've already discussed in the case of girls and women, boys and men who are raised without a mother, are not necessarily *motherless*. Rather, it is the *mothering* that has somehow run amuck and left these boys, and later their adult, masculine self in a vacuum of sorts.

Mothering can go astray in many ways, and we'll examine some case studies further on in this chapter. As a general rule, a mother who does not mother her sons well, may have any number or combination of the following issues:

- She did not have good parenting herself.
- She never learned how to love herself.
- She probably has poor self-esteem (no matter how accomplished or physically beautiful).
- She had poor role models; indeed, her own mother may have been cold and unfeeling.
- She may have little access to her own feelings due to all of the above.
- She may be both emotionally unavailable and very needy.
- She potentially lacks a self-reflective capacity.
- She is potentially reactive.
- She has poor boundaries.

- Due to her emotional unavailability coupled with neediness, she may be emotionally volatile in the sense that her son never truly knows when he can depend on her to be there for him, as she is so busy fulfilling her own unmet needs out there with any number of people, events, possessions, etc., and thus lacks the psychological wherewithal to be there for her son.
- She may have numerous addictions, although not necessarily to substances.
- She may be chaotic on many levels, or conversely, she may be a control freak or perfectionist in rigid, controlling ways in order to recapture some measure of serenity in a world that never felt safe to her.

Men who were children of mothers who in some major ways were not there for them, or whose mothers abandoned them, or who died at important stages of their lives, may occasionally find themselves attracted to the kind of woman who appears to be very sure of herself, very independent, perhaps not quite as young as the women his friends are attracted to, in short, a woman who can, on some level take good care of him. Careful, I'm not saying that she does or that she will - simply that she gives the appearance of being able to do this.

These men tend to have a yearning for warmth, closeness, and love that can be enormously attractive to women who come in touch with them. Yet, due to all the reasons we've already discussed, it often happens that when such men are given such warmth, closeness, and love, they begin to feel suffocated.

Yet I recall two couples, both in their early 40's where just the opposite happened. The husband's mother - in both cases - had been cold, critical, forbidding, even abusive on some levels, and the adult men craved warmth, love, affection, tenderness, and yet, both had married -

almost as if there were a spreadsheet formula or psychological protocol that they were following - *more than once* - women who were cold and rejecting.

Clinical case studies of the background and pattern of motherless men

"Jonathan" "You'll never measure up to your father"

- Successful father.
- Mother with no real accomplishments of her own - she is the father's right hand, hostess, companion, and helpmeet, but she lives her life vicariously through her husband.
- She admires him a great deal.
- He dominates her without being a boor, but he is the man of the house.
- He cherishes her, may load her with gifts, but she clearly comes after him in the food chain.
- The couple is generally already firmly established when the child is born, and often the child is an only child, but he may also be one of several siblings, often a middle child.
- In some instances I have observed, if the son is an only child, he comes as an afterthought.
- If he is one of several siblings, the couple may be striving for the "perfect" family.
- The son adores his mother, but she, although she loves him a great deal, seems to have eyes only for her beloved and adored husband.
- This boy admires his father tremendously, attempts to emulate him in everything, and tries to follow his footsteps.
- The pattern tends to be that no matter how accomplished he is, in his own eyes, somehow he has failed.

- He has not measured up to his father – not even in his mother's eyes - so she continues to regard him as a boy, even if he is a man.
- This will evidently affect his behavior in his adult relationships a great deal.

"Malcolm": "Abandonment"

- This boy is born into a family where the mother may be lacking in the ability to easily show her affection
- She may feel uncomfortable in the family milieu and may need to participate in many work or social activities in order to ameliorate this discomfort with the closeness of the family.
- Obviously the children, especially the sons, will suffer due to her lack of continuous presence.
- Once again the boy adores his slightly unapproachable mother.
- She may have a demanding career or job that maintains her away from him.
- She may devote herself to volunteer work or charities, or she may travel a great deal with the father - the point is, she is not there "enough" for the boy in the boy's eyes.
- In other words, he perceives that she abandons him, even though from her point of view she is actually very much there for him.
- He goes through the pain of real abandonment - as a small child - because of his perception of her lack of time and attention spent with him.
- The pattern tends to be that although he had nothing to do with what he perceives as her abandonment of him, or the lack of time she spends with him, he always feels as though if only he were a better boy, or if only he could please her more, so that she would love him more, she would not abandon him, or not spend so little time with him.

- He is not good enough − so he thinks − he somehow always fails to live up to his mother's expectations.
- This will evidently affect his behavior in his adult relationships a great deal.

"Richard": "Lovelessness and rejection"

- This mother is abusive.
- She may physically hurt her son, or she may stand by while the father does so and not defend the son.
- She may be cold and loveless, but not just with a little difficulty in expressing her emotions, but so cold and loveless that he knows deep in his bones that she does not love him.
- If she does not physically hurt her son, she may abuse him emotionally or psychologically, making sure he knows he is not loved and cared for.
- Or the abuse may be a combination of all three: physical, emotional, and psychological.
- I should say that this mother is not *sexually* abusive - for that to occur between mother and son, there is generally a totally different kind of relationship between the two than the one I am describing.
- The pattern again, depending on the degree of the abuse and utter lack of love and affection, tends to be that the son believes there is something wrong with him.
- Rejection and lack of self-esteem as well as rebellion can be typical feelings that arise throughout childhood and the teen years.
- This will evidently affect his behavior in his adult relationships a great deal.

"Damien": "Betrayal"

- In this case the mother tends to have a weaker personality than the father.

- The father may be quite dominant or authoritarian in the household.
- Frequently there may be a prolonged absence of the father, due to business, imprisonment, war, emigration to another country while the mother and son wait to be called once the father has established himself in the new country, typifies this particular situation.
- During the father's absence, especially if the son was very young, the son grows accustomed to being the mother's only "man".
- If family finances play a negative role, it may even happen that the young boy shares a bed with his mother due to a lack of space.
- So the boy becomes even more possessive of his mother than a normal child would.
- The love relationship between the two may be much more pronounced than it normally would due to the circumstances described.
- When the family then is called by the father to join him in the new country, or he returns from a long business trip, or a sojourn in prison, or from war, the young boy is rudely awakened.
- His father now replaces him in his mother's arms and her bed, and even though there has been nothing improper going on between mother and son, the son feels bereft and betrayed by his mother.
- He may also feel as though his father is an intruder, a usurper, someone who is stealing his mother.
- The pattern here tends to be that it revolves around betrayal - the son probably loves the mother a great deal, but after the initial act of betrayal there is always an uneasy feeling of mistrust.
- This feeling of insecurity; this need to defend the self undermines his confidence, as though the boy always has to conquer someone or something.
- This will evidently affect his behavior in his adult relationships a great deal.

"Victor": "I will spoil and pamper you - but you may not grow up"

- This mother is so loving one could never fault her with anything.
- She does everything for her young son.
- When he starts going to school she makes it her business to be part of any and all school committees in order to be closer to him.
- She makes certain other boys from the son's environment always want to come to his house, rather than sending him to their homes.
- She makes her home a place where everyone wants to come because in this way she is better able to 'control' her son's life.
- She helps her son with his homework, and if he forgets to do something, she sits up all night and does it.
- When he is a bit older, she takes care of his speeding fines.
- She is very concerned about his friends and therefore makes sure he begins to dislike those that she considers inappropriate by talking about them in such a way as to make him see them with other eyes.
- When he begins to see girls, she manages to get rid of those she does not approve of, and when there is one she likes, it is because she can either control her, or because in her she has an ally, i.e. a clone of herself.
- The pattern here tends to be that the son is always looking back at mommy to see if she approves; if she encourages him; if she is nodding her head and telling him he is OK.
- He has difficulty believing in his own judgement, and thus difficulty in crossing thresholds, in moving on in life, but of course because of his mother's strict controls with velvet gloves, at some point he will rebel.
- This will evidently affect his behavior in his adult relationships a great deal.

"Sean": "You owe me"

- This mother believes she has sacrificed herself for her son.
- She may do very little for him.
- She may show him little love and affection, but she never ceases to tell him how much he owes her for giving him life.
- She may have abused him physically, or particularly in the sense of making him feel ashamed of the fact that he is a man.
- She may have verbally denigrated men all his life, because men mistreat women, and because men are not to be trusted and so on, making it exceedingly difficult for him - as he grows up - to form an identity.
- She is an expert manipulator and constantly asks her son for "proof" of his love for her.
- The pattern here tends to be that the son feels he "owes" mother his life, his all; that he owes her all his time, because she gave him life, because she – or so she says – has done everything for him.
- He eventually feels he is in prison, and may not clearly see the way to get out. He may feel minimized or ridiculed in his masculinity.
- This will evidently affect his behavior in his adult relationships a great deal.

Typical Manifestations of Motherlessness & Fatherlessness

- Typically there is a major lack of self-love, self-esteem, true 'inner' (as opposed to 'outer' or persona-like) self-confidence, self-respect, self-approval, etc.
- They are often people pleasers in order to receive love, acceptance, affection, even respect and gratitude.
- These people may need to control their environment in ways that others might classify as overt perfectionism, although it is important to understand that this gives

them a sense of order in their inner chaos (note that this is very similar to a characteristic describing the mother of motherless men, and of course one of the reasons this pattern repeats itself in the two generations, is because the mother herself was not mothered well in her infancy and childhood).

- They are needy and insecure.
- They may be overly suspicious and even border on the paranoid.
- They may feel a great need to achieve and we might easily call them 'over-achievers' because it frequently gives them a sense of self due to the approval and admiration they receive from others when they reach their goals.
- Their fear of rejection induces them to many unhealthy behaviors, simply to ensure they will continue to be loved.
- They tend to have unhealthy boundaries and may often have become enablers and caretakers.
- Authority figures, rules, and restrictions may provoke them to unacceptable behavior.
- If they have gathered no insight about themselves - or until they do so - they may very well repeat the cycle of abuse with their own children.
- They tend to have difficulty in emotional expression.
- Often there is evidence of sexual dysfunction.
- Self-harming and/or eating disorders may form part of the profile.

Some characteristics of a functionally intact adult male or female

A functionally intact adult may not have grown up that way. What I am trying to say, is that he may have pulled himself out of the dysfunctional quagmire that was represented in his early years. He may have gone into therapy, or he may have recognized what happened to him and begun to work on himself. He may have been in a relationship that helped him to become more aware of his own issues emanating from his childhood, or he may have read a book, or taken a course at university, or participated in a workshop that opened his eyes to these unresolved matters.

Whatever the case, whether he grew up in a dysfunctional family, or in a somewhat healthier psycho-emotional environment, he has now come to a point at which he is able to demonstrate a fair share of the following characteristics, and as you will understand, it is crucial to be aware of this in order to know what to move towards via inner pictures, if you yourself are grappling with the issues described earlier in this chapter:

- He/she has learned (is learning) how to love him/herself
- He/she believes in him or herself.
- He/she achieves for the sake of achieving, and not in order to be recognized or praised.
- He/she has no need to control others.
- He/she finds it easy to trust others.
- He/she finds it easy to show affection and love.
- He/she does not manipulate others.
- He/she has no difficulty being transparent (open, honest, no "mixed messages") at all times.
- He/she knows he is responsible for everything he feels, thinks, says or does.
- He/she is aware of his reactions at all times, and knows there are always choices.
- He/she has no trouble maintaining healthy boundaries.

Chapter 7

Physical & Emotional Symptoms

Physical and emotional symptoms are some of the most important signs that tell you something is going on inside of you that requires tending. I've often said that with regards to the physical symptoms, they are like emails that your body is sending you with the urgent message that you need to do something *now*. The emotional symptoms are similar, and both their presence, as well as their absence - depending on the situation - indicates that something is occurring on deeper levels that requires your attention.

Clearly, however, unless you are already at least somewhat or even *very* aware of yourself, many of these symptoms may literally pass you by. In other words, you may not notice them at all because in some fashion they are simply part of the habitual background noise that goes on inside of you and has been there since you were very young.

Physical Symptoms

You may have noticed that when your partner is attempting to get very close to you - perhaps, from *your* perspective, far *too* close - that you feel a number of physical symptoms. These symptoms can range from a simple twinge in your stomach to great discomfort. Your partner becomes needy or overly clingy, or perhaps too physically affectionate in public, or demanding overt signs of love on your part, and almost as if by black magic, you feel the physical symptoms. You tend to have similar symptoms when your partner becomes - in your estimation - too emotionally demanding of you, or insisting on moving to the next step in your relationship or even committing to living together or getting married.

Please understand that this is a very different kind of discomfort than that felt by someone who is *not* emotionally unavailable, but simply not yet ready to move to the next level. The person who has no issue with emotional unavailability, and who is comfortable with his/her emotions, will not feel a rush of adrenaline, or fear, when being asked for greater affection, or to move to the next level. They may simply not want to do so, or for other, more rational reasons, decide they do not wish to further pursue a closer relationship with this person. Perhaps the relationship is still quite new and yet the new partner is already talking about marriage. The emotionally unavailable person, however, *will* feel that rush of adrenaline or fear, and will typically interpret is as being caused by the other, and hence being the fault of the other, and therefore perceives the other as a source of discomfort - whether physical or emotional.

Or you may have noticed that when your partner begins his/her *moves away* from you that you interpret as rejection and coldness or even abandonment, you notice similar physical symptoms.

These can be very different from person to person, but the following examples are some of the most typical ones:

- a twisting in the area of your stomach or the solar plexus
- a sensation of being stabbed in your heart
- an overly strong heart beat; a pounding heart
- a sense of physical suffocation, as though you can't breathe
- a tightness in your throat - you may find it difficult to speak
- a strong sensation of nausea
- noticeable waves of heat in the area of your chest, neck, or face

Emotional Symptoms or "Affect"

We all have normal emotions that we would expect of any human being in any number of different situations, but often our emotions - even if not *abnormal* - tell us much more than what happens to be occurring on the surface. Here are some examples:

- jealousy of a partner who nevertheless has proven to you over time that he/she is loyal
- dislike of someone you scarcely know
- fear invoked by impending change (a move to a new city or country, a new job, etc.)
- anger or indignation at someone whose opinion is contrary to yours on a subject such as finances, politics, or religion
- self-righteous judgement of someone that you feel has behaved in a morally reprehensible fashion

In each of these examples, the *apparent* reason for the emotion may be obvious; less obvious is the *true* - the underlying reason. Something inside of *you* - as opposed to what has just happened on the outside - is creating these emotions. Your emotions can be likened to a red flag: if something about this subject were not pushing a button in you (touching on some unresolved issue in you), you would not be experiencing these emotions in these specific situations. You would be able to contemplate them objectively from a position of inner equanimity, rather than emotional turmoil.

So both in the case of the physical symptom, as well as in the case of certain emotions, it is up to you to examine what is *really* going on - not as a result of what is happening *out there*; not by blaming something for the specific outer circumstances - but by closely looking at yourself - in order to understand the true meaning and significance of those symptoms. Only if you do that, will you be able to eliminate whatever is blinding you as symbolized by the symptoms, and hence find inner freedom.

Why Do These Physical Symptoms Manifest?

You will find a more integral explanation for this question in the following sections below, but just now I need you to understand that due to the interrelatedness between your psyche (mind & emotions), your spirit (soul), and your body, when your body signals distress just before, during, or after a situation involving interaction with another individual, especially an individual with whom you have a close relationship - although *also* with others - as said, it is as though your body were sending an email to the rest of you.

Clearly this is an email you need to pay close attention to and read carefully because it is in the *understanding and interpretation of the symbolic meaning* of this email, that you will find at the very least the beginning of understanding and potentially also the solution to many issues, including emotional unavailability and neediness.

The body has a language of its own. Not just the language of arms crossed in front of your chest, for example, to signify that you are, perhaps, not open to the conversation in which you are involved, or hands on your hips to signify, perhaps, that you are getting ready to do verbal battle, but a language of physical feelings.

We are all familiar with the heart in our throat syndrome when we are driving along an expressway and suddenly hear police sirens in the distance behind us. *Have I been speeding?* You ask yourself. *Will they stop me? Will I get a ticket?* And then again, we are all familiar with the subsiding of the adrenaline rush and our heart resuming its former quieter pace, when the police cars pass us in pursuit of someone else.

We understand why our heart was racing. We understand why we had the adrenaline rush, just as we also understand similar physical symptoms if someone shouts angrily at us - especially if it's unexpected. But we frequently tend to be *less aware of* and hence understand far less what is going on inside of us when we experience those other symptoms listed above. *Especially* if they arise in what we consider relatively normal relationship situations that we habitually blame on our partners as in: *he/she made me feel that I was under such pressure*, or: *he/she made me feel so rejected.*

All Those Things Your Partners Do to You

Let's look at this more closely. What did your partner just do or say? Your awareness of the actual words or gestures is of great importance in beginning to change your pattern. You generally tell yourself that you feel suffocated or uneasy or anxious because your partner is demanding that you do this or that. In other words, you *blame* your partner for how you feel. In your eyes, it is your partner who has caused those physical or emotional symptoms in you by his/her behavior.

But if you look at this interaction with your partner from the point of view that *your* reaction is caused by your childhood issues because the part of you that feels the symptoms is the part that simply never grew up to your current chronological age because of a deep-rooted fear of the pain that love and need and vulnerability cause, then you begin to see that by recognizing that part of you - that younger part that reacts subconsciously, then you may begin to grasp that it is your *younger self* that needs to be taken care of first. The resolution to your adult dilemma lies on a detour to your younger self. Without this detour to a subconscious and visceral world of feeling, you will probably attempt to resolve matters though your rational mind, and while it is indeed your rational mind that is needed to understand what is happening, the solution lies elsewhere. At least at the beginning.

Recognize the Origin of those Physical Symptoms

Therefore it is very important that you are aware enough to take notice of the physical and emotional warning signs that are telling you that you would be well advised to recognize that it's *your* issue and not your partner's (even if your partner has just done something you find wrong, or even something another person - not involved in your drama - would also deem wrong). Remember that this did not originate with your current partner, or a former partner, but in your own past. For much more about this subject see Chapter 14.

Chapter 8

Sex, Lust, Need & Unavailability

Often – but not always - the emotionally unavailable person is also unavailable sexually, or, if they have made some outward commitment, such as marrying, buying a house together, and/or having a child with the partner, they may - once the commitment is made - withdraw emotionally and sexually, finding it far too emotionally taxing to be engaged on more than one level. For them, simply living together may be enough. Becoming distant or somehow moving away from the partner sexually (sometimes interpreted as manipulative game-playing tactics by the needier person), or not being sexually responsive are furthermore ways of cutting off genuine relating and thus removing what many people with these issues consider to be threats.

Simply put, this might be necessary for some people because by cutting off genuine relating, no emotional expression is required. Engagement with the partner on meaningful levels is not required and that signifies that the emotionally unavailable partner feels safe. This - in some fashion - is another defense mechanism in order to *ensure* that feeling of safety from the potential pain of emotional vulnerability.

How good is your sex life? How often do you have sex? Have you stopped having regular sex because you've been married 10 years and your partner is no longer so stimulating? Or have you stopped because he's in andropause or because she's in menopause and because you never were that crazy about it to begin with? Or maybe you stopped having it with your last partner, but then you found someone new where the passion came alive again and now the pattern is repeating, and it's stopped being exciting once more.

What does all this mean? And more importantly, what can you do about it?

The *energy* that is inherent in sex makes it a much more important aspect of our lives than mere pleasure, although pleasure is obviously a massively contributing part of it. Twenty-first century socialization is such that we are primed from early adolescence on to expect fireworks from sex. We believe sex and all the pleasures it promises will be one of the most vital and essential experiences of our life – *as indeed it can be.*

However, due in part to this socialization via mass media (movies, television commercials, and glossy magazine ads, to name only a few), we come to expect something of our sexual lives that simultaneously *increases* its importance on levels that are perhaps inappropriate or less relevant, and *decreases* its importance in other, much more relevant areas. This ultimately creates a general population that is frequently dissatisfied with its sex life – but for all the wrong reasons, and without knowing what the solution could be.

What is sexual energy? Sexual energy is not only the passion that you feel (hopefully) as you engage in sex, but on other, much more transcendent levels, the doors that open energetically between you and your sexual partner during sex. This energetic exchange remains available for both individuals for a period of time after sex. Have you ever slept in the same bed as your partner and been drained the next day? Conversely, have you ever slept in the same bed as your partner and been refreshed the next day? If you are at all sensitive to the flow that can be established between two people after sex, you will have already connected the dots and realized that the way you feel the next morning does not *only* depend on expressed or unexpressed ardor, or the relative comfort of the mattress and the pillow, but just as much, if not more importantly, on the energetic exchange between the two of you.

Furthermore the importance of speaking clearly cannot be over-emphasized. This applies to sex as well. If you do not speak about it with your partner, you have little chance for the real energy inherent in it to come out. It may be wildly passionate for a time, but the energy you can access with it may not be available to you.

But speaking about sex with your partner is not what it is all about. You must make the *conscious decision to want to grow together with your partner*. This mutual endeavor, via the connection you have through the relationship you share makes the difference between a relationship that may ultimately fail, or lose its fervor, and a relationship that not only has a chance at long-term survival, but also one that – because of the energetic connection inherent in sex – does not eventually flounder and die a slow death of sexual strangulation. The essence of conscious growth in a relationship depends on the couple's desire to grow together psychologically, emotionally, and spiritually, as well as sexually. This implies conscious awareness of the self, conscious awareness of all of one's feelings, thoughts, actions, and reactions, and acceptance of the fact that each of us is responsible for all of these facets of ourselves. Such a *conscious link* between partners keeps sex alive in ways that go far beyond sex toys and fantasy games because it speaks to the *real – and eternal –* connection between the two individuals. My book *The Tao of Spiritual Partnership* deals with this topic in depth.

But let's go back to our sexual relationships the way they often play out long before we even begin to think about connecting on the levels I described above.

Imagine you had a mind-blowing passionate affair. It lasted five weeks, or six months, or two years. You each lived in your own place. Then you decided to move in together. Maybe you even marry. You were so much in love. It made sense to commit. But now, your once passionate partner who desired you so much doesn't want to make love anymore. He/she avoids you, shuns you, and you are bewildered, self doubt arises, you feel hurt, unloved, and finally angry. So you leave, or you threaten to leave, or you find yourself someone else who *does* find you desirable. Suddenly, magically, your partner wants you again. The passion is back. The old chemistry is flying once more. In time things settle down. Everyone is happy - or appears to be - just like at the beginning. *But it happens again. Your partner doesn't want to make love anymore.* What on earth is going on?

Are you a man, and when you were a child you were – in some fashion or another – abandoned by your parents? Perhaps you were ill and had to spend a lengthy period of time in hospital, and perhaps the hospital was too far from your parents' residence for them to visit you more than once a week. Perhaps your parents – and particularly your mother - were kind and caring, but you perceived that they simply did not love you enough for your needs. Perhaps an event occurred while you were still a child that caused you to feel rejected by your mother in a particularly important way.

Are you a woman, and when you were a child you were – in some fashion or another – abandoned by your father? Perhaps your parents – and particularly your father - were kind and caring, but you perceived that they simply did not love you enough for your needs. Perhaps your parents divorced and your father left and rarely saw you. Perhaps he was physically there, but emotionally absent. Perhaps he rejected you. Perhaps you felt he never gave you the approval you so avidly sought. Perhaps he (or another important male in the close family environment) abused you sexually, physically, psychologically, or emotionally.

Whatever the case, in the scenario both for boys and girls, the missing ingredient, or the essential point to realize, is that something has gone awry in the way the child views the love he or she receives from the parent. In other words, the child has not received – or perceived – a developmentally healthy *lesson* about love from the parent.

And what happens when you learn something incorrectly?

Think for a moment how you were taught to hold a pencil when you were learning how to write. Most of us learned it properly. Some didn't and you can see it in the way they hold a pen, or in the way they scrunch their fingers together. How about when you learned how to slice or dice vegetables? Do you julienne? Or do you chop and cut a mess of unequal misshapen pieces? And what about how you learned how to use Excel? Or sew? Or ride a bike? Or dance the tango?

So what happens when you learn something incorrectly? Don't many people continue to do whatever it is wrong again and again and again? Until something happens to make them want to change their method?

And this is exactly what happens when a child learns dysfunctional lessons about how love works. The child continues to "do it" incorrectly. Why? Because he or she believes that that is the right way to receive love. In essence, it shows the child that love means getting hurt.

So here you have a child who learned that love means getting hurt - whether the pain is in the heart or in the body is actually not so important. Pain of whatever kind hurts, and much of this kind of pain, however it originated, leaves noticeable impressions and trauma, but *before* the pain came, the child felt – even if only briefly – *real love.* The child experienced something that he or she believed to be the real thing. The love it felt for the parent was magnificent, the way love is meant to be, and the child reveled in it, the way most of us do when we feel we are truly loved and cherished. The child believed the parent reciprocated this love in the most wonderful and caring way. *The child felt safe. The child felt loved. The child felt secure.*

And then the blow fell.

Whether it came in the form of rejection or coldness or abuse or abandonment is not as important as the message the child gives itself in order to try to understand what happened. And although the content of this message may be varied, with multiple potential consequences, the message the child gave itself was that *love is not safe. Love is dangerous. Watch it! When you feel truly safe and loved, something bad will happen.*

So of course the child will wind up looking for love. That's only natural.

Fast forward. The child is now a teen or an adult, embarking on relationships. He is keenly interested in finding love and frequently looking for it in the guise of sex. Often this individual is – *or at least gives the appearance of being* - highly passionate. Sometimes this individual sees him or herself as more passionate than most other people due to what he experiences in his sexual relationships. He or she may believe sometimes, somehow, that sex is love. And when this individual finds another person with whom the sexual flame ignites in the way of great passions, then typically, frequently, this person falls desperately, frantically, obsessively, fearfully, longingly in love.

All of the adjectives in the last sentence that describe the state of mind of our protagonist as he or she falls in love tend – in some fashion or another - to form part of the scenario which is now choreographed. A dance begins. The individual often shows him or herself as a highly passionate, highly sexual person. He or she shows boundless desire for the partner, particularly during the phase of the relationship where the partner is not yet quite committed. *None* of this happens deliberately, or in a calculating fashion. It is an unconscious pattern in which sexuality plays a leading role, but not a scheming mindset designed to *catch* an unwitting prey.

The less accessible the partner, the more highly the flames of passion will leap, and eventually in some cases, the couple commits to a life in common. They decide to live together, to get married, have a child or buy a home together.

So now our protagonist has achieved what appears to have been the goal: love, a committed relationship, a life together. Finally there is this long-desired state of love. Love is corresponded. A long awaited state of circumstances has arrived, so now they live happily ever after, right? Well, possibly yes, but not, perhaps, without first going through some tough trials that involve the most intimate aspect of the couple's bedroom - the sexual relationship.

Now a phase begins that is generally misunderstood by both partners. Neither can explain how this once passionate person quickly turns into someone who shuns the marital bed, making up the most ludicrous excuses to avoid sex, or, if sex continues to play a part in the relationship, the partner who is turning off finds it more and more difficult to continue playing a role that is no longer tenable. In other words, the erstwhile passionate individual no longer wants sex. He or she may even find it disgusting, having a hard time keeping this fact from the bewildered partner, although frequently the turned off partner will do his or her utmost to make certain the other partner does not know how much sex has become repulsive, because *love has not necessarily diminished,* and there is no wish to hurt the shunned partner further.

In the meantime of course, the confused partner suffers a gradually decreasing sense of self esteem, at least as far as his or her sexuality is concerned. He or she may believe that sexual desire and hence the frequency of sex has waned because he/she is less attractive, less desirable, or because the partner has found someone else. They may also believe that the partner has become frigid or impotent; indeed, the person who no longer wants sex may believe this also. Occasionally they may seek out a new sexual partner, just to convince themselves that they can still *function.* Many things are imagined, but the crux at the heart of the matter is rarely realized, *particularly not by the partner who has turned physically cold.* And the solution never lies in exchanging one partner for another, because invariably the pattern will repeat itself until it has been resolved. Like most issues, this one must be resolved from within and not from without.

The truth of the matter – at least in some instances of the type of background described above – is the fact that the individual with the difficult childhood came to believe, back then, and on subconscious levels, that being safe in a loving situation is the threshold to some kind of pain - emotional pain, psychological pain, etc. When this person was a child, and felt safe and loved, something happened to cause this pain. The connection between feeling safe and loved on the one hand and pain or danger (this refers much more to emotional pain, and *not* physical pain) on the other hand, has been clearly established in the subconscious mind. So when this person finds him or herself in a safe loving situation, a type of inner panic button begins screeching a warning that danger is near, albeit on subconscious levels, and something has to be done to upset the applecart and avert the danger.

This is the moment that some of the people in this situation turn "cold" on their partners and sexuality wanes. It's almost as though by doing that, the dangerous connection (in their eyes) between love and potential loss of safety is successfully broken. They have been striving for just such a situation for so long, but nevertheless, they are sabotaging it in the most insidious way - insidious not only for their partner, but also for themselves. And of course no one knows what on earth is going on. Typically the individual who no longer desires the other continues to love that other very much - at least for a while. They feel tremendously guilty about not desiring them. The other partner feels rejected, but the one who is off sex, in time may begin to believe that it's actually due to the fact that the partner truly no longer is desirable. Or that their personal hygiene is off, or that their love-making techniques are no longer interesting, none of which of course have any relation to the real reason. Ultimately neither partner is looking for the answers inside. Ultimately it is such a difficult situation that many couples just give up. The guilt and the hurt can grow to enormous proportions.

So now what?

There are solutions and they begin with self-awareness and honesty *about* the self *to* the self. Much of the material in Chapter 14 will help to put you on the road to solving this. But I can't pretend the solutions are easy. Or even that there always are solutions. The dynamics of this particular psycho-emotional dilemma, whose almost invisible tentacles reach into an individual's sexuality, are difficult to disentangle. They require a great deal of awareness, not only on the part of the person who has gone cold, but also on the part of the partner. For some reason the rejected partner has also drawn this into his or her life, and so, on another level, this is a secondary dilemma that also needs to be faced, but that is that topic takes us beyond the scope of our current discussion.

If you are reading this and have recognized yourself or your partner, I urge you to seek help. Not because either of you is sick, but because this is a hard one to grapple with on your own. A very important element of the solution lies in removing pressure from finding the resolution as the solution is being sought. By that I mean that although the solution needs to be sought actively, it needs to be done in such a way that the partner who has gone cold *does not feel pressured to have sex for a time*. Another very important element is allowing love to live and flow despite the problem, in order that the partner who has gone cold begins to realize that he or she is loved *despite* the problem. For some people, on the receiving end of the sexual coldness this may be impossible, and in that case, the relationship has probably come to an end. But for those who are capable of continuing to love, there is hope for the relationship, and *hope for the eventual resurgence of passion*. And finally, the most important element of the solution lies in psychological and emotional awareness on the part of both partners about the dynamics of what is occurring, and to recognize that love – especially when our early lessons about it have been dysfunctional - is both the cause of the problem and the solution to the problem.

Chapter 9

Obsession, Possession & Control

The quality of all our relationships is a direct function of our relationship to ourselves. Since much of our relationship to ourselves operates at an unconscious level, most of the dreams and dynamics of our relationships to others and to the transcendent is expressive of our own personal psychology. The best thing we can do for our relationships with others, and with the transcendent, then, is to render our relationship to ourselves more conscious.
James Hollis

Obsession, possession, and both overt and covert or manipulative control form another pattern to which I am dedicating this entire separate chapter. As we've already seen in the chapter on patterns, every single relationship begins with a projection, even though you understand it as love, chemistry, infatuation, and any other number of names, and it is the case even when you are convinced that *this is the one, I've finally found my soul mate.* This applies even to people who are totally aware and conscious, but the difference is that they will recognize the projection very quickly and from that position of awareness, will then decide what to do about their burgeoning attraction to the other (also re-read the case example of Nina in the Foreword). However, when you aren't at that aware state yet, because of the nature of projections, where you often feel very attracted or repelled for reasons that at the beginning seem very clear, such as something you very much "love" about the other person, or something you very much "dislike" about them, it typically signifies that in those relationships where you do find yourself strongly attracted to someone quite quickly, in a way that goes beyond the mere physical or chemical attraction, you are almost certainly involved in a projection of your own psyche. Therefore most relationships of a close nature that you have tie into something that was important and most likely unresolved in your childhood.

We tend to seek the familiar which we find in our early childhood patterns which set the pace for future relationships, until we discover the patterns and sort them out. Here are some common elements that occur to many that may lead to a pattern dynamic in the psyche. You may find that your father or mother tended to:

- ignore you
- reject you
- criticize you
- judge you
- belittle you
- make fun of you
- show you off to his/her friends
- leave you alone for long periods
- say that things were always your fault
- made you feel that you had to be the responsible one
- made you realize that it was better not to speak up

- made you realize that it was best to always keep the peace
- made you realize that it was best to always try to make everyone feel good

As already stated, until you discover and recognize your patterns, you are attracted to precisely those individuals who will live out the pattern for you, or with whom you can re-live the pattern because it serves the purpose of making you come closer to knowing yourself and in that knowing, you come closer to being psychologically free.

If you have not yet done so, please now go back to Chapter 5 in order to complete the exercise there which can help you establish an overview of your relationship patterns.

Nevertheless, at the point at which the attraction happens, you're generally not aware of any of this in the least. All you know (and all that most people care about at that point) is that you are attracted to someone, and if you tend to be obsessive and if you have found yourself in previous relationships that began like this, you may also be aware of the fact that when you actually get into these relationships, you are *not free*. (Humanistic astrology – as opposed to predictive astrology – is an excellent tool for picking up on these patterns of relationships upon careful examination of the cross-aspects between the charts of the two people).

In this painful neediness that shows up as either trying to control another in an effort to assure yourself of your partner's love or allowing yourself to be controlled by another, in an effort to make sure that he/she will continue to love you, there is generally a terrible lack of self esteem and self-love. All of this makes for extremely difficult relationships.

Here are some characteristics of people who confuse love with obsession, and who therefore *erroneously* believe that because they feel or do any of the following, that it means that they are in love:

- They can't get a love interest out of their mind - no matter how hard they try.
- They are deeply into the relationship long before a reasonable amount of time has passed so that they might get to know the other person.
- They try to feel better about the self through the person they have fallen in love with.
- They may use money, sex, emotions, and substances, to exact control over another.
- Their methods of trying to control a partner may include using emotional or psychological abuse.
- They check up on their partner and continually make him/her account for their whereabouts.
- They may spend money far beyond their means trying to find or keep love or even just the *illusion* of love.
- They may stalk, harass or even become violent towards a partner.
- They continually obsess in their thoughts over a partner, trying to figure out yet even more bizarre means to control him/her at any cost.

What love really is remains much of a mystery to many of us. Its very enigmatic nature is what often spurs us on in the quest to find that elusive pot of gold at the end of the rainbow to which we aspire. Our intentions tend to be good, and we are basically almost all aware of the fact that love can have different faces at different moments of a relationship. However obsession is a different, destructive form of love that needs understanding and avoiding and ultimately surpassing.

Key to this understanding whether you are in love or obsessed with someone and vice versa is this: when you are obsessed you find it nearly impossible to function as a person on a daily basis without thinking about the other.

The obsessed person aims at getting all your attention, or, if you are the one who is obsessed, you focus on getting all their attention. The one who obsesses will make it difficult or at least uncomfortable in some fashion, for the other to keep in normal touch with friends and family, or to continue with outside interests - sometimes even when they include the possessive partner, because when people confuse love with obsession, they will do nearly anything to keep the "love object" a figurative prisoner and locked up in the relationship. When you love, however, there is mutual support, caring and giving. Healthy love is the opposite of controlling. It not only is independent, but it also encourages independence on the part of the partner.

Some things to consider:

- Identify how you attempt to control others (e.g., emotional, sexual, financial manipulation, etc.). This requires above all, great self-honesty and awareness. If you have already done the exercise to help discover your relationship patterns, you will be that much closer to truly seeing yourself. Remember that the self-reflective process is something that will take you not only to greater self-understanding, but also eventually to a much higher measure of inner well-being and freedom, which ultimately leads to a higher level of being.
- Are you able to forgive others?
- Are you able to forgive yourself?

For people who confuse love with obsession, it is common to struggle with some kind of addiction. In order to cope with your pain (or to run from it), you may have learned to soothe yourself with any number of not-so-healthy mechanisms, including, but not restricted to alcohol, drugs, food, and/or sex. This may apply most particularly during difficult times, when an object of obsession causes you to experience anxiety or emotional distress.

Healthy self-soothing when you are faced with a situation that looks as though it might be your undoing is not always learned in childhood, hence the incidence of so many adults who use mechanisms that are toxic on many levels. This is often called self-medicating, not only because so many people have relatively easy access to drugs (both prescription and other), but because many other addictions that are *not* drugs, have a similar soothing effect - albeit only for a time. In the next chapter we'll take a closer look at self-soothing and addictions.

The biggest and most important thing you can do in this process of helping yourself – whether you are the one who confuses obsession with love, or whether you are the one whose partner is trying to control: *become aware* of what is happening. Don't blame the other. There is *never, never, never* any point in that. Understand that *both* of you are in this *dance* in order to release childhood patterns, throw away old (and very heavy) baggage, in order to be able to grow in magnificent new directions. There lie freedom, peace, and inner harmony.

Chapter 10

Self-Soothing & Addictions

A Closer Look at Self-Soothing

When life becomes difficult, when rocks are thrown our way, when we don't know where to turn, when crises threaten to undo us – emotionally, financially, physically, professionally, and so on – we generally resort to something that will help us get through the difficult period. That is obvious and normal. We would be counter-productive, if we didn't do that. But what happens to us when we lose our way? We lose ourselves. And when we have lost ourselves, we have typically listened to advice (from ourselves or from others) that told us that the best way to calm down, or to feel better, was to soothe the self by feeling or thinking or doing something that allowed us to lose sight of whatever was bothering us.

So we turn to our work and become work-aholics, or we turn to drugs, serial relationships, a frenetic social life for the mere sake of rubbing shoulders or having something to do every evening and weekend just to avoid being alone, we turn to gambling, to prescription medication readily supplied to many by their well-meaning doctors, to the quest for eternal youth, to films that gives us an adrenaline rush, to sports that give us an adrenaline rush, to risky sex that gives us an adrenaline rush, or we become news junkies (that gives us another kind of adrenaline rush), or we become obsessed by the hue of our lawns, or by the number of our published articles in peer-reviewed journals, or by the value of our stock portfolios, or the letters after our name, or the books in our bookcases, or the sermons we preach from the pulpit on Sunday mornings. Whatever we turn to, *if it is something that causes us to turn away from the self, it is, in essence, causing us to lose our way.*

There is nothing wrong, in and of itself, with many of the above activities. It is when they are used to soothe the self, in other words, to ease an *inner condition* that we find ourselves unable to deal with because our inner world is unable to face the turmoil without resorting to something external, that the soothing activities cause us to lose the way. Losing the way literally means losing the connection to our true self.

What Are Your Addictions?

As stated, we use our addictions to soothe the self when we know of no other way to do it. I can just hear you saying: *I don't have any addictions. I don't drink, I don't smoke, I don't snort cocaine, and I certainly don't shoot heroin. I don't have any eating disorders and I don't gamble.*

- How about work? Have you ever had your partner complain that you spend too much time there?
- How about shopping? Did you ever cringe when the credit card bills came in at the end of the month and you realized that once again you had spent far more money than you have?
- Now how about *judging other people*? You do that more than just a bit? Like quite often? So that's an addiction. Judging other people is something we can get addicted to. If you try to stop you will notice that it is almost as hard to do as saying good-bye to your cigarettes. And while you're doing it, you can avoid thinking about your own issues.
- Then there's criticizing others.
- And stereotyping others.
- And being a fitness buff far beyond just being healthy about your body.
- Making money is a good one. This is an addiction that masks as something totally different such as being responsible or taking good care of your family.
- Socializing to the point of not wanting (or being able) to be alone.
- Being a news junkie.
- *Remaining young* - better said: *wanting* to remain young. So the addiction is going after whatever it is you believe will keep you young: creams, clothes, injections, surgery, retreats, sports, etc. None of these things by themselves are wrong, it's the desperate and continued and addictive search to remain young that keeps you from your life and your soul.
- Complaining?
- Feeling blue - now how's that for an addiction?
- Feeling that you are a victim.
- Not letting go of old wounds.
- How about being addicted to another human being? Can't be without them? Need their presence? Feel like

something is terribly wrong when they are not totally happy with you? This generally means someone we *think* we are in love with, but it could also be a child or a friend or anyone - stalkers of celebrities are an extreme example of this type of addiction.

- Blaming others. This is a big one. You are allowed to get off scot free, as long as you have someone to blame. And as long as you do, you don't really live your own life, connect to your true inner self, and you certainly have no way to learn how to sooth yourself in healthy ways.

- Living at any time *other than the present*; always moving into the past or the future in your thoughts. This addiction belongs to most people, at least until they wake up and become aware. We are always waiting for *that* to happen, or for this *other thing* to happen. Or we are always off in our nostalgic past, when things were so much better. Or, conversely, we live in the fear of our future (stress, worry) or in the pain of our past. *But we don't live in the present.* And so we are addicted to living in this other time that is not *now*.

- Addicted to hanging on to bad feelings. We don't release them, we don't forgive those who are connected to them, often because we believe we would no longer be who we are (or, *who would I be without my wounds?*), if we were to let go of those bad feelings. So we are addicted to them.

- Being addicted to gossiping. It's a very bad habit. Just as all the others depicted here, it keeps you from having to look at yourself.

- Needing - being addicted to - being needed - to doing something to help others. Maybe you volunteer at a charity or soup kitchen, or maybe you are the proverbial wonderful friend who solves everyone else's problems and organizes all the events. Just doing it is cool. But doing it because you are addicted to the look of

gratitude you get, or to the fact that you know the others need you, now *that* is an addiction.
- Social power. Being addicted to someone else's social power. Basking in the reflection of *their* sun. Rubbing shoulders with them, their social contacts, and the remainder of their entourage.
- Not forgiving. This is also an addiction.
- Excusing others for their bad behavior. Not calling the shots when you should. Having unhealthy boundaries.

No, no, you say. *Those things you're talking about are not addictions. If I judge or criticize another person, I have a good reason.*

- *Look at those racists in that African country.*
- *Or look at the lack of humanitarianism in the members of the regime of Myanmar after the cyclone hit.*
- *Or look at my boss - he is so unethical - he simply takes all the credit for work we've all done as a team.*
- *And what about my sister's daughter? She's nuts - taking drugs and going out with those tattooed guys that wear earrings.*
- *And speaking of earrings - what about those teenage girls that get a diamond inserted into their belly button?*
- *And don't get me started on those women that let themselves go after they hit menopause.*
- *And the pastor at my church! He has such an ego. All he wants to do is hear himself speak, so his sermons are far too long, And so boring.*

So - you continue telling me - *you can see I have very good reasons to judge others but that's not an addiction and I certainly don't do any of those other things you listed further up!*

Right. I'm sure you don't. But you judge *others* for doing those things. And furthermore, you don't seem to be able to *stop* doing so. All I'm trying to point out to you is that you have an addiction of judging other people. What does this addiction help you cover up in yourself? Oh, I don't mean bad behavior. I mean you cover up your own inner issues so *you* don't have to look at them. Not taking a careful look at your own issues keeps you safely unaware. And this judging of others – or *any* addiction helps you do that.

Ok, you say, *maybe you're right. Since I have read this, I actually tried to stop judging or criticizing people – even if it was just in my mind, and I realized that it would be quite hard to do.*

As long as you are addicted – to anything – you will not be able to become *what you truly can become*. You will be a fragmented personality. And the reason is because as long as you have addictions – of any kind – you are using the addictions to live your life for you. You use them to *cope*. You use them to cover up any difficult feelings. You use them to soothe yourself. You use them, in other words, to live your life for you, because without them, you are not able to. Your addictions live your life for you because they make choices for you. And as long as you don't recognize it, nothing changes. So how can it change?

This is not rocket science. If you've been reading the chapters in this book, you'll know at least one or two of the steps: *Become aware* of your addiction/s. *Make the choice* to make different choices each time you become conscious of falling back into your addiction/s. In other words, you make the choice to become responsible for *all of you*. Becoming responsible for all of you literally means *owning* all of what you think, feel, say, and do. *Owning it, means you deal with it in the moment you think, feel, say, or do it, rather than using an addiction to deal with it.*

Let me say that again: *Owning it means you deal with it in the moment you think, feel, say, or do it, rather than using an addiction to deal with it.* And while we will be taking a much closer look at this in Chapters 12, 13, and 14, this is precisely what you will have to work on very closely if you are battling with emotional availability or neediness because in the arena of 'owning your addictions' - even if those addictions consist of *blaming your partner for how you feel* - is where you will find your solution to this dilemma.

By applying some will power and tenacity to this process, you will become stronger and stronger in this department, and then *you will do it automatically because the addictions will no longer be controlling your choices.* And you won't need them to soothe yourself. Your neural pathways will have literally changed. And then you are on the road to self responsibility and above all, inner freedom and joy.

But at this point in your quest, while you are not at all yet certain whether you're really interested in doing this, what is of much more immediate importance, and much more useful to your daily life, is understanding that we typically do all of this soothing and losing the self simply because we have no clue how to deal with whatever it is that is causing our need to be soothed in other, healthier ways. And the whole point of this book, of course, is to show you that once you begin to learn how to be in charge of all those parts of you that threaten to fall apart or dissolve into fear, stress, panic, or pain, you don't really need to soothe the self in those unhealthy ways at all anymore, because you will find yourself, no matter what happens, in a place of awareness from which you will be able to deal with all of those states. You'll come to a point, if you follow through on the information in this book, where you will be your own witness; you'll be the observer of yourself at all times, and especially when you are in a difficult place emotionally. And as you learn to do that, and begin to feel the empowerment that such behavior and awareness gives you, you will come closer and closer to your true self, because you will feel more and more filled with an inner sense of well-being that now, perhaps, is only part of your life occasionally. But it's meant to be part of your life at all times!

And having said that, you will also come to realize that there is enormous value – precisely in life's difficult moments – to have a meaning in life that acts as a firm oak upon which you can lean, and the meaning in life is, of course, what you do with your life, how you live your life, the thing to which you dedicate your life. But that is very different from using your life purpose activity to *ignore* the self, to move away from the self, in the same way a bomb shelter, so to speak, allows you to hide away from life's nuclear bombs. The true purpose of a meaning in one's life is very different, *precisely because it allows you to deal with the bombs, not to hide from them.*

Soothing the self has many faces. And where we numb ourselves, we lose our path to the place where we are capable of great love of the self. Remember, an individual who loves the self, who *knows* that he/she loves him or herself, *simply would not numb the self.* Because it would be like having a huge mansion, and living only in a small section of the basement, as opposed to having access to all the magnificent reception rooms, the library, the solarium, and the screening room! Numbing the self means that you have cut yourself off from a part – or many parts - of yourself. By wishing to avoid something, and hence numbing the self, you have no contact with a portion of yourself, just as when you are anaesthetized, even if it's just local anesthesia, there is a part of you that you do not feel.

What is important here to remember is the fact that *what* you use to soothe yourself is just as important as *how* you use it. Clearly, using alcohol, drugs, gambling, indiscriminate shopping, overeating or not eating, self harming, risky sexual behavior and so on, are some very unhealthy ways to soothe yourself, i.e., to deal with emotions that you don't know how to handle. And therefore, by plunging yourself into study, physical exercise, or work, you are absolutely using a much healthier way to soothe yourself. But if this healthier way is used to numb yourself to parts of you that are feeling things you don't know how to handle, then this healthy way of self-soothing has just become unhealthy. And so a marriage may be destroyed just as much due to alcohol abuse as due to work abuse (or physical abuse – violence), and the relationship between a parent and a child may lose the potential richness of connection just as much due to frenetic social activity (which might be called networking by some), as due to drug abuse.

If, on the other hand, as you plunge yourself into work or study or a creative activity, or something physical such as training or practice in your chosen sport, in order to soothe yourself, while recognizing that you are doing it to allow a healing to take place in order to bring you to a new inner space from the current crisis, some time down the road, whether hours, days, weeks, or even months, then your approach – the *how* you are going about the self-soothing – has just taken on a very healthy hue. The important difference is that from the outset you are *aware* of what you are doing, why you are doing it, and that once you feel less in need of soothing, you already know in advance, that you will come back to your inner center. Soothing yourself under such premises literally means that each time you do this, you actually have a chance to grow and furthermore, to grow closer to your true self, as opposed to growing more numb and more distant from your true self. The process is analogous to taking an aspirin for a headache or fever, and taking it several times over the course of a day or two until the physical symptoms abate, and then, of course, you stop because you know the aspirin is no longer necessary, and you also know, that if you continued taking it, *you would be harming yourself*. Similarly, when you soothe the self, if you are aware of what you are doing, you either discontinue the self-soothing once you have come to a place inside where you are capable of managing life again without the self-soothing mechanism, or you do continue, but recognizing that now it is simply a healthy activity (e.g., jogging) as opposed to something you *need* to do in order to feel soothed about your inner turmoil.

There are so many ways of understanding how this happens. We are socialized, not only by our parents and school system, but also by everything we see around us in society: billboards, commercials, movies, novels, other people we may have taken on as role models, etc., into believing that our lives consist in doing well at school, becoming successful, being reasonably decent, taking reasonable care of our health, getting married, having children, and growing old. Very little – not even organized religion – gives us another kind of understanding of what we need to do in order to be healthy and vibrant on levels that go far beyond those included in the above description.

So what are we meant to be doing?

I believe it starts - or *should* start - by cultivating a connection to the self. Do you remember reading about being 'connected' to your partner in the chapter on sex? That kind of connection between partners begins with *first* establishing a connection to the self. And that of course implies understanding what or who the self is. Is my "self" the part of me that says "I am angry" when something that makes me angry happens? Is my "self" the part of me that wants to be loved by my partner? And is my "self" the part of me that suffers when my partner does not love me in the way I want? Is my "self" the part of me that gets tired in the evening, or that feels kind of blah in the morning? Is my "self" the part of me that wants to make a good salary or a killing on the stock market, and is it also the part of me that enjoys a good movie? What exactly is my "self"?

What it certainly is *not* is the part of you that is afraid, that is angry, that dies. The self does not die. Ever. So the language you want to use with and about the self must of necessity be different than the language you may use when you refer to those other parts that do get angry, afraid and so on, the parts that do die. We could call those parts, as many authors do, the ego. The unaware self. The ego is the self that is not aware of itself. Sorry, I'm not trying to play with these words as much as trying to get you to see and understand what the real self, the aware self, is.

Have you ever been furious about something, perhaps you were just in traffic, and some idiot nearly caused you to crash and total your car? Although all is well, you are now livid. As you scream at the other driver, there is a part of you that is actually observing you harangue and beleaguer him. A part of you that might be amused to see how totally beside yourself you are. Interestingly, this part of you is not angry at all. If you have ever had such an experience, let me tell you that the part that was angry is the ego, and the part that observed was the self / soul, or non-local consciousness.

Here's another example. It is highly likely that when you and your partner decided to join your lives together, was a poignant moment, to say the least. Perhaps as it was happening, and as you realized that the two of you were truly making that monumental decision, filling you with joy, there was a part of you that was off to one side, observing yourself. As it happened, you observed yourself hand-in-hand with your partner, skipping down the street, a song in your heart and the flush of happiness on your cheeks. Again, the part of you that was living the immediate emotion was the ego, and the part that observed was the self / soul.

And one more example: you've just been in or witnessed a horrific car crash. Or you've just seen the twin towers being dissected by a plane. Or you just heard the news of JFK's assassination, or you just saw the tragedy in Haiti after the earthquake, the devastation in Thailand after the tsunami, or Miami after Hurricane Andrew. You are in shock, horrified, perhaps even petrified, you feel numb, glazed, filled with fear and disbelief. *And you realize that a part of you is noticing the part that is in shock.* Again, the part that was feeling the shock and fear was the ego, while the part that observed it was the self / soul.

If you are stymied by my examples, and have never – at least not consciously – had such an experience, perhaps as you go through the process of becoming more aware, especially as you follow the indications in Chapter 14, you will find that soon you do have such an experience in the emotion of some moment. Keep an eye out for it, because it *will* happen.

Soothing the self can take many disguises. Loving the self is soothing. But the road towards loving the self so that it can be, so to speak, our self-soothing mechanism of choice, is not simple *because of the way we have been socialized.* Most people don't realize how everything else depends on our love for our "self", and therefore, how absolutely necessary it is to come to a place where we begin that process. In Chapter 14 much more detailed information is offered about loving the self, and for now it is sufficient to say that when our self-soothing mechanisms ultimately lead towards this road of loving the self, then they are healthy. When they don't lead there or when they are used independently of any kind of self-love, then they are not.

Chapter 11

What About Relationships?

Relationships are the arena in which you can grow most quickly. Relationships are the arena in which you can most learn about yourself. Relationships are wonderful tools, not only for love, joy, happiness, and satisfaction, but for speeding up the coming to recognition about all your issues, *if you so desire*. In other words, when relationships start to go sour, or when they lose their early rosy-colored hue, as they are wont to do, at that point is the place when you can begin to use them alchemically, to transform yourself, or, to put it into the words of renowned mythologist Joseph Campbell:

"through the alchemical cooking [...] the gold is brought out. And the gold is your own spiritual life [...]. The ordeal is a gradual clarification and purification of your life."

We tend to believe that relationships only exist to make us happy, to complete us, and to make our lives better, and if they do not fulfill these ideals, we tend to quickly discard them. Both psychologically and spiritually, however, the real purpose of relationship goes far beyond that, as stated above, because it is precisely through the problems and difficulties that you encounter in your intimate relationships, that you can grow the most, and furthermore, grow most rapidly.

However, this only happens if you are willing and capable of looking at yourself *before* you look at your partner with blame. It isn't a question of taking on the blame yourself - perhaps your partner has truly behaved atrociously or unacceptably - but of looking at what it is within yourself that has drawn you to this or that partner, and once you see that which you consider unacceptable, and which you have not been able to *change* in your partner over weeks (or decades) of trying, then you must ask yourself *what is it in me that has caused me to hang on for weeks (or decades) despite finding this type of behavior atrocious or unacceptable, or even just very annoying?*

It is the honest answer to questions such as these in the throes of relationship difficulty (furthered by having completed the exercise about your patterns in Chapter 5), that leads you to insight into the self and consequently, to the potential for growth. So the answer to those questions – if they are to lead to growth – will never be about the *other* nor will they have to do with blaming the other, they will only concern the self.

Here are some typical answers that concern the *other* and that therefore do *not* lead to the kind of growth that is the promise of all relationships, *unless you decide to do something about the part of yourself that says these things about the relationship*:

- My partner needs me so I have to stay.
- My partner is such a wonderful person inside, and I *know* that if I love him/her enough, and that if I show him patience and understanding, that wonderful part that I can see will eventually shine through.
- I am afraid of what he/she might do if I take a stand about this issue.
- I am afraid of what he/she might do (to him/herself, or to me) if I leave.
- I couldn't do this (a new type of behavior as opposed to whatever has been done in the past or up to this point in the relationship) to my partner.
- I've done that (showing some healthy boundaries) in the past and it has not changed anything in the way my partner treats me. He/she will never change.
- My partner is inconsiderate, rejecting, emotionally unavailable, needy, aggressive, violent, controlling, obsessive, abusive, rude, unfaithful, etc.
- My partner will get very angry if I do this (react in this new way).
- My partner would never understand that kind of behavior.
- My partner will never forgive me if I do this (react in this new way).

All of these examples show that the person who is saying or thinking them, could be learning something new from the problem that has arisen in the relationship, or that has existed in the relationship for a long time already, but because of the things this person is saying or thinking, it always has to do with the other, i.e., there is always either an element of a) *not being able to do this to the other* or b) *of blaming the other*. There is no looking at the self to see what is going on inside in order to try to understand one's own role in the dance. Because there always is a dance. When couples have come to see me and I begin to unravel their particular "dance" for them – by which I mean the steps each one of them takes in order to maintain a specific status quo or *dynamic* in the relationship - instead of changing things - they then often begin to understand how *subconsciously both members of the couple are somehow invested in keeping everything the same,* although on the surface, both may be quite livid!

And before you start thinking: *oh no, another subconscious thing that I am never going to get at without attending a very expensive workshop or buying some gadget that will cost a lot of money or going through years and years of therapy,* let me reassure you, that although what keeps you in this "dance" may be subconscious, you can quickly bring it to consciousness by beginning to become aware. There is that word again, that has been so stressed and reiterated in this book already. By becoming aware of yourself at every moment of every day on all possible levels: physical, psychological, emotional, spiritual, you will soon be able to comprehend what keeps you in the dance. Awareness alone will not pull you out of the dance, but it is a beginning; a very important beginning of just about everything that ails you.

Here's part of what happens: when something goes wrong in a relationship, you often tend, as stated, to believe it is the other person's fault. You may then attempt to reason, cajole, manipulate, or force the other person to change, perhaps back to the way you thought they were before, or simply to conform to whatever you believe would be a better form of behavior, a behavior that would suit your own purposes better. Naturally you don't necessarily look at it like that, but if you analyze any past relationship difficulties you may have had, much of the above is what probably happened. And by the way, however it was that your partner was before (or how you thought he/she was before), generally has much more to do with your *own* projections and needs, than with the reality of your partner.

Carl Gustav Jung had much to say about the *anima and animus,* the inner and hidden feminine side of a man and the inner and hidden masculine side of a woman, respectively. These hidden parts of yourself are what tend to attract you to your important life partners *and it is in the unveiling of these hidden bits, bringing them to consciousness, that you are able to begin to deal with your relationship issues and that you begin to understand that what you blame so much on your partner, or what pushes your buttons so much about your partner, has less to do with your partner, than with earlier circumstances in your own life that set the stage for the dance.* In other words, it has to do with your inner opposite gender self – anima or animus. June Singer, a Jungian analyst, wrote an entire book about the fact that there are four people in every relationship: the physical man and woman and the inner man – *animus* – of the woman, and the inner woman – *anima* – of the man, all of which play major roles in the unfolding of the relationship. All of this applies equally to same-gender relationships, by the way.

Going back to your attempt to get your partner to behave the way you want him/her to, you then either achieve your partner's acquiescence, or find yourself faced with an impasse. In the case of the former, all is well until you have another contretemps, at which point this entire scenario may repeat itself, but in the case of the latter, you may now spend weeks, months, years, or even decades, trying to convince your recalcitrant partner that he/she is at fault, and that they need to change. There may be recriminations, tears, insults, threats, punishing silences, and so on. If the two of you do not separate or divorce, all of this may, if nothing changes, eventually morph into resentment, apathy, depression, a debilitating and poisonous atmosphere in the home, or a deep-rooted pain on your part since you want your partner to change – all of which, of course is blamed on him/her because he/she is doing the so-called "bad" thing or not behaving the way you want him/her to behave or even wanting him/her to revert back to behaving the way you believe he/she was before, "when we met".

Unfortunately the problem with this scenario is that, as stated earlier, while it may very well be true that the "bad" partner is showing unacceptable behavior, or being atrociously unkind, rejecting, inconsiderate, or showing outright cruel behavior, the other partner, the one who considers that all that is going badly in the relationship is the "bad" partner's fault, has never stopped to look at the self and ask *why do I allow this? What has brought me to this point in this relationship?*

When I ask that question in my private practice of such a partner, the answer is typically: "Oh, I don't allow it, but my partner pays no attention to me. I've told my spouse / partner over and over that I don't want this, but he/she never changes one iota. I've begged and pleaded and cried and shouted and ranted and raved."

And while this is generally the absolute truth, it still does not take into consideration *why the aggrieved partner allows it*. And of course the kind of allowing I am referring to has to do with this: what *issue* is there inside of you that means that you are unable to change whatever it is that is going on? And when I say "change", I clearly am not referring to changing your partner - that is never anyone else's responsibility. The only responsibility you have is to change yourself.

Here are just a few common examples of what that issue in you that prevents you from seeing your part of the dance, might be:

- Lack of self love, self respect and self esteem
- Lack of conscious awareness
- Fear of being alone
- Emotional neediness
- Unhealthy boundaries
- Co-dependency
- Dysfunctional parenting
- Perception of having received insufficient love in childhood

All of these points (and many others) tie in directly with the first one, the most important of all, and the one that generally underlies all of the other reasons: you have not yet become connected with your true inner self. A lack of self love, a lack of self respect, and a lack of self esteem, all create such a fundamental problem in your life, and permeate everything else, that it can safely be said, that if you work on that one issue first, and only on that, eventually all other issues will resolve themselves. *Isn't it wonderful to know that?*

In any of the above-listed examples, if one of the partners is willing to look at an issue, and actually recognizes one as being such, he has now arrived at a new place inside. The possibility for real inner change now exists. As this inner change progresses, beginning with self-love, not only does the personality grow and expand, but also the soul because through this course of action the individual commences the road that brings him closer and closer to his true inner self, the one he ideally wants to connect with, the one that he truly is, as opposed to the one that suffers so much and so needlessly. In so doing, he automatically begins to experience a much higher level of inner well-being.

So there you have it: one example of how a relationship difficulty can eventually bring both partners, and more typically *one* of the partners, to greater self-knowledge and self-understanding. The lesson to be learned here is not how to figure out what all the different examples might be, because then we would have to write books and ever more books only about that, but to realize that when a problem arises in a relationship, it is up to each person to look inside, as opposed to blaming something or someone outside, *no matter what has transpired*. And in this process of looking within, seeds will be sown, buds will emerge, and oak trees will begin to dot the inner landscape.

Now let's look at the other side of the coin. Let's say you have begun the above-described process, or you are already familiar with it. You now know that relationships do not exist to make you happy (although they may, indeed, be the source of much happiness), but that your happiness is your own responsibility. You also know that relationships do not exist to fulfill your needs, but that you are responsible for fulfilling your own. Therefore, knowing this automatically means that as you move towards that inner goal, you will gradually come to a relationship (whether it's the one you are currently in, or a new one) from a position of *independence*, as opposed to one of dependence.

When you *need* the relationship to supply you with happiness, or when you *need* the relationship to fulfill any of your needs, then you are dependent on the other person for your well-being, which therefore means that in the moment that the other person does not behave the way you would wish them to, you are no longer happy or fulfilled. But when you are in charge of your own happiness, and when you are in charge of fulfilling your own needs, then, of course, you come into the relationship as an independent human being who does not *need* the other in the traditional sense of the word and who realizes and recognizes that when those inner needs arise, they are not to be placed in the lap of the other, but they must be resolved in the self. This by no means signifies that partners don't help each other along this road, but *that* kind of support - grown from an understanding of the need for growth in the self — is very different from depending on the partner for those things.

How many times have you not fallen into the trap of believing you love someone because you need them? And yet it is this very need that makes you dependent on the other person, and hence you are no longer free. Freedom in a love relationship does not imply less love, on the contrary, the quality of love that comes from a position of independence, as opposed to one of dependence, is far superior, as anyone who has experienced it, will attest. Coming from a position of dependence means you are together out of neediness of some kind, as opposed to coming from a position of independence, which means you complement each other. Rather than needing, the major descriptor is complementing.

That brings you to an entirely new partnership level that we can label as spiritual which is also discussed in Chapter 15 and which has a bearing - for those who care to look at this aspect of the subject of this book - on emotional unavailability and neediness. However, at this point, and before having worked on the actual issues, what follows is *not* yet a place where you will find yourself. I merely offer it as insight into what *is possible* once you do the work. (For much more about this topic also see my book *The Tao of Spiritual Partnership*).

Spiritual Partnerships

Some of the ways to define spiritual partnerships are these:

- You complement each other as independent individuals who know they are fully responsible for themselves, as opposed to needing each other and hence continually entering the *dance* I referred to earlier, that brings about so many of our blind reactions.
- You are each invested in working on yourselves, alone, as well as within the parameters of the relationship, in order to grow into the richness you know you have within.
- You are both aware of the fact that one of the best ways towards bringing about this growth, is through a conscious and aware relationship with a loving partner.
- You are fully conscious about *wanting* to do this, to behave this way in this spiritual partnership, because you know it will lead you to yourself, and ultimately to your soul. There is nothing religious about these ideas. There is nothing abstemious about this. There is nothing in this spiritual partnership that does not allow you to live all the love and sexual and sensual richness that you may

desire. Indeed, a spiritual partnership will lead you to greater richness *and* depth than you may have ever dreamed possible because there is no reason for passion to die the way it tends to in blind and reactive relationships!

- You both recognize the fact that the ego often rears its ugly head, wanting to be right, wanting to be more powerful, wanting things its way, and hence using manipulation as a tool to keep the partner under control, and that in order to circumvent the ego, so that ultimately each of you is in charge of your own ego, as opposed to the ego being in charge of each of you and hence in charge of the relationship, you both do your utmost to remain aware at all times in order to – from a position of awareness – be able to thwart the ego.

- This means that when either of you comes under the grip of those typical emotions that cause havoc in relationships, such as jealousy, insecurity, fear, anger, impatience, etc., you will make the conscious effort (which will require some discipline at the beginning), to remind each other of your goal: to remain aware, and to *not fall into the typical relationship traps of reactive blindness.*

- You both recognize that healthy boundaries are one of the relationship's priorities, and that in order to maintain such healthy boundaries, both of you will need to learn to respect the other *as well as the self.* You may – especially at the beginning – often forget about respecting these boundaries, and hence, precisely because this is the nature of a spiritual partnership, you will remind each other with love, tact, and compassion that your boundaries have been transgressed. When you do so, contrary to what will then occur in a blind and reactive relationship, the partner who is being reminded will be grateful for the reminder, and even if he finds himself momentarily caught up in a "blind" reaction, he will be able to catch himself simply because this is what he *consciously* wants to do, and because it's what you both signed up for, so to speak, when you agreed to enter this spiritual partnership.

- You are both aware of the necessity to grow your own love for yourself in order that the relationship may be more loving. Because of this, you will no longer tolerate your own moods, for example, recognizing that they are a sign of an unaware individual who has not assumed responsibility for his/her own inner well-being, nor will you tolerate the moods of the other. However, not tolerating means that you will each kindly, lovingly, and gently remind the other – when the need arises – that by having a mood he/she has forgotten about loving the self.

In a nutshell, in a spiritual partnership you most certainly will continue to run into snags. You continue to wish certain things were different. You may continue to - but perhaps less frequently, and certainly with much more awareness about your own role in it - feel jealousy, and anger, neediness, and emotionally unavailability, and all those other emotions that typically make our relationships so fraught with problems.

But there is one enormous difference: you are aware that you are in the relationship – the spiritual partnership – not only to love, but in this process of love, to grow through whatever comes up for the two of you in the relationship. You are also aware of the fact that by dealing with whatever comes up by looking at the self - *each of you* looking at the self – at *your own* self - you come to an entirely different way of dealing with those problems that arise. By so doing, you grow the self. Growing the self simply means you love the self enough to do the things (as enumerated here) that will help you enrich your well-being on many levels.

Chapter 12

For the Emotionally Unavailable Person

You know by now that if you are emotionally unavailable it is *not* because you deliberately chose to be like this, but because something happened to truncate your ideally healthy psychological and emotional development in childhood. The immediate consequence of this was that you built this significant defense mechanism that affects much of what you do without your conscious knowledge. You also know that once you become aware of what happened, you can begin to dismantle that defense mechanism in order to live a life that becomes gradually freer of these emotional constraints. So now let's examine in more detail what exactly drives the emotionally unavailable person.

Defining the Emotionally Unavailable Person: The Partner of the Needy Person

What does neediness tell you about *you* if you are *with* a needy partner? To begin with, much as you may protest that you hate being needed, smothered, suffocated, etc., it is, in fact, your partner's *neediness*, that gives you a sense of yourself. Due to his or her neediness - most especially at the beginning of the relationship - you are able to, for a time, feel good about yourself, because it makes you feel strong, powerful, and in control.

It also makes you feel loved and desired. There is a headiness associated with being needed so much - at least at the beginning.

Frequently a needy partner may initially appear to be very self-sufficient (as they often are, as long as they are not 'in love', and hence their 'neediness' button has not been activated), very much in control of their own life, and it is not until a closer relationship has been established, that you discover that they are, indeed, needy, as they begin to cling to you. During their 'independent phase' you will have pursued the needy partner endlessly in order to ensure that they are truly there for you. Once they have been ensnared, so to speak (and realize that this is not generally a question of inherently 'bad' or 'calculating' people, but of unresolved issues, as we have seen, that have created these emotional dilemmas and dramas), you begin to withdraw.

The pursuit of the needy partner can be heady, mainly because at that point you may believe them to be difficult to get, independent or unattainable, and there is a large element of sexual chemistry in this mix. Once the needy partner begins to show his/her neediness, much of the sexuality may wane, but this also explains what happens if the needy partner gets upset and leaves, or appears to be getting interested in a new partner: the sexual aspect of the relationship becomes electrified for you again, as you regain interest in winning your needy partner (who appears to have become independent again) back into your bed, your home, your life. Much of this is touched on in Chapter 8, and it also explains in part the push-pull dynamic of these relationships.

Other ways of defining the person who has a relationship with a needy individual, appear to be nearly the same as the person who has a relationship with an emotionally unavailable person (also see the next chapter).

To begin with, it is highly probable that there were issues with cool or rejecting or critical or absent parents on your side, as you read in the detailed discussion offered in Chapter 3. This means there may have been unmet or disappointed emotions on your part, leaving you feeling bereft and alone, like an abandoned child.

Therefore, you probably learned a dysfunctional model of love, where love was never freely given, or where it came at a price of some kind - whether that was acquiescent behavior, submissiveness, or the feeling of absolute impotence in the face of whatever was happening - but you accepted this as the status quo due to your lack of understanding and knowledge as a child.

Furthermore, since most of this remained unconscious, it may take a number of relationships and much pain before you begin to realize that perhaps a part of the solution lies in you, as opposed to being out there, in your partners, in those relationships you get into time and again, thinking that *this time it will be different.* What you tend to be aware of with this dysfunctionality is the physical and emotional distress, often a kind of *fight-or-flight syndrome* (Chapter 7) that arises when someone needs you too much, or becomes too emotionally intrusive or demanding.

But - until you become conscious of all that this book is addressing - you will tend to interpret the physical or emotional distress as the fault of your needy partner, because he/she is not behaving the way you would like him/her to behave. Consequently blame is placed firmly on the shoulders of the needy partner by you because you feel far too much is being demanded of you in the emotional arena.

What Can the Emotionally Unavailable Person Do?

First of all, this depends in large measure on your desire to change. Sometimes clients come in saying that they want to be able to offer more to their partner; that they are aware of the fact that they give so little emotionally, that they perceive that they are somehow stunted, even crippled, and that they want to be done with that. They are, in other words, scarred.

Who doesn't have scars? Whose body – other than a baby's - is unblemished? Who can report having lived a life that left no scars on the psyche, the heart, or the soul?

But what, in actual fact, is a scar? It's a mark left somewhere after a wound has been inflicted. So scarring implies wounding, and wounding implies pain. And when we look at our physical scars, we are reminded of an event that took place at some point in the past that caused the scar to form. But many physical scars neither continue to cause us pain, nor do they cause us to engage in painful memories just by looking at them. There is one thing however. The skin where the scar is visible is no longer unblemished. Something has changed in its appearance. Hence the scar.

Our emotional, psychological, or spiritual scars are somewhat different. We can't see them just by looking for them. Sometimes the only way we know they are there is by the absence of something. For instance, people who have little contact to their emotions are deeply scarred. We can't see puckered skin. But we *can* see the consequences of the wounding - the dysfunction in the emotional expression. Such a scar might be likened to the scar an amputation of a limb leaves. A prosthetic limb can be purchased. The body can learn how to use it, and a nearly normal range of movement can once again be established. With emotional scarring this is also possible - as long as the person who becomes aware of his or her scarring by the *absence* of something else, is *willing* to learn to use the prosthesis in order to regain a normal range of movement - in this case - is willing to learn how to connect to the emotions again, in order to regain a normal range of feeling.

Is this frightening? Not a doubt! Does it require courage to embark upon such an undertaking? Not a doubt! Is it easy? Absolutely not! Does it require practice and constancy? Unquestionably! Is awareness of the self a pre-requisite? Yes! Will it offer inner freedom and growth? Absolutely yes! Is life without it possible? Of course. But the range of movement will be so limited that the person so scarred will appear to be a cripple.

By now you will have understood that if you are emotionally unavailable, it means you are scarred. How deep those scars reach depends on many of the factors we've discussed.

Therefore, just as for the needy person, your *first step is to become aware.* As you become aware, you begin to look at the fear and the pain – both your own and that of your partner. All this requires more self-honesty than many are willing to give because being honest *about* yourself *to* yourself is never easy, especially if you are used to hiding behind the defenses that you have perfected and honed over the years.

At this point it helps if you decide to make use of that ability that we all have but don't always invoke: our right to choose at every moment of every day, and in every situation of any kind. So we can choose our reactions, our actions, our thoughts, and our words and gestures, but we *must remember to remain aware for this to have a hope of happening.*

You can also choose to change what you feel. I know that sounds almost impossible, but it's not. *Choosing to choose* to behave differently is one of the most powerful tools for change in the life of the emotionally unavailable or needy person.

Then do what you would do for any new skill you wish to perfect: practice, practice, practice (it may not make it perfect immediately, but it *will* make you change very quickly, at least *some* of the time). Most particularly, observe your body at all times - use the mind-body communication service! (Also refer to Chapter 7).

We'll be taking an in-depth look at all the steps you'll need to take in order to resolve the issues of emotional unavailability and neediness in Chapter 14. However, at this point, I would like to ask you to begin to practice taking some simple steps to move you into a direction where you begin to realize that *you* can be in charge of how you feel, as opposed to letting others or circumstances in your life be in charge of that. Although this practice is not what will directly resolve your neediness or emotional unavailability issue, it *does* form a very important and integral step to get you there. Learning how to be in charge of the state of your inner world - in other words, being in charge of how you feel - is paramount to this process.

Do you ever wake up in the morning feeling as though life isn't nearly as good as it could be? Ever wake up wanting to pull the covers back up and stay there until tomorrow? Even when you have spent the major portion of your life living in what many would consider one tropical paradise after another, as I have, there are still mornings a person can wake up and ask: "*Is this all there is?*" Or: "*How can I face this day ahead of me?*" Or: "*What? Another shabby day in paradise?*"

Right. Been there. Done that. We all know the feeling. So what is my point?

The point is that the capacity to change this feeling on a day-by-day basis is literally in your hands, and what's more, once you start, and especially once you see what a difference you can make to the quality of your feeling state during the rest of the day, you begin to realize the immense power inside of you to determine the state of your being even when circumstances are not to your liking or out of your hands.

So when you first wake up and feel less than good, ask yourself, on a scale of 1-10, with 1 being the lowest, or worst, and 10 the best, or highest, where your state of being lies. In other words, what is the reading on your energy barometer? How do you know? Simply answer with the number that immediately comes up. In other words, let your subconscious answer, rather than your conscious mind, and that means allowing the number that you immediately think of to be the answer. So let's assume that number is four. Just keep that on the back burner for a moment.

So the first thing you can do, after you have taken the subjective assessment, is to take stock of your body. Ask yourself where in your body you feel anything that may be causing distress or disharmony. I am not referring to physical pain, but to those things that are the body's language to let us know that something is not in perfect running order in our world. For example, do you have butterflies in your stomach (solar plexus, adrenal glands, third chakra)? Or is your solar plexus tight and hard with tension? Are you slightly nauseous? Perhaps you have a lump in your throat (thyroid gland, fifth chakra), have a sore throat, are suffering from chronic laryngitis, or must clear your throat frequently before you speak. Perhaps your heart (thymus gland, fourth chakra) hurts, or feels constricted and tight - I mean a real, physically felt pain or constriction, which happens to some people when their feelings have been harshly trampled on. Or perhaps your breathing (lungs, fourth chakra) is shallow, or fast, or restricted because of some felt nervousness, tension, or fear. All of this should only take a few seconds.

Next, take stock of your feelings. Has something been making you feel sad, worried, angry, jealous, heartbroken, frustrated, or anything else that you might classify negatively? Again, this should only take a few seconds.

Next, quickly scan your mind for negative self-talk that has been going on lately. What are you telling yourself that might somehow be influencing the body and emotional conditions you have just looked at? Note that I am not asking you to do anything about any of these states; I merely ask that you take note. And once again, this should only take a few seconds.

Okay, so now you know that on a scale of 1-10 you feel you are at four, and you know where your body, your emotions, and your mind are at, at least right now, on this particular morning, another *shabby* day, as we said earlier, in paradise.

So what do you do to quickly raise that number in order to feel better? I don't mean raise it to a whopping 10 right here and now, but to raise it enough for you to feel the difference, *so that in future you will feel powerful rather than impotent* when it comes to how you feel when you first wake up.

You know the value of physical exercise, right? I'm not referring to its merits from the weight-loss point of view, but because exercise increases the flow of serotonin to the brain (mood neurotransmitters that increase flexibility and happiness), and raises the levels of endorphins (the body's natural opiates). In other words, *exercise makes you feel better.* I know, I know - it's hard to exercise before work. Long before I speak to you about the benefits of mindfulness, I'd like to encourage you to do the brief 15-walk described in Appendix A on a daily basis. Does it mean getting up just a bit earlier to do it? Give it a try - it might just be the most valuable 15 minutes you have during your entire day, among other things, because it will *help to positively set your day for you.*

If you truly don't have time for the walk first thing in the morning, do it at another time during the day or early evening while there is still daylight, and in the meantime, right now, in the morning, practice the much briefer Gratitude Exercise described in Appendix B, which you can furthermore continue doing on a regular basis throughout your day, *every* time you notice yourself slipping into a lower mood because it takes just seconds each time.

What else? Here is something easy that could also take place in the hectic mornings of our hectic society. Depending on who is around you while you're getting ready in the morning, you might be able to do this next thing at home as well. If you spend some time driving to work on your own (even if it's just a short five-minute drive), perhaps you can do it then, or during your lunch hour, or later in the day. Think of it like having your daily vitamin shot of feel-good talks. From today on, make a point of collecting inspirational and motivational audio and/or video talks (freely available on the Internet: two marvelous sources are YouTube and TED Talks and also have a look at Appendix D for more ideas). The thing to do with them is to download them and convert them to something you can listen to in your car or on your cell phone so that you always have a good supply of them with you wherever you are, so that you use those little pockets of time most of us have during the day for this purpose. If you are not technically savvy and don't know how to do this, hire a teenager for a few hours to teach you. Your goal is to listen to any given talk for 10-20 minutes once or twice a day and then continue listening to the same talk (assuming it is longer) the next time. Only *you* can know which speakers or topics resonate with you. You will quickly come to recognize their power to raise your energy. Later you won't need them, but right now they are an invaluable tool.

Now assuming you have done at least some of the things I have suggested, measure yourself on that scale of 1-10 again. Remember: don't think about it. It's not meant to be a logical answer based on statistics. Just use your instinct. What number are you at now? Perhaps a 4.5 or a 5? Not a huge change, but nevertheless, a change. And YOU

DID IT. Just by changing some of what you do and how you do it. Realize that it was not necessary to remain at the lower energetic level you were at. It was possible to make a better day for yourself. This is very empowering, especially as you apply it again and again, every day, and as often every day as is necessary.

Next, I would ask that you run that scan over yourself again – your body, your emotions, your mind. What has changed? Perhaps the tight knot in your solar plexus has eased, perhaps the messages you send yourself now contain more positive than self-sabotaging thoughts, or perhaps you are breathing with greater freedom. Again. YOU DID IT.

So if you have been able to increase your feeling of 5well-being from 4 to 4.5 or 6 on a scale of 1-10, does that not imply you can do it on a greater scale if you try? Does it not imply that it is *up to you* whether or not you are going to have a good day? Does it not imply that when you wake up feeling *blah*, it is in your hands to do something about it? Does it not imply that you are not impotent in the face of however it is you feel? And therefore, does it not imply that the power is in your own hands, and not out there somewhere? So what are you waiting for? Go and grab some of that power for yourself *from inside of you*, and make a difference in your life, and by the ripple effect, in the lives of others.

Finally, please don't expect to climb Mount Everest in a day: remind yourself be good to yourself taking the first small steps, forgive yourself for mistakes you are bound to make, and remember, the child who is learning how to walk may appear to fall frequently, and just not put it all together into a cohesive whole – until one day, he not only no longer falls, but is walking perfectly, as though it had formed part of his repertoire all of his life. Understand that applying this process to yourself on a daily basis as your work on your other issues, will help get you there more quickly.

Chapter 13

For the Needy Person

Now let's move our focus to the needy person, the one who tends to be (at least until these issues are resolved) the *partner* of an emotionally unavailable person, what being that partner that tells you *about yourself*, if you are indeed in a relationship with an emotionally unavailable person, and what you can do about it. I might add, that the reason I wish to focus on the partner is because it is *typically* the partner of the emotionally unavailable person that comes to see me - at least at first - as opposed to the reverse. This is the partner who wishes for things to change because of the pain he or she feels. Only rarely is it the emotionally unavailable one who comes into my office for the initial session, although I have had a number of surprises.

Before going anywhere else in this chapter, I would like to encourage you to read (or re-read) the pages in Chapter 12 about choosing to change what you feel, starting with a body scan, because if you are able to do that, you will have come a long way towards understanding one of the pillars that sustain the process by which you will be able to resolve your neediness issue, and that process is laid out in great detail in Chapter 14.

Defining the Needy Person: The Partner of the Emotionally Unavailable Person

To begin with - just as in the case of the emotionally unavailable person - it is highly probable that there were issues with cool or rejecting or critical or absent parents on your side, as you read in the detailed discussion offered in Chapter 3. This means there may have been unmet or disappointed emotions on your part, leaving you feeling bereft and alone, like an abandoned child.

Therefore, you probably learned a dysfunctional model of love, where love was never freely given, or where it came at a price of some kind - whether that was acquiescent behavior, submissiveness, or the feeling of absolute impotence in the face of whatever was happening - but you accepted this as the status quo due to your lack of understanding and knowledge as a child.

Furthermore, since most of this remained unconscious, it may take a number of relationships and much pain before you begin to realize that perhaps a part of the solution lies in you, as opposed to being out there, in your partners, in those relationships you get into time and again, thinking that *this time it will be different.* What you tend to be aware of with this dysfunctionality is the physical and emotional distress (Chapter 7) that arises when someone keeps you too much at arm's length, is too distant, does not engage in healthy ways with you, or rejects you in so many different ways even though you are in a relationship.

But - until you become conscious of all that this book is addressing - you will tend to interpret the physical or emotional distress as the fault of your emotionally unavailable partner, because he/she is not behaving the way you would like him/her to behave. Consequently blame is placed firmly on his/her shoulders by you because you feel you are continually being *kept in the cold,* so to speak in the emotional and/or sexual arena by your emotionally unavailable partner and therefore are feeling all this distress.

What does emotional unavailability tell you about *you* if you are with an emotionally unavailable partner? To begin with, although you clearly do not enjoy being held at arm's length, or being treated in a somewhat, uninterested, or even slightly rejecting fashion, there is, in fact, something about your partner's *unavailability* that gives you a jolt of adrenaline - at the beginning. There is something about the emotional distance of your potential partner - most especially in the very early stages of the relationship - that excites you, especially if it comes immediately following the period of time during which the emotionally unavailable partner actively pursued you, as they tend to do right at the beginning, which allowed you to, for a time, feel good about yourself, because it made you feel strong, powerful, and in control. And while this excitement about their unavailability may initially appear primarily sexual in nature to you, there is a strong - albeit unconscious - element of reconnecting with your unresolved childhood issue or pattern with your parent in that excitement (which has absolutely *nothing* to do with sexuality, of course, nor is it, as we have seen, the *fault* of your partner).

It also makes you feel loved and desired. There is a headiness associated with attaining the unattainable - or at least you probably believe you have attained him or her - at the beginning.

Frequently an emotionally unavailable partner may initially appear to be quite needy (as they often are, until they are *sure* of someone, but of course once that happens, their 'unavailability' button gets activated), and not very independent in their own life at all, and it is not until a closer relationship has been established, that you discover that they are, indeed, quite unnervingly and painfully unavailable, as they begin to distance themselves from you.

During their 'needy' phase they will have pursued you - the needy partner - endlessly in order to ensure that you are truly there for them. Once you have been conquered, or have fallen in love with them, (and please realize that this is not generally a question of them being inherently 'bad' or 'calculating' people, but of unresolved issues, as we have seen, that have created these emotional dilemmas and dramas), they begin to withdraw.

To dissect it a bit further: you are strongly attracted to what you subconsciously *feel* to be their unavailable part due to your own childhood patterns (hence often the most incredible sexual chemistry enters the mix); but at this point you are not *consciously aware of this part* of their character. However, that unavailable part that you somehow viscerally recognize, and that reconnects you to something from your infancy or childhood, but that is hidden (not necessarily consciously, because they too, are part of the dance) at this early stage under the other face of the unavailable person: their needy face, when you are then pursued by this person, you feel powerful and good about yourself.

Other ways of defining the person who has a relationship with a needy individual, appear to be nearly the same as the person who has a relationship with needy person (also see the chapter prior to this one).

The dysfunctional model of love you learned as a child, in turn may have created a deep well of neediness,

neediness, neediness, and more neediness as we saw in the chapter by the same name.

The neediness in turn created a lack of healthy boundaries - *basically causing you to accept most types of unacceptable behavior, just as long as you received some form of love, acceptance, or approbation in return*. Of course, you may have occasionally exploded, when you had enough, but you never actually set the boundaries. You let things go, you accepted what should not have been accepted, you felt resentment, it went on for too long, then you exploded, and then eventually things went back to normal and the cycle would repeat itself. Poor boundaries are implicit in a lack of self-respect, self-worth, and very particularly, self-love.

For needy people there tends to be a desire to fuse or merge with a new partner almost immediately after the relationship has started. This frequently creates a loss of identity and little differentiation from the partner (you tend to take on their interests, activities, and friends, as opposed to continuing to develop your own).

Furthermore, of course, there tends to be *addiction* to the partner which implies withdrawal symptoms of the worst kind if and when the partner leaves, and in all likelihood your coping or self-soothing mechanisms were never learned in a healthy way, so you will use methods to calm yourself down that work against you (see Chapter 10).

Nevertheless, *under no circumstances* am I suggesting that you, who have as a partner an emotionally unavailable person, are to blame. All I am saying is that you have not yet accepted responsibility for your own well-being, which is a huge topic (touched on in Chapters 10 and 11 and in greater detail in Chapter 14). Without being responsible for your own well-being – *no matter what the outer circumstances* – you will always be at the mercy of those outer circumstances, including how you react to a partner such as the kind described here, who appears to make life miserable, painful, and difficult.

Chapter 14

A Do-It-Yourself Manual:
Let's Fix It!

Without a doubt, until you become aware of the patterns in your life, their origin in your childhood, the difficulties you have with attachment and commitment, being emotionally unavailable or not, as well as being needy, or the difficulties you have with possession and obsession, as well as awareness about how they continue to repeat and self-perpetuate, it will be very difficult, if not downright impossible to resolve these issues. Nevertheless, bearing in mind that you have come this far in the book, I will assume that you have indeed become aware of your patterns and have an over-arching desire to change these matters in your life.

If for some reason you are not able to discern the childhood origin of your issues, you have at the very least come to the realization that the mere fact of your emotional unavailability and/or neediness can be likened to a high fever, in the sense that the fever signals that your body has an infection *even if you are currently unable to discern the origin or cause of the infection*, and that this infection needs tending. Similarly, your emotional unavailability and/or neediness in relationships are clear red flags that indicate that you have relationship issues and patterns that are *your* responsibility to tend to, even though you may not yet be aware, as said, of the origins. As long as you can accept the possibility that their origins lie in your infancy and childhood, even if the patterns have not yet revealed themselves to you, then you are in the best position to begin to understand that the physical and emotional symptoms discussed in Chapter 7 - that arise at certain moments in such relationships - come from the child-that-you-were, with its fears and pain, and *not* - at least originally - from the adult-that-you-are. It is, however, the adult who must implement the changes in order for this to be resolved by *allowing the child* to feel safe and thus - finally - be able to begin its process of growth and maturation.

As with any issue, you can work on different areas of yourself one by one, or skip randomly from one to another and thus possibly find yourself working on several simultaneously, but however you do it, know that as you focus on one area, all others are being affected by that as well because they are all inter-related, and when one improves, the positive effects are felt in the others as well.

There are some very clear steps you can take, once you've discerned your patterns, and once you've assimilated the material in this chapter. However, those clear steps will *not* be clear for you until you have, in fact, taken a close look at all that follows and have begun to make it part of the fabric of your daily life. If I could tell you the number of both men and women who have found it within themselves to take these steps, you would possibly be astonished, especially if you are still very much mired in the issues, and furthermore have 'heard' or read that these issues are nearly impossible to change. But take heart from that. If those individuals can and have changed, so can you.

The specific steps to be taken can be found at the end of this chapter. If you go there now to *peek*, understand that in order for them to give you results, as said, you *must* first make a number of significant changes. They do not have to take months and years to be accomplished, but they must be looked at first, otherwise the 'specific steps' will not makes sense to you and you will find it nearly impossible to implement and maintain them.

Here are the main sectors that will require close attention, focus, and work if you wish to resolve your emotional unavailability and neediness:

1. Being Aware & Self-Aware
2. Choosing & Agreeing to be Self-Responsible
3. Parenting the Self
4. Recognizing There is Always a Choice
5. Learning to Love & Soothe Yourself
6. Creating Healthy Boundaries
7. Choosing to be Transparent & Vulnerable
8. Checking For Physical Symptoms & Emotions as They Arise
9. Choosing & Intending to Forgive
10. Changing the Narrative: Creating a New Self-Dialogue
11. Intending to Live Differently

Let's examine each of these points separately:

1. Being Aware & Self-Aware

As you can imagine, in order to be able to deal with your emotional unavailability and neediness, you must give serious consideration to learning how to be aware. Much of what happens in you when you have the reactions you are familiar with comes from a place of *unawareness*. What this means, is that although you may be fully *aware* of a physical symptom or of emotions arising, what you are in all likelihood *not* aware of, is *how* these arose. This signifies learning to pay close conscious attention not only to yourself and your physical or emotional symptoms, but also paying close conscious attention to everything your partner is doing and saying (without blaming or judging at this point), as well as paying close attention to your own inner self-dialogue.

We are neither born conscious, nor are we typically socialized into being conscious. Rather - at least initially - we become a bit like sheep (yes, yes, me too). Most of us conform to peer pressure and to precepts established by mass media, at least for a while. And so we are asleep. And if we don't wake up, we won't be able to overcome emotional unavailability and neediness.

The sooner you realize that the best way to live your life is by truly becoming acquainted with yourself, the sooner you will have crossed one of the biggest hurdles in life. Why are you here? Is it just to become successful, well-known, or wealthy, and surround yourself with socially and professionally relevant people and to acquire many things? To worry about remaining young and beautiful? To *be* more, or to *know* more, or to *have* more than other people that you know?

Or could it be that while some of the above is certainly valid, the real reason you are here, in fact, is quite different? Could we perhaps say that you are here to become more closely acquainted with yourself? Such a process of becoming conscious also signifies that you come closer to being able to resolve issues that have plagued you all your life.

But let's say you are already on that road. Maybe that's precisely the reason why you picked up this book. You caught a glimpse of what could be - the way all of us do as we begin to awaken. And you want more of it. So now what? How does it happen?

Being conscious and remaining conscious require practice, otherwise you quickly fall back into oblivion. How did Nadal, Federer, or Djokovic rise to be the number one player in tennis? How does a beginning golfer become good? How did Picasso create his paintings? You know the answer, of course. It was practice, and practice and more practice. Some discipline. And it was a firm belief in the value of what was being done and motivation to continue doing it - over and over and over again. Here's another way of looking at it: when you have a chipped tooth or a sharp edge on a molar, you know that your tongue goes there incessantly until eventually a very sore spot develops on it. It hurts. You wince each time your tongue goes there again in its unbidden and automatic way. So you start becoming conscious of your action. You stop your tongue half way to the tooth. You remember not to do it because you now have a vested interest in not doing it. And so eventually what had become an automatic habit stops because you chose to grow in awareness.

Becoming aware of the need to become conscious and then remain conscious as much as possible all day long and each and every single day that follows, is similar. Practice, discipline, intention, remembering to do it (or setting up reminders for yourself throughout your day, your house, your car, your office), and having a vested interest in the outcome of no longer succumbing to your automatic and blind ways of being all form part of the road to awareness.

Here are a few examples of being blind, especially in the emotional and relationship arena:

- Your partner says something that you consider cold or rejecting. You place the blame for how you now feel on his/her shoulders. Being conscious would mean that you would take responsibility for how you feel despite the cold or rejecting words. By not realizing (being conscious of) that it is in your hands, you are fettered to reacting to whatever others do blindly and reactively and so you are not free.

- Your partner is making you feel you are being smothered due to his/her clingy and needy behavior. You've received numerous calls and texts all day, and now that you are at home, he/she wants your undivided attention, seemingly not understanding that you are tired and need some space. You are close to boiling at this point and clearly need to show him/her that you won't tolerate such neediness, and so you turn to ice. Being conscious would mean that you would take responsibility for how uncomfortable you feel despite your partner's clinging to you or his/her needy manifestations. By not realizing (being conscious of) that it is in your hands, you are fettered to reacting to whatever others do blindly and reactively and so you are not free.

- At a gathering of social acquaintances, you may have noticed how simple it is to become aware of others' failings. This person goes on and on. That one has garlicky breath. Another one always talks about his/her health. A fourth keeps looking over your head to see if someone more important than you has arrived. Another clings to you in fear of standing alone, a sixth invariably pulls out photos of the children, and that one over there, that you're trying to avoid, all too often tells you what your political opinions ought to be. Not a big deal, you might say, and it certainly is not. But what is a big deal, is that in all of this you have not seen your own. You are still completely blind to your own shortcomings, I mean. You remain blind to the only one that you can, in fact, do something about: you. But in order to do so, in order to bring about changes within yourself, you'll need to cast that eagle eye towards yourself instead of outward.

As already outlined, this requires becoming conscious and aware of the moments in your relationships when you become emotionally unavailable and/or needy, as well as growing in awareness about how it happens that you experience certain distressful physical sensations and feelings that cause you to react in emotionally unavailable or needy ways.

Especially at the beginning of your work on yourself; it can be quite difficult. The truthful look at the self is always much harder and requires greater courage than the look outside, at all those others in our lives. But if we do it - if we take that look at the self - we must learn how to do it with love. Likewise, remember to keep loving the self in mind at all times because when mistakes happen, when you believe you have failed, recognize that - as Richard Bach put it - they can all just be called *unexpected learning experiences*.

In order to help yourself in the process of becoming conscious and aware, as well as being self-aware, here are some of the most important aspects to bear in mind:

- Use a strategy of any kind to remember to be aware (one very simple one is to put up some post-it's in your house and office - on the mirror, the laptop screen, the fridge, etc., and to write on them 'what am I thinking'? or 'what am I feeling'?. Each time you glance at one of them, you will momentarily be jolted into awareness. If this happens 20 times a day, you will have had 20 brief moments of awareness. A muscle of sorts begins to be built, a new neural pathway forms. You don't need to do this for a long time - just long enough to make it a habit, so that you will, indeed remain aware at all times). If you prefer that others don't see such 'strange' post-it's, you could simply write a different quotation by a favorite writer on each of them, but you would know that each time you notice them, it is to make you remember to be aware and to check for your thoughts and feelings. Remember that if you are not aware of yourself as much as possible, you won't *catch* those moments when your issues flare into being. Therefore, without awareness it will be nearly impossible to do anything about those issues.

- Take the mindfulness walk once a day (see Appendix A). It will help you begin to become aware of how often during the course of your day your thoughts take charge of you. When that happens, you are not aware and certainly not in charge of how you feel. Unbidden thoughts can be worse than Chinese water torture. That - putting it bluntly - is a highly unhealthy way to live, but quite simple to change.

- Use the gratitude exercise (see Appendix B). It will help you process difficult thoughts and feelings in order to bring you to a place of inner balance and equanimity. What you're looking to achieve is a state of inner well-being, or at least, as said, inner balance, no matter what the circumstances. This requires remaining aware of yourself and your state. It also requires recognizing that being in charge of this is your own responsibility, and that the sooner you take on this responsibility, the sooner you will find yourself living a life of freedom as opposed to one where you depend on someone or something external for your inner well-being and happiness.

Practice as often as you remember and you will notice that your ability to remain aware improves rapidly.

2. Choosing & Agreeing to be Self-Responsible

With this point the connection to your emotional unavailability and neediness becomes apparent quite quickly. *If* you really want to get to the bottom of this issue, and *if* you choose to be self-responsible, you need to also *agree* to be self-responsible. Agree? With whom? The short answer is: *with yourself.* If you don't, you might as well drop this book into the nearest trash container. Being, choosing, and agreeing to be self-responsible means you will never again blame someone else for anything at all, even if they - or circumstances - are theoretically at fault. The reason you would not blame them or circumstances is because you would know that you take on full responsibility for your inner world and your reactions to absolutely everything. So if you feel suffocated and pressured by your needy partner, or scared, and abandoned, or rejected by your emotionally unavailable partner, rather than blaming him/her, you *own* your inner reactions to all of this and take responsibility for them. It's *not* about what your partner does or says, but about *your* inner reaction and what you subsequently do.

As children, our parents often admonished us: *be responsible! Take responsibility for what you do.* And we took it to mean that if we had chores or homework to do, then we needed to be responsible about completing those tasks, and not dawdle, or worse, procrastinate so much that in the end they never got done, and we wound up with real emergencies on our hands.

When he was still quite young, I used to say to one of my sons (I found the saying in a long-forgotten article): *your lack of planning does not constitute my emergency* when he would come to me in the 11th hour with a paper that had not been written, or a project that had not been properly planned.

But this is not what *claiming responsibility for the self* is really all about.

One thing is to be responsible out there in the world, as described above, and another thing is to claim responsibility for the self. Both *types* of responsibility form part of responsible behavior, but the latter is much less understood, and even less implemented in an individual's life. We pay little attention to it because the world at large gives it little merit, it is not talked about as something valuable to achieve, such as having an outstanding academic record, getting a prestigious position in an important firm, or becoming financially successful in the world.

To claim responsibility for the self literally signifies to *decide to be responsible for all that goes on within the self*. Not, let me hasten to add, for *all that happens to the self*. You cannot control that. If you live in a police state and are arbitrarily arrested, or if you live in an area often devastated by hurricanes, or if you live in a third-world country with raging hunger and poverty, or if you are of the *wrong ethnic or religious origin* (according to the powers-that-be) and are subject to harassment or worse, it is clear that you are unable to claim responsibility for that class of events.

But you can - without the slightest doubt - claim responsibility for the way in which you react to all of that, and therefore, you can claim responsibility for the way you feel about all of it, for the state of your being in the midst of such havoc and chaos, and therefore, in a nutshell, you have control of your life. *As long as you are in control of what goes on inside of you, what happens on the outside carries much less weight.* Imagine the potential freedom this would give you. Imagine a world where you are free to choose how you feel, think, and react. Imagine a world where your inner well-being lies in your own hands.

You can take this into the arena of much more normal external events or experiences and understand how - with this new understanding - you can begin to take control of much of that which ails and plagues you *by claiming responsibility for the self.*

- your boss just passed you over for a promotion
- the bank declined your request for a loan
- the person you love just walked out on you
- the girl you asked out for a first date said she already has a boyfriend
- it rained the entire week you spent in Bali

- seven publishers rejected your manuscript
- your college application was put on waitlist
- one of your best clients moved over to the competition
- you had a reconciliatory dinner with your partner and the two of you wound up having a fight

In each of these examples something *external* to the self causes frustration, heartbreak, pain, annoyance, anger, or any number of other unhelpful emotions. And so we explain our negative emotions to ourselves by blaming them on the event or the person. *Obviously we feel that way because of what happened.*

**Being Self-Responsible Implies 'Agreeing' to Be So

If you don't agree to do this - if you don't agree to be self-responsible, it simply won't happen. Agreeing means that you will put your every intention behind the desire and push to become responsible for the self. You will attempt to continually be conscious of it. And of course being responsible for the self means accepting responsibility for everything you think, feel, say, do, and how you react in the face of the behavior of others or any other outer circumstance in your life and in the world at large as illustrated in the examples above.

As long as you do not take on such a responsibility, you will continue to blame other and outer circumstances for how you feel and what you do and how you react. *I can't help it*, you may say; or *I've been given a raw deal*; or *I just can't trust anyone after having been treated that way.*

There is a bit of the victim in not taking on this responsibility for the self, or a bit of hanging on to your wounds and pain, because of course as long as you can blame another or a circumstance for something in your life, no one will expect you to do anything about it. And so you can remain in your comfort zone. But not only does that mean that you would stagnate, it also means you would not be able to ever have a growth relationship: a truly adult and mature - or spiritual - partnership.

If your partner upsets you in any way, you must first ask yourself the question whether any of this is mirroring something about yourself back to you.

If your partner is abusive, obviously that is not your responsibility, but it is very much your responsibility what you then decide to undertake with regards to his/her abusive behavior, i.e., discussing it, going into therapy, making the decision to remove yourself from the situation, or perhaps even reporting it to the police. But apart from all of the above, if you intend to be consciously responsible you need to try to understand how you entered into a relationship with an abusive person; what parts of you subconsciously responded to something in this individual when you met, because clearly something did, even though at that point it was not evident that he/she was an abusive person, although there generally tend to be clues of some kind that can be recognized retrospectively. You will recall what we discussed about patterns in relationships being a repetition of something that happened in childhood, in order to finally put a problem to bed, i.e., to resolve it on the level of the psyche and the spirit, and this is precisely what it referred to.

If your partner continually crosses boundaries, again, obviously that is not your responsibility but it is very much your responsibility what you then decide to undertake with regards to his/her boundary transgression. You will need to consciously recognize how much you allowed it, and which part of you needed for it to be allowed, i.e. what needs were getting fulfilled by permitting this boundary transgression. Did it allow you to see yourself as a victim? Did it allow you to feel needed? Did it allow you to feel magnanimous (even while feeling resentful)?

The topic of boundaries is vast, which is why it is also addressed at some length in Chapters 4, 5, and 6 of this book, and in section 6 of this chapter. Boundaries are strongly linked to issues with poor self-love and hence neglecting to resolve your own unhealthy boundary issues will negatively impinge on any positive results you are seeking with regards to your relationships. It is not easy to emerge from the depths of lifelong poor boundaries, but they must be faced and surmounted if you wish to live a vibrant and rich life filled with the ever-present possibility of inner well-being. Your relationships can serve as the crucible in which you can learn to do this.

If you notice that due to an interaction of any kind with your partner you feel a negative emotion (anger, fear, jealousy, pain, despondency, etc.), it is very much your responsibility how you deal with your own feelings. First and foremost - long before you look at your partner, and see what needs to be changed there, you need to look at yourself. What is it in you that has caused you to lose your inner balance? It is your responsibility to regain that inner balance, no matter whether your partner cleans up his/her act or not. Clearly I'm not saying that your partner should be absolved of responsibility, but it's his or her choice to take on responsibility as you are doing, and it is not your responsibility to try to change the other. Furthermore, it is also possible that your partner has not, in fact, done anything at all, but that you nevertheless have had a negative reaction. Especially in such an instance, you need to be particularly careful in unraveling what is going on, if you want to live a conscious relationship. It is far too easy to blame another for your own negative feelings and that is why, the moment blame enters the picture, you need to be so aware of what might be going on in you in relationship to your partner more than what your partner just said or did. Clients often admit reacting negatively as far as their feelings are concerned, merely on the basis of a change in expression on the partner's face, or perhaps a small sound made by the partner. And while it is true that sometimes facial expressions and sounds express covert criticism, disapproval, and so on, it is also true that if that is the way it is being interpreted plus reacted to, then you are allowing yourself to be manipulated on the basis of your beliefs or thoughts, as opposed to reacting consciously on the basis of a choice you make after something has been said or occurred, after you have had some inner dialogue about it, and after you have sought to regain a measure of inner peace and balance (all of which can happen in seconds, as you gain practice in using this particular muscle), which again brings us full circle to the need to being fully responsible for the self.

3. Parenting the Self

The third point in our "do-it-yourself manual" is crucial if you are emotionally unavailable or needy because in some fashion you lacked one or more of the components of ideal parenting and in order that you may begin to heal your issues, you will need to find a substitute parent. And the best substitute parent for yourself is you.

So I'm going to assume that you were not parented in a healthy way. I'm not asserting your parents were bad parents - just that they were not the *adults* they should have been, and therefore created some of the issues you are currently trying to resolve. Compassion is a wonderful tool to use as you contemplate those parents of yours, who themselves in all probability did not have 'adult' parents, and who therefore were at the mercy of all their own unresolved issues as they parented you.

Clearly, it's not about bashing anyone's parents, simply about recognizing the fact that in order to 'make up' for some of that which you did not receive as a child, you might have to give it to yourself as an adult. Hence: parenting the self.

Take a moment to consider how it might have been if you had been parented by two people who truly were mature adults. As you can imagine, I'm not talking about their chronological age when you were born and growing up, but about the sad and yet undeniable fact that most of us are not parented by adults. And most of us are not adults *either* when we become parents. This is due to a lack of psycho-emotional maturity, a lack of living a life of conscious awareness, a lack of having made the conscious decision to take on full responsibility for ourselves in all ways, including what we feel and think, what we say and do, and how we react to any and everything and also due to our socialization, no matter in which corner of the global community we were raised. That's a tall order, as we have already seen in great detail in this chapter, and yet, that is precisely what changes for your children, when you begin to parent yourself, and by so doing, begin to love yourself and put into practice all the things we are discussing here.

What then happens is that you - the parent (assuming you are one) - begin to have the capacity to be an *adult* parent for your own children, as opposed to being another child in the household with all its needs and reactivity and ego. *Do you understand what this means not only for yourself, but most specially, for your children?* It totally changes the panorama.

A child who has been parented by an adult in the sense we are discussing here, is a child who feels above all secure and protected, and very much loved. Such a child has no attachment issues, and on the risk of stressing the obvious, such a child would never have developed emotional unavailability, neediness, poor boundaries or a lack of self-love.

We could therefore say that by parenting yourself you change the way you deal with and relate to your children by becoming self-loving, self-aware, and self-responsible. That signifies that when they push your buttons, for example, the awareness you have achieved *because* you have practiced loving yourself means that you will *not* become reactive. Rather, you will remain in the loving, kind and compassionate position of the *adult* who has chosen to learn to love himself in order that he will be capable of loving his children in the way they deserve (which will include healthy boundaries and specific limitations).

As you will have come to understand, parenting yourself implies learning to love yourself, and by so doing, taking very good care of yourself.

Please also refer to section 5 about self love in this chapter where more aspects of poor parenting and parents who themselves were not parented properly are discussed.

Further help yourself by practicing the helpful *Little Child Exercise* that leads not only to self-love, but also to making the part of you that has not fully 'grown up' begin to feel safe enough to attempt to do so (See Appendix C).

4. Recognizing There is Always a Choice

When you are emotionally unavailable or needy - just as when you have any other unresolved issue - you may tend to initially look at it from a position of "*well this is how I am. There's nothing I can do about it.*" Therefore, until you fully recognize that at every step of the way you *do* have a choice, you will not be capable of making the necessary inner changes in order to move on.

People are sometimes amazed at the freedom the mere acceptance of this concept brings into their lives: knowing that there is always a choice, no matter the circumstances, because where choice is never lost is in one's own inner reaction to any event. Oh, at first they may balk at the idea, giving many instances in which - according to them - there are no choices, but there truly are no such instances.

- If your picnic is spoiled by rain you can choose to think differently about it being spoiled and decide to have fun indoors.

- If you are not accepted at the college or job of your liking, you can choose to think differently about the outcome based on new plans that may open another set of doors.
- If you lose your job you can choose to think in ways that are not negative, even if only based on the fact that the more positive you keep your outlook, the better energy you will emanate, and the greater your possibilities for finding another position become.
- If you are jailed for 28 years like Nelson Mandela, or forced into Auschwitz like Victor Frankl, you can choose how to react inside, even if that choice is one of the hardest things you have ever done in your life.
- If your partner or children or others who are close to you behave in what you might label as hurtful ways, you can choose how to react, especially in order to maintain an inner state of harmony and peace - this is taking good care of and loving yourself - and only then attempt to engage in the hope of finding a resolution.

Therefore, based on these examples, you can at least consider the possibility of always having a choice, no matter what your outer (and inner) circumstances. However, obviously making such a consideration part of your life and part of your relationship is not something that will happen just because as you are reading this you now agree with it. You will need to practice it each and every time you are confronted with difficult situations and in so doing, will also be practicing remaining conscious and accepting full responsibility for all you think, feel, say, and do. Without this kind of thinking and behaving, solutions of the kind we are seeking in this book will forever remain out of your grasp.

If you are willing to give over control of your state of well being to an event or another person it is tantamount to saying that you are not in control of your own well being. You might ask: *How can I be in control of it when these things happen to me? The way I feel is totally dependent on what just happened. Anybody would feel that way under those circumstances.* Nevertheless, there is another way of looking at it - if only you will try. *You* can be in control of your state of well being by *deciding to be.* It's as simple as that.

Make the decision that when things happen that would normally upset you, you will, in future, look at all the possibilities, all the alternatives of reaction at your disposal. Of all of these alternatives, one of them is always going to be:

- I can choose not to get upset
- I can choose to remain calm
- I can choose to keep my cool
- I can choose to remain in a good mood
- I can choose to refuse to let this person or event bother me
- I can choose to look at this as a learning situation and take something positive from it in order to advance to the next place in my life
- I can choose to grow from this
- I can choose not to worry (because worrying never solved anything at all)
- I can choose to smile
- I can choose to walk away from this situation
- I can choose to let this person be the way they are, realizing that their way of thinking, or their behavior says nothing at all about me
- I can choose to believe in my own value as a wonderful human being
- I can choose to laugh
- I can choose to shake hands
- I can choose peace

The examples of the choices you can offer yourself are endless, but if you make certain that your choices are always roads that take you to a good state of being, that enhance your well-being, and that serve you in some way, you are truly taking control, and claiming responsibility for the self. The goal of all of this is - contrary to what many of us learned in our early years - that *we must first take care of ourselves*. This is not selfishness. This is not egotistical behavior. This is recognizing that the better your inner state of well-being is, the higher your energetic frequency is (when you are happy your energetic frequency is high, when you are depressed or distressed, it is very low), and therefore the greater the possibilities are that you will have a positive impact on your world. The ripple effect of your very state of being – if it is energetically high - will be good for others, and in your own small way, you will be helping to change the world in a positive manner. Recognizing you always have a choice is an integral part of this process.

5. Learning to Love & Soothe Yourself

As long as you do not love yourself, you need to seek love for yourself in others. As long as you seek love for yourself in others, you get a glimpse of heaven through them. It's a heaven you could create yourself, but until you become aware of the psychological and spiritual dynamic that is occurring, you have no inkling of this potential for heaven in your very own self. Therefore feeling so good when you see love expressed for yourself in others, and feeling so devastated when that love is withdrawn, should give you a major clue to what is really happening. But what you see out there in films, commercials, books and talk shows, not to mention the reality shows, tabloid press, and social media, simply feeds this erroneous conception of how love is meant to work.

Think of it like this: if I am hungry, but don't know how to supply food for myself, and you are offering delicious food, it makes sense that I get it from you. But what happens when you disappear, or offer your store of food to another person instead of me, or simply say I can't have any more of your food? I'll starve to death. I'll suffer. Unless I can quickly find another food supplier. Or - and this of course is the correct alternative - unless I learn how to supply food for myself. So now I no longer need you. (Note: this book is not about learning how not to need others, but about understanding that as long as you don't love the self, your need for others will lead you down many rocky paths.)

Let's take the analogy one step further. You supply me with meat and fish and I supply you with fruits and vegetables. Both are necessary for our survival, and if either is withdrawn or lost, the other will suffer. And again, if I learn how to hunt and fish in order to supply myself with meat and fish, I no longer need you, and if you learn how to start a garden in order to supply yourself with fruit and vegetables, you no longer need me. But here's the thing: what if we meet when we already know how to do all of this and we begin a relationship based not on each supplying the other with a necessary dietary ingredient, but based on simply loving and enjoying each other's company? Do you see how this changes the parameters of the relationship? Or what if one or both of us begins the process of figuring out how to get our own supply of the required food when our relationship has already been on-going for some time, and hence we stop needing it from our partner. That too, will change the parameters of the relationship. It might mean that our food supply partner decides they also want to learn how to get their own supply, or it might mean they want things to go back to the old *I need you … you need me* status quo. Either way, the relationship is no longer the same.

And that is basically how it works if one of the two in a relationship begins to become conscious and begins to take responsibility for making the choice of loving the self at all times. Now that you supply that so very necessary ingredient for yourself, you no longer need your partner in that very dependent way, and so we have the beginning of a relationship based on complementarity rather than on need; on freedom rather than on chains, and on independence rather than dependence.

The significance of this is that you make a priority of this love for the self in ways that we don't typically consider, mainly because - as stated earlier - we are not raised this way by our families, nor are we socialized this way by our environment. You may take your own inner energetic reading (*how do I feel?*) first thing when you wake up in the morning in order to gauge what you may need to do in order to bring yourself to a place of inner balance (also refer to Chapter 12 for more specific information on this subject). You do this because you love yourself and consider this kind of taking care of yourself as part of your daily routine, just as you would brush your teeth. You take this very seriously because you know that if you don't, a relationship soon disintegrates into blindness again, a state of not being aware. You may need to do this throughout the course of your day on numerous occasions when life gets in the way and threatens to throw you off-course, and so you need to adjust your inner settings. You do this because you love yourself and consider this kind of taking care of yourself as part of your daily routine, just as you would check your temperature if you are developing a fever, and then, if necessary, take aspirin or go to see the doctor.

Also, clearly, loving and caring for yourself and making a priority of your inner state of well-being, and having made the decision that you wish to live a conscious relationship, means that when issues arise with your partner that threaten to make you feel pain or anger or anything negative at all, you will first and foremost - as part of this love for yourself - ensure that you bring yourself into a state of inner balance before reacting to whatever just happened.

The things you may do in order to correct your inner state, your negative emotions and your inner balance because of this love for yourself could be likened to what a loving parent does for a child that has hurt itself and comes crying for comfort, except that in this case *you are your own loving parent*. We learn to mother and father ourselves in ways that perhaps never happened when we were children. If they had, this whole process might just be a bit easier on us. But however it was then, what you can do now is not so difficult. You may do a mindfulness exercise (see Appendix A), a gratitude exercise (see Appendix B), and you may learn how to correct your self-talk. Above all, you will begin to treat yourself as the beloved that you are, learning to forgive yourself, learning to soothe yourself in healthy ways, being kind to yourself, and continually seeking inner balance and inner well-being. (For more about self-soothing, also see Chapter 10).

Judging by much of the self-help literature available today, by the clients that walk through my door, and by typical current events in the news about people and their relationships and their pain, loving yourself appears to be one of the hardest things for most of us to do.

As we've already seen, loving and caring for yourself is simply not generally very high on our list of priorities, nor is it always instilled in us as we grow up. Only once we begin to realize that it just might be one of those things that is actually holding us back, and we begin to try to work on it, do we realize how potentially difficult it is to achieve. There are many reasons why we don't love ourselves, most of which are absolute myths, but which we often firmly believe. What follows represents only a few of these reasons:

- There's *nothing lovable* about me
- I'm a *bad* person
- It's a *sin* to love oneself
- It's *selfish* to love oneself

- The Bible says *love thy neighbor*
- I've spent so much time *not loving me*, that I don't know how to begin
- I'm so *ashamed* of myself
- How can I love myself if I don't *like* myself?
- I'm so *afraid* to love myself
- It *hurts* so much to love myself
- I'm *not good enough* to love myself
- My mother/father/partner *told me I'm useless / worthless/stupid/clumsy/*fill in the blank
- I'm *not worth it*
- I'll love myself *when I get a promotion, lose 20 pounds, make a million dollars, get him/her to love me, etc.*

Let's backtrack a moment. How did you get to this place where you find yourself unlovable, or afraid to love yourself, and so on? Were you born like this? Look at a baby. It may scream when it wants food or is uncomfortable, but wouldn't you say that when it does that, it is manifesting its supreme belief in its *right* to be fed or comforted? And who does that? Only someone who instinctively (we're not even talking about being rational here, merely instinctual) believes he or she is lovable. When a toddler comes up to your knee, sticky fingers on your clothes, and looks trustingly into your eyes, he or she believes he has a right to be there and hence believes he or she is lovable.

But – what happens when the baby is not fed or comforted, and just ignored until it cries itself to sleep? Or the toddler gets yelled at, pushed away, and told in no uncertain terms that he is not wanted there because he is dirty, or disgusting, or bad. You get the picture. I won't go into the hundreds of scenarios – more or less dysfunctional, and many of them take place in great homes - I could describe, because you're probably aware of your own, or at least, you've heard lots of the scenarios that bring about a lack of self-esteem, a fear of *being you*, a lack of self-respect and self-confidence, and so on.

Fast forward a few years. You now have a child – youngster – teen – young adult – who finds it hard to say what he or she wants. Or prefers. Or what opinion she has about a particular subject. Or what she's feeling. And because she *finds it hard* to say things of this nature, she allows others to say or do things that are not right, that are unacceptable, maybe just not *quite* right, but nevertheless, something *not right is being allowed*. All of that describes behavior by a person with little or no self-love and with poor boundaries as opposed to healthy ones. And before you jump at me, I'm not talking about hard-core abuse, it can be much less; it can even just be something she *perceives.* Partially this behavior stems from her assumption that by saying what she wants or prefers, etc. (as opposed to what the other person is saying), she will not get what she most wants: love and appreciation, that commodity that somehow was missing part of the time when she was little, so it is better to say nothing, because then she just might get some love; some few crumbs of love.

So we now have a person with low self-esteem, or a lack of self-love, or respect, and hence we have a person with poor boundaries. And this of course perpetuates into adult life *as long as it is not recognized and dealt with as an unresolved issue*. And it can do untold damage to the unfolding of the life of the person involved. His or her lack of belief or love in the self is forever perpetuated by the people chosen to participate in the life, because these are *precisely the sort of people* who are able to enact the kind of behavior that persons with poor boundaries should object to, or speak up about, and yet they do not.

The subject of boundaries is fraught with misunderstanding. Poor boundaries, or entirely missing boundaries *always* speak of a lack of love for the self, and while this may appear logical to the discerning reader - if such an emotionally weighted topic can be described as logical - it is the difficulty in going about loving the self when there have not been healthy models to build on in childhood, that creates what often appears to be an insurmountable Himalayan summit.

When a client visits me and recounts what many may consider unspeakable acts committed by the spouse or partner, while it may be true that the partner leaves much to be desired, what is also true is that the client sitting in despair or self-loathing in my office, has not had the benefit of a childhood that taught him how to take good care of the self.

We learn how to love the self by imitation. We observe how we are regarded and cared for by others. We see the reflection of love for us in our parents' eyes. These factors alone - when they are done in a loving and healthy fashion - are enough to give us the strength, courage, and knowledge to love and care for the self.

When, however, they are missing, or done only sporadically or depending on some mood, or not done at all, the lesson we learn is very different indeed. Here are some scenarios involving parents that depict how we miss out on learning those very important early lessons:

** Parents Who Have Not Learned To Love Themselves

Such a parent is incapable of teaching you the fundamental skill of how to love yourself. You're going to have to wing it - perhaps when you are still quite young, or as a teen, or perhaps not until late in life. But it's clear you will need to learn it on your own, without that vital parental support. *Why did they not learn to love themselves?* Easy: they - just like you - did not have the appropriate role model although you have a great advantage. You've been digging, searching, asking, and reading material such as that contained in this book. So you have an inkling of what is wrong. They may have never managed to get to this point - and remember - it has nothing to do with their level of education. This is, in some ways, very visceral. And it ties in strongly with both of the next two points.

The first point - the issue of poor boundaries - will have reared its ugly head frequently throughout their lifetime, either because they themselves allowed others to trespass their boundaries, or because they did it to others. *Oh, you had not realized that people with poor boundaries are often the greatest trespassers of others' boundaries?* It's simply two sides of one coin.

And the second point - lack of self-reflection - is a sort of corollary of the first. A person who does not reflect on the self - and such reflection implies being aware - is a person who has little real understanding of the dynamics of his/her own poor boundaries and his/her own lack of self-love.

Back to the parents who did not learn to love themselves. Have compassion. If they are still alive, try to imagine what it must have been like for them. Forgive them. And if they are no longer here, forgive them as well. Forgiving and self-love are very inter-related. (Also see section 8 in this chapter on forgiving).

But you *do* understand, don't you, that if the model you are copying has not learned how to walk, you may not learn how to do so until much later in life. And in this case, the issue is self-love. If you don't see it happening at home, the degree of difficulty in order for you to learn it augments considerably. You will need to become self-reflective and aware in order to get to the place where you will begin to consider and then understand that it is your own responsibility to start the process.

Parents With Poor Boundaries

Such a parent allows others (in particular your other parent, or their partner, should it not be your other parent, as well as their own parents, friends and offspring) to step on their boundaries, all the while describing themselves as *peacemakers*, or someone who likes to keep a harmonious home. Or they may take another tack and continually complain about how poorly they are treated, they may cry, shout, explode or become depressed because they consider themselves victims, but in the end, nothing changes, because they *never* learn how to implement healthy boundaries. Never forget: someone with poor boundaries, who is being mistreated in some way by another, *plays their own role in the drama* and must learn to take responsibility for their own side of this tango. It is never enough - and in fact, of little use - to blame the partner, because for things to change, it is the person with poor boundaries who needs to change, *whether the other changes or not*. (Note: domestic violence and physical abuse fall outside the scope of this book).

However, such a parent may also be acting out the other side of the coin, where they are the ones who trespass boundaries.

Either way, a child who grows up in such a household, will not learn anything at all about healthy boundaries: quite the contrary - this child may learn a great deal about painful twinges in the region of the solar plexus *each time* its own boundaries are trespassed, but never knows and understands what to do about them. It may also learn to become - by observation - an expert manipulator. Clearly, such a child will not learn how to appreciate and love itself.

**Parents Who Lack Skills of Self-Reflection

Such a parent is simply not aware. Think of it. If you are not aware you do not reflect about the self. If you do not reflect about the self, you are not aware. The habit of self-reflection tends to appear when a certain level of awareness of the self arises over and above the mere fact of how others impact on one's life. Introspection evidently forms an essential part of self-reflection, as does some kind of ability to separate the ego from the self. (Also see Chapter 10).

A parent who is mainly reacting to outer stimuli in the form of events, people, conversations, and activities, is not self-reflective. Therefore such a parent will not be able to choose self-responsible reactions. A child who sees this pattern of *reactivity* does not learn the art of self-reflection from a role model, as would ideally happen, but rather, if such a child learns it at all, it is because the child begins to question such reactivity on the part of the parent, perhaps first in the guise of thoughts such as: *I never want to be like that*.

Some areas that need to be touched on in self-reflection are:

- the intention *and desire* to be aware enough to be able to be reflective
- noticing how you are *perceiving* whatever it is that is happening
- noticing how you are *reacting* to whatever is happening
- noticing how you are *interpreting* whatever is happening
- noticing the *inner dialogue* that occurs alongside all of the above
- remembering that there is *choice* involved throughout this entire process
- being *willing* to make good choices

Loving the self and caring for the self is a process that may take a lifetime, but as soon as you consciously start doing it, you will immediately notice positive changes, not only in how you feel about yourself and your world, but very probably also with respect to your physical health. Loving and caring for the self can have a beneficial impact on every single arena of your life. All it requires is that you begin.

6. Creating Healthy Boundaries

For the creation of good boundaries we might say that many things have to fall into place. However, the most important one is to be aware that your poor boundaries are not caused merely by an inconsiderate or abusive partner, but *also* by a lack of decision on your part to begin to make some changes. Poor boundaries are the foundation for a lack of healthy self-love and by beginning to shore up that poorly-built foundation (created generally, as said above, by a combination of poor role models in the early phases of life, and partners subconsciously chosen to exacerbate an already difficult inner issue), self-love will surely arise similar to the mythical phoenix that arises from the ashes, and all it requires is the first step of inner awareness to begin to take you there.

Having healthy boundaries means that you have established visibly defined limits to the types of behavior by others (partners, children, colleagues, friends, etc.), which you consider acceptable or permissible, and that you have clearly indicated the kinds of consequences that will befall the perpetrator, should those boundaries be ignored or violated.

So what does that mean? Simply said, it means that you place a value on yourself. It means you *honor* yourself. It means you hold yourself in such high esteem, and that you love and respect yourself so much that you would "do" this for yourself.

Having established a boundary, a consequence merely states, "If you do not respect this boundary that I have established, then such-and-such will happen." Boundaries need not be harsh or resemble an ultimatum, but they might have to, depending on the circumstances, as these examples indicate:

- To a spouse if both of you work: If you refuse to do the shopping, I will not have time to cook dinner and we will have to eat sandwiches (this should only apply if you like sandwiches and the other person does not because consequences are not meant to cause *you* problems or difficulties, only the other person - see the next example in this sense as well)

- To an older teenage son or daughter: When you smoke marijuana in this house, you place us at legal risk and it is a fire hazard. Therefore if you do it again, you will not be allowed to use the car for one month, but since I will not be able to drive you around, you will have to walk or use public transportation. If after that time you use marijuana again, it may happen that we will need to consider whether you may continue to live in this house.

- To a person you are dating: When you phone me at the last minute without having previously made plans with me, expecting me to drop everything in order to see you, it makes me feel as though I have no importance in your eyes, so if you do it again, I will not be available to see you.

- From one woman to another: When you blow me off two hours before a dinner engagement with me in order to go on a date with a man who has just given you a last-minute call and invited you on a date, you make me feel as though you do not value our friendship, so if that happens again, I will have to re-think our relationship.

- To a chronically late employee: When you arrive late, you make the entire production line lose time, so if you continue to do it, I will begin to dock your pay by half hour increments. If it is then repeated, you will lose your job.

- To a partner who frequently lies, particularly about important things: When you lie to me, I feel as though you place no importance on my feelings, so if you do that again, I will have to re-think our situation / want a trial separation from you.

- To an emotionally abusive partner: When you do such-and-such, it is very hurtful to me, so if you behave like that again, I will have to remove myself from this relationship.

Don't forget the basic tenet of establishing boundaries: if consequences are not set up, then there is no boundary. However, you might want to *explain* your feelings to the other person first, as in these examples, in order that he/she understands what the specific behavior does to you, your family, your health, your safety, your business, etc.

Setting boundaries is one of the first steps to psychological health because by doing this, you are clearly telling yourself that you are loved (by yourself), that you are worth it, that you care for yourself, and that you will not allow others to do unto you, as you would (hopefully) *not* do unto them.

Clearly, boundaries are an important issue and everyone who has poor ones needs to learn how to establish healthy ones.

But there is also another variation on the same theme. Start by gauging how you feel when certain things are said or done to you. You *know* when you are feeling good and when you are not. The times that you do not feel good pursuant to someone's behavior or words, are the times that something needs to be done. Use your feelings as a barometer in order to *correct as needed*. I'm not talking about correcting the other person's behavior. Hopefully that will happen. But what I really mean, is for you to correct you own behavior. In other words, begin by speaking up. Begin by indicating that what has just been said or done is not acceptable. Begin by indicating in no uncertain terms (this can be done courteously and calmly), that when you are treated in such a way, or spoken to in that way, you feel hurt, or denigrated, or angry, or sad, or whatever. State clearly that you wish not to be treated that way again, nor spoken to that way again. And decide on a consequence if the behavior is repeated, i.e., if your expressed desire is ignored. It is very important that you choose a consequence that you are capable of carrying out (don't say you will leave the relationship, if you feel you will not be able to do that), and that will furthermore bother you less, or cause less of an upset in your life, than it will bother the other person. This is *not a punishment; it is a consequence for the person who has no respect for your boundaries.*

What you are attempting to do by all of this is not only to get the other person to understand that you will no longer tolerate or accept this behavior, but more importantly, *you are showing yourself – perhaps for the first time in your life – that you are worth speaking up about, and that your respect for you is more important than being accepted, or loved, or approved of, by another – no matter who the other is.* I don't mean to pretend that this is easy. I also don't mean to pretend that it can happen all at once, or that, even if you manage it once, you will manage it again each time thereafter. It's a learning curve, like so much else in life. But I promise you this: if you begin to make a practice of this – using your feelings as a barometer – you *will* begin to feel better about yourself. You *will* begin to empower yourself. And you *will* begin to love yourself. And that is worth gold.

7. Choosing to be Transparent & Vulnerable

We like to be in control. Being in control means that the borders of our comfort zones remain intact; there is no need to cross over into unknown territory. Being in control also means that no one carries more weight than we do in a given relationship. It may even mean that we are the one who calls the shots - in the arena of emotions and needs. Furthermore, it means we don't find ourselves being vulnerable, exposing ourselves to unfamiliar - *and feared* - emotions that we may have spent years avoiding in prior relationships. Being in control offers a measure of security, it keeps us well within the safe confines of the known, the status quo, the comfort zone where no reaching and stretching is required.

Does the mere idea of being emotionally vulnerable with another individual scare you so much that you retreat as fast as your racing heart will permit in order to find another person who feels safer to you because they do not bring out these feelings? This - as you know - is one of the telltale signs of emotional unavailability and neediness because the connection to your own emotions is thin, if not totally lacking. You fear emotions not only in yourself, but also in others. In some fashion emotions are like a foreign language that so many others know how to speak, but you do not, or if you've learned to wear a smooth veneer for social purposes, you probably always feel like an imposter. And because emotions create such inner havoc, you tend to retreat from them, but in so doing, attract into your life *precisely* those people who will *most* push the buttons that relate to these issues with emotions.

If you are unaware of the fact that the healthiest way to fulfill your emotional needs is by first *caring for yourself*, then you will forever be condemned to fulfill them via others as we have seen throughout this book. And that is not only how you get into trouble, but how you become enslaved to your need for others in your life to behave in specific ways so that you can get those needs fulfilled and therefore feel good. If your partner, for example, is in a bad mood one day, if you have not yet figured out how to take care of yourself and fulfill your own needs, that bad mood will throw your day (and how you feel inside) into a tailspin and consequently threaten to curtail any chance you have at feeling good *until your partner is once again in a better mood.* Why? Because you will assume the bad mood is somehow connected to you. How you feel - under such circumstances where you are not yet loving yourself and taking good care of yourself - is indelibly intertwined with your partner's moods and behaviors, and hence you depend on your partner to be in a good place in order for you to feel good. Is there anything positive about that? Would it not make more sense that you take care of how you feel without relying on anyone else? But that requires learning how to love the self.

Have you ever had a date with someone who was rather nice, and who seemed to like you a lot as well, even going so far as saying that seeing you again would be a pleasure, but you heard no more until several weeks later? And then suddenly you found missed calls, text messages, even, perhaps, some flowers, and finally you met again for another date which again turned out to be as enchanting, if not more, as your first date. He/she continued calling, you saw each other another three or four times in succession - clearly, you had hit it off, and then, just as suddenly as this particular and exciting *hurricane* had arisen, it subsided again. This time, however, compared to the earlier, solitary date, you feel upset. Nervous, perhaps, as well, worried about - as is to be expected - *why on earth have I not heard from him/her*? You've tried to get in touch with no results, your calls go to voice mail, and your texts remain unanswered. And then, a week later, it starts up again. You have another couple of great meetings, and during the third, you are blithely informed that a trip is coming up, it had been planned since before you met, and so your new person of interest will be gone for several weeks, hiking in the Himalayan lowlands. You begin to get the feeling that you are *so much more into this* than the other person, who somehow seems to stand slightly aloof of it all, and you wonder what is going on.

And of course what *is* going on is a case of mixed messages. You are being told - when the other person seeks out your company assiduously and perhaps even fervently - that you are sought after, and then - after only a short period - you get the *other* message: *what did you say your name was? Have we met?* The question of course is: why are you still there?

About two weeks after the trip to the Himalayas was over, you get a call again expressing great interest in seeing you, and indicating that he/she just knows how fascinated you will be to hear about everything that happened on the trip. *And by the way, I was thinking about you in Nepal and so I brought you an antique carved prayer bracelet from there.*

You feel pushed and pulled and you are also beginning to feel rather annoyed, perhaps even resentful. But curiously, you make few moves to confront your slippery friend, and fewer still to have a serious talk with yourself that this can't possibly be *healthy*.

So again, what is really going on?

Your new-found partner of sorts, whom you have now been seeing for several months dancing to the on-off rhythm I've described, is, of course, behaving in a way that those of you who have already shored up your listing boundaries to a healthy degree, will recognize as being unacceptable. This is the conduct of an emotionally unavailable person who does not have a healthy connection with his/her own emotions, and hence has difficulty with the emotions of others. Not only may he/she not have a healthy connection to his own inner emotions, but *there may not be any connection to them at all*.

By keeping you on stand-by mode with this on-off behavior, this person does not need to talk to you of his/her intentions. It is more than likely that there is *at least* one other person being dealt with in similar fashion, if not more, at the same time as you. You are *all* kept dangling, so to speak, by the recurring and overt interest expressed in you, then you are discarded like a toy one has grown bored with, until the interest pops up again. By not expressing his/her *real* intentions, you are kept in the dark, in suspense, but at the same time, you are kept interested enough, chafing at the bit, so to speak, so that you won't give up. The reason this person needs to do this (whether consciously or subconsciously) is because this way he/she is always emotionally *safe*.

Should you, by any chance, get tired of it and leave, there is, as said, at least one other egg in the basket, perhaps several. The reason this offers emotional safety, is because this way the person who is keeping you dangling never needs to speak openly to you about how he/she feels, hence never needs to feel vulnerable, and hence no matter what happens on your side; no matter what *you* decide, he/she always has another proverbial lap to fall into. This kind of person *attracts people like you and you are attracted to people like this.* This is one of the faces of emotional unavailability.

Now: what about you? *Why are you in this situation?* Why did you not take off and leave this person weeks, if not months ago, once you began to see what was happening? Isn't it true that by the second time you spent several 'dates' together a part of you had already bonded to this person? Isn't it true that a part of you already felt the need for him/her, which you then translated into some version of great attraction or even love? And isn't it also true that you either decided you would be able to change him/her, or that he/she would change of his/her own accord upon realizing how *good* the two of you are together? *This is your clue. It's your red flag.*

Here is what you are doing: instead of looking after *yourself*, instead of questioning a person who plays (even if it's a subconscious game and not one done deliberately and with malicious calculation) such a game with you (for *whatever* reason), instead of caring enough about yourself to question this whole scenario and ask yourself if you really want to be exposed to it - at least without first having some *real* dialogue with the other party, and instead of recognizing that you are probably following a well-trodden path that you have walked on before in your life in other relationships, you are simply *forgetting about your psychological, emotional and spiritual health and well-being* and are going ahead with this pattern once again. That simply means that you would do well to think about your boundaries and your self-love. But it also means that this person is in your life for a reason: wake up to what you are *not* doing for yourself, and by not doing it (loving yourself and taking good care of yourself), you are looking for love in the wrong places.

If you will learn to love yourself first in a *healthy* way you will begin to find your way out of this pattern. You will see that being vulnerable is no longer the frightening thing you had taken it to be because you will have learned that no matter how you are hurt, you have the inner wherewithal to come back to a place of well being and equanimity.

**Getting Hurt

We learn quickly in life that love can hurt. Perhaps it's not even truly love, but we *think* it is. First with our parents, who may love us dearly, but hurt us nevertheless due to their own lack of understanding about love, and occasionally the source of our pain comes through parents who don't love us and then hurt us emotionally, or psychologically, or physically, and evidently such hurting leaves indelible marks.

But when we get hurt in our later love relationships, we begin to have different reactions. Who hasn't been through relationship pain? Who hasn't curled up into a ball (even if it's inside your head) with the pain that some element of a relationship has caused? Who hasn't wished that a portion of the life lived could be erased, could be forgotten, that by magic some form of amnesia would take over the brain, just to not remember whatever it is that is causing the pain?

So what can be done? How do you deal with this?

Alcohol, recreational and prescription drugs, religion, praying, meditating, panic attacks, hyperventilating, spending large pockets of time on social networking sites, shopping, gambling, sex, frenzied social activity, numbness sought in movies, books, etc., are some of the self-soothing mechanisms people use to self-medicate in times of such relationship pain as we saw in Chapter 10.

None of it really takes you anywhere. None of it is really of any lasting use. Oh, it may get you through the worst of your pain, but it doesn't really help you deal with whatever the underlying issue may have been. The problem is not so much that there is relationship pain that was apparently caused by the actions of another person, but that you are reacting with such intensity and such pain.

You see, when another person behaves in a way that hurts you, or does something that goes far beyond hurt, and that leaves a deep-seated mark on you in such a way that you feel that you might never be the same again, then this is telling you that there is something inside of you – beyond the pain caused by the other – that needs attention. Basically what that means is that a good portion of your pain has to do with elements of yourself that have not yet been worked on by you, and that is why the actions of the other hurt so much. In other words, those same actions by the other would be perceived very differently by a person who has already begun the process of working on themselves.

One of the things that needs to be looked at is your awareness of yourself and what it is that brought you to the place you are currently at. Another piece of the puzzle has to do with the choices you make at every step of the way: choices that you make when you act, react, feel, and think. Awareness - being fully conscious of yourself - and making choices are two of the most important tools you can have in the quest for your own inner freedom, although there are others, such as keeping healthy boundaries and choosing happiness.

But what is a frequent reaction when we get hurt by another in a relationship? We resolve never to let that happen again. We resolve this perhaps with a stiff upper lip or with bottomless resentment welling up inside of us. Either way, what we are doing is looking at the other as the fount of our pain, rather than - as said above - looking at ourselves. And so when we find that next relationship, we keep a portion of ourselves in check. We ensure that we will never again allow ourselves to get hurt. What kind of a relationship do you think will ensue? Clearly it will *not* be a relationship that brings about joy and growth. Instead, it will stunt and blunt and eventually - although not in the ways you are attempting to protect yourself from - you and your partner will both be hurt.

If you hide behind the cover of continual work commitments, have a multitude of friends (often of your own gender) with whom you insist on spending a great deal of time, or simply always maintain a veneer of reserve, even with your closest and dearest, you are ensuring that others can never really get close to you. You simply don't let them.

And of course that means that it's almost impossible to have a conversation of any emotional depth with you; others may says it feels like struggling to grasp a slippery, wet fish if they try talking about emotions with you.

However, if you were to brave out into uncharted emotional territory, by allowing yourself to feel the trepidation and fear this brings on, *you are granted an invaluable opportunity to discover new facets of yourself, to enrich yourself, and to stretch and grow beyond your present limits*. Thus did Columbus discover the New World, so did man step on the moon, and so can you begin to express emotionally.

Not risking stepping outside the comfort zone in those delicate matters of the heart; always taking the safe road, or looking for paths you are familiar with, all spell the death of emotional growth, psychological insight, and innovation of the self. They also signify an unwillingness or fear of looking inward, because to do so is automatically a step outside of the boundaries of the comfort zone. Where, but in the confines of the not-yet-explored self, will we find such riches? Jung wrote: *There is no coming to consciousness without pain* and Joseph Campbell was to echo that later with these words: *The cave you fear to enter holds the treasure you seek.*

When your comfort zone is narrow, and when you decide not to expand it, in particular when someone who has entered your life has scratched at the outer edges of that zone, making you feel the familiar fear (which you may explain to yourself as *someone wanting to take over your life*), you may pull up a figurative drawbridge, making it impossible for anyone to cross the moat in order to get closer to you. Pulling up the drawbridge, or *closing your heart*, means that once again you have closed yourself off. This applies not only to others, or perhaps one specific other, but also to yourself. As long as you fear emotional involvement (and write it off as something else), and as long as you refuse to allow yourself to get emotionally involved in the healthy ways this book is discussing, you will not easily be up to the task of overcoming the twin syndrome of emotional unavailability and neediness. The moat without a drawbridge serves not only to keep others out, but also yourself, and if you can't get in, you will not be able to solve these issues.

** Trust

Trust can be a tricky dilemma in the best of relationships. We must trust when we do not know what our partner is doing, we must trust when we do not know where and in what company our partner is. We must trust that our partner will not spill our deepest secrets to the world, and above all, we must trust that our partner will not deliberately harm us when they know that our heart is in their hands.

Quite another aspect of trust is the trust we have within ourselves in the knowledge that *no matter what happens*, we will be able to deal with it. In other words, we trust our innate ability to maintain our inner balance and a modicum of well-being despite outer events. Most of us can't even begin to imagine what this is, until we have done some of the work proposed in this book.

But this latter kind of trust, of course, generally only comes after quite some acquaintance with pain, particularly the pain that arises in most relationships at some point or another. And that implies that in order to actually allow ourselves to enter those relationships that come *prior* to having achieved inner trust in our own ability to quickly find inner balance, we must somehow be able to trust the other. Because if we don't, we will either not enter new relationships, or only enter those that seem secure (we have the upper hand), or that offer another kind of compensation (such as the case of a woman who might have married a man, some generations ago - and perhaps even today - that will clearly provide for her financially, but will not be faithful). *Real* trust in an - as yet unknown or unproven partner - exposes us, makes us vulnerable, and presents us with genuine emotional risk.

Another issue to be contended with regarding trust is the fact that we may have been burned once or twice, and have now decided (and you can read about this type of decision in hundreds and thousands of forums all over the world by disgruntled, hurt, deceived, disappointed, and abandoned lovers) that we will *never* again allow someone the possibility of hurting us that way again. You know the all-too-familiar story.

But that is *precisely* the wrong way of going about this. Hardening the heart against vulnerability, trust and a new partner will either forever keep us from a truly emotionally satisfying, enriching, and growth-producing partnership, or will throw us unwittingly back into precisely the same type of painful thing again, because we have not examined what happened, except under the out-of-focus microscope of blame.

Blame, as already addressed in this book does not allow us to grow. It keeps us forever anchored in a high-security prison with fortified walls of steel until we decide to look at matters differently. Whether we were badly treated by the partner that brought about the pain is not truly the important question. Much more important than that is whether we have decided to look at what it is in us that leads us into those relationships and then to take the decision - from a position of awareness - to tackle that part of ourselves in order to grow beyond that place in our lives so that we no longer need to face that issue in a subsequent relationship.

The 'thing' that lives in us that brings us into relationships that create pain in our lives, is not something we need to blame *ourselves* for either. None of this needs to be about blame at all. Not blame with regards to the partner, nor blame with regards to ourselves. It needs to be about growth and self-understanding. That can *only* happen if we chose to become aware.

**Recognizing That Growth May Come About Though Vulnerability

We've already said much about vulnerability. Its most important characteristic for our purposes is the fear we may feel when we contemplate being vulnerable in a love relationship because that fear may ultimately wake us up to the recognition that *precisely by walking towards the fear, we may overcome it*. By embracing it, it may become our friend. By courageously looking it in the face, it will help us grow and in the growth, it will help us connect to our own emotions that we have held at arm's length for so long, just as we have held those others who wish to be part of our emotional lives at arm's length.

What is needed, rather than running away or controlling or suppressing or any other resistance, is understanding fear; that means, watch it, learn about it, and come directly into contact with it.

Vulnerability and the fear that often accompanies it can become our friends as long as we are able to give the possibility that they may form part of the Ariadne's thread that can lead us out of the labyrinth a chance.

Case Studies of Vulnerability, Unavailability & Neediness

In this section we will examine a number of typical case studies illustrating how individuals begin to experience the fear of becoming vulnerable (although it should be stated that at times these very similar scenarios are quite legitimate reasons for someone with a healthy connection to his or her own emotions to decide to cut off a burgeoning relationship):

I begin to feel too good when I'm with you ... there's danger there.

Teddy and Charlene started seeing each other and a few months later Teddy realized that Charlene was possibly quite close to being his ideal woman. She was classy, elegant, intelligent, independent and sexy all in one package. She seemed to understand him very well, and he found himself more and more comfortable speaking to her about almost any subject at all. And she seemed to think the world of him. She was tender and loving and quite clearly found his company immensely enjoyable. So what went wrong? Teddy found that the more he enjoyed being with her, the more he started feeling antsy. Something in his gut told him that danger lurked just around the corner. He knew the feeling from somewhere and he was not about to wait for disaster - emotional disaster with *his* emotions winding up in the wringer - to happen. And so he began seeing her less, avoiding her calls, and most of all, he began seeing someone else, because he knew from past experience that the new woman would take his mind off Charlene. Clearly Teddy's early attachment process with his parents or one of his parents had been fraught with some kind of difficulties. Whatever Teddy had experienced in those initial years of life, it had caused him to regard emotional closeness as a warning sign for danger. And he acted upon it each time he felt it. The only times he actually got himself into relationships was when he felt that he had the upper hand: financially, emotionally, intellectually or sexually, or a combination thereof. In other words, he allowed himself to enter committed relationship status, when he was *certain* that his partner would not abandon or otherwise hurt him, because of the partner's greater need of him than his of her. One final point: almost all of this took place subconsciously. It was only in therapy, when Teddy's relationship patterns were being analyzed, that he saw it. And it was only then that he had enough awareness to be able to make a conscious choice about the new direction in which he could tread.

Your desire to connect with me makes me feel suffocated.

April and Matthew met shortly after his 29th birthday. Matthew was unlike most of the men April had met before because he seemed to be so very much in touch with his own emotions - perhaps a bit too much. However, at the beginning it was a pleasure to speak to someone who was so open in so many ways that involved himself, his emotional self and his inner self. He was so obviously willing to share those parts of himself, as opposed to tightly guarding himself against opening those doors. At some point there came the time - and in hindsight April was able to pinpoint the moment precisely to the weekend they went away to celebrate her birthday - when he clearly wanted more from her on that emotional level, and began to openly ask her to share of herself in the same way he was doing. She parried and sparred as much as she could; protecting herself from these emotional demands, but Matthew became more and more insistent. As he did so, April began to feel he was suffocating her with those demands, and very shortly thereafter began to stop seeing him as much, stopped taking his calls, and one day simply told him that she had moved on. And she felt so relieved when she did so, as though she had escaped from a spider web. But who was the fly and who was the spider? Once again, in the case of April we have someone who must have had early attachment issues with one or both of the parents. What those issues were is much less important than the fact that April needs to be able to begin to see in her relationship patterns (also see the chapter on patterns) that while she very much basks in the early glow of emotional sharing on the part of a new partner, she always balks once demands are made of her to reciprocate. And interestingly, she tends to do quite well with partners who live in another city, or even another country, or with partners who are married, although in those instances she will often refer to her regret that the relationship cannot prosper further due to geographical distances or prior martial commitments.

Your desire to connect with me makes me believe you want to control me: Version A.

Spencer and Liz had met at a summer party in her brother's house. Spencer was ten years older than Liz and they soon started seeing each other several times a week. She was perhaps slightly more taken with him than he with her, but all in all they seemed to be very happy together. Since Spencer had a much larger place than Liz, when they spent weekends together, they would go there, and soon Liz began pointing out things that could be done to make the place more amenable, more efficient and above all, more feminine. Spencer began to feel the first twinges of discomfort. Although Liz worked in a high-profile real estate agency and was considered very successful, in particular given her age, she tended to be less deeply involved in her work than Spencer, who was an investment banker. And so it happened that Liz began calling Spencer more and more often on the days they did not see each other. She simply wanted to connect, say hello, and perhaps mention whatever she had been doing that day, and in all fairness, did not in fact call more often than once a day, but Spencer began to feel that she was checking up on him. It came to a point that he asked her to stop calling him so frequently because combined with the changes she kept suggesting for his home and then the calls, he felt she was trying to control him. She retreated slightly wounded, at his clear rejection of her greater attempts at intimacy, and he began to feel guilty. That made him feel even more controlled, and so he began to back off, and finally told her he wanted to cool it. The relationship was over. Spencer's early home life had included not only a very domineering mother, but also a mother who was not the best at making him feel loved and secure. For him Liz's behavior - while he did not necessarily recognize that parts of it reminded him of his mother - took him to an emotional danger zone and so he fled.

Your desire to connect with me makes me believe you want to control me: Version B.

In this case it's not only your desire to connect with me, but the fact that you seem to be leaving your life aside in order to spend time *only* with me. Julia and Antonio met when they were already in their 40's. Both had been in several unsuccessful long-term relationships although Antonio bemoaned the fact that he simply couldn't understand why, because he had always given his all to his partners. When they met, both had been alone for several years. Julia was a professional body builder who took her work very seriously and Antonio was a journalist for a local paper who had begun working out at the gym where Julia trained.

Julia was often out of town and when they met, Antonio had been working on a major national story and therefore was only around on weekends for the first few months of their relationship. However, when he finished the story and returned home full-time, Julia began to realize that he no longer showed any real interest in his friends nor in any other activities she had believed he participated in, and only wanted to spend time with her. At the beginning, a part of her was flattered, but she soon realized that more than being a delight, his need for her presence was becoming a burden that made her feel guilty, angry, suffocated and pushed all at the same time. The more he insisted on spending greater chunks of time with her, or on traveling with her when she had weekend shows to attend, the more she pushed him away.

His reaction was to become very sad and depressed, and he would often ask her what was wrong, because all he wanted was to be able to love her. Eventually, of course, this sent her over the edge and she ended the relationship. It may be very easy for you to recognize the dysfunctionality of Antonio's reaction in this relationship, but if you had a bird's-eye view of Julia's past relationships, you would see that Antonio's desperate and unhealthy need for Julia closely mirrored the behavior of her other partners. So the question becomes: why did she attract that kind of partner into her life? Or: why was *she* attracted to that kind of partner? Did she never see the early clues to what was going on? Was she totally blind to it? And if so, why? One possible answer is simple: if we are looking at partnerships through the spiritual window, as situations in our lives that have the potential to help us grow, then obviously we must have as partners *precisely* those people who will most bring up our own issues *through their individual issues.* Julia believed Antonio was an emotionally independent man, who spent much of his time away due to the article he was working on in the early months of their relationship. She did not notice - in those early days - that he rang a bit too often because in those days she enjoyed the attention because he was far away and could not make demands on her. She also did not notice that when he spoke to her on the phone, he would often mention friends and activities, but when he was actually home, he never spent time with any of those friends, nor participated in any of those activities. She simply wrote it down to a desire to be with her, bearing in mind they had little time, as she also trained many hours every day. And so, the part of her that actually feared emotional closeness and the vulnerability that accompanies it was not alert to any of the needier characteristics of Antonio until he returned home for good. She ended the relationship, feeling he wanted to control her, feeling manipulated, and feeling totally justified in leaving him. And Antonio, of course, believed that once again, he had given his all to someone who simply could not appreciate the extent of his love.

It should be pointed out that in all of these examples, the scorned partner may *also* have issues of his own, based on the premise that if he were attracted to these particular people who have fears of vulnerability, he himself has issues that tie in closely with that. In other words, by not having his emotional demands fulfilled, he also may come to a recognition about something in himself that will permit him to grow, if he so decides.

It also needs to be reiterated that most of this is not conscious - on *either* side. The person who has vulnerability issues *recognizes* a feeling; an uncomfortable, or perhaps even scary feeling that has *nothing* to do with the adult, and everything to do with the child that this adult once was. In the recognition of the feeling, which tends to be subliminal, the adult only knows that there is something about the partner that is suddenly no longer good because of that feeling. If the feeling begins to arise more and more frequently, they decide it is the partner's fault, and therefore they need to move on *in order to get rid of that feeling*, never realizing that the feeling arises from their own connections to difficult emotional attachments from their earliest childhood and that the arising of those feelings is the beginning of the possibility of resolving them once and for all.

8. Choosing & Intending to Forgive

By forgiving we begin the process of severing our energetic connection to our past pain, trauma, abuse and hurtful memories of any kind. Without forgiving, it is extremely difficult, if not impossible to sever that connection, and that means that each time we think about the past pain or event, or each time it is somehow jogged back into our memory, we will not only suffer, but the strength of the pain can even increase, because we continue to give attention to it. Clients who endured a painful childhood, or relationship trauma due to deception or abandonment, or any other kind of hurt at all, and who tell me that they are unable to move beyond the pain, almost always also admit - once I ask the question - that they have not been able to forgive the party that injured them. They may often have tried, but with limited or no success whatsoever.

Understanding how to forgive most often lies at the crux of the matter. For most of us the idea of forgiving is somehow entangled with condoning what happened, and yet *nothing* could be further from the truth. By forgiving another for whatever way they have transgressed against us, we are healing ourselves. Ultimately, the act of forgiving is for the person who is doing the forgiving. It is, one might say, a kind of agreement with the self, in which one chooses and decides to *intend* to forgive what was done, with the understanding that in so doing, the self will be able to move forward beyond the point of the pain and its memory.

Each time the memory of the transgression or pain arises in your mind, think: *I intend to forgive, even if right now I don't yet know how.* In so doing, you weaken the neural pathways in your brain and the energetic connection to the pain, as opposed to strengthening them by continuing to think about whatever it was that happened. This simple and brief little exercise - consistently practiced - will eventually bring you to the place where you will *know* you have forgiven.

In *Rewiring the Soul* I used an example from the press: an American couple traveling in Italy with their young son, found him taken from them by a sniper's bullet. These grieving and bereft parents had many choices about how to react. Choices that anyone would have understood might have been anger, bitterness, and a desire for revenge. Instead, they chose to donate all the organs of their son's body to other families with children who needed them. In so doing, they were able to begin a process of forgiving and healing.

Many of us have seen instances in film and even on the evening news of a parent whose child (small or adult) was taken from them by a murderer, where the parent publicly announces - perhaps in court at the trial of the person who killed the child - that they forgive this murderer. *How*, we ask, *can they do this*? I believe, as do numerous other authors, that this is part of the process of healing. To forgive means to heal the self.

So far, all I've mentioned have been highly charged memories of difficult events. How does this apply to relationships? It's easy to understand how partners reach a point of so much past detritus of resentment for smaller or larger injuries, that the relationship becomes so bogged down, and one or the other is continually harping back to what the other did at some point this morning, yesterday, last week or five years ago, that there seems to be little possibility of salvaging the initial feelings of love.

And that is precisely where a conscious, loving, responsible and spiritual partner (or one who wishes to move in that direction) will realize that forgiving *must* be part of the plan. It is required thinking. Therefore when past problems surface, they must evidently first be addressed. If there are disloyalty issues, broken promises, shirking of responsibilities and so on, these *must* be addressed. The partner who feels the other is behaving improperly needs to discuss these matters with the other, but always from a self-aware point of view. As mentioned already, it is not a question of looking for someone to blame for any feelings of pain. First, you must take responsibility for your own feelings, but then you need to examine what you have done to share your feelings about the matter with your partner in an adult and mature fashion, i.e., not with anger, blame, or manipulation. Do you perhaps need to inspect your boundaries and how you handle them? Have you and your partner ever really discussed these matters in ways that were not argumentative, but objective and rational? Have you ever - in the past - come up with a plan, a guideline of sorts to help you maneuver through the rocky waters of a growing relationship?

But once this has been tended, or once this road has at least been embarked upon, a next major step is to consciously forgive past transgressions your partner may have committed, in order that *you* may come to healing. It's about *your* healing. It's about the realization that from this point forward your are each responsible for your own thoughts, feelings, words, deeds, and reactions, and that it is no longer kosher to blame the other, *even when their behavior leaves much to be desired*. This point is perhaps always one of the most difficult to grasp. How can you possibly not blame the other when their behavior has been so blatantly inconsiderate or unfair or outright cruel? You see, as we discussed earlier, it is never about *them*. It's always about *your* reaction to it or them. What you now decide to do or implement once this behavior has occurred, is very much *your* responsibility. How they continue to act or react is *theirs*. Somewhere in there, real and transparent communication between the two partners needs to have taken place as indicated above, but at some point one or both need to begin to consciously assume responsibility for the self, including being willing to *intend* to forgive.

A small note about what Eckhart Tolle calls the *pain body*, and Chris Griscom calls the *emotional body*. One of the principal reasons - according to these authors - that we continue going back to past pain *before* we recognize the need to forgive and *before* we begin to consciously *intend* to forgive (or even when we're focusing on being in charge of our thoughts that float in and out of our mind, as long as we are not aware), is because of our great familiarity with the pain, the thoughts and the feelings that are connected, glued, we might say, and stuck to it.

This great familiarity with pain makes us feel, when our thoughts go down the road they have traveled on so frequently already, to the painful moment in our history, in some fashion that we are *at home*. Not in a loving or warm and comfortable home, because of course, it hurts immensely, but a home nevertheless because *we know it well*. We have been here so often that when our thoughts turn in this direction, we find it nearly impossible to withstand the pull; the nearly *seductive* urge to follow that route once more.

And so we give in to that urge. We don't fight it. We go over the same sad material one more time. In so doing, of course, all neural pathways associated with that event and all its memories, become that much stronger by virtue of the continual reinforcement of those memories and thoughts. However, once conscious of this dynamic, we are now in a position to fight this. Each time our thoughts and feelings go down that well-trodden path again, we are now capable of beginning an inner dialogue of negation; an inner dialogue in which we firmly refuse to go down that road again. We may need to fight this battle several times before we actually achieve our goal, but once accomplished for that first time, it will become easier each time that follows. We will find ourselves feeling strangely elated, lighter, and empowered. And that process will begin to erode the neural pathway associated with the memory, and the pain body or emotional body that was erected around this particular theme, begins to crumble. The new habits in turn, will create another set of neural pathways capable of enhancing our inner well-being in totally novel ways, simply because we are no longer going down that same old path of disenfranchisement.

Clearly if both partners are not on the same wavelength, and if only one of them has accepted the relationship as growth-oriented, then matters will not necessarily be easy. Possibly the partner who is not yet on that track, will observe the changes in the other with astonishment, and then notice an inner urge, a desire, to move in that direction as well. On other occasions, the partner who has not yet begun the *journey* towards such a partnership will insist on returning to the earlier status quo. What then ensues is very individual to each situation, but as you can imagine, in this latter case, the partner who has begun to grow, will find it exceedingly difficult to return to an earlier strait-jacket way of thinking and behaving, and hence this may be the breaking point in the relationship that then culminates in a separation or divorce.

Forgiving is as essential to a conscious partnership, as water is to plants. Choosing not to forgive, or believing that you do not have the capacity to forgive means that in some fashion you have not yet set yourself on the road to the different ways of new thinking as postulated in this chapter. Learning how to forgive is more a matter of intention, as stated, than a matter of knowing how to do it. Once the intention is set, you can begin. *Especially* if you recognize that it forms part of your growth process.

9. Checking For Physical & Emotional Symptoms As They Arise

Remember what was pointed out in Chapter 7 and refer to it. With your growing sense of awareness, you will pick up much more quickly on physical sensations that are not comfortable, as well as on distressing emotions that you are used to blaming on your partner.

This is a very important step because your physical and emotional symptoms are most often the trigger for all your previously blind, reactive, blaming, or automatic behavior, and by *recognizing* them with full awareness as they appear, you will be able to implement the next step where you change the narrative and create a new dialogue when they appear.

10. Changing the Narrative: Creating a New Self-Dialogue

The importance of this step cannot be over-emphasized. What you tell yourself *from now on* each time you feel the inner turmoil - whether at a physical level, or an emotional one - whenever your partner does something that you would normally blame him/her for, is paramount to moving yourself forward. You have the power in your hands to change these subconscious reactions that have been part of you for so long. They became your defense mechanisms at a very young age, and by now are probably very strong indeed. For this reason you need to move forward with patience in the understanding that this will not happen overnight, but I promise you this: each and every time you *do* in fact change the narrative and practice a new self-dialogue when the inner turmoil arises, you move yourself a step closer to the resolution. Will it take ten times of doing it? Twenty? Fifty? One hundred? The answer is that each case is different, but the answer is also that each time you do it you will notice a lessening of the turmoil.

So let's examine the turmoil. Something has happened. Your partner has said or done something that brings up the familiar physical sensations or distressing emotions. Your initial instinct; your go-to reaction is to blame your partner and either withdraw or pursue.

Here is how you might begin to change the narrative and use another inner dialogue:

- First, you tell yourself that what you are feeling on any level has much less to do with your partner than with you. This part of the changing narrative in your head is *crucial*. You need to tell yourself this over and over again, each time it happens.
- Next, you tell yourself that this has *nothing* to do with the adult that you are, but everything to do with the little boy or girl that you were. It came about because of the specific psychological and emotional conditions of your early infancy and childhood. *It came about subconsciously and blindly*, based not on rational fact, but on a defensive measure undertaken by the psyche of a child - you - who was reacting in pain.
- The only way this can change, is if you take this step on board. These reactions you have had all your life, that you have believed were caused by specific behavior of your partners, will only ever change, if you are willing to change the narrative: what you tell yourself about why this is happening. This step in your growth and healing process is further fleshed out starting on page 227.

11. Intending to live differently

The final step is about the intention. If you *intend* to carry this through, focusing on the different steps we've examined throughout this book and specifically this chapter, then you *will* succeed. Having an intention is simply telling yourself each and every time that you think of your dilemma, that you *intend* to resolve it by following these suggestions. And then when situations arise in your relationship, you *practice* - most particularly - the tenth step.

And with this intention, you no longer make any excuses for yourself. You no longer blame your partner - no matter what. You look inside. And you focus on the outcome that you are seeking by going through the new narrative even when no situation has arisen, simply to strengthen it in your mind for the moment when the need appears.

The 11 Steps:

So let's re-examine the headlines of the main sectors of your life that will require close attention and work if you wish to resolve your emotional unavailability and neediness:

1. Being Aware & Self-Aware
2. Choosing & Agreeing to be Self-Responsible
3. Parenting the Self
4. Recognizing There is Always a Choice
5. Learning to Love & Soothe Yourself
6. Creating Healthy Boundaries
7. Choosing to be Transparent & Vulnerable
8. Choosing & Intending to Forgive
9. Checking For Physical Symptoms & Emotions as They Arise
10. Changing the Narrative: Creating a New Self-Dialogue
11. Intending to Live Differently

I'm going to assume that to this point you have not yet begun to work on what I'm going to call *the heart* of your issues, although hopefully you have been practicing much of what has been laid out so far in this book. So now you are ready, willing, and able to begin the part that has always eluded you. You've examined your patterns, you have begun to practice being more aware and self-aware, you're choosing and agreeing to be more self-responsible, you are attempting to parent and care for yourself, you've come to understand (even if you don't always implement it) that you *always* have a choice, you're learning to love and soothe yourself in healthy and nurturing ways, and as a fundamental part of loving yourself you are also instilling healthier boundaries into your life. So far so good. You've read this whole book to get to this point.

Here now, is how I suggest you continue working with *the heart*, the core of your emotional unavailability and neediness. If you practice this, over and over each and every time you are put into a situation where it becomes germane to your growth, *even when it makes you feel very uncomfortable, and perhaps even afraid*, I promise you that much will change. At times it may happen gently, bit by bit, until you notice that the same distressing feelings and physical sensations are no longer occurring with the same frequency or strength on those occasions when they *always* used to bother you, and at times, growth may come in leaps and bounds, as you cross over thresholds you had long been avoiding. By doing this, you have an excellent chance to resolve these issues in such a way that your life will forever be better, and most importantly, contain far greater emotional freedom than you may have ever experienced.

For the Emotionally Unavailable Partner

Imagine you are *just* starting to feel pushed, pursued, suffocated, or emotionally intruded upon by your partner. In many instances, even before you discern the actual feelings, you are noticing one or more of the physical sensations that you have become accustomed to, and that you recognize from the past. Perhaps it happens frequently, perhaps not, or perhaps it's even happening before the relationship has properly evolved, and you are simply having dinner on a first or second date. Nevertheless, you recognize these feelings or physical sensations.

As *soon as you become aware* of them (and this is where the fact that you have been practicing having greater awareness and self-awareness will stand you in good stead, because you will be so much more ready to recognize these feelings or physical sensations in the moment that they arise), you need to examine *exactly* what you are thinking, because this will help you change the narrative - the "story" you have been telling yourself for so long - in order to create a new self-dialogue.

Potentially what you are thinking has much to do with *blaming* your partner (or your date for the evening) for being one of those people that *makes you feel this way* (and you already decided, long ago, that *this* is *not* a good way to feel). You don't like the tightening in your gut, or the twisting in your solar plexus, it heightens feelings of anxiety that are now swirling around inside of you - it may even provoke a *fight-or-flight* reaction - and it means - at least as far as you are concerned - that this person is simply *not good for you*.

OK. So far, probably not much is new, other than perhaps the fact that you are so much more conscious about almost always blaming your partner for these physical sensations and emotions.

So now you are going to begin to change the inner dialogue. You read about poor attachment and patterns in Chapters 3 and 4. You worked on discovering your own patterns in Chapter 5. You've understood how the parenting that you received was in all likelihood lacking (again, this is *not* about blaming your parents, but about understanding how you can move on), and so you have understood how you came to develop this very challenging defense mechanism of emotional unavailability.

Therefore, you understand that what you now need to do - in the moment of becoming aware of the physical and/or emotional symptoms in you - is to *change how you talk to yourself*; in other words, what you tell yourself about what is going on. In your narrative - which may have gone on over many decades - the part where you blame the other, your partner, is the part where you need to literally converse with yourself in order to say: *No. This is not about my partner. It's first and foremost about me. About a part in me that is still a little boy or girl that is getting scared of being hurt by love because of the things that happened involving love when I was small, and that made me fear the capacity of those that I love to hurt me. Here is where I always shut myself off inside and become distant, cool, aloof, or rejecting, until in the end - while I tell myself that I don't really need anyone - I feel very alone and unloved. Sometimes I quickly look for someone else to pursue (or perhaps I already have someone on the sidelines), until their needy side appears, and then I repeat the pattern of rejection and coolness, coming full circle to my own pain.*

What you want to do at this point is create a different narrative; one that will support you in your quest to move beyond your issue, and one that you can believe in. There are several parts to this *new* narrative, some of which we've already seen above, and that all simultaneously connect with caring for and loving yourself:

- The way I am feeling (physically and emotionally) is not about my partner.
- Furthermore, it's not about blaming my partner for anything at all (whether he/she has done something wrong or pushy or intrusive is not - just now - the point).
- It's about recognizing that what I am feeling on several levels has its origins in my childhood when I learned on subconscious and subliminal levels in totally *visceral* ways that love and emotional closeness bring pain in their wake, and that therefore, back in that subconscious, subliminal, visceral state, a part of me

'decided' that it was better to keep love and closeness at arm's length.

- What I am feeling - both physically and emotionally - is very much connected to fear, but in fact this fear emanates from a small child and *not* from my adult self.
- So these sensations and feelings belong to my little boy/little girl self that in some fashion still is alive in me.
- The reason this happens is because that small part of me is *afraid* of trusting and being vulnerable.
- Another reason it happens is because the small child *never learned* how to love itself.
- The adult part of me needs to make that small part of me feel *safe and protected* (hence also the 'Small Child Exercise' referred to earlier which you can find in Appendix C).
- So apart from that exercise (which you would do well to practice once a day for at least a month - remember, it takes only a few minutes), you now need to *speak*, as it were, to your younger, small, frightened little self, and tell it that you - the adult part of you - will be protecting it, and taking good care of it from now on. This part of the narrative (that also forms part of the above-mentioned exercise), is crucial, because what you are attempting to achieve over the long term, is that your small, or younger self, which is the self that reacts these ways physically and emotionally, and that therefore did not grow up the same way your social, professional, academic, and physical self grew up, gets the chance to come to the chronological age *emotionally* to which the rest of you has already progressed. By doing this you literally show your younger, helpless self, not only that you are protecting it, and keeping it safe, but also that you *care enough about it* to do this and in so doing, you allow it to *begin the process* of what it never learned: *to love itself.*
- It is not because you are *childish* that your smaller self did not grow emotionally, but because it got stuck at

the place from which the pain originally came. That was the point at which defense mechanisms arose (including such a lack of self-love), and that is the point you now wish to venture beyond - emotionally speaking - and so you have to take that smaller self by the hand and make it feel safe by this inner dialogue and narrative from *you to you*, so to speak.

- This - in a nutshell - is how you, the one who is already an adult, simultaneously learn how to love yourself, as well as showing your younger self how to do it!

- The more you do this, the more the narrative will have a chance to work on the fears of the child. Understand that it is *precisely* by not running away from that which makes you feel uncomfortable or distressed in your relationship situations, and by addressing it in the ways described that you are allowing the smaller self that you were - and still are emotionally - to begin to feel safe. And feeling safe is something that increases, the more you continue with the new narrative. And at some point the child or small self will feel safe enough to grow.

For the Needy Partner

Imagine you are *just* starting to feel held at arm's length, rejected, or perhaps your partner is even threatening to abandon you. In many instances, even before you discern the actual feelings, you are noticing one or more of the physical sensations that you have become accustomed to, and that you recognize from the past. Perhaps it happens frequently, perhaps not, or perhaps it's even happening before the relationship has properly evolved, and you are simply having dinner on a first or second date. Nevertheless, you recognize the above-described feelings and/or physical sensations.

As *soon as you become aware* of them (and this is where the fact that you have been practicing having greater awareness and self-awareness will stand you in good stead, because you will be so much more ready to recognize these feelings and/or physical sensations in the moment that they arise), you need to examine *exactly* what you are thinking, because this will help you change the narrative - the story you have been telling yourself for so long - in order to create a new self-dialogue.

Potentially what you are thinking has much to do with *blaming* your partner (or your date for the evening) for being one of those people that *makes you feel this way* (and you already decided, long ago, that *this* is *not* a good way to feel). You don't like the tightening in your gut, or the twisting in your solar plexus, it heightens feelings of anxiety, fear, and even despondency that are now swirling around inside of you, and it means - at least as far as you are concerned - that this person is simply *not good for you*, but you know from past situations of a similar nature, that you will not be able to walk away despite your partner's cool, aloof, or rejecting attitude. *Something very painful keeps you there.*

You *also* have feelings (that you have had many times before), that once again insist that *you are not good enough.* That is why you are being held at arm's length, rejected, or abandoned. It also makes you want to pursue your partner even more, just to show him/her that you *are* valuable, but also in order for you to be able to *have* that which - when this person is "there" for you - *makes you feel so good*. What you 'get' from the other person is something you are meant to be supplying for yourself, as we have seen throughout this book, but until you fully understand the mechanism and go through the process being described here, you may continue to fall into that hole of neediness and yearning over and over again.

OK. So far, probably not much is new, other than perhaps the fact that you are so much more conscious about the part where you almost always blame your partner for these physical sensations and emotions.

So now you are going to begin to change the inner dialogue. You read about poor attachment and patterns in Chapters 3 and 4. You worked on discovering your own patterns in Chapter 5. You've understood how the parenting that you received was in all likelihood lacking in many ways (again, this is *not* about blaming your parents, but about understanding how you can move on), and so you have understood how you came to develop this very challenging defense mechanism of neediness.

Therefore, you understand that what you now need to do - in the moment of becoming aware of the physical and/or emotional symptoms in you - is *change how you talk to yourself;* in other words, what you tell yourself about what is going on. In your narrative - which may have gone on over many decades - the part where you blame the other, your partner, is the part where you need to literally converse with yourself in order to say: *No. This is not about my partner. It's first and foremost about me. About a part in me that is still a little boy or girl that is getting scared of being hurt by love because of the things that happened involving love when I was small, and that made me fear the capacity of those that I love to hurt me. Here is where I always pursue and run after whoever is rejecting me or keeping me at a distance and eventually come full circle to a place where I feel so very needy, so very bereft, and so very bad about myself. My despair is often boundless.*

What you want to do at this point is create a different narrative; one that will support you in your quest to move beyond your issue, and one that you can believe in. There are several parts to this *new* narrative, some of which we've already seen above and that all ultimately connect with caring for and loving the self:

- The way I am feeling (physically and emotionally) is not about my partner.

- Furthermore, it's not about blaming my partner for anything at all (whether he/she has done something distant, or cool or rejecting is not - just now - the point).
- It's about recognizing that what I am feeling on several levels has its origins in my childhood when I learned on subconscious and subliminal levels in totally *visceral* ways that love and emotional closeness bring pain in their wake, and that therefore, back in that subconscious, subliminal, visceral state, a part of me 'decided' that if I wanted love, I had to chase it, run after it, do whatever it took in order to get it.
- What I am feeling - both physically and emotionally - is very much connected to fear, but in fact this fear emanates from a small child and *not* from my adult self.
- So these sensations and feelings belong to my little boy/little girl self that in some fashion still is alive in me.
- The reason this happens is because that small part of me is *afraid* and yet *craves* to be loved.
- Another reason it happens is because the small child *never learned* how to love itself.
- The adult part of me needs to make that small part of me feel *safe and protected* (hence also the 'Small Child Exercise' referred to earlier which you can find in Appendix C).
- So apart from that exercise (which you would do well to practice once a day for at least a month - remember, it takes only a few minutes), you now need to *speak*, as it were, to your younger, small, frightened self, and tell it that you - the adult part of you - will be protecting it, and taking good care of it. This part of the narrative (that also forms part of the above-mentioned exercise), is crucial, because what you are attempting to achieve over the long term, is that your small, or younger self, which is the self that reacts these ways physically and emotionally, and that therefore did not grow up the same way your social, professional, academic, and physical self grew up, gets the chance to come to the

chronological age *emotionally* to which the rest of you has already progressed. By doing this you literally show your younger, helpless self, not only that you are protecting it, and keeping it safe, but also that you *care enough about it* to do this and in so doing, you allow it to *begin the process* of what it never learned: *to love itself*.

- It is not because you are *childish* that your smaller self did not grow emotionally, but because it got stuck at the place from which the pain originally came. That was the point at which defense mechanisms arose (including such a lack of healthy boundaries and lack of self-love), and that is the point you now wish to venture beyond - emotionally speaking - and so you have to take that smaller self by the hand and make it feel safe by this inner dialogue and narrative from *you to you*, so to speak.

- This - in a nutshell - is how you, the one who is already an adult, simultaneously learn how to love yourself, as well as showing your younger self how to do it!

- The more you do this, the more the narrative will have a chance to work on the fears of the child. Understand that it is *precisely* by not running away from that which makes you feel uncomfortable or distressed in your relationship situations, and by addressing it in the ways described, that you are allowing the smaller self that you were - and still are emotionally - to begin to feel safe. And feeling safe is something that increases the more you continue with the new narrative. And at some point the child or small self will feel safe enough to grow.

Evolving Every Day

So far so good. But to instill all of this even more in your daily life, you now need to talk in a totally transparent fashion with your partner about what is going on inside of you when the physical sensations or distressing feelings arise in situations where you are either feeling suffocated, pushed, or kept at a distance and rejected.

That means that you have to shore up your courage and trust your partner to be able to hear you and not wish or decide to hurt you despite your vulnerability and open honesty about these very difficult subjects. Presumably you will have been focusing on potentiating your feelings of self-love, which will now stand you in good stead as you go through this part of the process where you communicate in such an open and trusting manner with your partner.

So if you are able to do this in the very moment that it's happening, while you are still mulling over the new narrative, then you might tell your partner that right now you feel smothered or rejected and that what you'd really like to do is leave the room, or that you feel so very hurt, but that you want him/her to understand that *you* know that it has *nothing* to do with him/her; that it is, rather, something to do with you and your past and your emotional make-up. You might then explain much of what we've been examining in this book, in order to bring your partner to the same page, so to speak.

(If your partner is clearly manipulating you for his/her own benefit, being cold and rejecting, or being intrusive despite repeated boundary talks by you, clearly, other decisions may need to be taken by you, but for the sake of clarity, I am focusing on the partner who essentially wishes to resolve this as much as you do, and who may even be willing to take on board that he has his own work cut out for him).

This applies, by the way, even if you are just beginning a new relationship, after having read this book. Because of what you now know, and because of how you now change that inner narrative when you become aware of the physical symptoms and feelings, you can gently begin to explain some of it to this new partner, as opposed to simply falling back into your old modus operandi. Will this scare the new person off? Perhaps. But if it does, you may well be better off without them.

The fascinating part about doing something like this is that it will frequently bring you closer to your partner. Simply having this kind of a conversation will by no means signify that the issue is resolved, or even that the two of you will eventually live together happily ever after. It does mean, however - by mere virtue of the fact that you are willing to talk in this new way - that *you* are on your way to healing your issue. If your partner begins to understand that he/she is with you because he himself has an issue, and then begins to try to unravel it, as you are doing, then not only will he/she have an opportunity of resolving it, but you two, as a partnership, will not only potentially weather the storms you have been through, but arrive at the new port safe and sound, in better shape, perhaps, than ever before.

Chapter 15

Some Considerations on the Soul

If you consider a discussion about the soul (which is also called "non-local consciousness" by a growing number of sources, to refer to that which transcends the boundaries of the physical body and its normal sensory mechanisms) in what at first glance appears to be a book with a purely psychological basis, please feel free to omit reading this chapter.

For those who are interested in further thoughts about that eternal element of the self with regards to the dilemma presented in the particularly difficult issue of emotional unavailability and neediness, you may find what follows eye-opening.

However you are inclined, with respect to the topic of the soul, please bear in mind that this chapter is largely composed of personal beliefs that under no circumstance do I wish or intend to force on anyone, as well as an accumulation and synthesis of much reading over nearly five decades in this field, including my own integral, holistic (body, mind, and soul) work with clients in more traditional psychotherapy, but also my work in the field of past life and between life regression therapy.

What I wish to focus on, however, is not so much past lives, as what happens when we reach the state that many refer to as the 'in between lives' state. Let's examine some basic concepts first:

The Eternal Validity of the Soul

What a concept! The first time I read about it in the more spiritual (as opposed to organized religion) manner thanks to a book by Jane Roberts titled *Seth Speaks: The Eternal Validity of the Soul*, I was moved - and simultaneously excited - beyond words. In my 20's, I had already read a great deal, but to have it expressed and laid out like that resonated with me on such a deep level, that I felt as though I had 'come home'.

Finally! Here was someone speaking the language I knew that I also spoke, but was just having a bit of difficulty remembering clearly. I'd call this an eternal language that so many people have woken up to during the course of their lives. As you hear it spoken, you feel an excitement building inside of you, as you realize you are connecting with something that - you now know - has been with you always. You crave to hear more of it, and you may realize with profound yearning, that it is not so readily available - at least at the beginning of learning to speak the language again. So you fervently seek out books, speakers, documentaries, seminars, retreats, as well as video and audio clips that give you that feeling of connection again, and feel so deeply blessed when you find them. Until the day comes when you realize all you really need to do to find this connection, is to look within. Mindfulness and meditation are but two possible paths that take you there.

And by the way, this language; this inner connection is *not* about past lives. That is simply *another* one of the numerous paths to get there, but by no means the only one, nor is it a *required* - or even recommended - path. There are no real rules here that I know of, other than perhaps: *love yourself and remain mindful*. As a child and young teen I had already felt this connection by reading books - mainly novels at that early time in my life - that had little or nothing to do with past lives, but that *did* have much to do with the spirit.

Assuming you believe that the soul is eternally valid, or perhaps you simply resonate with the idea, or perhaps you've noticed that whenever you hear or read concepts related to the idea, something in you jumpstarts, then you will agree that if the soul is indeed eternally valid, it stands to reason that you are not your body. As Pierre Teilhard de Chardin (a Jesuit priest) once famously wrote: *We are not human beings having a spiritual experience. We are spiritual beings having a human experience.*

And if you are not your body, then there is something that goes far beyond your body which is - we might say - on a level far superior, and certainly not as finite as your body.

Up to this point we could say we remain on the same page as the position taken by many of the world's organized religions. Indeed, Teilhard de Chardin was not necessarily talking about the spiritual experience in the way we are discussing it here, although his statement ties in beautifully with our subject matter.

However, as we continue, we distance ourselves more and more from many organized religions - for whatever reasons that may be - bearing in mind the numerous conspiracy theories out there trying to tell us that the 'bad' churches took many of these beliefs away from us. It's not my intention here to travel even one centimeter down that road, but it *is* my intention to offer some thoughts about the many ideas and beliefs that are based on this eternal validity of the soul.

Much of it has to do with growth. And how can anyone - even an eternal soul - grow exponentially without experiences? And so, if this life is the only one we'll ever live, we only have a very tiny chance at growth, and then we'll have to wait a very long time indeed for that famous Resurrection Day in order to discover whether we had been given a good grade!

Imagine you were only permitted to go to that first year of school once, and if you did not learn how to write, read, and do those early sums, they told you: *ok, you failed miserably, so now you can neither repeat the year, nor can you pass on to the next grade.* That would be a rather wretched - not to mention desperate - state of affairs. Repeating a year, as onerous as it might be, nevertheless gives us the chance to improve whatever it was that did not work out well the first time around, or that we had difficulty learning, or perhaps were too lazy to apply ourselves to, and by improving, we then have the opportunity of moving on to that next level or grade.

Then, once you do reach that next level, you might carry on slowly, learning whatever the lesson plans bring you, and simply move from one level to another, or, you might, depending on how much you apply yourself, skip a level, *because of how much you already learned on the prior level*, or you might choose - especially at the university level - to take on extra credits or material, in order to accomplish much more than usual in a short period of time *so that you would be able to move on more quickly.*

As you pass from one level to another, and become more accustomed to applying yourself fully to whatever tasks, challenges, and goals you are faced with, you may understand *how* you can move forward more quickly. You may realize, for example, that if you give up going out on Friday nights and use those hours to read or study, that you move forward much more quickly and easily.

On the other hand, if you don't apply yourself, or if you forget what you learned one year or in one subject area by the time you get to the next one, obviously it will take you a great deal more time to move on. In many ways this analogy can be applied to the notion of past lives.

Past Lives

The concept of more than one life made visceral sense to me even when I was a child. Later, after much reading, I found myself at Chris Griscom's Light Institute in Galisteo, New Mexico (read the story of this experience in my book *Rewiring the Soul: Finding the Possible Self*) in order to *examine* my own past lives.

The experience was life-changing to say the least. Paradigms shifted and I came into an entirely new understanding (for me) about what I was doing here in this particular lifetime. Not, I hasten to add, from the point of view of any 'purpose' for being here in the greater scheme of things, or in the eyes of the world, but simply from the point of view of the continued growth of my own self. I also realized that the multiple lives I had experienced, of which I was able to glimpse salient portions in the facilitated sessions, served one main purpose: my growth; my greater connection to my inner, or higher self - in a word - my greater connection to my soul.

I began to understand that I could make very conscious and deliberate choices about how I reacted to any given circumstance in my life in order to move this process forward in a much more accelerated fashion. The more quickly I 'learned' my many lessons, the more quickly I could move on to even greater challenges and rewards. Just like in school.

Karma

A question I have often asked myself since I first became aware of the concept of karma is whether it is ever possible to climb off the seemingly interminable wheel. Is it just cause and effect, or is there more involved? Many volumes have been written about this subject, with minds much wiser than mine pondering it. What seems clear to me is that once a given lesson is learned, and once it has been reinforced enough in order for it to have become part of the very fabric of your being, you may never need to tread down that particular path again.

Between Lives

Anyone who believes in past lives and who stops to think for a moment, will come to the realization that from the moment you die in one lifetime, to the moment you are born in the next, a great deal of time may pass. Counted in our mundane terms here on earth it might be as little as seconds or minutes, weeks, or months, or as long as years, or even centuries.

Many subscribe to the notion of the 'simultaneity of time', which we might boil down to the idea of everything occurring at once, and hence *all your lifetimes* would occur at the same time, and therefore what happens in one may affect what happens in all others, but I must tell you that this concept has proven to be quite mind-boggling, and I must simply accept that at this point in my life while I ponder on it frequently, I have not been able to understand it in such a way that I would feel free to even attempt to explain it any further.

So assuming there is a space of some sort between dying and being born again, and assuming you aren't playing the harp as you sit on a diaphanous cloud waiting for the bell to ring and announce your new birth, the between life state, as shown by numerous researchers and therapists in their work with their own clients and research subjects, appears to be a place and time where many interesting things occur.

To begin with it is here where choices about the conditions and people in your next life appear to be made, allowing for a stretching and deepening of the notion of free will. And it appears that those conditions are chosen not for their loveliness or how they might bring you to a state of well-being and happiness in the mundane sense of the word, but rather, for their potential to create growth in you. It also appears that the individuals with whom you experience situations and relationships are often people with whom you have a prior connection on the soul level. Yes, you may have lived out many lives with one or another, over and over again, but the connection I'm referring to, is on the soul level, as opposed to the earthly one. And so of course it brings up the possibility that these soul connections *agree* to act out roles for each other - often very difficult, frustrating, painful, even abusive and violent roles - in order to move the growth of one of the two (generally the one on the receiving end of the stick) on more quickly.

That brings me to the notion that it could very well be precisely the people who *harm* you the most in a given lifetime - particularly those who form part of your personal life (as opposed to the drunk driver who causes your death) - who carry the strongest soul connection with you, as perhaps they are the ones who *love you enough on that soul level* to be willing to do to you that which will carry your growth forward.

Clearly, I have no 'scientific' proof for any of this, nor do any of the hundreds of psychiatrists, psychologists, researchers, and other practitioners, who subscribe to these notions. Nor is - as stated - my intention to convince you of anything; merely to lay out ideas for you to consider or discard, as you wish.

Decisions Made to Accelerate Growth: A Deliberate Choice of Events for the Coming Life

All of the above begs the question: who exactly is it who *decides* how you will grow during each lifetime? And who *decides* what will happen during that lifetime? Who *decides* which people will be part of your life, who *decides* who will be your parents, siblings, who *decides* which person (or people) you will marry, and who *decides* who will be your children? God? Destiny? Your spirit guides? Or could it be yourself - *your eternal self*? Along with many other authors who write about these topics, I subscribe to the latter belief. We each - along with, perhaps some wise guidance - *choose* the events and people of our lives in an in-between life state, that place we inhabit in some fashion while we are between one incarnation and another.

If we choose the people and the events, it literally implies we also choose whether those events will be hard, easy, or nicely balanced, and that brings us back to the notion of learning more quickly the more challenging the experiences are. Is it not possible that for a given lifetime you might decide - in that in-between lives state - that you wish to make greater progress, and hence deliberately choose a number of situations to grapple with during the next lifetime in order to move yourself more quickly up the ladder of understanding, growth and remembering?

Perhaps you choose to be born with a stammer and to be bullied on the school playground. Perhaps your father dies early of an unexpected illness or in a car crash, and your mother has financial difficulties in coping, and so from a very young age you are left to your own devices. Perhaps you find a mentor, or a mentor finds you, and things begin to improve, although they are still hard. Perhaps you get your career on track, and eventually fall in love - despite the ongoing stammer - and get married and have a couple of children, and it all looks so rosy. You are even able to help your aging mother live a more dignified life. But then it begins to fall apart again. Your wife has an affair and wants out of the marriage. She's taking the children with her and moves out of state. You are bereft. What now happens - psychologically, emotionally, and spiritually, as well as on an external level - will to a large degree determine your growth factor in that specific lifetime.

Emotional Unavailability & Neediness & the Soul

And that of course brings us full circle to the topic of this book: the very difficult and painful relationships that ensue when you are emotionally unavailable or needy, as well as the parental connections you have probably had that brought you to that place in your psycho-emotional development where those issues came to life.

I speculate that you choose a parental and early home life situation which serves to bring about these psycho-emotional challenges that create the defense mechanisms described throughout the course of this book, and similarly you also chose a partner or partners that will further augment the difficulties you experience through your relationships with them. Why? Why would you choose such life situations? You choose them in order to grow. Because, as said, the frustration and pain such relationships bring to your life is one of the greatest reasons you may try over and over again to understand their dynamics and thus eventually find your way out of the labyrinth into a totally different kind of relationship where such issues no longer need to be brought to the table.

Therefore it is my contention that the particularly painful and frustrating dynamic represented by emotional unavailability and neediness - if you choose to work with it - may be a brilliant gem in disguise whose presence in your life - and psyche - exists in order to offer the growth of your soul through the personality that you are in this lifetime, the potential momentum to move forward in leaps and bounds.

Appendix A

15-Minute Mindfulness Walk

Choose a time, during daylight hours when you can walk unimpeded, on your own, for 15 minutes. Start by focusing on the beauty around you, whether this is beauty you see, smell, hear, taste or touch. When you do this, also allow yourself to feel gratitude for whatever it is you are perceiving with one or more of your senses. This brings you into the present moment, allowing your mind to be still. Then do it again, by noticing something else, and again, feel the gratitude. Try to continue doing this for the entire 15 minutes. If at one point you realize your thoughts have wandered off to your worries or past pain, or just everyday problems, don't get annoyed with yourself. Simply pull yourself back to noticing beauty again until your 15 minutes are up.

Just as in the beauty and gratitude exercise of Appendix B, new neural pathways are formed and strengthened each time you practice the mindfulness walk. This exercise and the beauty exercise build on each other, and when both are used in conjunction with one another, this section of your brain that has a great deal to do with inner well-being, and the speed with which you can 'switch' over to it, especially when thought are torturing you, will grow in strength even more quickly. You will not only become more conscious and aware, but you will also become much more in charge of your inner well-being and harmony.

Appendix B

Brief Beauty & Gratitude Exercise

While this exercise is very similar to the mindfulness walk in Appendix A, it differs in that it can be done at any time, in any place, and in less than one minute, and without anyone actually noticing that you are doing it. Whenever you need to find a momentary space of inner peace (and the more often you practice this exercise, the more quickly and strongly the sensation of peace will come to you), simply do this exercise.

Look about you. Find something beautiful, preferably nature, but it can be anything. Perhaps you see a tree, a cloud, or a flowering bush. Perhaps you see sunshine, or drops of rain, or a snowflake. Perhaps you look at a plant in the room in which you find yourself, a painting, a rug, or an object you admire. Focus on this thing of beauty, really letting yourself see it, and then allow yourself to feel gratitude for having it in your life at this moment. As you feel the gratitude, notice a small sensation of peace in your solar plexus.

Each time you do this, a new neural pathway in your pre-frontal cortex begins to form and strengthen. Therefore, each subsequent time you do it, you will notice the sensation of peace a bit more, and it may last a bit longer.

Furthermore, the more you practice this at *any* time during your day, the more it will begin to permeate your life at odd moments, when you are *not* practicing it, but when you might need that moment of peace and inner calm.

Appendix C

Connecting to Your Younger Self

Here is an exercise which may help you begin to care for yourself in the ways we have been discussing here. Variations on this exercise have been around for years, and can be found in many books.

If you have it, take out a photograph of yourself from when you were about five or six years old. Next, if you have a child of that age yourself, or friends (or neighbors) with a child that age, have a look – *really* have a look at that young, lovely and wonderful child so that you can appreciate how innocent the eyes, how *small* the child, how much it needs the protection and love of the adults in its life, how fresh the skin, how lovely, beautiful, and wondrous this little person is. If you have no such child in your life, simply have a good look at one in your supermarket, or neighborhood playground or park, etc. This part of the exercise that I have just described about the photograph and the flesh-and-blood child only needs to be done once.

When you have all of that set clearly in your mind, go to your bedroom, or any other place where you will not be disturbed for about five minutes (it's a short exercise, but you should try to do it every day for at least one month). Take a cushion, sit down, and place the cushion on your lap. Close your eyes, and in your mind's eye imagine that the cushion is you when you were little. Again, in your mind's eye, imagine hugging your younger self, caressing your own little self's cheek, touching your hair, saying *I love you so very much*, telling your younger self:

- *You are so beautiful / handsome*, in other words telling your younger self what a good-looking child you are.

- *That dress is so pretty / you look so good in that t-shirt* (or whatever might be appropriate, given your gender and your memories of the way you dressed), the point is to *lovingly compliment* something about the way you; i.e., your younger self looks. This will often make you - the adult - feel tearful.

- *What a gorgeous drawing ... I'm going to put it up on the fridge / what an amazing paper airplane you made / sandcastle you built* or whatever is appropriate, given your memories of what you used to do as a child. The point is to *admire* something you; i.e., your younger self has created.

- *You know, I am always going to take care of you and protect you and never let anything bad happen to you. I'm going to do that because I love you so very much* (the point is to instill a sense of safety in you; i.e., your younger self).

- That's basically it. Now you can hug and kiss your younger self good-bye – in your mind's eye - and say *see you again tomorrow.*

Now here's the important thing: you have just promised your younger self that because of your love for yourself, you will always take care of and protect yourself. So now you have left the room where you did this exercise, and gone back to your normal life. And a few hours later your spouse screams at you ... that's just the way your spouse is. Or your teenage son or daughter has just again been rude to you. Or the person you are just beginning to date and with whom you are out having dinner, is checking out all the other men / women who are entering the restaurant, taking his / her eyes off you each time the door opens.

Any of the above that apply (or any others you can think of) create that twisting feeling in your gut. *And you do nothing.* What do you think your younger self is going to figuratively say to you tomorrow when you get back together again? *I can't trust you. You promised to take care of me, and look what you did. You let me feel so bad again.*

Let me reiterate this very important thing to understand: when you have poor boundaries you learned at an early age not to "be yourself" because doing that was dangerous. Being yourself might simply have meant expressing dismay, or hurt, or that you didn't like something. What you did instead was to walk on eggshells around certain people, or you pushed yourself into the background in many different ways, in order to mold yourself into whatever you thought you needed to be in order to be accepted, approved of and loved. It was dangerous to truly express yourself (whether that meant showing others that you loved to paint or sing, or whether it meant saying that you preferred not to accompany your parent to the store, or whether it meant that you didn't want to listen to anyone shouting, but couldn't say so), because if you did, you ran the risk – as said – of not being accepted, approved of, and loved. And so you lived in a twilight zone of unease, anxiety, stress, fear where you may have felt many things, *but you most certainly did not feel protected.*

This is what is called learning a dysfunctional form of love. It's also what happens when we don't learn healthy ways to love ourselves. You might say it's a stunting or crippling process of the pure love nature that a child is born with – and lest you think I'm out on a vendetta against parents, please remember to be compassionate. After all, they (your parents, my parents, *and* you and I as parents ourselves) were often not taught any differently when they/we were children.

Now however, when you begin to "grow" your relationship with your younger, stunted self, and you make a promise of taking care of your younger self, protecting it, cherishing it, loving it, *you must keep that promise if you wish your younger self to eventually grow up to where the rest of you is*. And it will only do so, *if it trusts you!* When we fear for our emotional safety, and therefore take on protective measures such as those described above (and there are many other manifestations as well, but in this chapter I am concentrating on poor boundaries), in order to ensure that we receive a modicum of love and approval, or at least avoid outright rejection, the part of us that takes on the protective measures remains in some fashion child-like and stunted, and this is why, when similar buttons are pushed as we grow older and become adults, we may find ourselves reacting in ways that don't seem to be in accord with the rest of our personality.

We may have developed into highly sophisticated, intelligent, cosmopolitan and professionally adept individuals in most other areas of our lives, but in this one – the one where our emotional safety is at risk – we remain somehow childlike, fearful, withdrawn, perhaps even infantile in our reactions to others, at least with regards to how we react when being faced with the fact that our boundaries are being trespassed. Our *emotional self* has not grown up the same way the rest of us has.

Therefore, once you have begun the exercise of meeting with your younger self on a daily basis, it is very important that you begin to take steps to show this anxious, scared, younger part of you that you are not only to be trusted, but that you come through with what you promise. And so, when boundaries are crossed, and when another says or does something that you recognize – among others because of the twisting in your gut – as a crossed boundary that you need to say something about, say it. Just say it. Say *that is not acceptable*. Say it in a courteous tone of voice. Say that you can no longer accept being treated or spoken to this way. And give a consequence if your request is not met. Having established a boundary, a consequence merely says, "If you do not respect this boundary that I have established, then this will happen."

Appendix D

Sample Talks

As already indicated in the text, TED Talks (simply Google it), or YouTube are invaluable resources for inspirational and motivational talks of the kind I am recommending to you.

If you're not familiar with TED, do look under some of the categories listed on the main site in order to find topics you may consider interesting. The talks are all between approximately four and twenty minutes in length.

Specifically in YouTube, you might look for talks by some of the following speakers, in order to see who resonates with you (as you search for these people, on the right sidebar you will notice many other speakers elaborating on similar topics are shown there). Also, not all these speakers are freely available on YouTube; some talks - if they interest you - will have to be purchased:

- Wayne Dyer
- Deepak Chopra
- Eckhart Tolle
- Caroline Myss
- Joseph Campbell
- Bruce Lipton
- Gregg Braden
- Matthieu Ricard
- Chris Griscom
- Rudolph Tanzi
- Clarissa Pinkola Estés

- Thich Nath Hanh
- Bernie Siegel
- Steven Covey
- Marianne Williamson
- Pema Chödrön
- Ram Dass
- Jon Kabat-Zinn
- Dan Siegel
- Andrew Harvey
- Tom Campbell
- Rupert Sheldrake
- James Hillman
- Marion Woodman

Also visit one of my blogs: Rewiring the Soul (identical to the title of my first book), and on the left sidebar you will find a list of numerous links, some with an asterisk. Those are links that I've collected over the years that also provide material to inspire, motivate, and stimulate you.

Bibliography

In the print version of *Rewiring the Soul* I included about 40 pages of Bibliography prefaced with the following words:

Why does a book as deceptively simple as this one require such an extensive bibliography? It doesn't. Nevertheless, these books are a portion of those that have shaped my life and in so doing have shaped my thoughts and my understanding. And it is in the shaping of these that this book could be written so simply and so directly. Psychology, neuroscience, biology, sociology, history, politics, religion, spirituality, philosophy, mythology, dreams and fairy tales, body work, metaphysics and esoteric thought, motivational books, biographies and autobiographies all form part of this mélange, as well as some journals of certain writers or thinkers and several dozen novels that have also been included because they too, were significant.

I have returned over and over again to some of these books, as one returns to old and loved friends; friends that are beloved because of what has been shared and because of the support that has been given, and what has been learned. Sometimes, however, I return to a book, no longer certain if I remember it, and then I see the highlighting, the underlining and the scribbled notes on *precisely* those passages that still resonate with me now, and that reminded me then, when I first read them, of what I really already knew. *Just as you do.* It's not really important if you look at this list at all. But perhaps you'll enjoy doing so.

Emotional Unavailability & Neediness: Two Sides of the Same Coin is built on those books as well, because as I say above, these books shaped me and my thinking. But I hope you understand that in order to keep the publishing cost of this book down, those many pages will not be included again.

However, you can access them all here online by going to this link: http://mupri.me/F020b which will automatically open an Adobe Acrobat pdf file of the Bibliography or by using the QR Code embedded here:

ABOUT THE AUTHOR

Gabriella Kortsch, Ph.D. (Psychology) is also the author of the bestselling *Rewiring the Soul* (2011), *The Tao of Spiritual Partnership* (2012), and *The Power of Your Heart: Loving the Self* (2013). She works in private practice with an international clientele in southern Spain using an integral focus on body, mind and soul. Also an international speaker and radio broadcaster, she teaches workshops, posts on her blogs, and publishes a monthly newsletter in English and Spanish. She has three sons.

Contact details for Gabriella Kortsch, Ph.D. are as follows:

Websites: http://www.gabriellakortsch.com

http://www.advancedpersonaltherapy.com

Blogs: http://www.rewiringthesoul.com

http://www.taoofspiritualpartnership.com

http://www.powerofyourheart.com

Email: info@advancedpersonaltherapy.com

Made in the USA
Middletown, DE
13 September 2020

Michael A. Mancini

Integrated Behavioral Health Practice

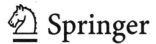 Springer

Michael A. Mancini
School of Social Work
Saint Louis University
Saint Louis, MO, USA

ISBN 978-3-030-59661-3   ISBN 978-3-030-59659-0   (eBook)
https://doi.org/10.1007/978-3-030-59659-0

This Springer imprint is published by the registered company Springer Nature Switzerland AG
The registered company address is: Gewerbestrasse 11, 6330 Cham, Switzerland

I dedicate this book to my parents for their grace and tolerance; to Becky for giving me strength, courage, and hope; and to Sofia for giving me joy.

Preface

The healthcare field has moved decidedly toward the integration of behavioral health services that are empirically supported, trauma-informed, and recovery-oriented. In integrated care, behavioral health and primary care professionals work collaboratively with clients to provide evidence-based health, mental health, and addiction interventions in a coordinated, systematic, and cost-effective manner. Behavioral health professionals provide screening, assessment, and interventions designed to prevent, detect, and address mental illness, addiction, and health conditions induced or exacerbated by trauma, stress, and economic disadvantage. Integrating behavioral health services with health services can increase access to behavioral healthcare by co-locating primary care and behavioral healthcare professionals in the same setting. This can increase ease of access to care and reduce the burdens that can interfere with patients' ability to follow-up on treatment recommendations. The integration of behavioral health and primary care has been driven by the increasing prevalence of behavioral health issues in the general population as evidenced by rising rates of addiction, mental illness, violence, and suicide, and the realization that untreated trauma can have significant negative health and mental health consequences.

Healthcare consumers in the United States, particularly Black, Indigenous, and Persons of Color (BIPOC), have historically received inadequate access to behavioral healthcare due to the separation of behavioral and primary care services. The implementation of the Patient Protection and Affordable Care Act (PPACA) has spurred an increased focus on inter-professional education and integrated behavioral healthcare to address health disparities due to inequitable access to healthcare and other social determinants of health such as adequate income, stable housing, employment opportunities, food, safety, and healthy environmental conditions. A significant barrier to providing integrated behavioral healthcare is a workforce lacking in professionals who are adequately prepared to practice in integrated care settings. Indeed, few clinical texts adequately reflect the new practice realities that face social workers and other behavioral health practitioners. This text seeks to respond to this need by providing readers with the latest evidence-based practices and interventions for common behavioral health disorders as well as issues related to suicide and violence. The proposed text invites graduate-level social work, psychology, and counseling students to consider how to best implement behavioral health assessment and treatment practices that are evidence-based, trauma-informed, and recovery-oriented.

Despite the promises of the Affordable Care Act, healthcare delivery in the United States remains inequitable, inefficient, and costly. The COVID-19 pandemic has exposed the inequities in access to healthcare and other social determinants of health that drive health disparities. Black, Indigenous, and Latinx Americans are far more likely to die from the coronavirus in large part due to pre-existing health conditions that result from inequitable access to political power and resources such as safe housing, health care, food, employment, and adequate income. These inequities are the result of a long history of racist policies that have segregated BIPOC communities and denied them power and access to the resources necessary for health and prosperity. Universal healthcare and integrating health, behavioral health, and social services represents one policy change that could have an important impact in reducing health inequities. In order to ensure equitable access to healthcare and other social determinants of health, changes must be made to *how* healthcare is delivered. The fragmentation that exists in health, mental health, addiction, and social service systems must be addressed to ensure coordinated, efficient, and equitable delivery and distribution of services and resources. One way to reduce health inequities and costs and improve health is to provide social care as part of health care. The integration of social workers and other behavioral healthcare providers into healthcare teams as a means to assess and address social determinants of health has been identified as an important public health strategy to improve healthcare delivery.

This book will prepare graduate-level students in social work and other helping professions to provide integrated behavioral health services in community-based health and mental healthcare settings that are evidence-based, recovery-oriented, person-centered, and trauma-informed. This book is divided into 11 chapters that address the core practice areas of integrated behavioral health practice. In Chap. 1, "Integrated Behavioral Health Service Models and Core Competencies," I define the core elements of integrated behavioral health practice and identify specific models and practice competencies that comprise this approach to care.

In Chap. 2, "Intersections of Social, Behavioral, and Physical Health," I review the prevalence of several behavioral health disorders and issues such as depression, trauma, anxiety, suicide, and violence in the United States for different groups and provide information on the co-morbidity of these disorders with other health conditions. In this chapter I also outline an ecological systems approach to frame biological, psychological, and social factors found to be important determinates of risk and resilience for common behavioral health disorders at individual, familial, institutional, and societal levels.

In Chap. 3, "Models of Change and Well-Being from Behavioral Health Disorders," I review several theoretical practices models of recovery and well-being and models of how people change health behaviors. I do so to provide guidance to behavioral health providers on how they can (re)create contexts that empower clients and promote health. In the first part of this chapter, I review three major theories of recovery and well-being that include: (1) The Model of Mental Health Recovery; (2) The Model of Subjective Well-being; and (3) The Model of Psychological Well-being. In the second part of this chapter, I review three theories related to understanding how people change health-related behaviors such as substance use and other risk behaviors. Three major theories will be reviewed, which include: (1) The Transtheoretical Model of Change; (2) The Health Belief Model; and (3) The Theory of Reasoned Action.

In Chap. 4, "Behavioral Health Screening and Assessment," I provide an overview of screening and assessment practices that are person-centered, strength-based, holistic, and recovery-oriented. This chapter will focus on assessment and documentation areas that include: (1) screening for common behavioral health issues such as depression, anxiety, stress, trauma, suicide, and substance use; (2) assessing personal strengths and capacities that lead to health; (3) past and current problems in the functional domains of health, mental health, substance use, interpersonal relationships, employment, and daily living; and (4) assessing social determinants of health.

In Chap. 5, "Person-Centered Treatment Planning," I review the specific areas of person-centered treatment planning, which include: (1) case conceptualization; (2) developing goals and objectives; (3) selecting interventions; and (4) progress notes and documentation.

Violence is an increasingly relevant aspect of behavioral health practice in primary care and behavioral health settings. In Chap. 6, "Integrated Behavioral Health Approaches to Interpersonal Violence," I explore the epidemiology of intimate partner violence and community violence in the United States. I then review screening, assessment, and intervention strategies for intimate partner violence (IPV) and community-based violence (CBV).

In Chap. 7, "Trauma-Informed Behavioral Health Practice," I explore the impact of trauma and adverse childhood events (ACEs) on health and well-being. This chapter includes epidemiological data on the prevalence of trauma and adverse childhood events and the impact of these experiences on health. I provide an overview of trauma-informed care practices and review the most relevant and evidence-based practices in regard to trauma screening, assessment, and intervention. This overview will include several evidence-based treatment strategies for trauma that include prolonged exposure therapy, cognitive processing therapy, Eye Movement Desensitization and Reprocessing Therapy (EMDR), and Trauma-Informed Cognitive Behavioral Therapy (TF-CBT).

In Chap. 8, "Screening and Assessment for Depression and Anxiety Disorders," I review the signs and symptoms and diagnostic criteria of major depressive disorder, adjustment disorders, and several anxiety disorders including generalized anxiety disorder, social anxiety disorder, panic disorder, agoraphobia, and obsessive-compulsive disorder.

In Chap. 9, "Brief Approaches to Treating Depression and Anxiety," I explore cognitive behavioral-based treatments and other evidence-based approaches for depression and anxiety. Specific treatments to be discussed include: (1) behavioral activation; (2) identification and reframing of negative thinking patterns; (3) developing problem-solving and other coping skills; (4) exposure-based therapies; and (5) relaxation and mindfulness-based stress reduction approaches. Other approaches that can be effective for both conditions include illness management skills, family psychoeducation, and positive psychological interventions.

In Chap. 10, "Screening, Assessment and Brief Interventions for Substance Use," I review screening and assessment practices and tools for substance use. I then provide an overview of brief interventions that can be used in time-limited clinical encounters. Specific skills and practices associated with brief motivational interventions will be provided.

In Chap. 11, "Stage-Based Treatment Approaches for Substance Use Disorders," I review three sets of interventions found to be effective in substance use disorder treatment: (1) harm reduction approaches; (2) motivational interviewing; and (3) brief cognitive behavioral treatments.

The information in these chapters is designed to cover topics that are most readily experienced by behavioral health practitioners working with adult populations in integrated settings across primary care and behavioral health. As such, I do not cover other important areas in behavioral health practice such as serious mental illness, personality disorders, eating disorders, intellectual disabilities, services designed specifically for children and youth, or psychiatric medications. In most chapters, I provide detailed case examples designed to help readers apply the strength-based, person-centered assessment, treatment planning, and intervention practices covered in the book. I have attempted to construct these cases to be inclusive of multiple identities and to provide readers with cases that are complex and multi-dimensional in order to simulate the rich lives of the clients we all serve.

Saint Louis, MO, USA   Michael A. Mancini

Acknowledgments

I gratefully acknowledge all of the people that have contributed to this book. I would like to specifically thank the people that have shaped my understanding and informed my thinking about behavioral health practice over the years including my colleagues Shannon Cooper-Sadlo, Gabriel Carrillo, Craig Miner, Don Linhorst, Michael Vaughn, Brandy Maynard, Monica Matthieu, and Gary Behrman. I also would like to thank my students who have challenged and inspired me to be more inclusive, creative, and dynamic in my thinking about how I teach behavioral health practice. I would also like to thank the staff at Springer including Jennifer Hadley, Janet Kim, Brinda Megasyamalan and Sudha Kannan for all of their contributions and help in editing this text. Finally, I thank Dr. Norman White, whose memory and voice continues to urge me to center social justice in my work and daily life.

Contents

About the Author

Michael A. Mancini PhD, MSW, is an associate professor in the School of Social Work at Saint Louis University in Missouri. He is also co-director of the Doerr Center for Social Justice Education and Research. He received his PhD in Social Work from the University at Albany in New York in 2003. His research focuses on the evaluation and implementation of integrated behavioral health services in community-based mental health programs, hospitals, and schools. He has published in a range of social work and mental health journals including: *Community Mental Health Journal, Qualitative Health Research, Psychiatric Rehabilitation Journal, British Journal of Social Work, Journal of Social Work Education, Journal of Behavioral Health Services and Research,* and *the American Journal of Drug and Alcohol Abuse.* He has conducted professional development seminars on trauma-informed care and co-occurring mental health and substance use disorder assessment and treatment, and has taught graduate-level social work courses on clinical assessment, diagnosis, and treatment of behavioral health disorders for the last 20 years. As a practitioner, he has worked as a social work case manager, program specialist, and administrator in a variety of behavioral health settings.

Chapter 1
Integrated Behavioral Health Service Models and Core Competencies

1.1 Introduction to Integrated Behavioral Health Practice

The COVID-19 pandemic has demonstrated to the world the importance of health care systems that are adequately prepared to effectively provide universal, comprehensive health care to address co-morbid health and behavioral health disorders. The pandemic has also demonstrated the importance of maintaining a healthy population and the high cost of systemic health inequities that naturally lead to disparities in health. The implementation of the Patient Protection and Affordable Care Act (PPACA) spurred an increased focus on integrated behavioral health care (IBHC) and a promise to address disparities and other issues related to health care access (Andrews et al. 2013). Ten years since the passage of the Affordable Care Act that promise remains unfulfilled. COVID-19 has shown how disastrous the continued failure to fulfill that promise has been to millions of Americans, especially for Black, Indigenous and People of Color (BIPOC) who are more likely to be infected due to their employment as essential workers and difficulty to social distance and who are more likely to experience serious illness and death if infected due to a lack of access to adequate health care and other essential resources (Koma et al. 2020). For instance, Black Americans are over 3.5 times more likely to die from COVID-19 than their white counterparts. For Latinx persons, the likelihood of death is almost twice that of whites. This, despite the fact that Black and Latinx populations are, on average, younger than the White population and should therefore experience *lower rates* of death due to COVID 19 (Gross et al. 2020). Currently, early evidence suggests that Indigenous communities with poor access to indoor plumbing combined with long histories of systemic poverty, high rates of comorbid conditions, and poor health care access also face a higher risk of infection, transmission, and death (Rodriguez-Lonebear et al. 2020). According to more recent data through late May 2020, obtained from the CDC and reported by the New York Times, Black and Latinx persons are three times more likely to contract COVID 19, and twice as likely to die from the virus, compared to their white counterparts. Native people are

© Springer Nature Switzerland AG 2021
M. A. Mancini, *Integrated Behavioral Health Practice*,
https://doi.org/10.1007/978-3-030-59659-0_1

also far more likely to contract the virus than white people (Oppel et al. 2020). This has been found throughout the United States and does not take into account the recent surge in cases that began in June, 2020.

These disparities are the direct result of racist policies and systems that have led to the inequitable access to health care, wealth, and basic resources such as food, adequate housing, clean air and water, and other social determinants of health (SDOH) for generations of BIPOC persons (Chowkwanyu and Reed 2020). In addition, the chronic daily stress caused by racism, discrimination, overcrowding, police violence, and intentional and unintentional racist insults and assaults experienced by Black and Brown people can lead to "weathering" or advanced aging that can increase the risk for disorders associated with higher rates of death from COVID-19 such as cardiovascular disease, high blood pressure and diabetes (Chowkwanyu and Reed 2020; Geronimus et al. 2006; Sue et al. 2007). The experience of racism has also been linked to higher rates of depression and suicide risk (O'Keefe et al. 2015).

From a behavioral health standpoint, the high stress caused by the pandemic, associated lockdowns, and related economic and educational impacts has placed large segments of the population at higher risk for high stress, addiction, complicated grief, trauma, loneliness, interpersonal violence, depression, and anxiety. Furthermore, the lockdown has prevented large segments of the population with preexisting behavioral issues from receiving adequate health and behavioral health care. The result is likely to be a precipitous rise in new cases of behavioral health disorders and a worsening in pre-existing conditions requiring increased capacity in behavioral health care that currently does not exist. The rising complexity of social and health-related challenges requires solutions that traverse the full range of health and behavioral health professions (Gehlert et al. 2017). The high prevalence of behavioral health problems experienced in the population (i.e., nearly 50% the US population will experience a behavioral health disorder in their lifetime) and the complexities of health and behavioral health require a health care workforce such as social workers and other professionals who can provide behavioral health care in a variety of multidisciplinary settings (Kessler et al. 2005).

1.2   Defining Integrated Behavioral Health Practice

In this book, I define behavioral health practice as care that addresses the needs of persons with co-occurring mental health and addiction issues as well as other behaviors impacting health. Figure 1.1 displays the domains of integrated behavioral health practice. I will address persons receiving care in a variety of settings and from multiple service professionals. As a result, I will use the terms "clients" and "providers" to refer to behavioral health service recipients and professionals, respectively. Behavioral health practice includes comprehensive screening, assessment, prevention, and treatment of the full range of mental health and addictions issues (Peek 2013). Integrated car is an effective means to provide people with access to a range of behavioral health professionals and interventions (Thota et al.

Fig. 1.1 Integrated
behavioral health domains
of practice

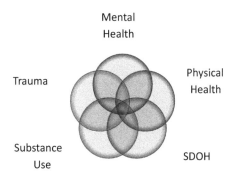

Mental
Health

Trauma

Physical
Health

Substance
Use

SDOH

2012). When behavioral health practice is fully *integrated* within health care settings, a team of multidisciplinary professionals provides holistic care for both medical and behavioral health issues. A comprehensive definition of integrated behavioral health and primary care was provided by the Agency for Health Care Research and Quality (2013):

> "The care that results from a practice team of primary care and behavioral health clinicians, working together with patients and families, using a systematic and cost-effective approach to provide patient-centered care for a defined population. This care may address mental health and substance abuse conditions, health behaviors (including their contribution to chronic medical illnesses), life stressors and crises, stress-related physical symptoms, and ineffective patterns of health care utilization." (Peek 2013; p. 2).

Figure 1.2 displays the central elements to integrated care. The National Integration Academy Council at the Agency for Health care Research and Quality identified five elements central to integrated care: (1) the deployment of collaborative, holistic, team-based health care designed to address the whole person (e.g., medical and behavioral health); (2) the implementation of universal screening and assessment protocols across health care settings; (3) the use of procedures designed to deliver efficacious, evidence-based treatments and interventions; (4) engaging in cross-disciplinary training and developing a workforce of health care professionals competent to practice integrated care; and (5) the coordination of organizational structures including communication systems, treatment plans, paperwork, records, and billing. Indeed, integrated care has also been defined as: "Tightly integrated, on-site teamwork with a unified care plan as a standard approach to care for designated populations. Connotes organizational integration as well, often involving social and other community services" (Peek 2013; p. 44). This includes the principles of multidisciplinary collaboration, and coordinated organizational practice structures, treatment plans, continuous quality improvement, training and payment, and billing systems (Peek 2013). Health and behavioral health organizations will need to implement professional development strategies that include coaching, alignment of organizational processes and procedures with integrated practices, and the establishment of communities of practice that can lead to organic and sustainable change across all levels of the organization (Mancini and Miner 2013). Achieving truly integrated care will also require a workforce capable of practicing in medical

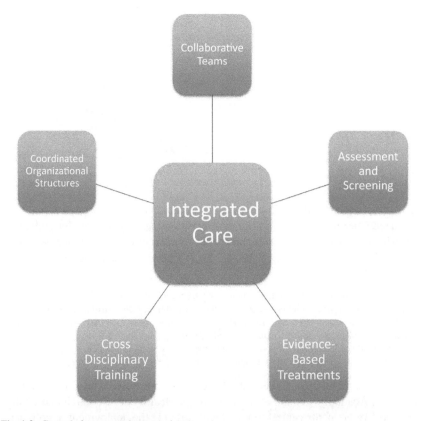

Fig. 1.2 Central elements to integrated care

and behavioral health realms and a health care system with the capacity to provide universal access to coordinated health care for all persons (Mancini et al. 2019).

1.2.1   The Need for Integrated Behavioral Health Practice

1.2.1.1   Comorbidity of Health and Behavioral Health Issues

Behavioral health conditions are common across populations. According to the 2018 National Survey on Drug Use and Health (NSDUH), almost a fifth of the US adult population had a mental illness in 2018 and over 21 million people over 12 years of age (1 in 13 people) needed treatment for either an alcohol or drug use (SAMHSA 2019). These stark numbers are almost certain to markedly rise considering that the long-term health and economic impact of the COVID-19 pandemic will be *generational*. While the current concern is focused on the capacity of health care systems to serve clients with physical illnesses, the behavioral health care system also faces the potential to be overwhelmed in the near and distant future.

Behavioral health and physical health conditions are commonly comorbid. Two diseases are comorbid when they co-occur in the same person and impact each other such as mental illness, substance abuse disorders, and chronic disease conditions (Santucci 2012). In 2016, 8.2 million (3.4%) persons had a co-occurring mental illness and substance use disorder. Adolescents also have high rates of comorbid substance abuse and psychiatric disorders (Hser et al. 2001). About half of persons who experience a mental illness will have a comorbid substance use disorder (Kelly and Daley 2013; Ross and Peselow 2012) and almost 70% of adults with a mental illness have a co-occurring chronic physical health condition. Persons experiencing poverty have even higher rates of comorbidity. In the U.S., almost half (49%) of Medicaid beneficiaries have a mental health condition and 52% of those with both Medicare and Medicaid have a mental health condition (Kronick et al. 2009). Behavioral health conditions such as depression, anxiety, substance use, bipolar disorder, and ADHD are commonly comorbid with physical health conditions such as diabetes, heart disease, hypertension, asthma, and obesity (Gerrity 2014; SAMHSA 2019; Young et al. 2015). For instance, Latinx persons with diabetes are more likely to experience comorbid depression than the broader population (Olvera et al. 2016). This co-occurrence of disorders leads to greater morbidity, mortality, functional impairment, and health care costs (Young et al. 2015).

1.2.1.2 Health care System Fragmentation

Health care consumers in the United States, particularly members of BIPOC communities and persons who are economically disadvantaged, receive inadequate access to behavioral health care due to the separation of behavioral and primary (physical) health care services and a limited number of providers of behavioral health services (CDC 2013; Cunningham 2009; Schoen et al. 2006). Less than half (41–43%) of persons with a mental health need over the age of 12 received mental health treatment in 2018, and only 11% who needed substance abuse treatment received care at a specialty facility (SAMHSA 2019). For persons with serious mental illnesses, a third did not receive any services (SAMHSA 2019). Further, adults and adolescents with mental health conditions are more likely to smoke, drink, and use substances than those without a mental health condition. Despite this, only a third of adolescents and almost half of adults with a co-occurring mental health and substance use issue received treatment for either disorder in 2018 (SAMHSA 2019). Providing integrated care can reduce inequities in behavioral health care access and the use of inefficient and costly emergency services because it can conveniently provide culturally competent behavioral health care in the same place as primary care. This reduces burdens on clients who lack child care services, transportation, or time and can increase overall access to services and needed referrals (Bridges et al. 2014; Corrigan et al. 2014; Mechanic and Olfson 2016; Reiss-Brennan et al. 2016; Woltmann et al. 2012),

The Institute of Medicine's seminal report titled *Crossing the Quality Chasm: A New Health System for the 21st Century* urged a redesign of health care in the United States and concluded that the current health care system in the United States was fundamentally inefficient, unsafe, fragmented, and unable to meet the health care needs of patients. The institute concluded that transformational change to the health care system was needed and, "that merely making incremental improvements in current systems of care will not suffice." (IOM 2001; p. 2). The authors of the report identified six aims for health care improvement that included making health care systems safer, more effective, patient-centered, timely, efficient, and equitable across race, gender, ethnicity, socioeconomic status, and geographic location. To achieve these aims, the authors identified the need for health care to be provided by a collaborative team of multidisciplinary professionals that provide patient-centered, holistic care coordinated across patient conditions, settings, and services over time (2001).

In another seminal report, Berwick and colleagues (2008) also highlighted the need for health care service transformation. As part of the Institute for Health Care Improvement (IHI), they identified the "triple aim" of health care to: (1) improve the health of the population; (2) improve patients' care experience (including quality, access, and reliability); and (3) reduce costs (Berwick et al. 2008; p. 760). Integrating health and behavioral health care can address these three aims (Mauer, 2009). Due to the lack of accessible, community-based behavioral health options, large numbers of people access behavioral health services through their primary care providers such as a family physician (Xierali et al. 2013). Co-locating primary care and behavioral health care professionals in the same setting can, therefore, increase access to behavioral health care and reduce the burdens that can interfere with patients' ability to follow-up on treatment recommendations (Xierali et al. 2013).

Indeed, the integration of behavioral health and primary care services carries vast potential in the prevention, detection, early intervention, and effective management of chronic diseases for patients with co-occurring behavioral and physical health problems (Croft and Parish 2013; Druss and Mauer 2010; Mechanic 2012; Shim et al. 2012). Integration of behavioral health and primary care has been shown to reduce depression symptom severity, increase coping skills, and has been associated with positive experiences of behavioral health care clinicians (Balasubramanian et al. 2017). The use of integrated care teams has been shown to significantly reduce emergency room utilization for persons with serious mental illness (Kim et al. 2017). Providing evidence-based integrated behavioral health treatment in primary care settings can also increase the likelihood that substance use disorders will be detected and patients referred for treatment (Chan et al. 2013), reduce psychiatric symptoms, improve functioning, and increase quality of care (Roy-Byrne et al. 2010). Integrated behavioral health care is also associated with higher referral completion rates at specialty mental health centers (Davis et al. 2016).

1.2.1.3 Health Inequity and Social Determinants of Health

Unfortunately, the pursuit of the triple aim has been inconsistent across the service landscape (Obucina et al. 2018). Further, the exclusive focus of the triple aim on improving population health through more efficient health care and reducing health risk behaviors runs the risk of ignoring the social determinants of health (SDOH) (e.g., lack of basic resources, housing, safety, income, education, and occupational endeavors) that drive health inequities and lead to poor health, particularly for people with behavioral health disorders (Bryan and Donaldson 2016; Kerman and Kidd 2019). Health care, therefore, must move beyond focusing exclusively on health indicators and adequately address the social determinants of health. Increasing transdisciplinary collaboration and integration of health and behavioral health care through collaborative care models and medical homes represents a key way to achieve this goal (Whittington et al. 2015).

Social determinants of health are the socioeconomic contexts that impact health such as income, political power, and access to various resources such as employment opportunities, food, healthy environmental conditions, transportation, quality K-12 education, safety, affordable and stable housing, and health care. Having equitable access to these determinants shape the health and quality of life of individuals and communities (CSDH 2008). Braveman and Gruskin (2003) defined health equity as:

> "the absence of systematic disparities in health (or in the major social determinants of health) between social groups who have different levels of underlying social advantage/disadvantage—that is, different positions in a social hierarchy. Inequities in health systematically put groups of people who are already socially disadvantaged (for example, by virtue of being poor, female, and/or members of a disenfranchised racial, ethnic, or religious group) at further disadvantage with respect to their health; health is essential to wellbeing and to overcoming other effects of social disadvantage." (p. 254)

Health inequity is the inequitable distribution of the conditions of health to groups that have differential access to wealth and power as the result of systemic issues such as racism, discrimination, income and wealth inequality, police violence and over-policing in BIPOC communities, unfair social policies, and environmental pollution among others that lead to health disparities in morbidity and mortality across race, gender, and class (Braveman and Gruskin 2003; Brennan Ramirez et al. 2008). We can improve health equity by reducing system fragmentation through transdisciplinary collaborations across health and behavioral health care organizations, communities, academic institutions, and local, state, and national governmental organizations. This requires community, policy, and system level change to improve the health of the community. (Braveman and Gruskin 2003; Brennan Ramirez et al. 2008; CSDH 2008). The impact of SDOH will be discussed in more detail in Chap. 2, and SDOH assessment practices will be discussed in Chap. 4.

1.3   Behavioral Health Care Integration

Behavioral health care integration exists along a continuum. Early work by Doherty (1995) and Doherty et al. (1996) conceptualized behavioral health care integration as existing across five levels of integration. These levels correspond to the amount of contact and collaboration between professionals. The levels range from complete separation of behavioral health and primary care services to full integration in which professionals work closely as part of a multidisciplinary team with a shared treatment plan, billing, and records system (Doherty 1995; Doherty et al. 1996). The Substance Abuse and Mental Health Services Administration later revised these levels to include six levels of integration (Heath et al. 2013).

Figure 1.3 displays the levels of integration for primary care and behavioral health. In Level 1, there is minimal or *no collaboration* between behavioral health and primary care services or systems. This level is characterized by a lack of communication or information sharing. In Level 2, behavioral health and primary care services are provided in separate settings and utilize separate professional staff and systems. At this level, professionals *occasionally* communicate or share information with one another on an as needed basis. In Level 3, behavioral health and primary care services are *co-located* in the same setting or facility. The co-location of care and familiarity of providers increases the likelihood of referral acceptance and follow-through. However, while behavioral health and primary care providers may occasionally communicate and share information on some patients, these providers make their own decisions regarding patient care, track and evaluate their own outcomes, and utilize separate care plans, billing systems, training schedules, and record systems. In Level 4, services are *co-located and there is closer collaboration* between behavioral health and primary care providers in the form of *shared communication, records, and billing systems* as well as cross-training opportunities.

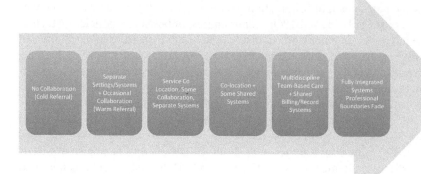

Fig. 1.3 Levels of integration

In this level, behavioral health specialists may be embedded within the primary care team or a behavioral health team may employ a nurse practitioner (Heath et al. 2013). Level four is where true integration begins.

Levels 5 and 6 demonstrate higher levels of collaboration. In Level 5, *multidisciplinary teams of behavioral health and primary care professionals engage in team-based care*. Providers clearly understand the roles of other professions and work together to design *collaborative care plans* for each patient. Communication, billing, and records systems may be partially integrated. The sixth and final level of integration indicates *full collaborative care in a multidisciplinary team*. The *boundaries of practice for behavioral health and primary care professionals begin to fade* as professionals begin to engage in *shared practices that focus on holistic care*. For instance, primary care professionals begin to provide brief screening and interventions for behavioral health issues, and behavioral health practitioners may screen for health conditions and assist in the management of chronic disease. Behavioral health and primary care practitioners work as a single health care team designed to address the whole person and this practice is applied to all patient populations. Records, communication, and billing systems are completely or almost completely integrated (Heath et al. 2013).

1.3.1 Common Integrated Behavioral Health Practices and Models

There are four practices that are crucial to providing quality integrative care. First, universal screening of all patients is a basic requirement for integrated behavioral health care. All clients should be screened in three areas: (1) common behavioral health concerns such as depressed and anxious mood, adverse events and traumatic stress, community and interpersonal violence, and alcohol and drug use; (2) common health indicators such as stress, heart rate, cholesterol, blood pressure, weight, BMI, and health risk behaviors (e.g., smoking, drinking, substance use, sedentary lifestyle, overeating, unprotected sex); and (3) social determinants of health (e.g., access to basic resources such as safe and secure housing, adequate food, childcare, transportation, safety, employment, and adequate income). In fully integrated behavioral health care settings, screening is a shared responsibility across team members. In partially integrated settings, the addition of a primary care provider (e.g., nurse practitioner) in behavioral health care settings, and/or a behavioral health care provider (e.g., social worker) in a primary care setting can be used to conduct screenings, assessments, counseling, and referrals.

Second, the deployment of peer providers that help people navigate the health care system and access and utilize services across medical and behavioral health systems is another important form of integrated practice. These providers may be health navigators, community health workers, peer specialists, or *promotodoras*. Peer providers provide a range of important, culturally and linguistically inclusive services that include: (1) promoting wellness; (2) increasing service access through client advocacy; and (3) engaging clients and keeping them connected to treatment through a robust therapeutic relationship.

Third, co-location of behavioral health and primary care services can reduce barriers to treatment. These barriers include poor transportation access, lack of trust, demands of family care obligations, and work schedules that often limit the ability of persons, particularly poor and BIPOC persons, to access health or behavioral health services. Short of utilizing fully integrated teams, co-location of services can be accomplished by employing or contracting with licensed behavioral health practitioners to provide culturally affirming and responsive services at health care sites or employing or contracting health care providers to provide health screening and intervention services at behavioral health sites. Co-location and coordination of behavioral health and primary care enhance access to both services by reducing or eliminating the need to travel long distances to multiple locations at different times. Case study 1.1 provides a descriptive example of how collaborative care can improve access to care and improve health outcomes.

Case Study 1.1: Inés and El Centro de Salud

Inés,[1] 33, emigrated to the United States from Central Mexico when she was 15 with her mother. She is married to Carlos, 36, and they have 2 young children, Carlos, Jr., 6, and Ana, 8. They currently live in a neighborhood with many other Latinx immigrants in a medium-sized Midwestern city. She works as a receptionist in a local community service agency for Latinx youth. She is also a volunteer counselor and runs a dance group for local children. Inés receives her health care from a local health clinic serving the Latinx community. She is able to walk to this clinic. The agency provides primary care services via a team of volunteer and paid physicians, nurses, social workers, and peer counselors. The agency is affiliated with a local university medical school and is a training site for social work, psychology, nursing, and medical students. All staff are bilingual. The agency provides primary care services seven days a week that include family medicine, wellness and prevention screening, vaccinations, diabetic and nutritional counseling, wellness services such as yoga, exercise and relaxation groups, a food pantry, and support groups for stress reduction, exercise, and developing wellness plans.

In order to provide behavioral health services to its clients and promote the mental health of its community, the clinic developed a collaborative with local mental health professionals providing child, youth, and adult mental health services for problems such as depression, intimate partner violence (IPV), anxiety, stress, PTSD, and addiction. The clinic has formal referral relationships with several mental health clinicians and agencies in the local community that provide bilingual and culturally competent care. The clinic also provides free office space to several bilingual counselors and social workers in exchange for providing individual and group counseling to the clients of the clinic. The clinic and providers within the collaborative also

---

[1] All names and other identifiers of this case have been changed to protect privacy and confidentiality.

engage in routine cross-training activities in order that clinic staff can implement more routine behavioral health practices (e.g., screening, assessment) in their work, while mental health providers can learn how to be more culturally fluent with the persons they serve. This promotes and ensures a pipeline of competent, culturally affirming behavioral health practitioners in the community. The clinic provides transportation, interpreter scheduling services, appointment reminder calls, and other administrative tasks in order to facilitate mental health care with collaborative providers. The clinic also conducts routine behavioral health screening, assessment, and brief interventions with patients. Those patients needing more intensive services are then referred to the collaborative for more advanced care.

The clinic also employs community health workers and peer counselors to provide system navigation services for persons needing referrals to community agencies. These "Guia's" or guides (1) provide transportation and interpretation services for clients, (2) accompany clients to health-related appointments outside the clinic, (3) help clients navigate payment and insurance forms and processes, (4) help clients get access to and navigate social services, and (5) provide wellness services by helping people develop wellness action plans around stress reduction, education about healthy relationships and parenting, diet and exercises, and how to maintain a healthy lifestyle.

Inés has several co-occurring health and behavioral health conditions that she has successfully controlled. She has diabetes and has a history of mild-to-moderate depressive episodes. She has also experienced several adverse childhood events (ACE's) (n = 5) that place her at an increased risk of several health conditions. Her ACEs include witnessing interpersonal violence, having a family member with a mental health and addiction disorder in the home, and experiencing sexual assault as a minor from a family member, which precipitated their leaving Mexico. She experienced partial PTSD symptoms for 15 years including hypervigilance, negative alterations in cognitions in mood (e.g., shame, guilt, anger, dissociation) and intrusive memories (e.g., flashbacks and nightmares). She also currently experiences occasional panic attacks when she is stressed. Inés receives comprehensive medical care from the clinic for a co-pay of $35. She does not have health insurance from her employment. During a visit 2 years ago she was screened for behavioral health symptoms as part of the clinic's initiative to provide more comprehensive behavioral health care "check-ups." It was at this screening that she realized she suffered from several mental health symptoms (e.g., depression, anxiety, and PTSD). She reports, "I thought everyone felt like I did. Tired, sad, nervous all the time. I thought this was normal. I figured, 'well, I went through a lot so I'm supposed to have these nightmares and anxious thoughts.' I thought what I went through was my fault and that I just shouldn't talk about it. My family certainly didn't want to discuss it. It was too hard for them to hear. So I just said to myself, 'Push it out of your mind, Inés, it's the past, it's over, get on with your life. Stop dwelling on it.'"

"After the screening and the talk with the social worker, who I love, she is the best, I realized that this wasn't normal and that I could get help. I went to a local social work provider who specializes in depression and trauma treatment. She provided me with education. She taught me relaxation skills. And after a while we did some cognitive processing therapy where I talked about what I went through and we examined my thoughts about it. I think differently now and I don't have the jumpiness and the nightmares anymore. She helped me realize it wasn't my fault. That I didn't deserve what happened to me. She is also Latina and we did therapy in Spanish, which was so, so helpful. I don't think I could have opened up with just anyone. She saved my life. I feel so much better now and my diabetes is under control. I have more energy. I sleep better. I'm a better Mom. I can't thank her and the clinic enough. They gave me transportation to therapy sessions and back to work. The therapy was not very expensive because of the collaborative. I could afford it. If it was expensive and I couldn't get a ride to the clinic I probably would have just gave up on it. That clinic is amazing and I hope to do some dance groups for the kids there soon."

The above example demonstrates the power of integrated care. While not completely integrated, the clinic in the example provided Inés with behavioral health and physical health services and were (1) culturally-tailored to her needs, (2) comprehensive, (3) coordinated, and (4) person-centered. The clinic also provided care that was inexpensive, easily accessible, and accommodated Inés's transportation needs. The clinic addressed her needs in relation to trauma, depression, and anxiety resulting in improved health and well-being. The agency also facilitated the development of a community of providers that are more person-centered and culturally competent.

Analysis

Contrast the above case example to what Inés could expect in a more usual care scenario where care is not integrated, but separate, uncoordinated, and fragmented.

How likely would it be that Inés would be able to become aware and develop an understanding of her behavioral health symptoms and get access culturally competent, affordable and accessible behavioral health care?

What level or stage (e.g., 1–6) of integrated care would you place El Centro de Salud (See Fig. 1.3)?

How likely would it be that Inés would just continue on as she was and think, "Hey, just get over it and move on"?

And what would Inés's health look like over the long term as a result of not getting the care she needed and deserved?

1.3.2   Two Integrative Practice Models: Health Homes and Collaborative Care

1.3.2.1   Health Homes

Approximately 68% of persons with a behavioral health condition also have one or more chronic health conditions (Alegria et al. 2003). The Health Home Model is defined explicitly in Section 2703 of the Affordable Care Act (ACA). Health homes are designed for recipients of Medicaid with two or more chronic health conditions. These conditions usually include a behavioral health condition (e.g., serious mental illness and/or addiction disorder) and one or more chronic health conditions (e.g., diabetes, cardiovascular disease, hypertension). The model is designed to serve persons with complex behavioral and physical health care needs by providing comprehensive care and case management through a multidisciplinary team of health care professionals (Alexander and Druss 2012; Mauer 2009). Health homes provide collaborative, person-centered care based on clients' preferences, needs, and values. Clinical decisions are based on objective screening, assessment, and monitoring data that are routinely collected on clients receiving services. Health home professionals rely on a shared care plan and integrated records and billing systems. Interventions that are provided are evidence-based. Health homes also routinely monitor outcomes and treatment responses in order to adjust care as needed and maximize effectiveness (Alexander and Druss 2012). Health homes focus on holistic health, or *whole health*, which include addressing health/primary care needs, mental health, substance use, and social support and other social determinants of health such as housing, nutrition, accessing basic needs, and income support through the provision of case management services.

1.3.2.2 Collaborative Care

The collaborative care model represents an effective means of providing high-quality integrated care in order to systematically manage chronic, complex comorbid health conditions (Katon et al. 1995, 1996). This model is based on the chronic care model developed by Wagner et al. (1996, 2001). In this model, care is provided by a multidisciplinary team of primary care providers that include a team leader or care manager (i.e., usually a nurse or social worker), psychiatrist, and a range of behavioral health professionals including social workers, counselors, psychologists, community health workers, and peers (Butler et al. 2009; Bower et al. 2006; Thielke et al. 2007). Team members provide consultations and work collaboratively to meet the individual needs of patients through case management and stepped care (i.e., providing treatments such as psychotherapy or medications of increasing intensity or dosage slowly to meet patient needs with the least amount of intervention). For instance, in stepped care a person with depression may first receive cognitive behavioral therapy. If symptoms persist, a low-dose antidepressant medication may be added in order to achieve additional treatment response. Ongoing screening and assessment measures are used to inform clinical decisions. Interventions are evidence-based and treatment outcomes are identified and systematically reviewed through a process of continuous quality improvement in order to optimize performance, increase accountability and enhance patient care. To implement this model effectively requires system and organizational integration that includes data sharing, cross-training, and professional development opportunities and ongoing performance review.

The Collaborative Care Model represents the highest level of integrated care and has shown positive outcomes for primary care patients with depression and anxiety problems in a range of settings compared to usual care (Archer et al. 2012; Thota et al. 2012; Unützer 2002; Unützer and Park 2012). A systematic review found robust evidence that collaborative care reduces depressive symptoms, increases adherence and response to treatment, improves remission and recovery, and improves quality of life and satisfaction with care (Thota et al. 2012). Collaborative care models have also been found to be cost-effective (Katon et al. 2005; Schoenbaum et al. 2001).

1.4   Developing Integrated Behavioral Health Professionals

1.4.1   Core Competencies for Integrated Behavioral Health Practice

Several core competencies have been identified for integrated behavioral health practice. Professional competencies for Integrated Behavioral Health and Primary Care (IBHPC) have been identified by the SAMHSA-HRSA Center for Integrated Care (Hoge et al. 2014) and include nine core competencies routinely practiced by social workers and other behavioral health professionals (Fraher et al. 2018; Stanhope et al. 2015). These competencies are listed in Table 1.1. Integrated behavioral health competencies focus on several important areas of practice. First, these competencies require providers to be able to collaborate across disciplines and understand how to work together as part of a multidisciplinary team that uses a shared care plan to address the full range of health and behavioral health needs of clients. Second, providers are required to understand the intersections of health, mental health, and addiction and be prepared to screen and assess for health and behavioral health issues. Based on the results, providers engage and motivate clients to identify and achieve health and behavioral health goals through person-centered care plans (Stanhope et al. 2015). Third, providers are required to be competent in delivering culturally and linguistically relevant interventions that address health and behavioral health concerns. Fourth, providers must be able to assess and intervene competently to address social determinants of health such as housing, safety, food, income, transportation, and other socio-economic concerns of clients. Fifth, relevant providers and organizations across service systems need to effectively communicate and coordinate care to address the needs of clients within the population. And lastly, providers and organizations need to be engaged in a process of continuous quality improvement that involves monitoring and evaluating performance in order to adjust practices to improve targeted outcomes (Hoge et al. 2014).

1.4.2   Developing an Integrated Behavioral Health Workforce

Effective interprofessional and integrated behavioral health practice requires effective communication and collaboration skills (Sangaleti et al. 2017). There are many barriers to effective integrated behavior health practice. For instance, high caseloads

Table 1.1 Integrated behavioral health competencies and practices

Competency category	Competency	Practices and principles
Interpersonal communication	Providers are able to engage clients, build rapport, answer questions, provide information, and communicate clearly and effectively with clients, family, and other health care providers	Clear communication Engagement Empathic listening Acceptance, nonjudgmental attitude Culturally and linguistically tailored
Collaboration and teamwork	Providers are to effectively participate and function as a member of a multidisciplinary team of heath and behavioral health professionals, clients, and family members	Understanding and respecting disciplines and roles of other team members Use shared decision-making
Screening and assessment	Providers are able to effectively screen and assess for a range of health-related issues	Screen and assess for health risk behaviors, suicidality, harmful substance use, psychosocial functioning, psychiatric symptoms, trauma, violence, and social determinants of health
Care planning and coordination	Providers are able to develop holistic treatment plans that address health, behavioral health, and social determinants of health. Creating and utilizing a shared treatment plan that takes a holistic view of the person and deploys strategies such as patient service navigation, developing wellness plans, supporting consumers in effectively managing chronic disease conditions	Person-centered goals Whole health Coordinating evidence-based treatments Wellness recovery plans Navigating service systems Accessing resources Addressing systemic barriers Enhancing social determinants of health
Evidence-based interventions	Providers are able to utilize evidence-based interventions that are recovery-oriented to address a range of short- and long-term health and behavioral health issues	Motivational interviewing Cognitive behavioral therapies to address trauma, mental health, and substance use issues Case management Crisis intervention and safety planning Health promotion and illness prevention

(continued)

Table 1.1 (continued)

Competency category	Competency	Practices and principles
Cultural competence	Providers utilize services that are culturally and linguistically competent and tailored to meet the unique needs of the individual and are inclusive, equitable, and high quality	Identifying and dismantling racist structures and policies that contribute health inequities that drive health disparities Ensuring equitable access to high-quality care Addressing social determinants of health Ensuring providers are diverse and reflective of the community they serve Training to identify and eliminate implicit and explicit biases Adapting services to cultural norms of client community
System-oriented practice	Providers are able to operate effectively within the organizational structures of the health care system and setting	Effectively navigating the organization and system health care landscape Informing clients about how to access benefits and resources within the system Staying up-to-date with changing health care policy and practices
Practice-based learning and quality improvement	Providers are able to continually evaluate practice and engage in a process of continuous quality improvement to provide effective care that achieves positive health outcomes	Identify and implement evidence-based practices with fidelity Evaluating outcomes and client satisfaction with care. Using data to reduce errors and provide high-quality care Working with other team members to continually improve care
Informatics	Providers enhance and improve health care through the use of information technology	Integrated electronic records and billing Using telehealth technologies Application and/or web-based screening, assessment, intervention, and monitoring Ensuring confidentiality and privacy

and paperwork demands limit the time and energy providers have to listen, understand and respond to the needs and concerns of clients and their families. Fragmented billing, records, communication, and data sharing systems interfere with the ability of providers to communicate and coordinate care across client problems. A lack of understanding and respect for the roles of other professionals interfere with effective assessment and treatment of health and behavioral health issues in multidisciplinary settings (Ambrose-Miller and Ashcroft 2016). These barriers make it difficult for primary care and behavioral health care providers to provide holistic, person-centered care (Kathol et al. 2010; Miller et al. 2011). For instance, simple depression screenings in primary care sites continue to remain low (Akincigil and Matthews 2017), and recent data have demonstrated that a significant barrier to IBHC implementation is a lack of professionals competent in providing integrated care (Hall et al. 2015).

Over 110 million people in the United States live in one of the over 5000 designated areas with a shortage of behavioral health professionals (HRSA 2018). Currently, it would take an estimated 6628 professional to close this shortage (HRSA 2018). Addressing this need requires an increase in new and retrained behavioral health workers competent in transdisciplinary communication and collaboration (Cohen et al. 2015; Hall et al. 2015; Horevitz and Manoleas 2013; HRSA 2014). Enhancing the behavioral health workforce will require education and training initiatives that integrate primary care and behavioral health services within a framework that is collaborative and interprofessional, person-centered, strength-based, trauma-informed, and evidence-based, (Davis et al. 2015; Hoge and Morris 2004). It will also require the development of professional identities of primary care and behavioral health providers that are more open to transdisciplinary practice (Forenza and Eckert 2018; Gehlert et al. 2017). Professional education settings can contribute to more effective interprofessional education for primary care and behavioral health providers through a combination of clear roles and effective leadership (Jones and Phillips 2016). Early learning experiences that expose preservice providers to positive behavioral health role models can improve quality care (Lee and Del Carmen Montiel 2010). Mentoring relationships formed early in social work training through service-learning and clinical shadowing can also enable students to form relationships that help guide them through their postgraduation career choices (Allen et al. 2004; Mancini et al. 2019).

1.5   Summary and Conclusion

The current health care policy and practice landscapes are fragmented, inefficient, and inequitable, leading to disparities in health and well-being. The ongoing COVID-19 pandemic has laid bare the devastating impact of health and wealth inequities in BIPOC communities. The behavioral health needs of these communities and others in the coming years due to the pandemic and its economic and social effects will be enormous. Anything short of a revolution in how behavioral health care is provided will be inadequate. In order to meet the demand, behavioral health screening, assessment, and treatments must be fully integrated into primary care services in order to efficiently provide high-quality mental health and addiction services to persons in need. Collaborative care models represent one way forward. These models co-locate health and behavioral services and provide care through a team of multidisciplinary professionals who collaboratively coordinate and monitor care through shared treatment plans and records systems. These models currently exist, but are not sufficiently available to serve the needs of the population. We are past due on our promise of the Affordable Care Act to end health disparities caused by inequitable access to care. Integrated practice modalities such as the collaborative care model represent a commonsense way forward. But to provide these services at a scale adequate to the needs and demands of the population will require national policies that provide full, universal access to high-quality health care for all Americans.

References

Akincigil, A., & Matthews, E. B. (2017). National rates and patterns of depression screening in primary care: Results from 2012 and 2013. *Psychiatric Services, 68*(7), 660–666. https://doi.org/10.1176/appi.ps.201600096.

Alegria, M., Jackson, J. S., Kessler, R. C., & Takeuchi, D. (2003). *National Comorbidity Survey Replication (NCS-R). 2001–2003.* Ann Arbor: Inter-university Consortium for Political and Social Research.

Alexander, L. & Druss, B (2012). Behavioral health homes for people with mental health and substance use conditions: The core clinical features. SAMHSA-HRSA Center for Integrated Health Solutions.

Allen, T. D., Eby, L. T., Poteet, M. L., Lentz, E., & Lima, L. (2004). Career benefits associated with mentoring for protégés: A meta-analysis. *Journal of Applied Psychology, 89*(1), 127–136.

Ambrose-Miller, W., & Ashcroft, R. (2016). Challenges faced by social workers as members of interprofessional collaborative health care teams. *Health and Social Work, 41*(2), 101–109.

Andrews, C. M., Darnell, J. S., McBride, T. D., & Gehlert, S. (2013). Social work and implementation of the affordable care act. *Health & Social Work, 38*, 67–71.

Archer, J., Bower, P., Gilbody, S., Lovell, K., Richards, D., Gask, L., Dickens, C., & Coventry, P. (2012). Collaborative care for depression and anxiety problems. *The Cochrane database of systematic reviews, 10*, CD006525. https://doi.org/10.1002/14651858.CD006525.pub2

Balasubramanian, B. A., Cohen, D. J., Jetelina, K. K., Dickinson, L. M., Davis, M., Gunn, R., et al. (2017). Outcomes of integrated behavioral health with primary care. *The Journal of the American Board of Family Medicine, 30*(2), 130–139. https://doi.org/10.3122/jabfm.2017.02.160234.

Bower, P., Gilbody, S., Richards, D., Fletcher, J., & Sutton, A. (2006). Collaborative care for depression in primary care—Making sense of a complex intervention: Systematic review and meta-regression. *British Journal of Psychiatry, 189*, 484–493.

Berwick, D. M., Nolan, T. W., & Whittington, J. (2008). The triple aim: care, health, and cost. *Health affairs (Project Hope), 27*(3), 759–769. https://doi.org/10.1377/hlthaff.27.3.759

Braveman, P., & Gruskin, S. (2003). Defining equity in health. *Journal of Epidemiology and Community Health, 57*(4), 254–258.

Brennan Ramirez, L. K., Baker, E. A., & Metzler, M. (2008). *Promoting health equity: A resource to help communities address social determinants of health.* Atlanta: Department of Health and Human Services, Centers for Disease Control and Prevention.

Bridges, A. J., Andrews, A. R., 3rd, Villalobos, B. T., Pastrana, F. A., Cavell, T. A., & Gomez, D. (2014). Does integrated behavioral health care reduce mental health disparities for Latinos? Initial findings. *Journal of Latina/o psychology, 2*(1), 37–53. https://doi.org/10.1037/lat0000009.

Bryan, S., & Donaldson, C. (2016). Taking triple aim at the triple aim. *Healthcare Papers, 15,* 25–30.

Butler, M., Kane, R., McAlpine, D., Kathol, R. G., Fu, S. S., Hagedorn, H., & Wilt, T. J. (2009). *Integration of mental health/substance abuse and primary care*. Minneapolis: Minnesota Evidence-Based Practice Center.

Centers of Disease Control. (2013). CDC health disparities report. *Morbidity and Mortality Weekly Report (MMWR), 62*(Suppl. 3), 1–187.

Chan, Y. F., Huang, H., Sieu, N., & Unutzer, J. (2013). Substance screening and referral for substance abuse treatment in an integrated mental health care program. *Psychiatric Services, 64*(1), 88–90. https://doi.org/10.1176/appi.ps.201200082.

Chowkwanyu, M., & Reed, A. L. (2020). Racial health disparities and Covid-19 – Caution and context. *New England Journal of Medicine*, Downloaded on May 27th, 2020. https://doi.org/10.1056/NEJMp2012910.

Cohen, D. J., Davis, M. M., Hall, J. D., Gilchrist, E. C., & Miller, B. F. (2015). *A guidebook of professional practices for behavioral health and primary care integration: Observations from exemplary sites*. Rockville: Agency for Healthcare Research and Quality.

Commission on Social Determinants of Health (CSDH). (2008). *Closing the gap in a generation: Health equity through action on the social determinants of health*. Geneva: Final report of the Commission on Social Determinants of Health. World Health Organization.

Corrigan, P. W., Pickett, S., Batia, K., & Michaels, P. J. (2014). Peer navigators and integrated care to address ethnic health disparities of people with serious mental illness. *Social Work in Public Health, 29*(6), 581–593. https://doi.org/10.1080/19371918.2014.893854.

Croft, B., & Parish, S. L. (2013). Care integration in the patient protection and affordable care act: Implications for behavioral health. *Administration and Policy in Mental Health, 40*(4). https://doi.org/10.1007/s10488-012-0405-0.

Cunningham, P. J. (2009). Beyond parity: Primary care physicians' perspectives on access to mental health care. *Health Affairs, 28*(3), w490–w501. https://doi.org/10.1377/hlthaff.28.3.w490.

Davis, T. S., Guada, J., Reno, R., Peck, A., Evans, S., Moskow Sigal, L., & Swenson, S. (2015). Integrated and culturally relevant care: A model to prepare social workers for primary care behavioral health practice. *Social Work in Health Care, 54*(10), 909–938. https://doi.org/10.1080/00981389.2015.1062456.

Davis, M. J., Moore, K. M., Meyers, K., Mathews, J., & Zerth, E. O. (2016). Engagement in mental health treatment following primary are mental health integration contact. *Psychological Services, 13*(4), 333–340.

Doherty, W. (1995). The why's and levels of collaborative family health care. *Family Systems Medicine, 13*(3–4), 275–281. https://doi.org/10.1037/h0089174.

Doherty, W. J., McDaniel, S. H., & Baird, M. A. (1996). Five levels of primary care/behavioral healthcare collaboration. *Behavioral Healthcare Tomorrow*, 25–28.

Druss, B. G., & Mauer, B. J. (2010). Health care reform and care at the behavioral health—Primary care interface. *Psychiatric Services, 61*(11), 1087–1092. https://doi.org/10.1176/ps.2010.61.11.1087.

Forenza, B., & Eckert, C. (2018). Social worker identity: A profession in context. *Social Work, 63*(1), 17–26.

Fraher, E. P., Richman, E. L., Zerden, L. D. S., & Lombardi, B. (2018). Social work student and practitioner roles in integrated care settings. *American Journal of Preventive Medicine, 54*(6S3), S281–S289.

Gehlert, S., Hall, K. L., & Palinkas, L. A. (2017). Preparing our next-generation scientific workforce to address the grand challenges for social work. *Journal of the Society for Social Work and Research, 8*(1), 2334–2315.

Geronimus, A. T., Hicken, M., Keene, D., & Bound, J. (2006). "Weathering" and age patterns of allostatic load scores among blacks and whites in the United States. *American Journal of Public Health, 96*, 826–833.

Gerrity, M., Zoller, E., Pinson, N., Pettinari, C., & King, V. (2014). Integrating Primary Care into Behavioral Health Settings: What Works for Individuals with Serious Mental Illness. New York, NY: Milbank Memorial Fund. https://www.milbank.org/wpcontent/uploads/2016/04/Integrating-Primary-Care-Exec-Sum.pdf

Gross, C. P., Essien, U. R., Pasha, S., Gross, J. R., Wang, S., & Nunez-Smith, M. (2020). Racial and ethnic disparities in population level Covid-19 mortality. *medRxiv.* https://doi.org/10.110 1/2020.05.07.20094250.

Hall, J., Cohen, D. J., Davis, M., Gunn, R., Blount, A., Pollack, D. A., Miller, W. L., Smith, C., Valentine, N., & Miller, B. F. (2015). Preparing the workforce for behavioral health and primary care integration. *Journal of the American Board of Family Medicine, 28*, S41–S51. https://doi.org/10.3122/jabfm.2015.S1.150054.

Health Resources & Services Administration. (2014). *Behavioral health workforce education and training FY 2014 awards.* Retrieved from http://www.hrsa.gov/about/news/2014tables/behavioralworkforce/

Health Resources and Services Administration (HRSA). (2018). *Designated health professional shortage areas statistics: Fourth quarter of fiscal year 2018 designated HPSA quarterly summary.* Bureau of Health Workforce: Health Resources and Services Administration: US Department of health and Human Services. Retrieved October 22, 2018 from https://ersrs.hrsa.gov/ReportServer?/HGDW_Reports/BCD_HPSA/BCD_HPSA_SCR50_Qtr_Smry_HTML&rc:Toolbar=false

Heath, B., Wise Romero, P., & Reynolds, K. (2013). *A review and proposed standard framework for levels of integrated healthcare.* SAMHSA-HRSA Center for Integrated Health Solutions: Washington, DC.

Hoge, M. A., & Morris, J. A. (2004). Implementing best practices in behavioral health workforce education: Building a change agenda. *Administration and Policy in Mental Health, 32*(2), 85–89.

Hoge, M. A., Morris, J. A., Laraia, M., Pomerantz, A., & Farley, T. (2014). *Core competencies for integrated behavioral health and primary care.* Washington, DC: SAMHSA - HRSA Center for Integrated Health Solutions.

Horevitz, E., & Manoleas, P. (2013). Professional competencies and training needs of professional social workers in integrated behavioral health in primary care. *Social Work in Health Care, 52*, 752–787. https://doi.org/10.1080/00981389.2013.791362.

Hser, Y. I., Grella, C. E., Hubbard, R. L., et al. (2001). An evaluation of drug treatments for adolescents in 4 US cities. *Archives of General Psychiatry, 58*(7), 689–695.

Institute of Medicine. (2001). *Crossing the quality chasm: A new health system for the 21st century.* Washington, DC: National Academy Press.

Jones, B., & Phillips, F. (2016). Social work and interprofessional education in health care: A call for continued leadership. *Journal of Social Work Education, 52*(1), 18–29.

Kathol, R. G., Butler, M., McAlpine, D. D., & Kane, R. L. (2010). Barriers to physical and mental condition integrated service delivery. *Psychosomatic Medicine, 72*(6), 511–518. https://doi.org/10.1097/PSY.0b013e3181e2c4a0, https://www.ncbi.nlm.nih.gov/pubmed/20498293

Katon, W., Von Korff, M., Lin, E., Simon, G., Walker, E., Bush, T., & Ludman, E. (1995). Collaborative management to achieve depression treatment guidelines. *JAMA: The Journal of the American Medical Association, 273*(13), 1026–1031.

Katon, W., Robinson, P., Von Korff, M., Lin, E., Bush, T., Ludman, E., Simon, G., & Walker, E. (1996). A multifaceted intervention to improve treatment of depression in primary care. *Archives of General Psychiatry, 53*(10), 924–932. http://www.ncbi.nlm.nih.gov/pubmed/8857869

Katon, W. J., Schoenbaum, M., Fan, M. Y., Callahan, C. M., Williams, J., Hunkeler, E., Harpole, L., Zhou, X. H., Langston, C., & Unutzer, J. (2005). Cost-effectiveness of improving primary care treatment of late-life depression. *Archives of General Psychiatry, 62*(12).

Kelly, T. M., & Daley, D. C. (2013). Integrated treatment of substance use and psychiatric disorders. *Social Work in Public Health, 28*, 388–406. https://doi.org/10.1080/19371918.2013.774673.

Kerman, N., & Kidd, S. A. (2019). The healthcare triple aim in the recovery era. *Administration and Policy in Mental Health and Mental Health Services*. https://doi.org/10.1007/s10488-019-00997-0.

Kessler, R. C., Berglund, P., Demler, O., Jin, R., Merikangas, K. R., & Walters, E. E. (2005). Lifetime prevalence and age-of-onset distributions of DSM-IV disorders in the National Comorbidity Survey Replication. *Archives of General Psychiatry, 62*(6), 593–602.

Kim, J. Y., Higgins, T. C., Esposito, D., & Hamblin, A. (2017). Integrating health care for high need Medicaid beneficiaries with serious mental illness and chronic physical health conditions at managed acre, provider and consumer levels. *Psychiatric Rehabilitation Journal, 40*(2), 207–215. https://doi.org/10.1037/prj0000231.

Koma, W., Artiga, S., Neuman, T., Claxton, G., Rae, M., Kates, J., & Michaud, J. (2020). *Low-income and communities of color at higher risk for serious illness if infected with coronavirus.* Report of the Kaiser Family Foundation. Accessed on 5/8/20 at: https://www.kff.org/disparities-policy/issue-brief/low-income-and-communities-of-color-at-higher-risk-of-serious-illness-if-infected-with-coronavirus/#

Kronick, R. G., Bella, M., & Gilmer, T. P. (2009, October). *The faces of Medicaid III: Refining the portrait of people with multiple chronic conditions.* Center for Health Care Strategies, Inc.

Lee, C. D., & Del Carmen Montiel, E. (2010). Does mentoring matter in the mental health field? *Social Work in Mental Health, 8*(5), 438–454.

Mancini, M. A., & Miner, C. S. (2013). Learning and change in a community mental health setting. *Journal of Evidence Based Social Work, 10*(5), 494–504.

Mancini, M. A., Maynard, B., & Cooper-Sadlo, S. (Epub ahead of print, September 23, 2019). Implementation of an integrated behavioral health specialization serving children and youth: Processes and outcomes. *Journal of Social Work Education.* https://doi.org/10.1080/10437797.2019.1661905.

Mauer, B. J. (2009). *Behavioral health/primary care integration and the person-centered healthcare home.* National Council for Community Behavioral Healthcare.

Mechanic, D. (2012). Seizing opportunities under the Affordable Care Act for transforming the mental and behavioral health system. *Health Affairs (Millwood), 31*(2), 376–382. https://doi.org/10.1377/hlthaff.2011.0623.

Mechanic, D., & Olfson, M. (2016). The relevance of the Affordable Care Act for improving mental health care. *Annual Review of Clinical Psychology, 12*(1), 515–542. https://doi.org/10.1146/annurev-clinpsy021815-092936.

Miller, B. F., Teevan, B., Phillips, R. L., Petterson, S. M., & Bazemore, A. W. (2011). The importance of time in treating mental health in primary care. *Families, Systems & Health: Journal of Collaborative Family Healthcare, 29*(2), 144–145. https://doi.org/10.1037/a0023993.

National Healthcare Disparities Report. (2013). *Highlights from the 2013 National Healthcare Quality and Disparities Reports.* May 2014. Rockville: Agency for Healthcare Research and Quality. Retrieved from http://www.ahrq.gov/research/findings/nhqrdr/nhdr13/highlights.html

O'Keefe, V. M., Wingate, L. R., Cole, A. B., Hollingsworth, D. W., & Tucker, R. P. (2015). Seemingly harmless racial communications are not so harmless: Racial microaggressions lead to suicidal ideation by way of depression symptoms. *Suicide and Life-threatening Behavior, 45*(5), 567–576.

Obucina, M., Harris, N., Fitzgerald, J. A., Chai, A., Radford, K., Ross, A., et al. (2018). The application of triple aim framework in the context of primary healthcare: A systematic literature review. *Health Policy, 122*, 900–907. https://doi.org/10.1016/j.healthpol.2018.06.006.

Olvera, R. L., Fisher-Hoch, S. P., Williamson, D. E., & Vatcheva, K. P. (2016). Depression in Mexican Americans with diagnosed and undiagnosed diabetes. *Psychological Medicine, 46*(3), 637–646. https://doi.org/10.1017/S0033291715002160.

Oppel, R. A., Gebeloff, R., Lai, R., Wright, W., & Smith, M. (2020, July 5th). The fullest look yet at the racial inequity of coronavirus. *The New York Times.* Retrieved on July 7th at: https://www.nytimes.com/interactive/2020/07/05/us/coronavirus-latinos-african-americans-cdc-data.html

Peek, C. J. (2013). *The National Integration Academy Council. Lexicon for behavioral health and primary care integration: Concepts and definitions developed by expert consensus* (AHRQ Publication No.13-IP001-EF). Rockville: Agency for Healthcare Research and Quality.

Reiss-Brennan, B., Brunisholz, K. D., Dredge, C., Briot, P., Grazier, K., Wilcox, A., et al. (2016). Association of integrated team-based care with health care quality, utilization, and cost. *JAMA, 316*(8), 826–834. https://doi.org/10.1001/jama.2016.11232.

Ross, S., & Peselow, E. (2012). Co-occurring psychotic and addictive disorders: Neurobiology and diagnosis. *Clinical Neuropharmacology, 35*(5), 235–243. https://doi.org/10.1097/WNF.0b013e318261e193.

Roy-Byrne, P., Craske, M. G., Sullivan, G., Rose, R. D., Edlund, M. J., et al. (2010). Delivery of evidence-based treatment for multiple anxiety disorders in primary care: A randomized controlled trial. *JAMA, 303*(19), 1921–1928. https://doi.org/10.1001/jama.2010.608.

Rodriguez-Lonebear, D., Barceló, N., Akee, R., Carroll, S.R (2020). American Indian Reservations and COVID-19: Correlates of Early Infection Rates in the Pandemic. *Journal of Public Health Management and Practice, 26*(4), 371–377. doi: 10.1097/PHH.0000000000001206

Sangaleti, C., Schveitzer, M. C., Peduzzi, M., Campos Pavone Zoboli, E. L., & Baldini Soares, C. (2017). Experiences and shared meaning of teamwork and interprofessional collaboration among health care professionals in primary health care settings: A systematic review. *JBI Database of Systematic Reviews and Implementation Reports.* https://doi.org/10.11124/JBISRIR-2016-003016

Santucci, K. (2012). Psychiatric disease and drug abuse. *Current Opinion in Pediatrics, 24*(2), 233–237. https://doi.org/10.1097/MOP.0b013e3283504fbf.

Schoen, C., Davis, K., How, S. K., & Schoenbaum, S. C. (2006). US health system performance: A national scorecard. *Health Affairs, 25*(6), w457–ww75.

Schoenbaum, M., Unutzer, J., Sherbourne, C., Duan, N., Rubenstein, L. V., Miranda, J., Meredith, L. S., Carney, M. F., & Wells, K. (2001). Cost-effectiveness of practice-initiated quality improvement for depression: Results of a randomized controlled trial. *Journal of the American Medical Association, 286*(11).

Shim, R. S., Koplan, C., Langheim, F. J. P., et al. (2012). Health care reform and integrated care: A golden opportunity for preventive psychiatry. *Psychiatric Services, 63*(12), 1231–1233. https://doi.org/10.1176/appi.ps.201200072.

Stanhope, V., Videka, L., Thorning, H., & McKay, M. (2015). Moving toward integrated health: An opportunity for social work. *Social Work in Health Care, 54*, 383–407.

Substance Abuse and Mental Health Services Administration. (2019). *Key substance use and mental health indicators in the United States: Results from the 2018 National Survey on Drug Use and Health* (HHS Publication No. PEP19-5068, NSDUH Series H-54). Rockville: Center for Behavioral Health Statistics and Quality, Substance Abuse and Mental Health Services Administration. Retrieved from https://www.samhsa.gov/data/

Sue, D. W., Capodilupo, C. M., Torino, G. C., Bucceri, J. M., Holder, A., Nadal, K. L., & Esquilin, M. (2007). Racial microaggressions in everyday life: Implications for clinical practice. *American Psychologist, 62*(4), 271–286. https://doi.org/10.1037/0003-066X.62.4.271.

Thielke, S., Vannoy, S., & Unutzer, J. (2007). Integrating mental health and primary care. *Primary Care, 34*(3).

Thota, A. B., Sipe, T. A., Byard, G. J., Zometa, C. S., Hahn, R. A., McKnight-Eily, L. R., et al. (2012). Collaborative care to improve the management of depressive disorders: A community guide systematic review and meta-analysis. *American Journal of Preventative Medicine, 42*(5), 525–538. https://doi.org/10.1016/j.amepre.2012.01.019.

Unützer, J. (2002). Collaborative care management of late-life depression in the primary care setting: A randomized controlled trial. *JAMA: The Journal of the American Medical Association, 288*(22), 2836–2845. https://doi.org/10.1001/jama.288.22.2836.

Unützer, J., & Park, M. (2012). Strategies to improve the management of depression in primary care. *Primary Care, 39*(2), 415–431. https://doi.org/10.1016/j.pop.2012.03.010.

Wagner, E. H., Austin, B. T., & Von Korff, M. (1996). Organizing Care for Patients with chronic illness. *The Milbank Quarterly, 74*(4), 511–44. http://www.ncbi.nlm.nih.gov/pubmed/8941260

Wagner, E. H., Austin, B. T., Davis, C., Hindmarsh, M., Schaefer, J., & Bonomi, A. (2001). Improving chronic illness care: Translating evidence into action. *Health Affairs, 20*(6).

Whittington, J. W., Nolan, K., Lewis, N., & Torres, T. (2015). Pursuing the triple aim: The first 7 years. *Milbank Quarterly, 93*, 263–300. https://doi.org/10.1111/1468-0009.12122.

Woltmann, E., Grogan-Kaylor, A., Perron, B., Georges, H., Kilbourne, A. M., & Bauer, M. S. (2012). Comparative effectiveness of collaborative chronic care models for mental health conditions across primary, specialty, and behavioral health care settings: Systematic review and meta-analysis. *American Journal of Psychiatry, 169*(8), 790–804. https://doi.org/10.1176/appi.ajp.2012.11111616.

Xierali, I. M., Tong, S. T., Petterson, S. M., Puffer, J. C., Phillips, R. L., & Bazemore, A. W. (2013). Family physicians are essential for mental health care delivery. *Journal of the American Board of Family Medicine, 26*(2), 114–115.

Young, J. Q., Kline-Simon, A. H., Mordecai, D. J., & Weisner, C. (2015). Prevalence of behavioral health disorders and associated chronic disease burden in a commercially insured health system: Findings of a case-control study. *General Hospital Psychiatry, 37*(2), 101–108. https://doi.org/10.1016/j.genhosppsych.2014.12.005.113.

Chapter 2
The Intersections of Social, Behavioral, and Physical Health

2.1 Overview of Health and Behavioral Health Intersections

Behavioral health disorders in general, and depression, anxiety, and substance use disorders (SUDs) specifically, are a leading cause of disease burden worldwide (Vos et al. 2015; Whiteford et al. 2013). These disorders commonly co-occur with other chronic medical conditions such as diabetes, arthritis, pain, cancer, cardiovascular disease, hypertension, cerebrovascular disease, lung disease, stomach problem, and asthma in a dose–response relationship (Scott et al. 2016). For instance, depression, anxiety, and substance use are associated with higher risk ratios for all of the above disorders and risk for these physical conditions increases as the number of behavioral health comorbidities rises (Scott et al. 2016). This indicates that behavioral health conditions such as depression and anxiety may be precursors to physical disease (Stein et al. 2014; Scott et al. 2016). Behavioral health disorders also make treatment and management of medical disorders complicated and more difficult (Scott et al. 2016; Walker and Druss 2016).

   In order to address the comorbid nature of physical and behavioral health disorders, behavioral health treatment programs should seek to target comorbid physical conditions in all clients. Likewise, addressing behavioral health disorders in primary care settings that treat clients with chronic physical conditions is indicated. The above data make a strong case for integrated care that addresses both physical and behavioral health conditions simultaneously (Walker and Druss 2016). The combination of co-occurring disorders with high stress, early adverse childhood experiences (ACEs), and high-risk health behaviors such as smoking, drinking, substance use, sedentary life style, and obesity leads to high morbidity and increased risk for early mortality due to overdose, disease, accidents, and suicide. Integrating fragmented health care systems to provide integrated health and behavioral health care is an effective

M. A. Mancini, *Integrated Behavioral Health Practice*,
https://doi.org/10.1007/978-3-030-59659-0_2

means to increase access to care and mitigate the effects of comorbid conditions (Druss and Walker 2011). Doing so requires the use of theoretical models that consider the dynamic process that leads to comorbid conditions. Ecological models that conceptualize the complex interactions of various risk and protective factors at the individual, interpersonal, organizational, and community levels represent a comprehensive approach to understanding of the dynamic interplay of the various factors that influence health. In the next sections I will outline the epidemiology of common behavioral health conditions in the United States. I then review the various risk and protective factors that contribute to health and resilience through the lens of ecological systems theory.

2.2   Prevalence of Behavioral Health Conditions in the United States

2.2.1   Substance Use

Substance use in the United States is very common. In 2018, 165 million people (60% of the population) over the age of 12 reported using substances in the past month. Of that number, 47 million people reported tobacco use and 67 million reported binge drinking. In 2018, 43.5 million reported marijuana use, over 10 million people reported opioid misuse, and 5.5 million reported cocaine use (SAMHSA 2019). In 2018, almost 15 million people had an alcohol use disorder and over 8 million people had a nonalcohol related substance use disorder or about 8% of the general population over the age of 12 (1 in 13 people; SAMHSA 2019). Two million and 4.5 million people had an opioid use and cannabis use disorder, respectively (SAMHSA 2019). While over 21 million people 12 years of age and older needed treatment for either an alcohol or drug use disorder, only about 1 in 10 received care at a specialty facility (SAMHSA 2019).

The 12-month prevalence of substance use disorders (SUDs) in the US population is 3.7%. In any given year, White people are the most likely group to have a substance use disorder (4%). Black and Latinx persons have a 12-month prevalence rate of 3% and 3.6%, respectively. Approximately, 1% of Asian Americans have a SUD in any given year (Vilsaint et al. 2019). In another study using a large national sample, 12-month and lifetime prevalence for substance use disorders for the total population were about 4% and 10%, respectively (Grant et al. 2016). This study also found that in the United States, substance use disorders are most prevalent in men, White persons, and Indigenous populations, as well as younger persons and those never married. SUDs are commonly comorbid with a wide range of disorders including depressive and anxiety disorders, borderline and antisocial personality disorders, bipolar spectrum disorders, and PTSD. Unfortunately, treatment rates for persons with 12-month and lifetime SUDs were only 13.5% and 24.6%, respectively (Grant et al. 2016).

2.2.2 Mental Illness and Treatment

While mental illness is common and treatable, treatment rates are low indicting the need for increased service availability and access. In 2018, 48 million American had a mental illness and 11.4 million persons had a serious mental illness (SMI) (e.g., major depressive disorder [MDD], bipolar spectrum disorder, schizophrenia spectrum disorder). Furthermore, 14.4% of adolescents between the ages of 12 and 17, and 13.8% of young adults aged 18–25 had a major depressive episode (MDE) in 2018. About 10% of adolescents had an MDE with severe impairment. Less than half of adolescents (41.4%) and young adults (49.6%) received treatment (SAMHSA 2019). Of the nearly 47.6 million adults with a mental illness, less than half (43%) received mental health care in 2018 and a third of the over 11 million adults with a serious mental illness did not receive any mental health care (SAMHSA 2019). Nearly half of lesbian, gay, and bisexual (LGB) adults (44%) report any mental illness, and 38% of this number have a serious mental illness. Despite this, 30–40% of LGB adults with SMI did not receive treatment in 2018 (SAMHSA 2020).

2.2.3 Suicide

Suicide has become one of the leading causes of death in the United States. In 2017, approximately 47,000 people or 14.5 per 100,000 people completed suicide making it the tenth leading cause of death in the United States. Of that number, almost 24,000 suicides involved firearms (Kochanek et al. 2019). Suicide rates have increased in almost every state since 1999 with more than half of states experiencing at least a 30% increase during that time period. Perhaps most importantly, over half (54%) of people who completed suicide in 2016 did not have a diagnosed mental health condition (Stone et al. 2018). Furthermore, persons who complete suicide have often seen a behavioral health or primary care provider in the three months preceding their death, further indicating the need for integrated behavioral health care prevention, screening, and intervention services in health care settings (Luoma et al. 2002; Pearson et al. 2009; Pirkis and Burgess 1998).

In 2018, nearly 11 million adults over the age of 18 (4.3%) reported thinking seriously about suicide. Over three million made plans (1.3%) and nearly one and a half million made an attempt (0.6%; SAMHSA 2019). Rates of suicidal ideation and suicide attempts in lesbian, gay, and bisexual (LGB) young adults are more than twice that of the US population. Almost 27% of LGB young adults experienced suicidal ideation in the past year and 5.4% attempted suicide compared to 11% and 1.9% in the broader US population (SAMHSA 2020). Transgender and gender nonconforming (TGNC) persons have far higher rates of suicidal ideation and attempts than the general US population. In a large representative national sample, 40% of transgender adults reported a lifetime suicide attempt compared to 4.5% of the US population, and 7% had attempted suicide in the past year, which was nearly 12 times the rate of the US population (James et al. 2016).

American Indian/Alaskan Natives, older Non-Hispanic Whites, and military veterans also have suicide rates significantly higher than the general population. Experiencing physical and sexual violence also increases the risk for suicidal ideation and completion of suicide. Women are more likely to attempt suicide, but men are far more likely to die by suicide due to more lethal means (Curtin et al. 2016). For instance, in 2017 men accounted for 86% of all firearm-related suicides (CDC 2020a). Experiencing poverty, violence, and discrimination also contributes to increased suicide rates.

Research has indicated a significant rise in suicides and suicide attempts among Black youth requiring far more national attention (Lindsey et al. 2019; Price and Khubchandani 2019). Rates of suicide attempts, while declining in White youth by 7.5% from 1991 to 2017, have risen in Black youth by 73% to record highs. Suicide is the second leading cause of death for Black youth (13–19) behind homicide (Price and Khubchandani 2019). While rates of suicide deaths have increased 33% over the last 20 years for all groups, they have risen higher in Black youth. For instance, from 2001 to 2017 the suicide rate for Black males increased 60%. For Black females, suicides increased a striking 182%. The methods used in the vast majority of suicides in both groups were the two most likely to result in death: hanging and firearms (Price and Khubchandani 2019). Indeed, suicide injuries and deaths for Black males have drastically increased suggesting they are using more lethal means (Lindsey et al. 2019). The rise in suicides in Black youth can be tied directly to their likelihood of experiencing higher rates of trauma, discrimination, poverty resulting from economic inequity, and a systematic lack of access to culturally fluent health and behavioral health care. These findings call for immediate action in the form of policies designed to: (1) increase access to high-quality, affordable, and culturally tailored health and mental health care; (2) eliminate economic inequities; (3) enhance public awareness of suicide risk and protective factors; and (4) improve other social determinants of health in Black communities such as increasing access to safe and affordable housing, increasing employment and education opportunities, increasing access to food, and reducing violence and environmental hazards (e.g., lead, water and air pollution, vacant buildings) (National Partnership for Action: HHS Action Plan to Reduce Racial and Ethnic Health Disparities, 2011).

Despite the fact that most people who complete suicide do not have a diagnosed behavioral health condition, one of the primary risk factors for suicide is the presence of any psychiatric disorder, particularly major depression and bipolar spectrum disorders. Other risk factors include hopelessness, male gender, previous suicide attempts, PTSD, anxiety, family history of suicide, and alcohol and substance misuse (APA 2013; Hawton et al. 2013). Another important risk factor is access to firearms. The risk disparities between gun owners and nonowners are striking. In a large study of gun ownership in California, male and female gun owners had suicide rates three and seven times more than male and female nonowners, respectively. New gun owners were also 100 times more likely to die by suicide within the first 30 days of possessing a gun than nonowners (Studdert et al. 2020). An important aspect of this study is that gun owners and nongun owners completed suicides without a gun at roughly the same rate, suggesting that possession of a firearm led to more suicides and was therefore a likely driver of increased rates for gun-owners who may have otherwise not completed suicide.

This highlights the importance of reducing the prevalence of access to unsecured firearms as a key component of effective suicide prevention and the need for better tracking of gun sales and gun stocks (Studdert et al. 2020). In the early days of COVID-19, news reports documented a spike in gun and ammunition purchases with news images of long lines of people, almost exclusively men, standing outside gun stores. How many of those were new gun sales? While it is too early to tell at the time of this writing, yet another effect of COVID-19 may be an increase in suicide rates—especially given the stress, job losses, and economic burdens felt by tens of millions of Americans, compounded by rise in firearm ownership.

2.2.4 Depression

The lifetime and 12-month prevalence rates of major depressive disorder (MDD) in the United States are 17% and 6%, respectively (Karg et al. 2014; Kessler et al. 2005a). The lifetime prevalence of dysthymia is 2.5%, bipolar disorders (I and II) 3.9%, and of any mood disorder is 20.8% (Kessler et al. 2005a). Worldwide estimates place the lifetime prevalence of MDD at 12% (Kessler et al. 2011). In 2015, 4.4% of the world population (322 million) experienced major depressive disorder (WHO 2017). Major depressive disorder has one of the highest burdens of disease in the world and costs US economy approximately 200 billion dollars (Greenberg et al. 2015; Whiteford et al. 2013). MDD is the second leading cause of disability in the United States and worldwide (Ferrari et al. 2013; Murray et al. 2013).

Prevalence of MDD in women is approximately twice the rate as in men in the United States and worldwide (17% vs 9%; Hasin et al. 2005; Seedat et al. 2009; WHO 2017), which may be due to a combination of biological, psychological, and environmental circumstances such as higher rates of poverty, trauma, and stress (Kuehner 2017; Malhi and Mann 2018). For adolescents aged 12–17, the 1-year and lifetime prevalence rates for major depressive episode are 8% and 11%, respectively (Avenevoli et al. 2015; Perou et al. 2013). A significant and growing percentage of pediatric depression cases are undertreated or untreated (Mojtabai et al. 2016). Lifetime prevalence of depression in older community dwelling adults is less than younger adults (Kessler et al. 2010a, b), and depression prevalence appears to decrease over time (Byers et al. 2010). However, older adults in primary care settings and those with chronic medical comorbidities can have much higher depression rates than the general older adult population (Lyness et al. 2006; Schulberg et al. 1998).

Lifetime prevalence of major depression was 18% for Whites, 13% for Caribbean Blacks, and 10% for African Americans (Williams et al. 2007). Approximately 15% of the US Latinx population will experience a depressive disorder in their lifetime (Alegria et al. 2008). The 12-month prevalence of mood disorders in the Latinx population is about 11% (Vilsaint et al. 2019). While variations in socioeconomic factors such as education level and nativity may play an important role in racial differences in behavioral health prevalence rates, national lifetime prevalence rates for behavioral health disorders in Latinx immigrant populations are typically lower than that of non-Latinx Whites (Alegria et al. 2008; Vilsaint et al. 2019).

Rates of depression in the LGBTQ community are high. Depression is twice has high in LGB adults as in the general US population. Over 30% of young LGB adults and almost 20% of adults between the age of 26 and 49 have experienced major depression in the past year (SAMHSA 2020). For transgender and gender nonconforming (TGNC) persons, 38% reported serious psychological distress in the past month compared to 5% of the general US population (James, et al. 2016). In a large, random sample of over 1200 TGNC college students across more than 70 campuses in the United States, almost 80% of respondents met criteria for one or more behavioral health problems compared to 45% of cisgender students. Almost 60% screened positive for depression, 50% screened positive for an anxiety disorder, and over half reported nonsuicidal self-injury (NSSI; Lipson et al. 2019).

2.2.5 Anxiety

Anxiety disorders include panic disorder, agoraphobia, generalized anxiety disorder, and social anxiety disorder (APA, 2013). Anxiety impacts 3.6% of the population worldwide and affects 28.8% of the US population (Kessler et al. 2005a; WHO 2017). It is also ranked sixth in terms of disease burden and affects 264 million people across the globe (WHO 2017). Twelve-month prevalence rates for anxiety disorders in the United States are 12.7% for the total population, 13.4% for Whites, 11.6% for African Americans, 8.1% for the Latinx population, and 7.7% for the Asian population (Vilsaint et al. 2019). Anxiety disorders cause significant distress and impairment in day-to-day functioning and are often comorbid with each other and major depressive disorder. The lifetime prevalence rates of panic disorder, social anxiety disorder, and generalized anxiety disorder are 4.7%, 12.1%, and 5.7%, respectively (Kessler et al. 2005a).

2.2.6 Post-Traumatic Stress Disorder (PTSD)

The 12-month and lifetime prevalence rates of PTSD in the United States are 4.7% and 6.1%, respectively. Women have twice the lifetime prevalence rate as men (8.0% vs 4.1%) (Goldstein et al. 2016). The 12-month and lifetime prevalence rates of PTSD in the US Black population are 4.7% and 6.2%, respectively. Whites have similar PTSD rates at 4.8% for 12-month and 6.3% for lifetime prevalence. Asian and Pacific islanders in the United States have the lowest PTSD prevalence rates at 1.8% for 12-month and 2.3% for lifetime. Latinx persons have a 12-month prevalence rate of 4.2% and lifetime prevalence rate of 5.6%. Indigenous populations living on reservations have the highest PTSD rate of any racial, ethnic, or cultural group with lifetime prevalence rates ranging between 14% and 16% (Goldstein et al. 2016). Persons who experience sexual assault, other intentional interpersonal violence (vs accidents), poverty, mass conflict, war, and combat have higher rates of PTSD (Chivers-Wilson 2006; Steel et al. 2009; Resnick et al. 1993).

Lifetime prevalence rates for PTSD decrease as income increases with 9% of the population earning family income less than $20,000 experiencing PTSD compared to 3.9% of persons with family income over $70,000 experiencing PTSD (Goldstein et al. 2016). PTSD is associated with an increased risk of type 2 diabetes (Roberts et al. 2015) and hypertension (Sumner et al. 2016) in a dose–response relationship with more severe PTSD symptoms associated with a higher risk. Research also indicates that meaningful reductions in PTSD symptom severity scores can significantly reduce the risk for type 2 diabetes (Scherrer et al. 2019).

Latinx adults, particularly women, show high rates of experiencing violence and related psychopathology (Cuevas et al. 2012). A nationally representative sample of Latinx immigrants shows that 11% have experienced some form of political violence with 76% having also experienced other forms of trauma (Fortuna et al. 2008). These rates can differ in clinical samples where as much as 54% of Latinx clients have experienced political violence (Eisenman et al. 2003), and 60–75% have experienced some form of trauma (Holman et al. 2000; Kaltman et al. 2010). Clinical samples of Latinx women have shown high prevalence rates of trauma and related psychopathology (Labash and Swartz 2018; Mancini and Farina 2019). The cumulative burden of trauma can lead to higher rates of PTSD, depression, suicidality, anxiety, and alcohol and substance use (Bjornsson et al. 2015; Labash and Swartz 2018; Myers et al. 2015; Ulibarri et al. 2015).

2.2.7 Comorbid Mental Health and Substance Use

In 2018, 19 million adults had a substance use disorder. Of that number almost half (48%) had a co-occurring mental illness in the past year, and one in five persons with a mental illness had a co-occurring substance use disorder in the past year (SAMHSA 2019). Substance use disorders are commonly comorbid with a wide range of behavioral health disorders including depressive and anxiety disorders, borderline and antisocial personality disorders, bipolar disorder, and PTSD. Unfortunately, treatment rates for persons with 12-month substance use disorders is only 13.5% and 24.6% for lifetime SUD (Grant et al. 2016).

In 2018, 28% of persons with a serious mental illness (SMI) had a substance use disorder in the past year (SAMHSA 2019). Furthermore, for adults with any mental illness, 37% reported substance use and 31% reported binge drinking within the past year, while almost half (49.4%) of persons with SMI reported illicit drug use in the past year and a third (32%) reported binge drinking in the past year (SAMHSA 2019). Almost half of persons with co-occurring mental illness and substance use disorder did not receive any type of care in 2018 (SAMHSA 2019). For LGB adults with mental illness and SUD, 90% did not receive any treatment (SAMHSA 2020). Almost a third (31%) of persons with SMI and SUD did not receive any type of care in 2018 (SAMHSA 2019). For LGB adults with co-occurring SMI and SUD, 33% did not receive treatment (SAMHSA 2020).

2.2.8   Comorbid Health and Behavioral Health Conditions

Comorbidity or multimorbidity is the existence of two or more health conditions in the same person (Valderas et al. 2009). Comorbidity of medical and mental health conditions is common and often has a bi-directional relationship (Katon 2003; Scott et al. 2016). The 2001–2003 National Comorbidity Survey Replication (NCS-R) data indicated that about 25% of the adult population had a mental disorder, while almost 60% had a medical disorder. For adults with a mental health disorder, 68% had a comorbid medical condition, and for those with medical conditions, 29% had a comorbid mental health condition (Alegria et al. 2003). Major depressive disorder is commonly comorbid with a range of other psychiatric disorders (Zimmerman et al. 2008). The most common psychiatric disorders that are comorbid with depression are anxiety disorders such as panic disorder, agoraphobia, generalized anxiety disorder, and social anxiety disorder (Kessler et al. 2005b; Lamers et al. 2011). Lamers et al. (2011) found that for persons with depression, two-thirds had a comorbid anxiety disorder, and 75% had experienced an anxiety disorder at some point in their lifetime. Other psychiatric disorders that are commonly co-morbid with depression include post-traumatic stress disorder (PTSD), obsessive compulsive disorder (OCD), attention deficit hyperactivity disorder (ADHD), and substance use disorder (APA, 2013; Kessler et al. 2005b).

Research also indicates that the presence of a mental health disorder raises the risk of developing a range of chronic medical conditions including heart disease, diabetes, stroke, hypertension, arthritis, cancer, chronic pain, asthma, and lung disease (Favreau et al. 2014; Stein et al. 2014; Tully et al. 2015; Tully et al. 2013; Scott et al. 2016). Comorbidity between psychiatric diagnoses and these chronic diseases leads to greater morbidity, functional impairment, health care costs, and premature mortality (Colton and Manderscheid 2006; Dickerson et al. 2008; Druss et al. 2002; Eaton et al. 2008; Egede 2007; Katon 2003; Kessler et al. 2008; Kronick et al. 2009; Scott et al. 2016; Stein et al. 2006; Young et al. 2015).

For instance, persons with chronic illness may be at higher risk of depression and suicide (Gurhan et al. 2019). Compared to nondepressed patients in primary care settings, patients with depression are more likely to present with a wide range of medical conditions that include asthma, diabetes, cancer, kidney disease, arthritis, heart disease, and hypertension (Smith et al. 2014; Wang et al. 2019). Depression was also associated with a higher metabolic risk for factors that can lead to heart disease and type 2 diabetes such as high blood pressure, high blood sugar, high cholesterol and triglycerides, and obesity (Vancampfort et al. 2014). The presence of depression can also lead to negative outcomes and prognosis of medical conditions due to the metabolic and physical effects of depression, decreased adherence to treatment, and a higher liklihood of engaging in unhealthy behaviors. The prevalence of these comorbidities indicates the importance of behavioral health specialists and primary care providers working together to increase the quality of care by addressing the impact of co-occurring mental illness, chronic disease conditions, and substance use disorders in an integrated fashion (Croft and Parish 2013; Druss and Mauer 2010; Mechanic 2012; Shim et al. 2012). In the next sections I will review ecological models of health and human behavior that can help frame and understand behavioral health disorders from a psychosocial perspective.

2.3 Models of Health and Human Behavior

The numbers above are daunting and clear. Physical health and behavioral health are inextricably linked. Physical illness and behavioral health disorders are routinely comorbid. Addressing physical and behavioral health equally and simultaneously is the solution. From a public health perspective, the next questions to ask are: What leads to these problems in the first place? What factors place people at higher risk? What factors are protective? What enables some people to flourish despite experiencing many risk factors? How can the damage caused by these problems be mitigated or, better yet, prevented from occurring in the first place? In the next section, I will explore the risk factors that contribute to the emergence of health and behavioral health issues and the protective factors that contribute to resiliency in the face of these risk factors. Doing so will require the application of frameworks that position human behavior as the result of complex interactions between the individual and their physical and social environment—their ecology.

2.3.1 Ecological Systems Theory

Ecological systems theory frames human behavior as a relational intersection of the individual with their social environment across multiple levels including family and friends, neighborhoods, schools, faith groups, and other social organizations/systems (e.g., social services, health care, mental health, addictions, criminal justice), community, and culture. The person-in-environment (PIE) approach is a common theoretical model guiding social work practice that is rooted in Bronfenbrenner's ecological systems theory (Bronfenbrenner 1979) and the social ecology of resilience (Ungar 2011). PIE is also part of the Life Model of Social Work Practice put forth by Germain and Gitterman (2008). In ecological systems theory, understanding human behavior and development is a function of understanding how an individual, possessing genetic, biological, and psychological strengths and vulnerabilities, interacts with differing levels of their social and built environment. These interactions are bi-directional. Figure 2.1 displays the levels of this model.

Bronfenbrenner (1979) proposed five levels of interaction. (1) Microsystems represent the specific, close relationships a person has with others in their immediate environment. This includes close individuals such as family and friends as well as teachers, faith leaders, or neighbors. (2) Mesosystems connect individuals and their microsystems directly to other systems. For instance, a child's relationship with their teacher exists within their microsystem. However, that relationship also connects the child's family to the broader school system. The relationship between the child and to the broader school system through these networks represents the mesosystem. (3) Exosystems are the broader systems that have an impact on the person, but that the persons do not directly interact with, such as parent workplaces, peers, local neighborhood, or economic or political context. (4) Macrosystems are the outermost layer of influential systems. They are the larger socio-cultural contexts that impact the individual such as societal beliefs, the economy, policies,

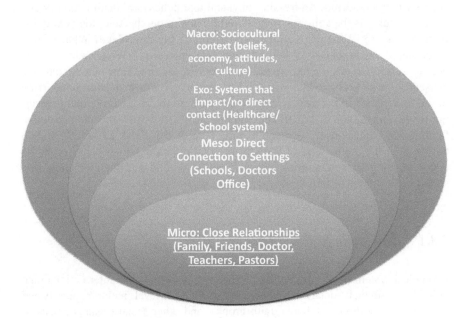

Fig. 2.1 Ecological systems model

attitudes, culture, and religion. These systems impact the services that a person may have access to, or resources that may exist in their environment. (5) The chronosystem is the influence of time on the individual's developmental trajectory. This can include external events (e.g., parental divorce, natural disasters) or internal developmental trajectories (e.g., adolescence). These five systems make up an individual's ecology. Human development and behavior is understood as the result of the dynamic interplay or interaction between the individual and these five systems across time (1979).

2.3.2 Stress–Vulnerability Models

The main tenet of the stress-diathesis model or the stress–vulnerability model is that genetic risk or vulnerability (e.g., diathesis) and environment (e.g., stress) interact to produce psychopathology (Genes X Environment; Monroe and Simons 1991). Figure 2.2 displays the elements of the stress–vulnerability model. For instance, a person may possess a genetic vulnerability or diathesis toward depression or schizophrenia. This model posits that when this person interacts with stressful

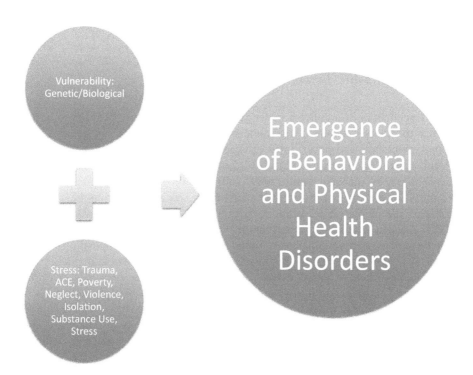

Fig. 2.2 Stress–vulnerability model

environments, they may develop the disorder if their stress level reaches a particular threshold. Psychopathology emerges when a person with a predisposition or vulnerability to a particular disorder encounters stress that activates the diathesis and leads to the emergence of symptoms (Colodro-Conde et al. 2018). Stress factors can include adverse life events such as divorce, relationship problems, exposure to interpersonal or community violence, chronic illnesses, injuries, and social determinants of health such as poverty, unstable housing, social isolation, and lack of safety. While many people in a population may be exposed to these factors, the experiences of these stressors can produce psychopathology in persons who hold a genetic vulnerability or risk.

The impact of these stressors can have multiplicative effects that go far beyond the sum of the experienced events (Colodro-Conde et al. 2018). An extension of the diathesis–stress model has emerged called the *differential susceptibility* theory. This model posits that individuals may be more susceptible or sensitive to positive *and* negative factors in their environment. This means that some individuals with a vulnerability to psychopathology may be less likely to develop problems if they are exposed to positive environments than others with the vulnerability (Belsky and Pluess 2009). In other words, some people are more prone to respond to positive environments than others. In the next section we will review the resiliency model and examine how risk and protective factors can influence human development and behavior.

2.3.3   Risk and Resilience
from a Bio-Psycho-Social Framework

Resilience has been a concept under study for half a century. Resilience is the ability to flourish despite being immersed in risk factors such as toxic stress, trauma, violence, and poverty that can increase the risk for negative behavioral health outcomes (Agnafors et al. 2017; Luthar 2003; Luthar et al. 2000; Rutter 1987, 2006; Werner and Smith 1982, 2001; Cicchetti 2010). Resilience is the result of the presence of protective factors that buffer a person from the risk factors that can increase the likelihood of experiencing negative outcomes (Rutter, 1987; Cicchetti 2010; Werner and Smith 1982, 2001). Risk and protective factors can be biological, psychological, or social and they are often in opposition to each other. A person's potential for resilience is the result of a dynamic interaction of these various factors. Early research examined the various correlates and processes that contributed to resilience in order to design resilience-promoting interventions that boosted protective factors and ameliorated the risk factors known to contribute to negative outcomes. More recent research seeks to understand the dynamic interplay between the biological, psychological, and social risk and protective factors and how these factors interact to produce resilience and well-being (Agnafors et al. 2017).

The ecological approach to resilience positions the ability of individuals to take advantage of the opportunities available in their environments as central to their health and well-being in the face of risks (Asakura 2016; Ungar 2011). This conceptualization of resilience moves the focus of research, policy, and practice away from the individual factors we know promote resilience and toward the study and implementation of programs and policies designed to develop and enhance contextual environments that promote resilience. A definition of ecological resilience offered by Ungar (2008) reads: "In the context of significant adversity, resilience is both the capacity of individuals to *navigate* their way to the psychological, social, cultural, and physical resources that sustain their well-being, and their capacity individually and collectively to *negotiate* for these resources to be provided and experienced in culturally meaningful ways" (p. 225). In other words, research on resilience should move away from analysis of predetermined outcomes, and focus instead on the *pathways* to resilience within a range of environmental contexts. Doing so will shed light on understanding the complexity and atypicality of resilience across cultural and socioeconomic groups. For instance, a process, trait, or behavior (e.g., aggression, callousness, emotional receptivity, democratic parenting) that is functional in one environment may not be so in another environment (Ungar 2011).

Viewing resilience from an ecological perspective requires understanding the dynamic complexities between physical and social environments and how individuals interact at micro (interpersonal), meso (organizational and systems), and macro (cultural and institutional) levels (Asakura 2016; Ungar 2011). This includes understanding the contextual qualities that promote resilience at each of these levels. Individual protective factors include the ability to problem solve and possessing self-efficacy. The most powerful protective factors that can help youth develop these traits include close, nurturing attachments to adult caregivers and other positive adult role models. Other important protective factors include being immersed in positive peer groups and being a part of schools and community groups that are properly resourced, staffed with competent and supported personnel, and that hold students to high expectations of behavior. Finally, living in communities that are safe, connected, stable, and that have equitable access to adequate resources (e.g., food access, health care, parks and recreation, transportation) promotes health and resilience in youth. These factors are identified in Fig. 2.3. The next frontier in resilience research is understanding how these protective factors interact with each other to produce resilience and identifying which factors can magnify or lead to the emergence of other protective factors. Answering these questions can provide local, state, and national governments information on where to invest resources to best promote resilience across levels. In the next sections, I will review the most prominent risk and protective factors involved in the emergence and prevention of behavioral health disorders.

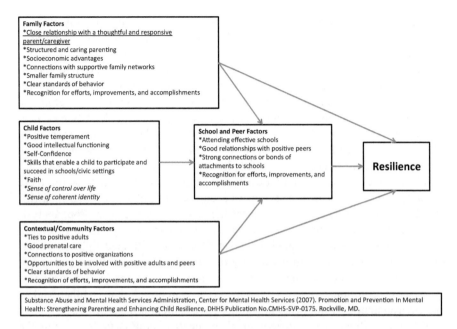

Family Factors
*Close relationship with a thoughtful and responsive parent/caregiver
*Structured and caring parenting
*Socioeconomic advantages
*Connections with supportive family networks
*Smaller family structure
*Clear standards of behavior
*Recognition for efforts, improvements, and accomplishments

Child Factors
*Positive temperament
*Good intellectual functioning
*Self-Confidence
*Skills that enable a child to participate and succeed in schools/civic settings
*Faith
*Sense of control over life
*Sense of coherent identity

School and Peer Factors
*Attending effective schools
*Good relationships with positive peers
*Strong connections or bonds of attachments to schools
*Recognition for efforts, improvements, and accomplishments

Resilience

Contextual/Community Factors
*Ties to positive adults
*Good prenatal care
*Connections to positive organizations
*Opportunities to be involved with positive adults and peers
*Clear standards of behavior
*Recognition of efforts, improvements, and accomplishments

Substance Abuse and Mental Health Services Administration, Center for Mental Health Services (2007). Promotion and Prevention In Mental Health: Strengthening Parenting and Enhancing Child Resilience, DHHS Publication No.CMHS-SVP-0175. Rockville, MD.

Fig. 2.3 Protective (buffering) factors that promote resilience

2.3.4   Common Risk and Protective Factors for Behavioral Health Disorders

Risk Factors   There are numerous bio-psycho-social factors that increase the risk for behavioral health disorders. However, there are several targeted risk factors that drive comorbidity in health and behavioral health disorders that could be a prime focus of integrated behavioral health practice settings. These include factors related to poverty and other social determinants of health and adverse childhood events. These factors are often interrelated and place a person at heightened risk for health and behavioral health problems. Youth who are immersed in high-risk environments marked by communities that have a lack of opportunities, high violence, drug use, poor functioning schools, and families with high stress, mental illness, violence, or drug use are at a higher risk for a range of health, social, and behavioral health problems. These factors are outlined in Fig. 2.4.

Due to their vast and differential impact on health, these factors should be key areas of assessment and intervention for integrated behavioral health settings. The combination of stress and high-risk health behaviors associated with these environments can also lead to a variety of negative health outcomes including chronic bodily inflammation, depression, suicidality, chronic disease, and premature death (Black 2006; Felitti et al. 1998; Honkalampi et al. 2005; Katon 2003). Four modifiable health risk behaviors have been identified that have a differential impact on

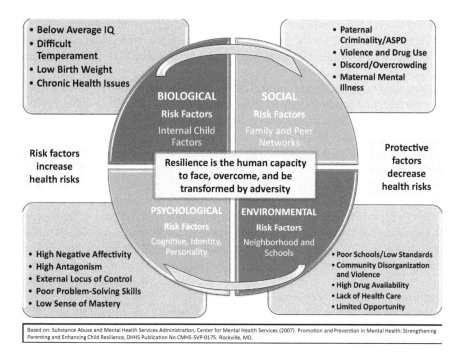

Fig. 2.4   Common risk factors for behavioral health problems

health: sedentary life style, smoking, alcohol and substance use, and poor nutrition (CDC 2020b). These behaviors can lead to, or magnify, the effects of health and behavioral health conditions. For instance, poor diet and sedentary lifestyle can contribute to higher rates of obesity in persons with mental health conditions who already face premature mortality rates two to four times the rate of persons without mental health conditions (Chwastiak et al. 2009; Eaton et al. 2008; Goodwin 2003; Simon et al. 2000). Routine screening, assessment, and the use of brief interventions in primary care and behavioral health settings to help people smoke and drink less, move more, and eat healthier food could substantially reduce morbidity and mortality in person with diagnosed behavioral health conditions.

Social determinants of health such as poverty are also associated with adverse health behaviors (Kronick et al. 2009) and increased risk for comorbid mental health and medical disorders (Harper and Lynch 2007; Lantz et al. 1998; Lorant et al. 2003). Adverse events experienced in childhood (ACEs) can lead to a range of negative behavioral health outcomes (Anda et al. 2006; Whitfield et al. 2003). For example, children exposed to interpersonal violence are at an increased risk for substance use, depression, and continued violence exposure, both as a victim and perpetrator, in adulthood (Briggs-Gowan et al. 2010; Carter et al. 2010; Chapman et al. 2004; Edwards et al. 2003; Whitfield et al. 2003). The experience of socioeconomic disadvantages and the toxic stress of racism in childhood has also been linked to a range of negative behavioral health outcomes (Reiss 2013). Children exposed to caregivers with behavioral health problems such as depression, substance use, or psychosis, or who lack adequate coping skills that interfere with healthy attachment are at risk for behavioral health outcomes in adulthood (Felitti et al. 1998; Goodman et al. 2011; Anda et al. 2006).

Experiencing early adverse events such as interpersonal violence, parental incarceration, parental death or divorce, close familial mental illness, or substance use can also lead to a range of chronic physical illnesses such as cancer (Brown et al. 2013), COPD; Anda et al. 2008), heart disease (Dong et al. 2004), and autoimmune diseases such as rheumatoid arthritis (Dube et al. 2009). Experiencing early childhood trauma can also lead to risk behaviors later in life such as smoking (Anda et al. 1999), alcohol and drug use (Dube et al. 2003; Strine et al. 2012), and obesity (Williamson et al. 2002). Rates of attempted suicide are substantially higher for persons who experience one or more ACEs compared to those who experience no ACEs and the risk increases as the experiences of ACEs increases in a dose–response relationship (e.g., more ACEs = more risk; Dube et al. 2001). It appears that experiencing adverse events in childhood can cause chronic over-activation of the stress response system that can lead to negative metabolic, cardiovascular, and other health-related outcomes (Felitti et al. 1998). Evaluation of these experiences should be a routine practice in primary and behavioral health care settings as they have implications for treatment. Figure 2.5 displays the ways in which toxic stress can impact health and behavioral health.

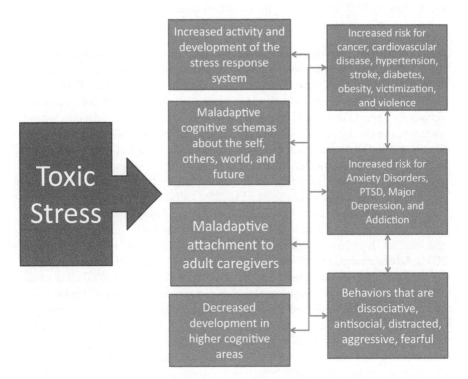

Fig. 2.5 How toxic stress impacts behavioral health

2.3.4.1 Protective Factors

There are several biological, psychological, social, and environmental factors that have been studied that have repeatedly led to robust effects at the micro, meso, and macro levels. Figure 2.6 outlines some of the most important protective factors at each of these levels. At the individual level, possessing good intellectual functioning (e.g., problem solving, cognitive flexibility, high IQ), competence in practicing pro-social behaviors (e.g., emotional regulation, social skills, emotional competence), a sense of self-efficacy, an internal locus of control, and an easy-going temperament have been associated with resilience in children exposed to high levels of risk (Agnafors et al. 2017; Garmezy 1983; Kim et al. 2013; SAMHSA 2007). There is also evidence of genetic factors, particularly involving the 5-HTT gene, that can protect against the development of depression in the face of increased risk (Agnafors et al. 2017; Clarke et al. 2010; Caspi et al. 2003). Familial factors that promote resilience include most notably caregivers who possess ability to adequately bond and develop health attachments with their children. This includes caregivers with good mental health and coping skills (Al-Yagon 2008; Huhtala et al. 2014; SAMHSA 2007) as well as positive caregiver support, clear expectations of behavior, and a positive home environment in which children are able to have routine positive interactions with loving caregivers (e.g., playing, reading; Donnon and Hammond 2007; Klebanov and Brooks-Gunn 2006; Sroufe et al. 2005; SAMHSA 2007).

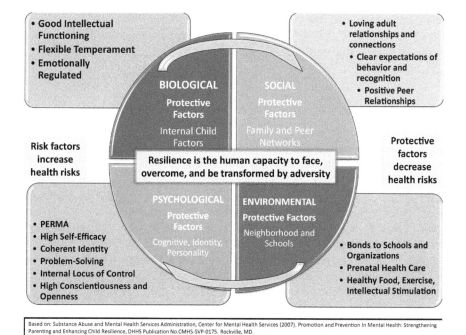

Based on: Substance Abuse and Mental Health Services Administration, Center for Mental Health Services (2007). Promotion and Prevention In Mental Health: Strengthening Parenting and Enhancing Child Resilience, DHHS Publication No.CMHS-SVP-0175. Rockville, MD.

Fig. 2.6 Common protective factors for behavioral health problems

In addition to individual and familial characteristics that promote resilience, several other environmental factors at the school and community level are important. From an ecological standpoint, increasing a child's access to positive ecological contexts that include healthy relationships with caregivers who are supportive, competent, and have high expectations of behavior, access to positive peer networks, and being a member of communities and schools that are cohesive, culturally sensitive, and that have high expectations of behavior and achievement are vital to child development and have been shown to enhance resilience (see Fig. 2.3; Donnon and Hammond 2007; Masten 2001; Masten and Coatsworth 1998; Robertson et al. 2003; SAMHSA 2007). These contexts are the most likely to nurture youth who are confident, good problem solvers, emotionally and socially competent, and have good self-control (Donnon and Hammond 2007; SAMHSA 2007). Furthermore, several other ecological contexts can promote resilience and offset risk factors such as low birth weight, the mental illness of one parent or caregiver, low IQ or difficult temperament in children. What promotes these protective factors is no secret—they are resources that have been inequitably distributed to middle- and upper-class caregivers and communities for generations, but denied to Black, Indigenous, and people of color (BIPOC) communities and/or communities that are poor through racist structures and policies. These resiliency promotive contexts include: (1) equitable access to resources for caregivers such as good prenatal care, child care, and pre-school; (2) adequate income for caregivers to meet their basic needs including nutrition, utilities, leisure, and transportation; and (3) stable housing in neighborhoods that are safe, healthy, and have playgrounds and green spaces (SAMHSA 2007). In short, the best way to reduce health and behavioral health disorders is the elimination of poverty and improvement of social determinants of health.

2.4 Social Determinants of Health and Health Equity

Poor neighborhood conditions including lack of transportation, poor quality housing, low-quality schools, high unemployment, and lack of safety have also been found to increase the risk of health and mental health conditions (Bitsko et al. 2016; Cutrona et al. 2005; Cutrona et al. 2006; Pickett and Pearl 2001). The health of a population is dependent on a variety of social determinants that include adequate income, safety, stable housing, health care, nutrition, education, and employment (Marmot et al. 2008; Schoeni et al. 2008; Woolf and Braveman 2011). Figure 2.7 categorizes social determinants of health into four broad domains focused on housing, income/financial resources, relationships, and safe and healthy environments. These social determinants of health (SDOH) are the economic, social, and physical conditions in the various places and spaces in which people exist that impact their physical and emotional health. Health-related social needs (HRSN) located in the various social and built environments or "places" in which people live (e.g., home, school, work, and neighborhood) over time have an enormous impact on health and well-being (Nuruzzaman et al. 2015).

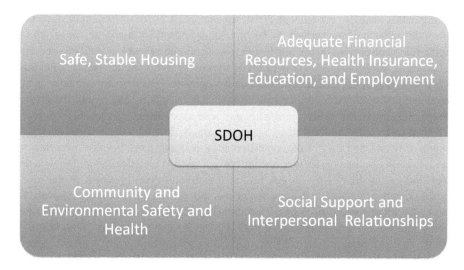

Fig. 2.7 Social determinants of health domains

The World Health Organization's Commission on Social Determinants of Health (CSDH) offers this widely adopted definition of social determinants of health: "The social determinants of health are the conditions in which people are born, grow, live, work and age. These circumstances are shaped by the distribution of money, power and resources at global, national and local levels. The social determinants of health are mostly responsible for health inequities - the unfair and avoidable differences in health status seen within and between countries" (CSDH 2008).

Addressing social determinants through the robust provision of social services can improve health and reduce overall health care costs (Bradley et al. 2017; Bradley et al. 2016). In the United States, states with higher rates of social service spending relative to health care have better health outcomes related to obesity, diabetes, cancer, cardiovascular disease, behavioral health, and asthma (Bradley et al. 2016). Similar findings were shown when comparing member nations in the Organization for Economic Co-operation and Development (OECD) as well those countries that have higher spending rates on social services relative to health care costs. The nations that spend more on social services have better health outcomes while spending *less* on health care (Bradley et al. 2017). As an example, the United States spends more than any other OECD country on health care, but does not do so on social services and experiences lower health overall and high health inequity compared to other OECD countries (Bradley et al. 2017; Marmot and Bell 2009). This demonstrates that spending on social services, particularly on education, income support, transportation, environmental health, public safety, and housing can improve health and lower health care costs (Bradley et al. 2016). For instance, investing in nutritional assistance, prenatal care, and early childhood education can lead to reduction in infant mortality and reduced blood pressure (Arno et al. 2009;

Campbell et al. 2014; Foster et al. 2010; Khanani et al. 2010). Programs designed to provide stable housing, access to healthy food, and utility assistance have led to reduction in obesity, diabetes, and health risks to children (Frank et al. 2006; Ludwig et al. 2011; Viola et al. 2013). Investing in improving evironmental health standards such as enhancing green spaces and tree canopies (i.e. shade), implementation of lead and pest abatement and improving water and air quality can reduce the prevalence of asthma, heat-related problems, and lead exposure.

Health inequities in the United States are largely driven by these social determinants of health and the results are differences in infant mortality, life expectancy, and disability burden between those who have access to resources and those who do not. Enhancing SDOH by improving the social conditions in which people live; addressing the inequitable distribution of income, power, and resources; and evaluating the effectiveness of policies through ongoing transdisciplinary research are important ways to promote health equity (CSDH 2008; Phelan et al. 2004; Marmot et al. 2008; Marmot and Bell 2009). Income inequality and poverty are associated with inadequate access to clean water, healthy food, health care, stable housing, cohesive communities, employment, education, and safety, and therefore play an important role in physical and behavioral health (Kondo 2012; Marmot 2005; Nuruzzaman et al. 2015). Lack of access to these resources and the associated experience of higher psychosocial stress, risky behaviors (e.g., drug and alcohol use, unsafe sex), and health and behavioral health issues can lead to a pathway to higher rates of morbidity and mortality (Kondo 2012).

Addressing these issues involves implementation and/or expansion of several policies that include ensuring that people have adequate access to clean water and air, sanitation, transportation, and stable, affordable, and safe housing. This also means the implementation and robust expansion of early childhood education, income support, employment, and nutritional assistance programs and the implementation of policies that ensure universal access to health care are vital components to reducing health inequities and enhancing the social determinants of health (Bradley et al. 2016, 2017; Phelan et al. 2004; Marmot et al. 2008).

2.4.1 Integrated Behavioral Health Practice and Social Determinants of Health

How health care is provided in the United States must change. The COVID-19 pandemic has laid bare the disastrous inequities that exist in the United States, particularly in the area of health. Black and Latinx Americans are far more likely to die from the coronavirus in large part due to preexisting health conditions that result from the above inequities. These inequities are not accidental. They are the direct result of a long history of racist policies designed to segregate Black and Brown communities and reduce their access to quality housing, education, employment, social services, and healthy environments. Access to universal health care is but one policy change that could have an important impact on reducing health inequities. But how health care and social care are delivered in the United States must also change. System fragmentation both within health care systems and across health care and social service systems must be addressed to ensure coordinated, efficient, and equitable delivery and distribution of services and resources. The provision of social care as part of health care represents one way to improve health care delivery and outcomes. The integration of social workers and other behavioral health care providers into health care teams as a means to assess and address social determinants of health has been identified as an important public health strategy to improve health care delivery (NASEM 2019). The inclusion of social workers in collaborative health care teams who are designated to specifically address social and behavioral health needs is vital to better incorporating and integrating person-centered care. Person-centered care is defined as patient care that prioritizes patient values, preferences, and goals to guide health care clinical decision-making that is both respectful and responsive to patient needs (IOM 2001).

As identified in Chap. 1, collaborative care teams that feature primary care providers and social workers that work together to address medical, behavioral, and social health needs represent an important opportunity to address the social determinants of health, reduce health inequities, and improve the health of patients. Collaborative care approaches that utilize interprofessional treatment teams of multidisciplinary professions to screen, assess, treat, and monitor patients for mental and medical conditions work best and are cost-effective (Bitsko et al. 2016; Butler et al. 2009; Bower et al. 2006; Katon et al. 2005; Schoenbaum et al. 2001; Thielke et al. 2007; Wagner et al. 1996, 2001). Two particular elements that are important are: *stepped care* and the use of *case managers* (Bower et al. 2006). In stepped care, clients receive successive interventions designed to address health and behavioral health problems and achieve positive outcomes. For instance, a client with depression may receive cognitive behavioral therapy to address symptoms. If symptoms persist, they may then receive additional interventions such as antidepressant medication to resolve remaining symptoms. Case managers provide wraparound services to clients to address factors associated with social determinants of health such as housing, employment, safety, benefits, food, and other social needs. These programs ensure clients receive multidimensional care with good follow-up to address health and behavioral health comorbidities (Druss and Walker 2011).

2.5   Summary and Conclusions

The connection between physical health and behavioral health is strong and bi-directional. One's health or morbidity in one domain has direct implications for their health and morbidity in the other. The current fragmentation of physical health and behavioral health services does not reflect this reality and leads to inefficient and ineffective care. Integration of these service systems can lead to lower costs and improved outcomes. But integration of physical and behavioral health practices is not enough. Several factors exist at the individual, interpersonal, and environmental levels that promote health. Likewise, several factors at each of these levels are known to increase risk for physical and behavioral health problems.

The single greatest influence on physical and behavioral health is one's access to power, resources, and social determinants of health. Increasing access to these resources and eliminating the inequities that plague the US health care system represent the most efficient, effective, and socially just way to promote health and well-being. This will require a fundamental redistribution of power and the creation and implementation of policies designed to eliminate economic and health inequities, experienced disproportionally by BIPOC communities, by expanding universal access to health, education, housing, income, and employment resources. This, coupled with the integration of health, behavioral health, and social care services, can more effectively address the social determinants of health required to achieve true health equity in all communities.

Case Study 2.1: Maria

Maria[1] is a 20-year-old cisgendered female Latinx college student attending a local University as a freshman. She is unmarried and not dating. She commutes to campus and currently lives with her mother and two younger sisters. She works evenings and weekends as a server in a busy restaurant. She and her family arrived in the United States about 8 years ago from Honduras and were granted asylum. She speaks two languages fluently. She is majoring in biology and plans on becoming a doctor.

She is speaking to you, a behavioral health specialist, because her doctor referred her to you because Maria complains of having trouble with sleep, anxiety, and mood fluctuations. The doctor thinks Maria needs some counseling and has prescribed her a sleep aid and an antidepressant, which Maria has not taken. She complains that she often experiences periods of being sad for no reason. At other times, she experiences bouts of intense anxiety bordering on panic. She states that she is terrified that she will be sent back to her home country. She and her family are currently trying to gain permanent citizenship, but she states, "who knows what's going to happen now. I can't sleep, I don't eat and then I eat junk until I'm full. I just don't feel well and I'm worried that all of this is just going to be for nothing." Maria is approximately 30 pounds overweight for her height. She exercises sporadically. She has used dieting to lose weight, but always struggles to keep the weight off. Her blood pressure is 132/82, her resting heart rate is 99, and her "bad" low-density lipoprotein (LDL) cholesterol is over the recommended limits by 25%.

Maria reports that she fled Honduras due to community violence. A local organized crime syndicate targeted her father who owned a restaurant for protection money; when he refused, they killed him and burned the restaurant down. The family had some savings and used it to go into hiding for a couple of months.

---

[1]All names and other identifiers of this case have been changed to protect privacy and confidentiality.

They then applied for asylum in the United States and went to live with Maria's aunt and two cousins. The family was later able to get an apartment and start rebuilding their lives.

Maria's mother lived with a man for a period of time when Maria was 17. Unfortunately, he became psychologically abusive to the whole family, yelling at Maria about her weight and appearance. He had several affairs with other women. He began physically assaulting Maria when he came home drunk. Maria's mother ended the relationship. Maria states: "he was real nice at first and treated me with respect but then he changed over time. It dawned on me one day that this isn't normal. I realized that he treated me just like my dad treated my mom and me. My dad would come home half drunk from the restaurant and he would berate us all and tell us what garbage we were and what a burden we were on him. He would slap my mom when she would intervene, he would slap us when we cried, and then he'd go and pass out on the couch. He would have affairs all around town and not even hide it. He would get into these bad states of mind. Sometimes, for months, he would be great. Sweet and kind. And then he would get real moody and start doing his 'crazy dad thing.' My mom says that he had a problem with his brain from his own dad who used to beat him up all the time. As bad as he was sometimes, losing him was the worst thing to ever happen to me. But I have my future career and my school and my mom and sisters and that's all I need now. It's just that I still have these nightmares sometimes and then I get all amped up for no reason. It's like I have to remind myself that I'm safe now—but sometimes I don't believe what I tell myself. I get moody and down. I don't like myself so much and I feel ashamed and I don't know why. Taking my nieces out to get clothes or something to eat makes me feel good. When I'm busy I'm OK. But when I'm alone I just freak out. I don't dare drink or do drugs—I'm too terrified what that might do to me. And those meds? I don't know—I'm afraid of that stuff too. I just wish I could calm down. What I want is to feel normal. I want to feel healthy. Instead I feel heavy, sluggish and sad except when I'm freaking out. I'm tired. I just don't feel good! How can I be a doctor when I don't feel good myself? What am I going to tell my patients? How are they going to listen to me and take me seriously when it's obvious that I don't even have my own stuff together?"

Analysis
- What is your preliminary conceptualization of Maria?
- What protective factors does she possess?
- What risk factors are present in her environment?
- How many ACES does she have?
- What are the potential consequences for her health and well-being?
- Based on the above, what are some potential areas of intervention to maximize Maria's health and well-being?

References

Agnafors, S., Goran-Svedin, C., Oreland, L., Bladh, M., Comasco, E., & Sydsjo, G. (2017). A biopsychosocial approach to risk and resilience on behavior in children followed from birth to age 12. *Child Psychiatry and Human Development, 48*, 584–596.

Alegria, M., Jackson, J. S., Kessler, R. C., & Takeuchi, D. (2003). *National Comorbidity Survey Replication (NCS-R). 2001–2003*. Ann Arbor: Inter-University Consortium for Political and Social Research.

Al-Yagon, M. (2008). Maternal personal resources and children's socioemotional and behavioral adjustment. *Child Psychiatry and Human Development, 39*(3), 283–298.

Alegría, M., Canino, G., Shrout, P. E., Woo, M., Duan, N., Vila, D., Torres, M., Chen, C. N., & Meng, X. L. (2008). Prevalence of mental illness in immigrant and non-immigrant U.S. Latino groups. *The American journal of psychiatry, 165*(3), 359–369. https://doi.org/10.1176/appi.ajp.2007.07040704

American Psychiatric Association. (2013). *Diagnostic and Statistical Manual of Mental Disorders, Fifth Edition (DSM-5)*. Arlington: American Psychiatric Association.

Anda, R. F., Croft, J. B., Felitti, V. J., Nordenberg, D., Giles, W. H., Williamson, D. F., & Giovino, G. A. (1999). Adverse childhood experiences and smoking during adolescence and adulthood. *JAMA, 282*, 1652–1658.

Anda, R. F., Felitti, V. J., Bremner, J. D., Walker, J. D., Whitfield, C., Perry, B. D., et al. (2006). The enduring effects of abuse and related adverse experiences in childhood: A convergence of evidence from neurobiology and epidemiology. *European Archives of Psychiatry and Clinical Neuroscience, 256*(3), 174–186. https://doi.org/10.1007/s00406-005-0624-4.

Anda, R. F., Brown, D. W., Dube, S. R., Bremner, J. D., Felitti, V. J., & Giles, W. H. (2008). Adverse childhood experiences and chronic obstructive pulmonary disease in adults. *American Journal of Preventative Medicine, 34*(5), 396–403.

Arno, P. S., Sohler, N., Viola, D., & Schechter, C. (2009). Bringing health and social policy together: The case of the earned income tax credit. *Journal of Public Health Policy, 30*(2), 198–207.

Asakura, K. (2016). It takes a village: Applying a social ecological framework of resilient in in working with LGBTQ Youth. *Families in Society, 97*(1), 15–22.

Avenevoli, S., Swendsen, J., He, J. P., et al. (2015). Major depression in the national comorbidity survey-adolescent supplement: Prevalence, correlates, and treatment. *Journal of the American Academy of Child and Adolescent Psychiatry, 54*, 37.

Belsky, J., & Pluess, M. (2009). Beyond diathesis stress: Differential susceptibility to environmental influences. *Psychological Bulletin, 135*(6), 885–908. https://doi.org/10.1037/a0017376.

Bitsko, R. H., Holbrook, J. R., Robinson, L. R., Kaminski, J. W., Ghandour, R., Smith, C., & Peacock, G. (2016). Health care, family, and community factors associated with mental, behavioral, and developmental disorders in early childhood – United States, 2011–2012. *MMWR Morbidity and Mortality Weekly Report, 65*(9), 221–226.

Bjornsson, A. S., Sibrava, N. J., Beard, C., Moitra, E., Weisberg, R. B. P., Benítez, C. I. P., & Keller, M. B. (2015). Two-year course of generalized anxiety disorder, social anxiety disorder, and panic disorder with agoraphobia in a sample of Latino adults. *Journal of Consulting and Clinical Psychology, 82*(60), 1186–1192.

Black, P. H. (2006). The inflammatory consequences of psychologic stress: Relationship to insulin resistance, obesity, atherosclerosis and diabetes mellitus, type II. *Medical Hypotheses, 67*(4), 879–891.

Bower, P., Gilbody, S., Richards, D., Fletcher, J., & Sutton, A. (2006). Collaborative care for depression in primary care—Making sense of a complex intervention: Systematic review and meta-regression. *British Journal of Psychiatry, 189*, 484–493.

Bradley, E. H., Canavan, M., Rogan, E., Talbert-Slagle, K., & Ndumele, C. (2016). Variation in health outcomes: The role of spending on social services, public health and health care, 2000-09. *Health Affairs, 35*(5), 760–768C. https://doi.org/10.1377/hlthaff.2015.0814.

Bradley, E. H., Sipsma, H., & Taylor, L. A. (2017). American healthcare paradox-high spending on health care and poor health. *QJM, 110(2)*, 61–65. https://doi.org/10.1093/qjmed/hcw187.

Briggs-Gowan, M. J., Carter, A. S., Clark, R., Augustyn, M., McCarthy, K. J., & Ford, J. D. (2010). Exposure to potentially traumatic events in early childhood: Differential links to emergent psychopathology. *Journal of Child Psychology and Psychiatry, 51(10)*, 1132–1140.

Bronfenbrenner, U. (1979). *The ecology of human development: Experiments by nature and design*. Cambridge, MA: Harvard University Press. (ISBN 0-674-22457-4).

Brown, M. J., Thacker, L. R., & Cohen, S. A. (2013). Association between adverse childhood experiences and diagnosis of cancer. *PLoS ONE, 8(6)*, e65524. https://doi.org/10.1371/journal.pone.0065524.

Butler, M., Kane, R., McAlpine, D., Kathol, R. G., Fu, S. S., Hagedorn, H., & Wilt, T. J. (2009). *Integration of mental health/substance abuse and primary care*. Minneapolis: Minnesota Evidence-Based Practice Center.

Byers, A. L., Yaffe, K., Covinsky, K. E., Friedman, M. B., & Bruce, M. L. (2010). High occurrence of mood and anxiety disorders among older adults: The National Comorbidity Survey Replication. *Archives of general psychiatry, 67(5)*, 489–496. https://doi.org/10.1001/archgenpsychiatry.2010.35

Campbell, F., Conti, G., Heckman, J. J., Moon, S. H., Pinto, R., Pungello, E., et al. (2014). Early childhood investments substantially boost adult health. *Science, 343(6178)*, 1478–1485.

Carter, A. S., Wagmiller, R. J., Gray, S. A., McCarthy, K. J., Horwitz, S. M., & Briggs-Gowan, M. J. (2010). Prevalence of DSM-IV disorder in a representative, healthy birth cohort at school entry: Sociodemographic risks and social adaptation. *Journal of the American Academy of Child and Adolescent Psychiatry, 49(7)*, 686–698.

Caspi, A., Sugden, K., Moffitt, T. E., Taylor, A., Craig, I. W., Harrington, H., et al. (2003). Influence of life stress on depression: Moderation by a polymorphism in the 5-HTT gene. *Science, 301(5631)*, 386–389.

Centers for Disease Control and Prevention. National Center for Injury Prevention and Control (2020a). Web-based Injury Statistics Query and Reporting System (WISQARS). (2012–2016). Accessed July, 2020.

Centers for Disease Control and Prevention (2020b) Chronic Diseases and Health Promotion. (2020b). www.cdc.gov/chronic disease/overview/. Accessed 28 Feb 2020.

Chapman, D. P., Whitfeld, C. L., Felitti, V. J., Dube, S. R., Edwards, V. J., & Anda, R. F. (2004). Adverse childhood experiences and the risk of depressive disorders in adulthood. *Journal of Affective Disorders, 82(2)*, 217–225.

Chivers-Wilson, K. A. (2006). Sexual assault and posttraumatic stress disorder: A review of the biological, psychological and sociological factors and treatments. *McGill Journal of Medicine, 9(2)*, 111–118.

Chwastiak, L. A., Rosenheck, R. A., McEvoy, J. P., Stroup, T. S., Swartz, M. S., Davis, S. M., & Lieberman, J. A. (2009). The impact of obesity on health care costs among persons with schizophrenia. *General Hospital Psychiatry, 31(1)*, 1.

Cicchetti, D. (2010). Resilience under conditions of extreme stress: A multilevel perspective. *World Psychiatry, 9(3)*, 145–154.

Clarke, H., Flint, J., Attwood, A. S., & Munafò, M. R. (2010). Association of the 5- HTTLPR genotype and unipolar depression: a meta-analysis. *Psychological medicine, 40(11)*, 1767–1778. https://doi.org/10.1017/S0033291710000516

Colodro-Conde, L., Couvey-Duchesne, B., Zhu, G., Conventry, W. L., Byrne, E. M., Gordon, S., et al. (2018). A direct test of the diathesis-stress model for depression. *Molecular Psychiatry, 23(7)*, 1590–1596.

Colton, C. W., & Manderscheid, R. W. (2006). Congruencies in increased mortality rates, years of potential life lost and causes of death among public mental health clients in eight states. *Preventing Chronic Disease, 3*, 2.

Croft, B., & Parish, S. L. (2013). Care integration in the patient protection and affordable care act: Implications for behavioral health. *Administration and Policy in Mental Health., 40(4)*. https://doi.org/10.1007/s10488-012-0405-0.

Commission on Social Determinants of Health (CSDH) (2008). Closing the gap in a generation: Health equity through action on the social determinants of health. In *Final report of the commission on social determinants of health*. Geneva: World Health Organization.

Cuevas, C. A., Sabina, C., & Bell, K. A. (2012). The effect of acculturation and immigration on the victimization and psychological distress link in a national sample of Latino women. *Journal of Interpersonal Violence, 27(8)*, 1428–1456.

Curtin, S. C., Warner, M., & Hedegaard, H. (2016). Increase in suicide in the United States, 1999–2014. *NCHS Data Brief, 241*, 1–8.

Cutrona, C. E., Russell, D. W., Brown, P. A., Clark, L. A., Hessling, R. M., & Gardner, K. A. (2005). Neighborhood context, personality, and stressful life events as predictors of depression among African American Women. *Journal of Abnormal Psychology, 114(1)*, 3–15.

Cutrona, C. E., Wallace, G., & Wesner, K. A. (2006). Neighborhood characteristics and depression—An examination of stress processes. *Current Directions in Psychological Science, 15(4)*, 188–192.

Dickerson, F., Brown, C. H., Fang, L., Goldberg, R. W., Kreyenbuhl, J., Wohlheiter, K., & Dixon, L. (2008). Quality of life in individuals with serious mental illness and type 2 diabetes. *Psychosomatics, 49(2)*, 109–114.

Dong, M., Giles, W. H., Felitti, V. J., Dube, S. R., Williams, J. E., Chapman, D. P., & Anda, R. F. (2004). Insights into causal pathways for ischemic heart disease: Adverse childhood experiences study. *Circulation, 110*, 1761–1766.

Donnon, T., & Hammond, W. (2007). Understanding the relationships between resiliency and bullying in adolescence: An assessment of youth resiliency from five urban junior high schools. *Child and Adolescent Psychiatry Clinics of North America, 16*, 449–472.

Druss, B. G., & Mauer, B. J. (2010). Health care reform and care at the behavioral health—primary care interface. *Psychiatric Services Washington DC., 61(11)*, 1087–1092. https://doi.org/10.1176/ps.2010.61.11.1087.

Druss, B. G., & Walker, E. R. (2011). *Mental disorders and medical comorbidity*. Robert Wood Johnson Foundation. The Synthesis Project. Synthesis Report # 21.

Druss, B. G., Marcus, S. C., Olfson, M., & Pincus, H. A. (2002). The most expensive medical conditions in America. *Health Affairs (Millwood), 21(4)*, 2002.

Dube, S. R., Anda, R. F., Felitti, V. J., Chapman, D. P., Williamson, D. F., & Giles, W. H. (2001). Childhood abuse, household dysfunction, and the risk of attempted suicide throughout the life span: Findings from the Adverse Childhood Experiences Study. *JAMA, 286(24)*, 3089–3096. https://doi.org/10.1001/jama.286.24.3089.

Dube, S. R., Felitti, V. J., Dong, M., Chapman, D. P., Giles, W. H., & Anda, R. F. (2003). Childhood abuse, neglect and household dysfunction and the risk of illicit drug use: The Adverse Childhood Experience Study. *Pediatrics, 111(3)*, 564–572.

Dube, S. R., Fairweather, D., Pearson, W. S., Felitti, V. J., Anda, R. F., & Croft, J. B. (2009). Cumulative childhood stress and autoimmune disease. *Psychosomatic Medicine, 71*, 243–250.

Eaton, W. W., Martins, S. S., Nestadt, G., Bienvenu, O. J., Clarke, D., & Alexandre, P. (2008). The burden of mental disorders. *Epidemiologic Reviews, 30(1)*, 1–14.

Edwards, V. J., Holden, G. W., Felitti, V. J., & Anda, R. F. (2003). Relationship between multiple forms of childhood maltreatment and adult mental health in community respondents: Results from the adverse childhood experiences study. *American Journal of Psychiatry, 160(8)*, 1453–1460.

Egede, L. E. (2007). Major depression in individuals with chronic medical disorders: Prevalence, correlates and association with health resource utilization, lost productivity and functional disability. *General Hospital Psychiatry, 29(5)*, 409–416.

Eisenman, D. P., Gelberg, L., Liu, H., & Shapiro, M. F. (2003). Mental health and health-related quality of life among adult Latino primary care patients living in the United States with previous exposure to political violence. *Journal of the American Medical Association, 290(5)*, 627–634.

Favreau, H., Bacon, S. L., Labrecque, M., & Lavoie, K. L. (2014). Prospective impact of panic disorder and panic anxiety on asthma control, health service use, and quality of life in adult patients with asthma over a 4-year follow-up. *Psychosomatic Medicine, 76*, 147.

Felitti, V. J., Anda, R. F., Nordenberg, D., Williamson, D. F., Spitz, A. M., Edwards, V., Koss, M. P., & Marks, J. S. (1998). Relationship of childhood abuse and household dysfunction to many of the leading causes of death in adults: The Adverse Childhood Experiences (ACE) study. *American Journal of Preventive Medicine, 14*(*4*), 245–258. https://doi.org/10.1016/S0749-3797(98)00017-8. PMID 9635069.

Ferrari, A. J., Charlson, F. J., Norman, R. E., et al. (2013). Burden of depressive disorders by country, sex, age, and year: Findings from the global burden of disease study 2010. *PLoS Medicine, 10*, e1001547.

Fortuna, L., Porche, M., & Alegria, M. (2008). Political violence, psychosocial trauma, and the context of mental health services among immigrant Latinos in the United States. *Ethnicity & Health, 13*, 435–463.

Foster, E. M., Jiang, M., & Gibson-Davis, C. M. (2010). The effect of the WIC program on the health of newborns. *Health Services and Research, 45*(*4*), 1083–1104.

Frank, D. A., Neault, N. B., Skalicky, A., Cook, J. T., Wilson, J. D., Levenson, S., et al. (2006). Heat or eat: The low income home energy assistance program and nutritional and health risks among children less than 3 years of age. *Pediatrics, 118*(*5*), e1293–e1302.

Garmezy, N. (1983). Stressors of childhood. In N. Garmezy & M. Rutter (Eds.), *Stress, coping, and development in children* (pp. 43–84). New York: McGraw-Hill.

Germain, C. B., & Gitterman, A. (2008). *The life model of social work practice* (3rd ed.). New York: Columbia University Press.

Goldstein, R. B., Smith, S. M., Chou, S. P., et al. (2016). The epidemiology of DSM-5 posttraumatic stress disorder in the United States: Results from the National Epidemiologic Survey on Alcohol and Related Conditions-III. *Social Psychiatry and Psychiatric Epidemiology, 51*, 1137.

Goodman, S. H., Rouse, M. H., Connell, A. M., Robbins Broth, M., Hall, C. M., & Heyward, D. (2011). Maternal depression and child psychopathology: A meta-analytic review. *Clinical Child and Family Psychology Review, 14*(*1*), 1–27.

Goodwin, R. D. (2003). Association between physical activity and mental disorders among adults in the United States. *Preventive Medicine, 36*(6), 698–703.

Grant, B. F., Saha, T. D., Ruan, W. J., Goldstein, R. B., Chou, S. P., et al. (2016). Epidemiology of DSM-5 drug use disorder: Results from the national Epidemiologic Survey on Alcohol and Related Conditions-III. *JAMA Psychiatry, 73*(*1*), 39–47. https://doi.org/10.1001/jamapsychiatry.2015.2132.

Greenberg, P. E., Fournier, A. A., Sisitsky, T., et al. (2015). The economic burden of adults with major depressive disorder in the United States (2005 and 2010). *Journal of Clinical Psychiatry, 76*, 155.

Gürhan, N., Beşer, N. G., Polat, Ü., et al. (2019). Suicide risk and depression in individuals with chronic illness. *Community Mental Health Journal, 55*, 840–848. https://doi.org/10.1007/s10597-019-00388-7.

Harper, S., & Lynch, J. (2007). Trends in socioeconomic inequalities in adult health behaviors among U.S. States, 1990–2004. *Public Health Reports, 122*(2), 177–189.

Hasin, D. S., Goodwin, R. D., Stinson, F. S., & Grant, B. F. (2005). Epidemiology of major depressive disorder: Results from the National Epidemiologic Survey on Alcoholism and Related Conditions. *Archives of General Psychiatry, 62*, 1097.

Hawton, K., Casanas i Comabella, C., Haw, C., & Saunders, K. (2013). Risk factors for suicide in individuals with depression: A systematic review. *Journal of Affective Disorders, 147*(1), 17–28.

Holman, E. A., Silver, R. C., & Waitzkin, H. (2000). Traumatic life events in primary care patients: A study in an ethnically diverse sample. *Archives of Family Medicine, 9*(9), 802.

Honkalampi, K., Hintikka, J., Haatainen, K., Koivumaa-Honkanen, H., Tanskanen, A., & Viinamaki, H. (2005). Adverse childhood experiences, stressful life events or demographic factors: Which are important in women's depression? A 2-year follow-up population study. *Australian and New Zealand Journal of Psychiatry, 39*(7), 627–632.

Huhtala, M., Korja, R., Lehtonen, L., Haataja, L., Lapinleimu, H., & Rautava, P. (2014). Associations between parental psychological wellbeing and socio-emotional development in 5-year-old preterm children. *Early Human Development, 90*(*3*), 119–124.

Institute of Medicine (2001). *Crossing the Quality Chasm: A New Health System for the 21st Century.* Washington, DC: National Academy Press.

James, S. E., Herman, J. L., Rankin, S., Keisling, M., Mottet, L., & Anafi, M. (2016). *The report of the 2015 U.S. Transgender Survey.* Washington, DC: National Center for Transgender Equality.

Kaltman, S., Green, B. L., Mete, M., Shara, N., & Miranda, J. (2010). Trauma, depression, and co-morbid PTSD/depression in a community sample of Latina immigrants. *Psychological Trauma: Theory, Research, Practice, and Policy, 2,* 29–31.

Karg, R. S., Bose, J., Batts, K. R., et al. (2014). *Past year mental disorders among adults in the United States: Results from the 2008–2012 Mental Health Surveillance Study.* Substance Abuse and Mental Health Services Administration, Center for Behavioral Health Statistics and Quality Data Review. http://www.samhsa.gov/data/sites/default/files/NSDUH-DR-N2MentalDis-2014-1/Web/NSDUH-DR-N2MentalDis-2014.pdf. Accessed 3 Mar 2020).

Katon, W. J. (2003). Clinical and health services relationships between major depression, depressive symptoms, and general medical illness. *Biological Psychiatry, 54*(3), 216–226.

Katon, W. J., Schoenbaum, M., Fan, M. Y., Callahan, C. M., Williams, J., Hunkeler, E., Harpole, L., Zhou, X. H., Langston, C., & Unutzer, J. (2005). Cost-effectiveness of improving primary care treatment of late-life depression. *Archives of General Psychiatry, 62*(12), 1313.

Kessler, R. C., Berglund, P., Demler, O., et al. (2005a). Lifetime prevalence and age-of-onset distributions of DSM-IV disorders in the National Comorbidity Survey Replication. *Archives of General Psychiatry, 62,* 593.

Kessler, R. C., Chiu, W. T., Demler, O., et al. (2005b). Prevalence, severity, and comorbidity of 12-month DSM-IV disorders in the National Comorbidity Survey Replication. *Archives of General Psychiatry, 62,* 617.

Kessler, R. C., Heeringa, S., Lakoma, M. D., Petukhova, M., Rupp, A. E., Schoenbaum, M., Wang, P. S., & Zaslavsky, A. M. (2008). Individual and societal effects of mental disorders on earnings in the United States: Results from the National Comorbidity Survey Replication. *American Journal of Psychiatry, 165*(6), 703–711.

Kessler, R. C., Birnbaum, H., Bromet, E., et al. (2010a). Age differences in major depression: Results from the National Comorbidity Survey Replication (NCS-R). *Psychological Medicine, 40,* 225.

Kessler, R. C., McLaughlin, K. A., Green, J. G., Gruber, M. J., Sampson, N. A., Zaslavsky, A. M., et al. (2010b). Childhood adversities and adult psychopathology in the WHO world mental health surveys. *British of Journal of Psychiatry, 197*(5), 378–385.

Kessler, R. C., Ormel, J., Petukhova, M., et al. (2011). Development of lifetime comorbidity in the World Health Organization world mental health surveys. *Archives of General Psychiatry, 68,* 90.

Khanani, I., Elam, J., Hearn, R., Jones, C., & Maseru, N. (2010). The impact of prenatal WIC participation on infant mortality and racial disparities. *American Journal of Public Health, 100*(*Suppl 1*), S204–S209.

Kim, J. W., Hye-Kyung, L., & Kounseok, L. (2013). Influence of temperament and character on resilience. *Comprehensive Psychiatry, 54*(7), 1105–1110.

Klebanov, P., & Brooks-Gunn, J. (2006). Cumulative, human capital, and psychological risk in the context of early intervention: Links with IQ at ages 3, 5, and 8. In B. M. Lester, A. S. Masten, & B. McEwen (Eds.), *Resilience in children* (pp. 63–82). Boston: Blackwell.

Kochanek, K. D., Murphy, S. L., Xu, J. Q., & Arias, E. (2019). *Death: Final data for 2017. National Vital Statistics Reports; vol 68 no 9.* Hyattsville: National Center for Health Statistics.

Kondo, N. (2012). Socioeconomic disparities and health: Impacts and pathways. *Journal of Epidemiology, 22*(*1*), 2–6. Epub 2011 Dec 10. https://doi.org/10.2188/jea.JE20110116.

Kronick, R. G., Bella, M., & Gilmer, T. P. (2009). *The faces of Medicaid III: Refining the protract of people with multiple chronic conditions.* Center for Health Care Strategies, Inc.,

Kuehner, C. (2017). Why is depression more common among women than among men? *Lancet Psychiatry, 4,* 146–158.

Labash, A. K., & Swartz, J. A. (2018). Demographic and clinical characteristics associated with trauma exposure among Latinas in primary medical care. *Journal of Ethnic & Cultural Diversity in Social Work*. https://doi.org/10.1080/15313204.2018.1449691.

Lamers, F., van Oppen, P., Comijs, H. C., et al. (2011). Comorbidity patterns of anxiety and depressive disorders in a large cohort study: The Netherlands Study of Depression and Anxiety (NESDA). *Journal of Clinical Psychiatry, 72*, 341.

Lantz, P. M., House, J. S., Lepkowski, J. M., Williams, D. R., Mero, R. P., & Chen, J. M. (1998). Socioeconomic factors, health behaviors, and mortality—Results from a Nationally Representative Prospective Study of US Adults. *Journal of the American Medical Association, 279*(21), 1703.

Lindsey, M. A., Sheftall, A. H., Xiao, Y., & Joe, S. (2019). Trends of suicidal behaviors among high school students in the United States: 1991-2017. *Pediatrics, 144*(5), e20191187. https://doi.org/10.1542/peds.2019-1187.

Lipson, S. K., Raifman, J., Abelson, S., & Reisner, S. L. (2019). Gender minority mental health in the U.S.: Results of a national survey on college campuses. *American Journal of Preventive Medicine, 57*(3), 293–301. https://doi.org/10.1016/j.amepre.2019.04.025.

Lorant, V., Deliege, D., Eaton, W., Robert, A., Philippot, P., & Ansseau, M. (2003). Socioeconomic inequalities in depression: A meta-analysis. *American Journal of Epidemiology, 157*, 2.

Ludwig, J., Sanbonmatsu, L., Gennetian, L., Adam, E., Duncan, G. J., Katz, L. F., et al. (2011). Neighborhoods, obesity, and diabetes—A randomized social experiment. *New England Journal of Medicine, 365*(16), 1509–1519.

Luthar, S. (Ed.). (2003). *Resilience and vulnerability: Adaptation in the context of childhood adversities*. Cambridge: Cambridge University Press.

Luoma, J. B., Martin, C. E., & Pearson, J. L. (2002). Contact with mental health and primary care providers before suicide: a review of the evidence. *The American journal of psychiatry, 159*(6), 909–916. https://doi.org/10.1176/appi.ajp.159.6.909

Luthar, S. S., Cicchetti, D., & Becker, B. (2000). The construct of resilience: A critical evaluation and guidelines for future work. *Child Development, 71*, 543–562.

Lyness, J. M., Niculescu, A., Tu, X., et al. (2006). The relationship of medical comorbidity and depression in older, primary care patients. *Psychosomatics, 47*, 435.

Malhi, G. S., & Mann, J. J. (2018). Depression. *Lancet, 392*, 2299.

Mancini, M. A., & Farina, A. S.J. (Epub ahead of print December 17, 2019). Co-morbid mental health issues in a clinical sample of Latinx adults: Implications for integrated behavioral health treatment. *Journal of Ethnic & Cultural Diversity in Social Work*, https://doi.org/10.1080/15313204.2019.1702132

Marmot, M. (2005). Social determinants of health inequalities. *Lancet, 365*, 1099–1104. https://doi.org/10.1016/S0140-6736(05)74234-3.

Marmot, M. G., & Bell, R. (2009). Action on health disparities in the United States: Commission on Social Determinants of Health. *JAMA, 301*(11), 1169–1171.

Marmot, M., Friel, S., Bell, R., Houwelling, T. A., Taylor, S., & Commission on Social Determinants of Health. (2008). Closing the gap in a generation: Health equity through action on social determinants of health. *Lancet, 372*(9650), 1661–1669. https://doi.org/10.1016/S0140-6736(08)61690-6.

Masten, A. (2001). Ordinary magic: Resilience processes in development. *American Psychologist, 56*, 227–238.

Masten, A. S., & Coatsworth, J. D. (1998). The development of competence in favorable and unfavorable environments: Lessons from research on successful children. *American Psychologist, 53*(2), 205–220.

Mechanic, D. (2012). Seizing opportunities under the Affordable Care Act for transforming the mental and behavioral health system. *Health 59 Affairs (Project Hope), 31*(2), 376–382. https://doi.org/10.1377/hlthaff.2011.0623.

Mojtabai, R., Olfson, M., & Han, B. (2016). National trends in the prevalence and treatment of depression in adolescents and young adults. *Pediatrics, 138*, 9.

Monroe, S. M., & Simons, A. D. (1991). Diathesis-stress theories in the context of life stress research: Implications for the depressive disorders. *Psychological Bulletin, 110*, 406–425.

Murray, C. J., Atkinson, C., Bhalla, K., et al. (2013). The state of US health, 1990-2010: Burden of diseases, injuries, and risk factors. *JAMA, 310*, 591.

Myers, H. F., Ullman, J. B., Wyatt, G. E., Loeb, T. B., Chin, D., Prause, N., Zhang, M., Williams, J. K., Slavich, G. M., & Liu, H. (2015). Cumulative burden of lifetime adversities: Trauma and mental health in low-SES African Americans and Latino/as. *Psychological Trauma: Theory, Research, Practice, and Policy, 7(3)*, 243–251.

National Academies of Sciences, Engineering, and Medicine. (2019). *Integrating social care into the delivery of health care: Moving upstream to improve the nation's health*. Washington, DC: The National Academies Press. https://doi.org/10.17226/25467.

National Partnership for Action: HHS Action Plan to Reduce Racial and Ethnic Health Disparities, 2011; and The National Stakeholder Strategy for Achieving Health Equity, 2011. Available from: http://minorityhealth.hhs.gov/npa

Nuruzzaman, N., Broadwin, M., Kourouma, K., & Olson, D. P. (2015). Making the social determinants of health a routine part of medical care. *Journal of Health Care for the Poor and Underserved, 26(2)*, 321–327.

Pearson, A., Saini, P., Da Cruz, D., Miles, C., While, D., Swinson, N., Williams, A., Shaw, J., Appleby, L., & Kapur, N. (2009). Primary care contact prior to suicide in individuals with mental illness. *The British journal of general practice : the journal of the Royal College of General Practitioners, 59*(568), 825–832. https://doi.org/10.3399/bjgp09X472881

Perou, R., Bitsko, R. H., Blumberg, S. J., et al. (2013). Mental health surveillance among children—United States, 2005-2011. *MMWR Suppl., 62*, 1.

Phelan, J. C., Link, B. G., Diez-Roux, A., Kawachi, I., & Levin, B. (2004). Fundamental causes' of social inequalities in mortality: A test of the theory. *Journal of Health and Social Behavior, 45*(3), 265–285.

Pickett, K. E., & Pearl, M. (2001). Multilevel analyses of neighbourhood socioeconomic context and health outcomes: A critical review. *Journal of Epidemiology and Community Health, 55*, 2.

Pirkis, J., & Burgess, P. (1998). Suicide and recency of health care contacts. A systematic review. *Br J Psychiatry., 173*, 462–474. https://doi.org/10.1192/bjp.173.6.462.

Price, J. H., & Khubchandani, J. (2019). The changing characteristics of African-American adolescent suicides, 2001–2017. *Journal of Community Health, 44*(4), 756–763. https://doi.org/10.1007/s10900-019-00678-x.

Reiss, F. (2013). Socioeconomic inequalities and mental health problems in children and adolescents: A systematic review. *Social Science Medicine, 90*, 24–31.

Resnick, M. D., Harris, L. J., & Blum, R. W. (1993). The impact of caring and connectedness on adolescent health and well-being. *Journal of Paediatrics and Child Health, 29*(Suppl 1), S3–S9. https://doi.org/10.1111/j.1440-1754.1993.tb02257.x.

Roberts, A. L., Agnew-Blais, J. S., Spiegelman, D., Kubzansky, L. D., Mason, S. M., et al. (2015). Posttraumatic stress disorder and incidence of type 2 diabetes mellitus in a sample of women: A 22 year longitudinal study. *JAMA Psychiatry, 72*(3), 203–210.

Robertson, E. B., David, S. L., & Rao, S. A. (2003). *Preventing drug use among children and adolescents: A research-based guide for parents, educators and community leaders* (2nd ed.). Washington, DC: National Institute on Drug Abuse.

Rutter, M. (1987). Psychosocial resilience and protective mechanisms. *American Journal of Orthopsychiatry, 57*, 316–331.

Rutter, M. (2006). Implications of resilience concepts for scientific understanding. *Annals of the New York Academy of Sciences, 1094*, 1–12.

Scherrer, J. F., Salas, J., Norman, S. B., Schnurr, P. P., Chard, K. M, …, Lustman, P. J. (2019). Association between clinically meaningful post traumatic stress disorder improvement and risk of type 2 diabetes. *JAMA Psychiatry*. https://doi.org/10.1001/jamapsychiatry.2019.2096. [Epub ahead of print].

Schoenbaum, M., Unutzer, J., Sherbourne, C., Duan, N., Rubenstein, L. V., Miranda, J., Meredith, L. S., Carney, M. F., & Wells, K. (2001). Cost-effectiveness of practice-initiated quality improvement for depression: Results of a randomized controlled trial. *Journal of the American Medical Association, 286(11)*, 1325.

Schoeni, R. F., House, J. S., Kaplan, G. A., & Pollack, H. (2008). *Making Americans healthier: Social and economic policy as health policy.* New York: Russell Sage Foundation.

Schulberg, H. C., Mulsant, B., Schulz, R., et al. (1998). Characteristics and course of major depression in older primary care patients. *International Journal Psychiatry in Medicine, 28*, 421.

Scott, K. M., Lim, C., Al-Hamzawi, A., Alonso, J., Bruffaerts, R., Caldas-de-Almeida, J. M., Florescu, S., et al. (2016). Association of mental disorders with subsequent chronic physical conditions: World mental health surveys from 17 countries. *JAMA Psychiatry, 73(2)*, 150–158. https://doi.org/10.1001/jamapsychiatry.2015.2688.

Seedat, S., Scott, K. M., Angermeyer, M. C., et al. (2009). Cross-national associations between gender and mental disorders in the World Health Organization World Mental Health Surveys. *Archives of General Psychiatry, 66*, 785.

Shim, R. S., Koplan, C., Langheim, F. J. P., et al. (2012). Health care reform and integrated care: A golden opportunity for preventive psychiatry. *Psychiatric Services, 63(12)*, 1231–1233. https://doi.org/10.1176/appi.ps.201200072.

Simon, G. E., VonKorff, M., Rutter, C., & Wagner, E. (2000). Randomised trial of monitoring, feedback, and management of care by telephone to improve treatment of depression in primary care. *British Medical Journal, 320*, 7234.

Smith, D. J., Court, H., McLean, G., et al. (2014). Depression and multimorbidity: A cross-sectional study of 1,751,841 patients in primary care. *Journal of Clinical Psychiatry, 75*, 1202.

Sroufe, L. A., Egeland, B., Carlsn, E. A., & Collins, W. A. (2005). *The development of the person: The Minnesota study of risk and adaptation from birth to adulthood.* New York: Guilford.

Stone, D. M., Simon, T. R., Fowler, K. A., Kegler, S. R., Yuan, K., Holland, K. M., Ivey-Stephenson, A. Z., & Crosby, A. E. (2018). Vital Signs: Trends in State Suicide Rates - United States, 1999–2016 and Circumstances Contributing to Suicide - 27 States, 2015. MMWR. *Morbidity and mortality weekly report, 67(22)*, 617–624. https://doi.org/10.15585/mmwr.mm6722a1

Steel, Z., Chey, T., Silove, D., Marnane, C., Bryant, R. A., & van Ommeren, M. (2009). Association of torture and other potentially traumatic events with mental health outcomes among populations exposed to mass conflict and displacement: A systematic review and meta-analysis. *JAMA, 302(5)*, 537–549. https://doi.org/10.1001/jama.2009.1132.

Stein, M. B., Cox, B. J., Afifi, T. O., Belik, S. L., & Sareen, J. (2006). Does co-morbid depressive illness magnify the impact of chronic physical illness? A population-based perspective. *Psychological Medicine, 36(5)*, 587.

Stein, D. J., Aguilar-Gaxiola, S., Alonso, J., et al. (2014). Associations between mental disorders and subsequent onset of hypertension. *General Hospital Psychiatry, 36*, 142.

Strine, T. W., Dube, S. R., Edwards, V. J., Prehn, A. W., Rasmussen, S., Wagenfeld, M., Dhingra, S., & Croft, J. B. (2012). Associations between adverse childhood experiences, psychological distress, and adult alcohol problems. *American Journal of Health Behaviors, 36(3)*, 408–423.

Studdert, D. M., Zhang, Y., Swanson, S. A., Prince, L., Rodden, J. A., Holsinger, E. E., & Miller, M. (2020). Handgun ownership and suicide in California. *New England Journal of Medicine, 382*, 2220–2229.

Substance Abuse and Mental Health Services Administration. (2019). *Key substance use and mental health indicators in the United States: Results from the 2018 National Survey on Drug Use and Health* (HHS Publication No. PEP19-5068, NSDUH Series H-54). Rockville, MD: Center for Behavioral Health Statistics and Quality, Substance Abuse and Mental Health Services Administration. Retrieved from https://www.samhsa.gov/data/

Substance Abuse and Mental Health Services Administration. (2020). *The 2018 National Survey on drug use and health: Lesbian, Gay, & Bisexual (LGB) Adults* (HHS Publication No. PEP19-5068, NSDUH Series H-54). Rockville, MD: Center for Behavioral Health Statistics and Quality, Substance Abuse and Mental Health Services Administration. Retrieved from https://www.samhsa.gov/data/

Substance Abuse and Mental Health Services Administration, Center for Mental Health Services. (2007). *Promotion and prevention in mental health: Strengthening parenting and enhancing child resilience.* DHHS Publication No. CMHS-SVP-0175. Rockville, MD.

Sumner, J. C., Kubzansky, L. D., Roberts, A. L., Gilsanz, P., Chen, Q., et al. (2016). Post-traumatic stress disorder symptoms and risk of hypertension over 22 years in a large cohort of younger and middle aged women. *Psychological Medicine, 46*(15), 3105–3116.

Thielke, S., Vannoy, S., & Unutzer, J. (2007). Integrating mental health and primary care. *Primary Care, 34*(3), 571–592.

Tully, P. J., Cosh, S. M., & Baune, B. T. (2013). A review of the affects of worry and generalized anxiety disorder upon cardiovascular health and coronary heart disease. *Psychological Health & Medicine, 18*, 627.

Tully, P. J., Turnbull, D. A., Beltrame, J., et al. (2015). Panic disorder and incident coronary heart disease: A systematic review and meta-regression in 1131612 persons and 58111 cardiac events. *Psychological Medicine, 45*, 2909.

Ulibarri, M. D., Ulloa, E. C., & Salazar, M. (2015). Associations between mental health, substance use, and sexual abuse experiences among Latinas. *Journal of Child Sexual Abuse, 24*(1), 35–54.

Ungar, M. (2008). Resilience across cultures. *British Journal of Social Work, 38*, 218–235.

Ungar, M. (2011). The social ecology of resilience: Addressing contextual and cultural ambiguity of a nascent construct. *American Journal of Orthopsychiatry, 81*(1), 1–17.

Valderas, J. M., Starfield, B., Sibbald, B., Salisbury, C., & Roland, M. (2009). Defining comorbidity: Implications for understanding health and health services. *Annals of Family Medicine, 7*(4), 357–363.

Vancampfort, D., Correll, C. U., Wampers, M., et al. (2014). Metabolic syndrome and metabolic abnormalities in patients with major depressive disorder: A meta-analysis of prevalence and moderating variables. *Psychological Medicine, 44*, 2017.

Vilsaint, C. L., NeMoyer, A., Fillbrunn, M., Sadikova, E., Kessler, R. C., et al. (2019). Racial ethnic difference in 23 month prevalence and persistence of mood, anxiety, and substance use disorders: Variation by nativity and socioeconomic status. *Comprehensive Psychiatry, 89*, 52–60.

Viola, D., Arno, P. S., Maroko, A. R., Schechter, C. B., Sohler, N., Rundle, A., et al. (2013). Overweight and obesity: Can we reconcile evidence about supermarkets and fast food retailers for public health policy? *Journal of Public Health Policy, 34*(3), 424–438.

Vos, T., Barber, R. M., Bell, B., Bertozzi-Villa, A., Biryukov, S., Bolliger, I., et al. (2015). Global, regional, and national incidence, prevalence, and years lived with disability for 301 acute and chronic diseases and injuries in 188 countries, 1990–2013: A systematic analysis for the Global Burden of Disease Study 2013. *Lancet, 386*(9995), 743–800. https://doi.org/10.1016/S0140-6736(15)606.

Wagner, E. H., Austin, B. T., & VonKorff, M. (1996). Organizing care for patients with chronic illness. *Milbank Quarterly, 74*(4), 511–544.

Wagner, E. H., Austin, B. T., Davis, C., Hindmarsh, M., Schaefer, J., & Bonomi, A. (2001). Improving chronic illness care: Translating evidence into action. *Health Affairs, 20*(6), 64.

Walker, E. R., & Druss, B. G. (2016). A public health perspective on mental and medical comorbidity. *JAMA, 316*(10), 1104–1105. https://doi.org/10.1001/jama.2016.10486.

Wang, F., Wang, S., Zong, Q. Q., Zhang, Q., Ng, C. H., Ungvari, G. S., & Xiang, Y. T. (2019). Prevalence of comorbid major depressive disorder in Type 2 Diabetes: A meta-analysis of comparative and epidemiological studies. *Diabetic Medicine, 36*(8), 961–969. https://doi.org/10.1111/dme.14042.

Werner, E. E., & Smith, R. S. (1982). *Vulnerable but invincible: A longitudinal study of resilient children and youth.* New York: McGraw-Hill.

Werner, E. E., & Smith, R. S. (2001). *Journeys from childhood to midlife: Risk, resilience, and recovery.* Ithaca: Cornell University Press.

Whiteford, H. A., Degenhardt, L., Rehm, J., Baxter, A. J., Ferrari, A. J., et al. (2013). Global burden of disease attributable to mental and substance use disorders. Findings from the global burden of disease study 2010. *Lancet, 382*(*9904*), 1575–1586. https://doi.org/10.1016/S0140-6736(13)61611-6.

Whitfield, C. L., Anda, R. F., Dube, S. R., & Felitti, V. J. (2003). Violent childhood experiences and the risk of intimate partner violence in adults: Assessment in a large health maintenance organization. *Journal of Interpersonal Violence, 18*(2), 166–185.

Williams, D. R., González, H. M., Neighbors, H., et al. (2007). Prevalence and distribution of major depressive disorder in African Americans, Caribbean blacks, and non-Hispanic whites: Results from the National Survey of American Life. *Archives General Psychiatry, 64*, 305.

Williamson, D. F., Thompson, T. J., Anda, R. F., Dietz, W. H., & Felitti, V. J. (2002). Body weight, obesity, and self-reported abuse in childhood. *International Journal of Obesity, 26*, 1075–1082.

Woolf, S. H., & Braveman, P. (2011). Where health disparities begin: The role of social and economic determinants—and why current policies may make matters worse. *Health Affairs (Millwood), 30*(10), 1852–1859.

World Health Organization (2017). Depression and Other Common Mental Disorders: Global Health Estimates. Geneva: License: CC BY-NC-SA 3.0 IGO.

Young, J. Q., Kline-Simon, A. H., Mordecai, D. J., & Weisner, C. (2015). Prevalence of behavioral health disorders and associated chronic disease burden in a commercially insured health system: Findings of a case-control study. *General Hospital Psychiatry, 37*(2), 101–108. https://doi.org/10.1016/j.genhosppsych.2014.12.005.113.

Zimmerman, M., McGlinchey, J. B., Chelminski, I., & Young, D. (2008). Diagnostic co-morbidity in 2300 psychiatric out-patients presenting for treatment evaluated with a semi-structured diagnostic interview. *Psychological Medicine, 38*, 199.

Chapter 3
Models of Change and Well-Being from Behavioral Health Disorders

3.1 Overview to Theories of Change and Well-Being

The ultimate goal of integrated behavioral health practice is to help people achieve a state of well-being. Well-being is dynamic and multidimensional. It involves individual behavior change, a sense of personal self-efficacy and empowerment, positive interpersonal relationships and support, access to basic resources and treatment, and opportunities for meaningful engagement in the community. All of these factors interact and reinforce each other to lead to whole health. Providers of behavioral health services play varying roles in promoting each of these areas in the way they engage with clients, how they assess their needs, and how they plan and treat identified areas of intervention. This chapter will help providers understand how people change and what psychosocial factors promote and hinder their recovery and wellness. It will outline the practices that lead to recovery and wellness as well as the practices that can get in the way of progress.

In the first part of this chapter, I review a set of theories focused on recovery and well-being. The first theory in this set, the mental health recovery model (Slade 2009; Leamy et al. 2011; Mancini 2006; Mancini et al. 2005), proposes that recovery from behavioral health disorders is a multidimensional process that involves developing insight, a positive sense of self, social support, wellness skills, and developing a sense of meaning and purpose in one's life (Leamy et al. 2011; Mancini 2003, 2006; Mancini et al. 2005, 2008). The second theory in this set is the theory of subjective well-being. Subjective well-being (Diener 1984) is a theory that posits that well-being is comprised of three concepts: (1) high life satisfaction; (2) high positive affect (feeling good); and (3) limited or low negative affect (feeling bad). The third theory is the theory of psychological well-being (Ryff 2014). This theory views well-being as the achievement of a life of meaning and personal growth. I discuss how these theories can orient providers toward practices that enhance recovery and well-being, and to avoid practices that can interfere with their clients' pursuit of health.

© Springer Nature Switzerland AG 2021
M. A. Mancini, *Integrated Behavioral Health Practice*,
https://doi.org/10.1007/978-3-030-59659-0_3

In the second part of this chapter, I review three theories that help us understand the process of how people change health-related behaviors. The first theory is the transtheoretical model of change (Prochaska et al. 1992), which posits that people go through a series of stages as they consider change and that interventions should be tailored to match a person's particular stage of change. The second is the theory of reasoned action (Ajzen and Fishbein 1980), which posits that behavior is the result of intention, attitudes, and norms regarding a particular target behavior. The third theory of change that I review is the health belief model (Janz and Becker 1984), which posits that people change their behaviors to the degree they understand the amount of risk they are exposed to, and how much control they have to reduce their risk exposure. At the end of each section, I identify common practices and interventions that are relevant to each set of theories. For instance, I provide an overview of practices and interventions that are recovery-oriented and focus on helping people achieve a state of well-being beyond symptom remission. I also provide an overview of interventions that are stage-based, that is, interventions that are responsive to, and aligned with, a person's particular stage of change and that are most likely to be effective in helping people take up the behaviors that promote health and leave unhealthy behaviors behind.

3.2   Theories of Recovery and Well-Being

Well-being has been the focus of research and inquiry for much of recorded history. The Buddha described well-being as a state of joy and emptiness embodied as freedom from suffering rooted in craving and desire. The Buddha believed that we all have the power to achieve joy and well-being in the here and now. All we have to do is change how we think. Or perhaps more precisely, stop thinking so much about the past and the future and just focus on the present moment—letting go of desire and grasping to achieve a state of loving kindness toward oneself and all beings. This concept is the root of positive psychology and cognitive behavioral therapy—two theoretical approaches to practice that are central to this text.

More recently, Aristotle explored two types of well-being: hedonic and eudemonic. He characterized *hedonic* well-being as simply the experience of pleasure and the absence of pain. This is most closely aligned with the psychological concept of *subjective well-being* (Diener 1984). Aristotle characterized *eudemonic* well-being as a type of happiness rooted in an authentic, functional life characterized as possessing a deep sense of meaning, purpose, competence, and quality relationships. This is most closely aligned with the concept of *psychological well-being* and the *mental health recovery model* (Ryff 2014; Slade 2009). In this section, I review each of these models in order to demystify well-being, identify the contexts that contribute to establishing well-being, and to frame our practice moving forward in this text.

3.2.1 The Recovery Model

3.2.1.1 Recovery Overview

The emergence of the recovery model approximately three decades ago dispelled long held myths about the chronicity of serious behavioral health disorders. Since that time, the mental health recovery model has been a vision guiding behavioral health service development for persons with serious psychiatric disabilities, such as major depression, anxiety, schizophrenia spectrum disorders, and bipolar spectrum disorders. The recovery model is comprised of at least three strands of scholarship. One area of scholarship emerged from the convergence of results of several longitudinal studies that discovered that recovery from severe forms of psychiatric distress was common and expected (Harding et al. 1987). The second area of scholarship was on the emergence of evidence-based, recovery-oriented practices within the field of psychiatric rehabilitation that were found to lead to positive outcomes for persons with serious mental illness. These psychiatric rehabilitation treatments were found to help improve outcomes in the areas of employment, independent living, co-occurring substance use disorders, social skills, family relationships, and wellness skills (Anthony 1993; Drake et al. 2005). The third area of influence was the rise of the consumer, survivor, ex-patient (CSX) movement. This is a diverse, multifaceted social justice movement comprised of former and current recipients of mental health services and their allies. Engaged scholarship and activism from this movement led to the widespread recognition of the stigma, oppression, and human rights abuses endured by persons with psychiatric disabilities. The CSX movement continues to fight for mental health policies and service systems based on human rights, self-determination, and choice among a wide range of professional and non-professional treatment alternatives (Chamberlin 1988; Deegan 1997).

The concept of mental health recovery consists of complex and overlapping perspectives and orientations (Davidson et al. 2009; Slade 2009). Two domains of recovery have emerged. The first domain is *clinical* recovery. Clinical recovery is rooted in the medical model of illness. This form of recovery is defined as the achievement of a set of objective, measurable clinical outcomes, such as stabilization or remission of psychiatric symptoms or reduced psychiatric hospitalizations (Davidson et al. 2009; Slade 2009). A second domain of recovery and the focus of this section has been labeled *social or personal recovery* (Slade 2009). This model of mental health recovery is rooted in personal accounts from persons with lived experience of psychiatric disability and recovery and position recovery as a complex, multidimensional, and subjective journey of growth, healing, and transformation (Leamy et al. 2011; Mancini et al. 2005). This process involves overcoming the social and functional impacts of mental illness to achieve a positive sense of self and a life of purpose, hope, empowerment, meaningful relationships, authenticity, self-determination, and holistic well-being (Anthony 1993; Leamy et al. 2011; Mancini et al. 2005; Mancini 2006; Slade 2009). One of the most widely cited definitions of recovery is one offered by Anthony (1993). He describes recovery as:

"...a deeply personal, unique process of changing one's attitudes, vales, feelings, goals, skills, and/or roles. It is a way of living a satisfying, hopeful, and contributing life even within the limitations caused by illness. Recovery involves the development of new meaning and purpose in one's life as one grows beyond the catastrophic effects of mental illness." (pg. 17)

In this perspective, recovery is more than an outcome that results from the application of specific interventions or practices. It is a process of (re)establishing one's life and place in the world. Recovery involves more than symptom management. It is the development of pursuits, interests, and relationships and the sense of mastery and self-efficacy that follows. It is living life on one's own terms and embracing the personal responsibility that comes with that level of autonomy and self-determination (Mancini 2007).

3.2.1.2   Factors That Facilitate and Hinder Recovery

Several elements comprise the recovery process. Figure 3.1 displays the main processes that comprise recovery that will be discussed below. The first element is that recovery is a process of moving from a psychological place of exclusion, internalized stigma and despair to a place of inclusion, hopefulness, and well-being (Dell et al. In Press; Mancini et al. 2005; Mancini 2006). Systematic reviews have identified several components of the recovery process. Ellison et al. (2018) synthesized systematic and other literature reviews and found that recovery was conceptualized as emerging from empowerment, person-centered practice, meaning and purpose, and hope for the future. Likewise, other reviews on recovery have found broad

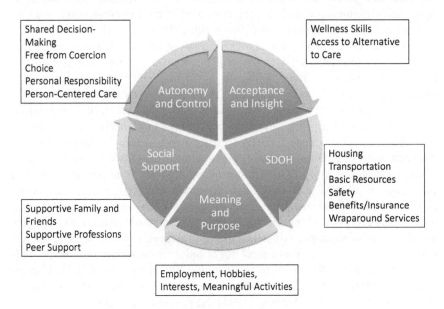

Fig. 3.1 Domains of recovery (Based on Dell et al. In Press)

support for the CHIME framework of recovery (Dell et al. Under Review; van Weeghel et al. 2019). The CHIME framework (Leamy et al. 2011) identifies five components of recovery: (1) *C*onnectedness with others through meaningful relationships; (2) *h*ope for the future; (3) development of a positive *i*dentity; (4) a sense of *m*eaning and purpose; and (5) *e*mpowerment (Leamy et al. 2011).

Recovery is largely a process of positive identity development or movement from a negative identity marked by internalized stigma, helplessness, and despair to an identity marked by self-efficacy, insight into one's illness and wellness, and acceptance of one's self. Persons diagnosed with behavioral health disorders often develop an internalized sense of stigma where they view themselves through the stigmatized lens of society (De Ruysscher et al. 2017; Leamy et al. 2011; McKenzie-Smith 2019; McCarthy-Jones et al. 2013). What leads to this negative sense of self is the experience of stigma from others, troubling symptoms, and lack of resources. For instance, a person with a behavioral health disorder struggles with confusing, scary, and debilitating symptoms. At the same time, they experience people withdrawing from them or communicating to them directly or indirectly that they are broken, deviant, incapable, and sick. Stigma for persons with behavioral health disorders is severe. This is even more true for Black, Indigenous, and People of Color (BIPOC); Transgender and Gender Nonconforming (TGNC) persons; and Lesbian, Gay, and Bisexual (LGB) persons with psychiatric disabilities. Stigma is not an abstract concept. A person with psychiatric disabilities can lose their autonomy over their affairs, be physically restrained and assaulted, have their children taken away, experience abandonment by their family, and experience harsh, disabling, or ineffective treatment from oppressive healthcare providers and systems. Persons with psychiatric disabilities can internalize stigma and oppression and become lost to themselves. How, then, does one (re)develop a sense of confidence, self-efficacy, and self-worth? How does one develop a sense of hope for the future? How does one believe in themselves again (or for the first time)? In other words, how does one enter into recovery? Several factors contributing to recovery have been identified.

Social Support Social isolation is the single most impactful risk factor preventing recovery in persons with behavioral health disorders. Positive relationships with family, friends, intimate partners, and peer and non-peer professionals have consistently been found to be a determining factor in recovery because they help people feel connected to the world and give people a sense of belonging. Positive relationships communicate to the person that they are valued and important. Relationships are also sources of practical support that include money, transportation, food, shelter, and connections to employment. Most importantly, relationships contribute to an internal sense of connection, which is a vital ingredient for recovery (De Ruysscher et al. 2017; Leamy et al. 2011; Lovell 2019; McCarthy-Jones et al. 2013; Temesgen et al. 2019).

Meaning and Purpose The development of meaning and purpose through relationships, activities, and the pursuit of positive social roles has also been identified as an important component of recovery (Clarke et al. 2016; De Ruysscher et al.

2017; Leamy et al. 2011; McKenzie-Smith 2019; McCarthy-Jones et al. 2013). The experience of mental illness can result in a life that is isolated and devoid of meaningful goals, functional roles, and pursuits. Recovery involves becoming a part of something bigger than one's self through developing pursuits through hobbies, professional development, employment, education, activism, volunteering, and participating in other enriching activities and groups (Mancini et al. 2005; Mancini 2006).

Autonomy and Control Autonomy, control, and personal responsibility are core elements of mental health recovery model (Clarke et al. 2016; De Ruysscher et al. 2017; Leamy et al. 2011; McCarthy-Jones et al. 2013). Autonomy and control mean having the freedom to make informed treatment decisions and life choices. Recovery cannot occur in environments where a person is helpless, powerless, coerced, paternalized, abused, or denied the liberty to make decisions about their life (Dell et al. In Press; Leamy et al. 2011; Lovell 2019; McKenzie-Smith 2019; McCarthy-Jones et al. 2013; Temesgen et al. 2019; Wood and Alsawy 2018). Recovery involves a life in which a person exercises *personal responsibility* and *self-determination* in their personal choices, pursuits, behaviors, and decisions. To have autonomy is to have power, to have control over one's fate and to be able to make decisions about one's life and treatment. Personal responsibility is about being accountable for the decisions one makes. It is about taking the necessary steps that either lead to recovery, or taking responsibility for the consequences of individual choices. This means that people can choose among a variety of treatment alternatives, are free to pursue their dreams and aspirations, and have control over the decisions of their lives in terms of where, with whom, and how to live.

Being a part of the mental health treatment system sometimes involves a loss of independence, being coerced into treatments and living arrangements, and enduring paternalism and false choices among a range of bad options. Treatment professionals sometimes encourage consumers to "play it safe" and avoid the stresses of work, independent living, and social networks and instead live less fulfilling lives in order to avoid relapses in symptoms. Advocates counter that recovery must be built around the pursuit of goals, taking personal responsibility for their actions and "getting a life" and all of which that entails. Recovery involves taking risks, reflection, and learning from successes and failures. Autonomy and control can be enhanced in treatment relationships with providers marked by collaboration, shared decision-making, and choice (Mancini et al. 2005).

Acceptance and Insight Becoming aware and enlightened about one's illness is one of the most important factors that lead to and maintain recovery. This enlightenment involves the development of insight into one's illness and acceptance of the illness as part of one's life that requires management and actions that promote and maintain wellness. Insight and acceptance are often initiated through access to person-centered and recovery-oriented services, settings, and providers. Recovery-oriented services are designed to serve a variety of bio-psycho-social domains of living, such as physical health, socialization, vocational pursuits, independent living, and psychiatric symptoms (De Ruysscher et al. 2017; Hine et al. 2018; Lovell

2019; McKenzie-Smith 2019; Ness et al. 2014; Ng et al. 2016; Richardson and Barkham 2020; Schön and Rosenberg 2013; Stuart et al. 2017; Temesgen et al. 2019; Woodgate et al. 2017).

Professionals that are recovery-oriented practice from a perspective of respect, collaboration, warmth, honesty, and are non-judgmental and supportive (Clarke et al. 2016; De Ruysscher et al. 2017; Lovell 2019; McCarthy-Jones et al. 2013; Slade et al. 2012; Woodgate et al. 2017). Peer providers represent important professionals in the development of acceptance and insight. Peer providers are persons who have a lived experience of mental illness and recovery and use that experience to help others with psychiatric disabilities. They can coach people on how to live with and manage the effects of the illness and are key sources of hope and insight (De Ruysscher et al. 2017; Mancini 2018; McKenzie-Smith 2019; McCarthy-Jones et al. 2013; Temesgen et al. 2019).

Developing insight and awareness is also dependent on having access to treatments and wellness strategies designed to manage symptoms and improve the person's ability to achieve and maintain holistic health (Dell et al. In Press; De Ruysscher et al. 2017; Kaite et al. 2015; Lovell 2019). While medications can be important strategies for wellness, it is important that clients have a relationship with professionals committed to shared decision-making and managing adverse effects from medication. Learning wellness skills and strategies from peer providers, supportive professionals, and through trial and error can lead to the development of an arsenal of effective strategies to maintain recovery.

Social Determinants of Health Recovery is not solely an internal process, but also requires access to resources, power, and safe environments. It is a process contingent on the dynamic interaction between the individual and their social and environmental contexts (Dell et al. In Press; Hine et al. 2018; Stuart et al. 2017; Wood and Alsawy 2018). It can only happen in an environment that is free from coercion, violence, and trauma and that include access to basic resources, services, opportunities, and connection (Clarke et al. 2016; Hine et al. 2018; Kaite et al. 2015; Lovell 2019; McCarthy-Jones et al. 2013; McKenzie-Smith 2019; Shepherd et al. 2016; Stuart et al. 2017). Inpatient and outpatient service settings and providers must operate from a trauma-informed lens and ensure clients feel secure and safe. Access to adequate income, affordable health care, transportation, adequate and stable housing, and basic resources such as clothing, food, and utilities provide the foundation to health and are essential to recovery.

3.2.1.3 Recovery-Oriented Practices That Promote Wellness

Recovery-oriented practice is characterized as being strength-based, person-centered, trauma-informed, and collaborative. Recovery-oriented practice and approaches are designed to engage clients and help them develop the skills, perspectives, and capacities needed to participate fully in the communities in which they choose to live. Recovery models focus on utilizing person-centered care dedicated to shared decision-making and engaging clients in treatments designed to help them achieve whole health (Adams and Grieder 2014; Berwick 2009; Stanhope and Ashenberg-Straussner 2018; Tondora et al. 2014). Several of these practices address social determinants of health such as housing stability, employment, safety, and access to basic resources as well as assist clients in developing the skills needed to live meaningfully in the community. Practices that address social determinants of health can improve health, increase care quality, and enhance client satisfaction while lowering healthcare costs (Andermann 2018; Kerman and Kidd 2020). Recovery-oriented approaches that meet these aims include supported employment (Kinoshita et al. 2013) and housing-first programs (Tsemberis et al. 2004) that can facilitate access to basic resources and lead to the development of meaning, purpose, and autonomy through employment, independent living, and recreational and volunteer pursuits.

Another recovery-oriented approach mentioned earlier includes services provided by peer professionals who have a lived experience of mental illness and recovery and use their personal stories and perspectives to help others in their recovery journeys (Mancini 2018, 2019). Peers build authentic and supportive relationships with clients and use their shared experiences to create a sense of hope and empowerment by providing a counter-narrative to the stigmatized stories people have developed about themselves. These counter-narratives help to dismantle the effects of internalized oppression often experienced by persons with behavioral health disorders (Mancini 2019; Mancini 2018). The utilization of peer-provided services may also promote better treatment engagement, social connections, and insight by helping people learn how to accept and manage their illness through the development of skills designed to promote well-being (Cook et al. 2013).

Families also play a vital role in the recovery process for persons with psychiatric disabilities. Family psychoeducation programs help families of persons with psychiatric disabilities develop a better understanding of behavioral health disorders and how these conditions impact the family and their loved ones. Family psychoeducation programs support families by: (1) increasing their knowledge about mental illness; (2), building their confidence, reducing their sense of isolation, and relieving stress; (3) providing them with the tools to understand what their loved one is going through and how to be better advocates and allies. These programs can improve family relationships, which can then lead to improved practical and emotional support for persons with behavioral health conditions (McFarlane 2016).

Recovery-oriented practices seek to help people with psychiatric disabilities achieve a holistic sense of well-being. As we will see, recovery-oriented approaches share several commonalities with theories of well-being that exist in the field of psychology. We turn to two of these theories, psychological and subjective well-being, next.

3.2.2 Theories of Well-Being

3.2.2.1 Well-Being Overview

Well-being has been a concept that has been studied in psychology for decades. The concept of well-being dates back to the third century when Aristotle conceptualized eudemonic and hedonic well-being. Hedonic well-being, or "feeling good," is the experience of positive emotion or pleasure and the avoidance of pain or negative emotion (Ryan and Deci 2001), while eudemonic well-being is the experience of a life rooted in meaning, achievement, and purpose. Psychological research has debated these to two forms of well-being for a long time. Hedonic well-being has been re-conceptualized as subjective well-being, while psychological well-being is a construct most aligned with eudemonic well-being. The field of positive psychology has been one forum where these debates have played out. We will not re-enact those debates here. Instead, we will consider the implications of subjective and psychological well-being for our practice and how they can help us assist the people we work with in their recoveries. It is important to understand the contextual factors that contribute to well-being so that providers can seek to educate their clients on how they can bring well-being about, and to know the social and environmental resources and contexts necessary to establish and maintain well-being.

3.2.2.2 Psychological Well-Being

As mentioned, the eudemonic view of well-being is living a life of meaning, purpose, and achievement (e.g., authenticity, truth, virtue, harmony, contemplation, personal development) (Ryan and Deci 2001). Psychological well-being (PWB) (Ryff 1989, 2014) is the view of well-being most closely associated with the eudemonic view of well-being. PWB is defined as living a functional life dedicated to meaning and personal growth (Ryff 1989). It is predicated on more than "feeling good," and involves six components including: (1) having a sense of purpose in life; (2) living life authentically and true to oneself (autonomy); (3) personal growth or living a life that maximizes one's talents; (4) environmental mastery or managing one's affairs with competence; (5) supportive, positive personal relationships; and (6) and self-acceptance or an accurate evaluation and acceptance of one's talents and shortcomings (Ryff 2014).

A person high in psychological well-being is autonomous; independent; unconcerned about how others see them; has a high level of self-efficacy in a multitude of domains; views themselves as continually developing; has a number of warm, trusting relationships with adults; has a sense of purpose in life; and has a positive view of themselves (e.g., self-esteem). In short, the person who experiences a high amount of psychological well-being is a person who is secure, independent, competent, engaged, purposeful, confident, and feels a sense of belonging as part of a community. A person low on psychological well-being is over-reliant on the judgment and evaluations of others, cannot manage their lives or take care of themselves, feels stuck, has few confidantes or trustworthy people in their lives, lack a sense of meaning or purpose in their lives, and lacks a general positive view of the self (Ryff 2014).

Research has also linked personality traits to psychological well-being. For instance, openness to experience was associated with personal growth, and agreeableness was associated with positive relationships with others. Extraversion was associated with mastery of the environment and conscientiousness was associated with purpose in life (Schmutte and Ryff 1997). Other variables are also associated with psychological well-being including optimism (Ferguson and Goodwin 2010), self-esteem (Paradise and Kernis 2002), and emotional regulation strategies (Gross and John 2003). Healthy behaviors such as proper exercise, good sleep, having a faith life, and having good friendships have been associated with increased psychological well-being and mental health more generally (Grzywacz and Keyes 2004). Further, those with high levels of psychological well-being have shown decreases in stress and inflammation via biological markers, such as cortisol and cytokine levels as well as better sleep and lower risk for cardiovascular disease (Ryff et al. 2004; Ryff 2014). Psychological (and subjective) well-being have both been shown to be associated with reduced risk for metabolic syndrome (Morozink-Boylan and Ryff 2015) and improved cardiovascular health (Boehm and Kubzansky 2012). Purpose in life has also been associated with reduced heart disease (Kim et al. 2012) and cerebrovascular disease (Kim et al. 2013). Major depression has been linked to low PWB (Keyes 2002).

3.2.2.3   Subjective Well-Being

The hedonic view of well-being is associated with the psychological concept of subjective well-being (SWB). Subjective well-being (Diener 1984) is associated with three concepts: (1) life satisfaction or how a person assesses their life as a whole and how satisfied they are with it; (2) positive affect or "feeling good"; and (3) the absence of negative affect or "feeling bad" (Metler and Busseri 2017). People who view their overall life as satisfactory and have a fair amount of positive affect and limited amounts of negative affect generally score highly on tests of subjective well-being. Personality traits positively associated with SWB include extroversion and agreeableness, while neuroticism was negatively correlated with SWB (DeNeve and Cooper 1998).

Research suggests that SWB and PWB are not dichotomous, but rather are components to a broader concept of well-being that also includes grit, hope, and a meaning orientation to happiness (Disabato et al. 2016). Research has found that hedonic and eudemonic well-being are largely correlated and are part of a broader concept of well-being that includes both experiencing pleasure and striving toward personal growth (Vittersø and Søholt 2011). In other words, subjective well-being (Diener 1984) and psychological well-being (Ryff 1989) may be parts of one overarching model of well-being. It appears that in regard to well-being, it is important have both a sense of satisfaction with life and a sense of meaning and purpose (2016).

Psychological and subjective well-being have parallels with the personal and clinical models of recovery discussed above. Subjective well-being may be more closely associated with clinical recovery due to its focus on reduction of negative symptoms and the improvement of positive affect. Psychological well-being, with its focus on meaning, relationships, and purpose, may be more aligned with the personal recovery model, suggesting that both may be necessary. Studies of depressed and anxious patients in symptom remission still showed low levels of PWB. This indicates that while reducing symptoms is important, it is not enough as a measure of recovery or well-being (Rafanelli et al. 2000; Fava et al. 2001; Ryff 2014). Well-being therapy in conjunction with cognitive behavioral therapy (CBT) provided sequentially after CBT has shown increases in PWB. Well-being therapy strategies have clients engage in tasks that help them focus on positive experiences and assist them in engaging in positive relationships and activities to encourage the elements of PWB (Fava 1999; Fava et al. 1998).

3.2.2.4   PERMA and Flourishing

Martin Seligman, a pioneer in the area of positive psychology, has proposed that human flourishing may be a combination of psychological and subjective well-being (2011). His model of well-being is comprised of five interrelated components using the acronym PERMA: (1) *P*ositive emotions (feeling good); (2) *E*ngagement or flow in activities; (3) positive, high-quality *R*elationships; (4) *M*eaning or a sense of being a part of something bigger than oneself; and (5) *A*chievement or grit in the face of frustrations (Seligman 2011). PERMA and SWB have been found to be highly correlated, suggesting that SWB may be an accurate way to measure well-being (or at least good enough) (Goodman et al. 2018). However, as Seligman has argued, measuring well-being is not the same as *building* well-being. He suggests that PERMA contains the elements that build well-being and are thus important concepts to consider when working with actual clients in practice (Seligman 2018). In this way, PERMA can be viewed as having clinical relevance in that the five elements are the building blocks of well-being rather than as a discreet form of well-being (Seligman 2018). Figure 3.2 outlines the main elements that comprise well-being from this perspective.

Several positive psychology interventions designed to enhance PWB, SWB, and reduce depression have been found to have positive and sustainable effects (Bolier et al. 2013). They suggest the importance of combining positive psychology interventions (PPI) with other problem-oriented interventions such as cognitive behavioral therapy, problem-solving therapy, and interpersonal therapy. These interventions include optimism and gratitude exercises (Boehm et al. 2011), practicing gratitude and counting blessings (Emmons and McCullough 2003), individual positive psychotherapy (Seligman et al. 2006), and other interventions such as active constructive responding, gratitude visits, life summary, and three good things exercises (Schueller and Parks 2012).

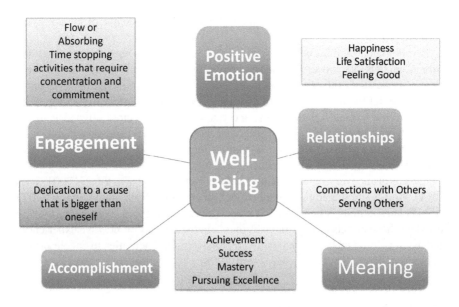

Fig. 3.2   Well-being

3.3   Model of Health Behavior Change

Achieving recovery and well-being often involves making changes in behavior away from unhealthy behaviors and habits toward healthier behaviors. This is often in areas where behavioral health providers can assist clients the most in their recovery journeys. Change involves several components including motivation, information, and support. In this section, I review three theories of health behavior change. The first theory is the transtheoretical model of change (Prochaska et al. 1992). This theory posits that people go through a series of stages in their motivation and intention to change. The second is the theory of reasoned action (Ajzen and Fishbein 1980), which posits that behavior is the result of a combination of intention, attitudes, and norms. The third theory of change is the health belief model (Janz and Becker 1984), which posits that people change their behaviors to the degree they are informed about their risk and susceptibility to a condition and how much confidence they have that they can change. In the sections that follow I will discuss the components of each theory and provide information about assessment and treatment practices relevant for each theory.

3.3.1 Transtheoretical Model of Change

The transtheoretical model of change (TTM) (Prochaska et al. 1992) has been one of the most utilized models of change in social work, medicine, public health, psychology, and addiction treatment. The central tenet of this model is that behavior change is dependent on people's readiness to change their behavior. The model has been used to understand and assess behavior change in relation to smoking, drinking, and drug use; adherence to medication; weight management; and diet adherence. The central concept of the model rests on the assumption that readiness to change progresses through a series of stages that include: *precontemplation, contemplation, preparation, action, and maintenance*. Providers can use these stages to inform treatment decisions and align selected interventions with a client's readiness to change resulting in a more effective approach to treatment (Prochaska et al. 1992). Table 3.1 outlines the stages of change and identifies stage-based practices that align with each stage.

A person in the *precontemplation* stage of change has no intention of changing their behaviors in the near future. People in precontemplation are often unaware that their behavior has health consequences, or are indifferent or unconcerned about the consequences of their behavior. A person in precontemplation is committed to the behavior and will actively resist efforts to change their mind or behavior. There is no ambivalence in their belief about continuing the behavior. If you asked a person about their intention to change a particular behavior their answer would be "No" or "I don't have a problem." There is little to no "change talk" and they have no intention to change (Prochaska et al. 1992). For instance, a client who is in precontemplation about their smoking may say when asked about their behavior, "I don't need to quit. I feel fine and my father smoked until he was in his 80s. I'm only 35 so I'm not worried about it." A person in precontemplation about their harmful drinking habits may state, "I work hard and I deserve to have a little fun once in a while. People need to just relax. I can handle my drinking. They have the problem, not me." People in precontemplation will often get defensive and resist suggestions to change behavior. People in precontemplation are *indifferent or resistant* to change.

Contemplation is a stage in which a person is seriously considering change in the next 6 months, but continues to weigh the benefits and risks of making a change in behavior. A person in *contemplation* demonstrates a degree of *ambivalence* toward change (e.g., not sure if they want to change or not) and acknowledges that they and/or their loved ones may experience negative consequences of a particular behavior. They may voice a desire to change, but admit that they don't know how to change or are unsure if they want to change. People in contemplation lack commitment and action around change (Prochaska et al. 1992). This stage is defined by *ambivalence*. A person may spend a long time in contemplation. In this stage a person may admit that they know they "should" (i.e., lose weight, exercise, eat healthier, stop smoking, reduce drinking, stop using drugs) and may intend to change in the future, but they have not made a plan, nor have they engaged in or committed any actions toward change. For instance, a person who screens positive for problem drinking

Table 3.1 Stages of change and stage-based interventions (Based on Prochaska et al. 1992)

Stage of change	Definition	Example	Stage-based interventions
Precontemplation	No intention to change behavior Commitment to behavior is high Ambivalence is low Little talk of change	Person says: I don't have a problem. They have the problem.	Outreach and engagement Empathic listening Build relationship Harm reduction Addressing practical needs Crisis interventions Continued assessment
Contemplation	Person has begun to consider change in the near future Ambivalence toward change is high in regard to confidence and/or importance No commitment to take action	Person says: I know I should probably stop (smoking, drinking, getting high, eating sweets), but I (like it, don't want to lose my friends, deserve to have a little fun…).	Motivational interviewing Brief motivational interventions Psychoeducation Build awareness of problem Decisional balance exercise Offer a menu of treatment options
Preparation	Person intends to take action soon and/or has taken initial steps toward action Seeking information May have set a date Intention is high	Person says: I need to do this. I'm tired and I need to make a change. I can't keep going on like this.	Motivational interventions Goal-setting/clarification Support client Consider and resolve potential barriers to success Provide access to treatment resources Problem-solving skill development Peer support/self-help Family support
Action	Committed to change Successful in modifying behavior for about 6 months. Person has achieved initial goals and/or clinical benchmarks Potential for relapse is high	Person may have quit smoking; lost weight; reduced or eliminated drinking, drug use, or other risk behaviors; and/or completed a treatment program.	Cognitive-behavioral treatments Skill development Substance abuse counseling Medication-assisted treatments. Relapse prevention Self-help/12-step programs Family support

(continued)

Table 3.1 (continued)

Stage of change	Definition	Example	Stage-based interventions
Maintenance	Person has sustained change for more than 6 months Continues make strides and consolidate successes Has accomplished goals for more than 6 months	Person has developed strong skills and a determined commitment to be well.	Continue relapse prevention. Continue self-help. Integration of healthy lifestyle behaviors into other areas of life

may acknowledge a need to cut down on their drinking for health or marital reasons, but may be concerned that they will lose friends or experience concern about giving up a favored activity despite its negative consequences. People in contemplation may be concerned about the amount of time, cost, effort, and negative consequences associated with engaging in an action or stopping an addictive behavior. As a result, they spend a lot of time considering the pros and cons of a particular action. In the example used above, a person in contemplation for their problem drinking may voice their ambivalence by saying things like: (1) "I know I should probably cut down, but I work hard and I think I deserve to blow off some steam once in a while"; or (2) "I would like to cut down, but I'm afraid I may lose my friends if I do." People in contemplation are *thinking* about change.

In the *preparation stage*, a person intends to take action soon (e.g., within the next month or two). It is a combination of the intention to take action and action itself in the form of small, incremental steps (Prochaska et al. 1992). Examples of small steps toward change can include cutting down on drinking or smoking, switching to a less harmful substance, eating healthier, exercising occasionally, researching or purchasing a gym membership, setting a date to change a behavior, setting up an appointment for treatment or a treatment consultation, or agreeing to go to therapy. This stage may also include people who have taken steps to change in the past year, but been unsuccessful in their attempts. In this stage, people are in a mixture of contemplation and action. They are *getting ready* for change and making small strides.

People in the *action stage* have successfully modified their behavior. Being in the action stage requires the achievement of certain criteria for a period of time that is less than 6 months. The action stage is defined by the achievement of advanced criteria through explicit change behaviors or efforts (Prochaska et al. 1992). They have entered and completed addiction or psychological treatment. They may have quit smoking, drinking, or drugs and have not used for several months. They may have successfully integrated a diet or treatment regimen into their routine. Or they have lost weight or achieved a particular clinical benchmark (e.g., cholesterol, glucose, T-cell, or blood pressure level). They are committed to change, have engaged in significant change efforts, and have achieved results. They are *doing* it.

In *maintenance* a person continues their change efforts and makes strides to consolidate and sustain gains (Prochaska et al. 1992). A person in the maintenance stage has achieved their criteria for at least six or more months and is now working on learning and executing relapse prevention efforts in order to maintain their gains. *They have done it and are trying to sustain and extend their gains.*

Three things are important to recognize in relation to the stages of change. First, a person may move backwards and forwards through the various stages of change. Successful attempts to change behavior typically involve relapse and repeated attempts to change. This is a normal part of the process and should not be considered as a failure, but as a learning opportunity. Relapse is an expectation and an opportunity to learn new strategies to gain future success. Second, each stage of change has a particular set of intervention strategies that are most effective. For instance, harm reduction, motivational and education strategies are most appropriate for persons in precontemplation (Mancini et al. 2008). In this stage, building awareness of the problem and ways to solve it, while also providing safer or less harmful alternatives to the behavior are important (e.g., needle exchange programs, carrying and knowing how to use Narcan, condom use). In contemplation, relevant approaches include brief interventions and motivational interviewing approaches that help people understand their ambivalence toward change and evaluate the pros and cons of continuing or changing the status quo. Helping motivate people toward making a decision about change would be the most effective approach in this stage. In preparation and action stages, a provider would use a combination of motivational interviewing strategies to continue to support change, and cognitive behavioral and other active treatment approaches to build skills and capacities to assist the person in their change efforts. Inpatient or outpatient treatment programs, self-help groups, cognitive behavioral approaches to therapy, nutritional support, and medication regimens are most effective in these stages. In maintenance, it is most important to give people the skills and tools to avoid relapse and maintain gains. This may also involve helping people change their lifestyles and environments, such as finding new social networks, moving locations, changing jobs, and establishing new routines to maintain health and prevent relapse. It may also involve learning new skills to manage cravings and avoid risky situations, learn assertiveness and problem solving skills in order to manage situations that can jeopardize their recovery, or learn new skills around employment, eating, sleeping, daily living, and relationships. It is important for behavior health agencies to integrate billing, records, assessment and treatment practices, and professional development activities that promote the routine and effective use of stage-based interventions when helping clients with behavioral health issues into their policies and procedures (Mancini and Linhorst 2010; Mancini and Miner 2013; Mancini and Wyrick-Waugh 2013).

Third, a person may simultaneously be in different stages of change for different behaviors. For instance, a person may be in preparation stage for their diabetes management plan, maintenance for past problem drinking behavior, and precontemplation for smoking marijuana. It is important to accurately assess a person's stage of change for each target behavior and adjust the approach for each target. A provider will have to blend approaches identified above to effectively address each target area. Also, if the engagement in one preferred behavior gets in the way of change efforts for other target behaviors, this will have to be made apparent to the client. For example, a person who actively wants to eliminate cocaine use and is in the action stage, but who also is in contemplation about their marijuana usage, may find that using marijuana triggers the craving associated with cocaine use. In this scenario it may not be possible for the person to successfully abstain from cocaine, while also using marijuana. This will need to be brought to light to the client and a plan of action developed.

3.3.2 Health Belief Model of Change

The origins of the Health Belief Model of Change (HBM) dates back to the 1950s, and was developed by social psychologists in the US Public Health Service as a means to develop a conceptual understanding of how a person chooses to engage in behaviors that promote health or help avoid disease (e.g., screening, immunizations, preventative medicine) (Rosenstock 1974). The health belief model has been widely studied and has a high degree of empirical support (Carpenter 2010). A person's beliefs regarding a particular target health behavior are influenced by several constructs. The first construct is the person's level of *perceived susceptibility* to the risk of developing a disease (Janz and Becker 1984). Perceived susceptibility to a disease can range from no susceptibility to high susceptibility. If a person believes that they are highly susceptible or at a high risk of developing a disease or condition, then they are more likely to take action to avoid that disease state. Alternatively, if a person believes that they are not likely to be susceptible to a disease (e.g., low risk), then they may not feel compelled to make healthy choices or follow advice related to healthy behavior. For example, a smoker may believe that they are not susceptible to lung disease if, for instance, a close relative was a heavy smoker and lived a long time without contracting lung disease.

The second construct that is important is the *perceived seriousness or threat* of the disease condition and the severity of the consequences of the disease (Janz and Becker 1984). If the person believes that developing a particular condition is a serious threat to one's health, then they will be more likely to engage in behaviors that help them avoid that particular disease state. If a person does not believe that a particular disease state is serious, then they will be less likely to engage in behaviors that are designed to avoid the disease state. For example, if a person does not believe that the flu is particularly worrisome, they will be less likely to get a flu shot. A person's *perceived threat* is the combination of their level of perceived susceptibility and perceived seriousness of the disease. The higher the perceived threat, the more likely a person is to engage in behaviors that lead to enhanced health and well-being. The lower the perceived threat, the less likely a person is to engage in behaviors that promote health or avoid disease. Perceptions of a person's susceptibility, seriousness, and threat toward a disease are contingent on education and awareness of the disease or condition (Janz and Becker 1984). Figure 3.3 outlines the main components of the health belief model.

Whether a person engages in healthy behaviors or in behaviors that reduce the risk to a particular condition also depends on the *perceived benefits and barriers* to taking action. If a person perceives that the benefits of taking a particular action are high and that the likelihood of taking that action will reduce the risk to a particular disease condition, then the person is more likely to take action. Likewise, if a person perceives significant barriers to engaging in a particular action, then they are less likely to take action. Barriers can include financial cost, access to resources, perceived side effects or risk of a particular behavior, inconvenience, lack of time, physical or emotional pain or loss, and loss of social and other benefits due to the behavior. Several modifying variables also influence whether a person will engage in a behavior. These can include demographic variables such as age, gender, race, and ethnicity as well as other social variables that include peer group influences, social class, education, and access to information and other healthcare resources.

In the HBM, *cues* or triggers to action are often required to prompt a behavior that promotes health. These cues can be internal or physical (e.g., pain, anxiety), external (e.g., media advertisement, news event, or health promotion education campaigns or communications), or interpersonal (e.g., messages or signals from loved ones, loved one experiencing a positive or negative health-related consequence of a target behavior). For instance, recent new stories discussing an outbreak of lung disease and death linked to vaping might cue a person to consider stopping the behavior. Another example might be if a person sees a news story close to home that involves an outbreak of COVID-19, they may be more likely to avoid crowds, wear a mask, or cancel travel plans. A person who sees a loved one or friends wearing a mask in public may be more likely to wear a mask themselves. A suspicious

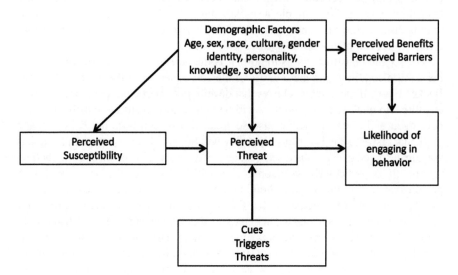

Fig. 3.3 Health belief model

mole might prompt a person to get a body scan and use more sunscreen regularly, especially if a loved one has developed skin cancer. A comment by their doctor that they may be drinking too much may initiate a person to reduce their drinking.

A final concept relevant to the HBM is the concept of *self-efficacy*. Self-efficacy refers to the *perceived ability or competence* of a person to engage in a particular health-related behavior successfully (Janz and Becker 1984). How well a person believes they possess the capability of engaging in healthy behaviors will influence whether they take action. In summary, according to the HBM, the decision to take action regarding one's health can include reducing or quitting substances, eating healthier, screening for health problems, wearing a mask, getting immunizations, engaging in safer sex practices, using seat belts and helmets, taking medication, engaging in exercise and stress reduction activities, or leaving an abusive relationship. Engaging in these actions rests on a dynamic interaction of several factors: (1) the presence of a cue or trigger to take action; (2) the perceived risk and seriousness of negative health consequences and susceptibility to disease; (3) the benefits and risks of taking action; and (4) the self-efficacy one possesses in their ability to successfully engage in taking action (Janz and Becker 1984). Modifying variables include age, sex, gender, and race/ethnicity as well as social factors such as peers/family, social class, education, and access to information and awareness. Practices that are important to helping people change behaviors or take action in the face of a negative health consequence include: (1) providing education about the susceptibility and risks associated with a disease; (2) informing, motivating, and coaching people about behaviors that they can do that are effective in reducing harm; (3) providing skills and resources designed to increase competence and self-efficacy around change behaviors; and (4) providing people with resources that can enable them to make changes such as assistance with income, transportation, insurance, and access to treatment, medication, or equipment (e.g., masks, helmets, nicotine replacement therapy, clean needles). Integrated care is one important area that can help people take action. Integrated care provides convenient access to education and awareness (information), tools, motivation, and assistance in taking action in one convenient setting.

3.3.3 Theory of Reasoned Action

The theory of reasoned action (TRA) is another social psychological theory of human behavior change (Ajzen and Albarracin 2007; Ajzen and Fishbein 1980; Fishbein 2008; Fishbein and Ajzen 2010). The central tenet of the TRA is that *intention* is the driving force of determining whether people will change their behaviors. Intention to perform a target behavior is also impacted by three components: *Attitudes, normative pressure, and perceived control*. Figure 3.4 outlines the main components of TRA.

Attitudes toward a particular behavior are determined by the beliefs that people hold about the behavior and its consequences—they can be instrumental (i.e., What are the costs vs. benefits?) or experiential (i.e., What have I experienced in the past?) (McEachan et al. 2016). This may be influenced by past attempts to engage in the behavior (outcomes) or learned beliefs about the positive or negative consequences of performing the behavior. For instance, how important are the perceived benefits of the behavior (health, happiness, social harmony, economic) compared to the perceived costs of performing the behavior (loss of pleasure, financial costs, social costs).

Normative pressure refers to what a person believes others think about the target behavior (Manning 2009). These pressures can be from one's peer group or a reference group. People can be influenced by what peers think about a behavior and whether they are performing the target behavior themselves. In order words, "What do others think about this behavior?" "What do they think I should do?" and "What are people close to me doing?"

And lastly, *perceived control* has to do with whether or not a person believes they have the autonomy, skills, and resources to perform the target behavior effectively (Yzer 2012). In other words, "Can I do it?" These three components lead to the intention to perform an act or target behavior. They are, in turn, influenced by a variety of variables, such as past experiences, demographics, personality, temperament, affectivity (e.g., risk aversion, conscientiousness, openness, surgency, negative/positive affectivity), attitudes toward risk and change, and exposure to media and other messaging.

The theory of reasoned action helps us to identify how to help people make a decision about a particular target behavior by helping us understand what is getting in their way. For instance, if a person does not have an intention to perform a

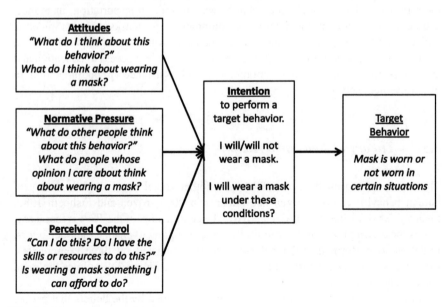

Fig. 3.4 Theory of reasoned action

behavior that is deemed healthy, or change a behavior that is unhealthy, what is the reason behind the lack of intention? Motivational interviewing approaches that help people explore the pros and cons of a particular behavior change may help people consider change. However, if a person has the intention to change, but lacks the skills and capacities to change, then skill development may be the better intervention. If perceived lack of self-efficacy is the problem, then a combination of information, skill development, rehearsal, and support may be in order. The deployment of peer providers can be useful in this situation because they act as role models that both inspire people and provide important practice advice and information. If a person lacks the resources to change a behavior, then interventions that provide more practical support such as income enhancement, recreational activities, medication, transportation, housing, or food access may be more appropriate. For instance, if a person has an intention to stop opioid use, but lacks the ability to cope with cravings and is surrounded by other users, then a combination of medications to control cravings; helping the person identify alternative activities during the day such as employment, treatment groups, or recreational activities; and helping the person change social circles may be the best approach to treatment. TRA, like other change theories, helps providers assess the factors influencing a client's intention and motivation to change and can, therefore, assist clients and providers in selecting appropriate, person-centered interventions.

3.4   Summary and Conclusion

Recovery and well-being are a dynamic process of whole health facilitated by positive relationships, access to basic resources, and treatment provided via warm, supportive relationships. Integrated behavioral health practice and person-centered care are wholly compatible with recovery-oriented practices and approaches that facilitate well-being. These approaches, when combined with an understanding of change theories, can help providers engage in assessment and intervention practices that match a client's particular intention to change. Unfortunately, many of our clients engage in behaviors that negatively impact their health and interfere with their ability to move toward well-being. This can be frustrating as a provider, but it is not always the case that a person doesn't *want* to change. They might lack the resources and capacity to change. Intention can be influenced by multiple factors. Clients may not believe change is worth it and would instead benefit from safer ways to continue their behaviors. They may lack the skills, resources, social support, and peer structures to encourage change, or they may need a change in scenery or access to other information from trusted sources such as peer providers. The above theories help providers in understanding the underlying factors influencing client behavior so that they can design interventions that help people make choices that lead to recovery, whole health, and well-being.

References

Adams, N., & Grieder, D. M. (2014). *Treatment planning for person-centered care: Shared decision making for whole health* (2nd ed.). Boston: Elsevier Press.

Ajzen, I., & Albarracin, D. (2007). Predicting and changing behavior: A reasoned action approach. In I. Ajzen, D. Albarracín, & R. Hornik (Eds.), *Prediction and change of health behavior* (pp. 1–22). Mahwah: Lawrence Erlbaum.

Ajzen, I., & Fishbein, M. (1980). *Understanding attitudes and predicting social behavior.* Englewood Cliffs: Prentice Hall.

Andermann, A. (2018). Screening for social determinants of health in clinical care: Moving from the margins to the mainstream. *Public Health Reviews, 39*, 19. https://doi.org/10.1186/s40985-018-0094-7.

Anthony, W. A. (1993). Recovery from mental illness: The guiding vision of the mental health service system in the 1990s. *Psychosocial Rehabilitation Journal, 16*(4), 11–23. https://doi.org/10.1037/h0095655.

Berwick, D. (2009). What "patient-centered" should mean: Confessions of an extremist. *Health Affairs, 28*(4), w555–w565. https://doi.org/10.1377/hlthaff.28.

Boehm, J. K., & Kubzansky, L. D. (2012). The heart's content: The association between positive psychological well-being and cardiovascular health. *Psychological Bulletin, 138*, 655–691.

Boehm, J. K., Lyubomirsky, S., & Sheldon, K. M. (2011). A longitudinal experimental study comparing the effectiveness of happiness-enhancing strategies in Anglo Americans and Asian Americans. *Cognition & Emotion, 25*, 1263–1272. https://doi.org/10.1080/0269993 1.2010.541227.

Bolier, L., Haverman, M., Westerhof, G., Riper, H., Smit, F., & Bohlmeijer, E. (2013). Positive psychology interventions: A meta-analysis of randomized controlled studies. *BMC Public Health, 13*, 119.

Carpenter, C. J. (2010). A meta-analysis of the effectiveness of health belief model variables in predicting behavior. *Health Communication, 25*(8), 661–669. https://doi.org/10.1080/1041023 6.2010.521906.

Chamberlin, J. (1988). *On our own.* New York: Mind Publications.

Clarke, C., Lumbard, D., Sambrook, S., & Kerr, K. (2016). What does recovery mean to a forensic mental health patient? A systematic review and narrative synthesis of the qualitative literature. *The Journal of Forensic Psychiatry & Psychology, 27*(1), 38–54.

Cook, J. A., Jonikas, J. A., Hamilton, M. M., Goldrick, V., Steigman, P. J., Grey, D. D., Burke, L., Carter, T. M., Razzano, L. A., & Copeland, M. E. (2013). Impact of Wellness Recovery Action Planning on service utilization and need in a randomized controlled trial. *Psychiatric Rehabilitation Journal, 36*(4), 250–257. https://doi.org/10.1037/prj0000028.

Davidson, L., Tondora, J., Staeheli-Lawless, M., O'Connell, M. J., & Rowe, M. (2009). *A practical guide to recovery-oriented practice: Tools for transforming mental health care.* New York: Oxford University Press.

De Ruysscher, C., Vandevelde, S., Vanderplasschen, W., De Maeyer, J., & Vanheule, S. (2017). The concept of recovery as experienced by persons with dual diagnosis: A systematic review of qualitative research from a first-person perspective. *Journal of Dual Diagnosis, 13*(4), 264–279.

Deegan, P. E. (1997). Recovery and empowerment for people with psychiatric disabilities. *Social Work in Health Care, 25*(3), 11–24. https://doi.org/10.1300/J010v25n03_02.

Dell, N. A., Long, C., & Mancini, M. A. (In press). Models of recovery in mental illness: An overview of systematic review. *Psychiatric Rehabilitation Journal.*

DeNeve, K. M., & Cooper, H. (1998). The happy personality: A meta-analysis of 137 personality traits and subjective well-being. *Psychological Bulletin, 124*, 197–229.

Diener, E. (1984). Subjective well-being. *Psychological Bulletin, 95*, 542–575. https://doi.org/10.1037/0033-2909.95.3.542.

Disabato, D. J., Goodman, F. R., Kashdan, T. B., Short, J. L., & Jardan, A. (2016). Different types of well-being? A cross-cultural examination of hedonic and eudaemonic well-being. *Psychological Assessment, 28*(5), 471–482. https://doi.org/10.1037/pas0000209.

Drake, R. E., Lynde, D. W., & Merrens, M. R. (2005). *Evidence-based mental health practice: A textbook*. New York: W.W. Norton & Company.

Ellison, M. L., Belanger, L. K., Niles, B. L., Evans, L. C., & Bauer, M. S. (2018). Explication and definition of mental health recovery: A systematic review. *Administration and Policy in Mental Health and Mental Health Services Research, 45*(1), 91–102. https://doi.org/10.1007/s10488-016-0767-9.

Emmons, R. A., & McCullough, M. E. (2003). Counting blessings versus burdens: An experimental investigation of gratitude and subjective well-being in daily life. *Journal of Personality and Social Psychology, 84*, 377–389.

Fava, G. A. (1999). Well-being therapy: Conceptual and technical issues. *Psychotherapy and Psychosomatics, 68*, 171–179.

Fava, G. A., Rafanelli, C., Grandi, S., Conti, S., & Belluardo, P. (1998). Prevention of recurrent depression with cognitive behavioral therapy. *Archives of General Psychiatry, 55*, 816–821.

Fava, G. A., Rafanelli, C., Ottolini, F., Ruini, C., Cazzaro, M., & Grandi, S. (2001). Psychological well-being and residual symptoms in remitted patients with panic disorder and agoraphobia. *Journal of Affective Disorders, 65*, 185–190.

Ferguson, S. J., & Goodwin, A. D. (2010). Optimism and well-being in older adults: The mediating role of social support and perceived control. *International Journal of Aging and Human Development, 71*, 43–68.

Fishbein, M. (2008). A reasoned action approach to health promotion. *Medical Decision Making., 28*, 834–844.

Fishbein, M., & Ajzen, I. (2010). *Predicting and changing behavior: A reasoned action approach*. New York: Taylor and Francis.

Goodman, F. R., Disabato, D. J., Kashdan, T. B., & Kauffman, S. B. (2018). Measuring well-being: A comparison of subjective well-being and PERMA. *Journal of Positive Psychology, 13*(4), 321–332. https://doi.org/10.1080/17439760.2017.1388434.

Gross, J. J., & John, O. P. (2003). Individual differences in two emotion regulation processes: Implications for affect, relationships, and well-being. *Journal of Personality and Social Psychology, 85*, 348–362.

Grzywacz, J. G., & Keyes, C. L. M. (2004). Toward health promotion: Physical and social behaviors in complete health. *American Journal of Health Behavior, 28*, 99–111.

Harding, C. M., Brooks, G. W., Ashikaga, T., Strauss, J. S., & Breier, A. (1987). The Vermont longitudinal study of persons with severe mental illness, I: Methodology, study sample, and overall status 32 years later. *American Journal of Psychiatry, 144*, 718–726.

Hine, R. H., Maybery, D. J., & Goodyear, M. J. (2018). Identity in recovery for mothers with a mental illness: A literature review. *Psychiatric Rehabilitation Journal, 41*(1), 16–28.

Janz, N. K., & Becker, M. H. (1984). The health belief model: A decade later. *Health Education & Behavior, 11*(1), 1–47. https://doi.org/10.1177/109019818401100101.

Kaite, C. P., Karanikola, M., Merkouris, A., & Papathanassoglou, E. D. (2015). "An ongoing struggle with the self and illness": A meta-synthesis of the studies of the lived experience of severe mental illness. *Archives of Psychiatric Nursing, 29*(6), 458–473.

Kerman, N., & Kidd, S. A. (2020). The Healthcare Triple Aim in the Recovery Era. *Administration and policy in mental health, 47*(4), 492–496. https://doi.org/10.1007/s10488-019-00997-0

Keyes, C. L. M. (2002). The mental health continuum: From languishing to flourishing in life. *Journal of Health and Social Behavior, 43*, 207–222.

Kim, E. S., Sun, J. K., Park, N., Kubzansky, L. D., & Peterson, C. (2012). Purpose in life and reduced risk of myocardial infarction among older U.S. adults with coronary heart disease: A two-year follow-up. *Journal of Behavioral Medicine, 36*, 124–133.

Kim, E. S., Sun, J. K., Park, N., & Peterson, C. (2013). Purpose in life and reduced stroke in older adults: The health and retirement study. *Journal of Psychosomatic Research, 74*, 427–432.

Kinoshita, Y., Furukawa, T. A., Kinoshita, K., Honyashiki, M., Omori, I. M., Marshall, M., Bond, G. R., et al. (2013). Supported employment for adults with serious mental illness. *Cochrane Database of Systematic Reviews, 13*(9), CD008297. https://doi.org/10.1002/14651858. CD008297.pub2.

Leamy, M., Bird, V., Boutillier, L., Williams, J., & Slade, M. (2011). Conceptual framework for personal recovery in mental health: Systematic review and narrative synthesis. *British Journal of Psychiatry, 199*, 445–452. https://doi.org/10.1192/bjp.bp.110.083733.

Lovell, T. (2019). *Recovery in forensic mental health services: A review and meta-ethnography of reported accounts of service user experiences.* (Doctoral dissertation, Canterbury Christ Church University).

Mancini, M. A. (2003). *Theories of recovery elicited from individuals with psychiatric disabilities.* (Doctoral Dissertation: State University of New York at Albany; Nelson A Rockefeller School of Social Welfare, Albany, N.Y.).

Mancini, M. A. (2006). Consumer-providers theories of recovery from serious psychiatric disabilities. In J. Rosenberg (Ed.), *Community mental health: Challenges for the 21st century* (pp. 15–24). New York: Brunner-Routledge.

Mancini, M. A. (2007). The role of self-efficacy in recovery from serious psychiatric disabilities: A qualitative study with fifteen psychiatric survivors. *Qualitative Social Work: Research and Practice, 6*, 49–74.

Mancini, M. A. (2018). An exploration of factors that effect the implementation of peer support services in community mental health settings. *Community Mental Health Journal, 54*(2), 127–137. https://doi.org/10.1007/s10597-017-0145-4/.

Mancini, M. A. (2019). Strategic storytelling: An exploration of the professional practices of mental health peer providers. *Qualitative Health Research, 29*(9), 1266–1276. https://doi.org/10.1177/1049732318821689.

Mancini, M. A., & Linhorst, D. M. (2010). Harm reduction in community mental health settings. *Journal of Social Work in Disability & Rehabilitation, 9*, 130–147.

Mancini, M. A., & Miner, C. S. (2013). Learning and change in a community mental health setting. *Journal of Evidence Based Social Work., 10*(5), 494–504.

Mancini, M. A., & Wyrick-Waugh, W. (2013). Consumer and practitioner perceptions of the harm reduction approach in a community mental health setting. *Community Mental Health Journal, 49*(1), 14–24.

Mancini, M. A., Hardiman, E. R., & Lawson, H. A. (2005). Making sense of it all: Consumer providers' theories about factors facilitating and impeding recovery from psychiatric disabilities. *Psychiatric Rehabilitation Journal, 29*(1), 48–55.

Mancini, M. A., Hardiman, E. R., & Eversman, M. H. (2008). A review of the compatibility of harm reduction and recovery-oriented best practices for dual disorders. *Best Practices in Mental Health: An International Journal, 4*(2), 99–113.

Manning, M. (2009). The effects of subjective norms on behaviour in the theory of planned behaviour: A meta-analysis. *British Journal of Social Psychology, 48*, 649–705.

McCarthy-Jones, S., Marriott, M., Knowles, R., Rowse, G., & Thompson, A. (2013). What is psychosis? A meta-synthesis of inductive qualitative studies exploring the experience of psychosis. *Psychosis, 5*(1), 1–16.

McEachan, R., Taylor, N., Harrison, R., Lawton, R., Gardner, P., & Conner, M. (2016). Meta-analysis of the reasoned action approach (RAA) to understanding health behaviors. *Annals of Behavioral Medicine, 50*(4), 592–612. https://doi.org/10.1007/s12160-016-9798-4.

McFarlane, W. R. (2016). Family interventions for schizophrenia and the psychoses: A review. *Family Process, 55*, 460–482. https://doi.org/10.1111/famp.12235.

McKenzie-Smith, L. (2019). *Recovery experiences of forensic mental health service users.* (Doctoral dissertation, Canterbury Christ Church University). http://create.canterbury. ac.uk/18413/1/Laura_McKenzie-Smith_MRP_2019.pdf

Metler, S. J., & Busseri, M. A. (2017). Further evaluation of the tripartite structure of subjective well-being: Evidence from longitudinal and experimental studies. *Journal of Personality, 85*(2), 192–206. https://doi.org/10.1111/jopy.12233.

Morozink-Boylan, J., & Ryff, C. D. (2015). Psychological well-being and metabolic syndrome: Findings from the MIDUS National Sample. *Psychosomatic Medicine, 77*(5), 548–558.

Ness, O., Borg, M., & Davidson, L. (2014). Facilitators and barriers in dual recovery: A literature review of first-person perspective. *Advances In Dual Diagnosis, 7*(3), 107–111.

Ng, F. Y., Bourke, M. E., & Grenyer, B. F. (2016). Recovery from borderline personality disorder: A systematic review of the perspectives of consumers, clinicians, family and carers. *PLoS One, 11*(8).

Paradise, A. W., & Kernis, M. H. (2002). Self-esteem and psychological well-being: Implications of fragile self-esteem. *Journal of Social and Clinical Psychology, 21*, 345–361.

Prochaska, J. O., DiClemente, C. C., & Norcross, J. C. (1992). In search of how people change: Applications to addictive behaviors. *American Psychologist, 47*(9), 1102–1114. https://doi.org/10.1037//0003-066x.47.9.1102.

Rafanelli, C., Park, S. K., Ruini, C., Ottolini, F., Cazzaro, M., & Fava, G. A. (2000). Rating well-being and distress. *Stress Medicine, 16*, 55–61.

Richardson, K., & Barkham, M. (2020). Recovery from depression: A systematic review of perceptions and associated factors. *Journal of Mental Health, 29*(1), 103–115.

Rosenstock, I. (1974). Historical origins of the health belief model. *Health Education & Behavior, 2*(4), 328–335. https://doi.org/10.1177/109019817400200403.

Ryan, R. M., & Deci, E. L. (2001). On happiness and human potentials: A review of research on hedonic and eudaemonic well-being. *Annual Review of Psychology, 52*, 141–166.

Ryff, C. D. (1989). Happiness is everything, or is it? Explorations on the meaning of psychological well-being. *Journal of Personality and Social Psychology, 57*, 1069–1081. https://doi.org/10.1037/0022-3514.57.6.1069.

Ryff, C. (2014). Psychological well-being revisited: Advances in the science and practice of Eudemonia. *Psychotherapy and Psychosomatics, 83*, 10–28. https://doi.org/10.1159/000353263.

Ryff, C. D., Singer, B. H., & Love, G. D. (2004). Positive health: Connecting well-being with biology. *Philosophical Transactions of the Royal Society of London: Series B Biological Sciences, 359*, 1383–1394.

Schmutte, P. S., & Ryff, C. D. (1997). Personality and wellbeing: Reexamining methods and meanings. *Journal of Personality and Social Psychology, 73*, 549–559.

Schön, U. K., & Rosenberg, D. (2013). Transplanting recovery: Research and practice in the Nordic countries. *Journal of Mental Health, 22*(6), 563–569.

Schueller, M. S., & Parks, C. A. (2012). Disseminating self-help: Positive psychology exercises in an online trial. *Journal of Medical Internet Research, 14*, e63. https://doi.org/10.2196/jmir.1850.

Seligman, M. (2011). *Flourish*. New York: Free Press.

Seligman, M. (2018). PERMA and the building blocks of well-being. *The Journal of Positive Psychology, 13*(4), 333–335. https://doi.org/10.1080/17439760.2018.1437466.

Seligman, M., Rashid, T., & Parks, A. C. (2006). Positive psychotherapy. *American Psychologist, 61*, 774–788.

Shepherd, A., Doyle, M., Sanders, C., & Shaw, J. (2016). Personal recovery within forensic settings: Systematic review and meta-synthesis of qualitative methods studies. *Criminal Behavior and Mental Health, 26*, 59–75.

Slade, M. (2009). *Personal recovery and mental illness*. London: Cambridge University Press.

Slade, M., Leamy, M., Bacon, F., Janosik, M., Le Boutillier, C., Williams, J., & Bird, V. (2012). International differences in understanding recovery: Systematic review. *Epidemiology and Psychiatric Sciences, 21*(4), 353–364.

Stanhope, V., & Ashenberg-Straussner, S. L. (Eds.). (2018). *Social work and integrated health care: From policy to practice and back*. New York: Oxford University Press.

Stuart, S. R., Tansey, L., & Quayle, E. (2017). What we talk about when we talk about recovery: A systematic review and best-fit framework synthesis of qualitative literature. *Journal of Mental Health, 26*(3), 291–304.

Temesgen, W. A., Chien, W. T., & Bressington, D. (2019). Conceptualizations of subjective recovery from recent onset psychosis and its associated factors: A systematic review. *Early Intervention in Psychiatry, 13*(2), 181–193.

Tondora, J., Miller, R., Slade, M., & Davidson, L. (2014). *Partnering for recovery in mental health: A practical guide to person-centered planning.* Hoboken: Wiley.

Tsemberis, S., Gulcur, L., & Nakae, M. (2004). Housing first, consumer choice, and harm reduction for homeless individuals with a dual diagnosis. *American Journal of Public Health, 94*(4), 651–656. https://doi.org/10.2105/ajph.94.4.651.

van Weeghel, J., van Zelst, C., Boertien, D., & Hasson-Ohayon, I. (2019). Conceptualizations, assessments, and implications of personal recovery in mental illness: A scoping review of systematic reviews and meta-analyses. *Psychiatric Rehabilitation Journal, 42*(2), 169–181. https://doi.org/10.1037/prj0000356.

Vitterso, J., & Soholt, Y. (2011). Life satisfaction goes with pleasure and personal growth goes with interest: Further arguments for separating hedonic and eudaemonic well-being. *The Journal of Positive Psychology, 6*(4), 326–335. https://doi.org/10.1080/17439760.2011.584548.

Wood, L., & Alsawy, S. (2018). Recovery in psychosis from a service user perspective: A systematic review and thematic synthesis of current qualitative evidence. *Community Mental Health Journal, 54*(6), 793–804.

Woodgate, R., Sigurdson, C., Demczuk, L., Tennent, P., Wallis, B., & Wener, P. (2017). The meanings young people assign to living with mental illness and their experiences in managing their health and lives: A systematic review of qualitative evidence. *JBI Database of Systematic Reviews and Implementation Reports, 15*(2).

Yzer, M. (2012). Perceived behavioral control in reasoned action theory: A dual aspect interpretation. *The Annals of the American Academy of Political and Social Science, 640*, 101–117.

Chapter 4
Behavioral Health Screening and Assessment

4.1 An Orientation to Behavioral Health Assessment

Screening and assessment are an important set of competencies that drive effective and efficient integrated behavioral health practice (SAMHSA 2020). In this chapter, I will review a behavioral health assessment approach that is holistic, person centered, strength based, and recovery oriented. First, assessments must consider the whole person. Holistic behavioral health assessments gather and synthesize the individual and social information necessary to develop a useful, person-centered and multidimensional treatment plan (Adams and Grieder 2014). One way to accomplish this is to utilize the person-in-environment perspective (PIE) that is rooted in the ecological systems theoretical model discussed in Chap. 2 (Bronfenbrenner 1979; Germain and Gitterman 1980, 2008). The PIE approach to assessment focuses on the bio-psycho-social aspects of health and functioning and views the individual as part of their broader environmental system or *ecosystem*. Providers using a PIE approach focus on the "fit" between a person's strengths, capacities, and resources and their social environment (Germain and Gitterman 1980, 2008). It is a comprehensive assessment method that goes beyond individual pathology to address various domains that impact functioning (Karls and O'Keefe 2008). An assessment process rooted in the PIE approach begins by engaging clients though rapport-building and development of a therapeutic alliance. It then blends screening and assessment of both individual and social determinants of health (SDOH) along with commonly comorbid clinical conditions to provide a comprehensive and person-centered assessment of the bio-psycho-social factors influencing a client's physical and behavioral health. This assessment can then be used to develop a multidimensional case conceptualization that then informs the treatment planning process. Figure 4.1 outlines each of the phases of the assessment and treatment planning process.

Behavioral health assessment has four interrelated processes. First, at the individual level it is important to screen each client for common behavioral health

© Springer Nature Switzerland AG 2021
M. A. Mancini, *Integrated Behavioral Health Practice*,
https://doi.org/10.1007/978-3-030-59659-0_4

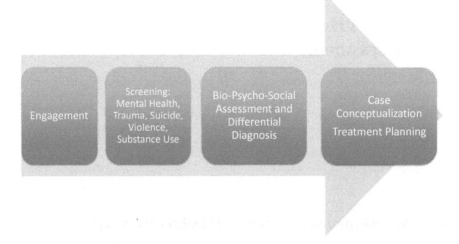

Fig. 4.1 Phases of assessment and treatment planning

symptoms and issues that impact behavioral health such as social determinants of health (SDOH), depression, anxiety, perceived stress, traumatic stress, violence, substance use, and suicidal behavior. Providers should also screen and assess for health issues and conditions that are commonly comorbid with behavioral health disorders such as diabetes, hypertension, inflammatory conditions, cerebrovascular, and cardiovascular diseases, as well as health risk behaviors such as obesity, sedentary lifestyle, and the use of tobacco, alcohol, and other substances. Health and behavioral health are closely connected and exert a strong impact on each other and overall health, making both areas an important focus of assessment and treatment (Karls and O'Keefe 2008).

Using the PIE framework, providers also assess and address relevant aspects of a person's social environment. As mentioned in Chap. 2, health is impacted by social determinants. Social determinants of health include factors such as housing quality, income, employment, social support, environmental conditions, transportation, safety, and the ability to meet basic needs such as food, rent, utilities, and medical expenses. Assessing for strengths and problems in each of these domains is an important part of any comprehensive assessment. Treatment planning that is based on a holistic assessment means addressing SDOH by helping client's access resources such as better housing, employment, financial resources, child care, transportation, food, and social support among other resources (Adams and Grieder 2014).

Second, effective behavioral health assessment requires an approach to communication with clients that is person centered. Person-centered approaches focus on the importance of client and provider relationships built on communication, trust, partnership, empathy, and support. Through these relationships, providers find common ground with clients and are committed to: (1) meeting client preferences and needs; (2) measuring client satisfaction with care; (3) improving quality of care and outcomes; and (4) reducing costs and making care more efficient (Stewart et al. 2000). A person-centered approach also requires providers to practice from lens of cultural competency and equity. This includes recognizing that clients who are Black, Indigenous, and People of Color (BIPOC) endure racism and discrimination that have an impact on health. This also means recognizing that clients who are members of the LGBTQ community have experienced discrimination that has similarly impacted their health. Ensuring that individual and agency practices are sensitive, competent, inclusive, equitable, open, and affirming is central to the person-centered approach.

Third, assessment approaches using a strength-based perspective explore how clients can use their skills, talents, capacities, and resources to deal with current problems and achieve their goals (Gottlieb 2014; Rapp and Goscha 2012). Strength-based approaches to assessment are inherently holistic and collaborative, making them compatible with person-centered approaches. The strengths perspective to assessment is an alternative to the diagnostic method of focusing solely on pathologies. This perspective can be blended with traditional diagnostic approaches to more fully capture a person's strengths, capacities, and vulnerabilities. The strength-perspective is perfectly compatible with the PIE and person-centered assessment approaches because it is holistic, collaborative, and provides a way to assess both problem areas and a person's talents, resources, coping skills, and future goals (Saleebey 1996).

And lastly, assessment should utilize a recovery orientation. The personal mental health recovery model, as outlined in Chap. 3, is a perspective that views recovery as a process or journey from a state of despair, isolation, and illness to a state of well-being. Recovery from this perspective moves beyond clinical outcomes such as symptom remission or reduction in hospitalization days, to include elements of subjective and psychological well-being such as: (1) a sense of happiness and satisfaction with life, (2) insight into one's illness, (3) a sense of belonging and connection through nurturing social relationships, (4) self-determination and empowerment as one learns coping skills and takes control of their lives, (5) the development of a sense of meaning and purpose as one takes up functional roles and activities, and (6) the positive sense of self-efficacy and mastery that develops from these sources of well-being (Dell et al. In Press; De Ruysscher et al. 2017; Leamy et al. 2011; Mancini et al. 2005; Mancini 2006, 2007; McCarthy-Jones et al. 2013; McKenzie-Smith et al. 2019).

Assessment practices oriented toward recovery share many similarities with person-centered care and are defined by several components. First, providers conduct assessments using a warm, engaging approach that is respectful, nonjudgmental, empathic, and welcoming (Davidson et al. 2009; Tondora et al. 2014). Providers take their time, ask questions in a sensitive manner, show concern, provide culturally affirming, fluent and competent care, and seek to engage clients in service. Second, providers are concerned about more than symptoms. They ask people about who is important to them; what activities give them meaning and joy; what interests, strengths, and talents they possess; and what troubles or concerns them about their lives in terms of health, relationships, safety, and access to resources. Lastly, providers consider a client's stage of change regarding a particular issue (Prochaska et al. 1992). Once problems have been initially identified and defined, it is important for service providers to offer clients a range of options to address the problem. Clients will be in various stages of change. Some may not be interested in addressing the problem at all or may not even recognize that a problem exists. Some clients will recognize the problem, but be ambivalent about how, or if, to address the problem. Some clients may be ready to take action. Given this range of perspectives, service providers should offer treatment options that can fit any one of these stages.

In the following sections, I will review the four areas of screening and assessment that can provide a comprehensive, detailed, and accurate portrait of a client's current situation and set the stage for the treatment planning process. These four areas are: (1) engaging clients and building rapport; (2) assessing for strengths and resources; (3) screening and assessment for common behavioral health symptoms, problems, and concerns; and (4) screening and assessment for social determinants of health (SDOH). Following this description, a review of important areas of documentation will be provided. A case study of Mr. Clarence Smith will be offered at the conclusion of this chapter.

4.2   Setting the Stage: Engaging Clients and Building Rapport

Assessment occurs at the beginning of the treatment partnership and continues throughout the relationship. During the early stages of assessment, it is important to take the time to create a welcoming, engaging, and empathic atmosphere. This is the time to engage clients in treatment and build trust and a solid rapport with them. Building rapport and trust with clients makes them feel safe and comfortable. This can lead to more honest and open conversations around experiencing discrimination, violence, and trauma as well as health-related behaviors surrounding drinking, suicidality, drug use, and sex that can be seen as intrusive and difficult to answer. Building good rapport and a strong therapeutic alliance during the initial visits and consultation is important in identifying and effectively treating behavioral health issues in clients because doing so can increase the motivation of clients to follow through with treatment recommendations leading to better treatment outcomes and higher satisfaction with services (Parker et al. 2020). Engaging clients in treatment and building rapport require providers and organizations to routinely engage in several practices that increase a sense of safety, respect, welcoming, warmth, empathy, hope, and optimism. I will review these areas next.

Creating WISE Service Environments That Are Welcoming, Inclusive, Safe, and Equitable

The people that walk through our doors have often experienced tragedy, oppression, poverty, despair, neglect, and abuse. They may be in pain. They may feel afraid. And they may be lonely. Despite these experiences, they have survived and they have decided to come see us for help. This is an honor and a responsibility. This may be your only chance to help them. Don't let clients walk away from you or your agency thinking that they made a mistake coming to see you. When clients knock on our door, we want them to feel welcomed and safe. We want them to feel like it was a good idea to come to see us.

Make your setting a welcoming place to be. Ask yourself, what are the first things a client experiences when they call or arrive at my agency? Is it a pleasant place to be? Are they acknowledged and treated with respect and courtesy? Was it easy to make an appointment? Making the clinical environment safe, comfortable, and welcoming can be the first step in building rapport with clients. For instance, having plants, artwork, and pleasant wall colorings, flooring, and comfortable furniture can be an important way to create a safe and comfortable environment. Ensuring that staff treat all clients equally and respectfully and implementing visible messaging about safety, confidentiality, cultural competence, and respect are important. It is also important to ensure that organizations are adequately staffed with providers and administrative personnel who are supportive, pleasant, trauma informed, patient, warm, and inviting on the phone when scheduling appointments or answering questions, upon arrival in the waiting area, in the exam room or therapy office, and all the way through discharge. This can increase clients' sense of safety and create a safer overall work environment for everybody. If you want to engage clients—then send the message: "We see you and we're glad you're here." Procedurally, it is important that providers have adequate time to conduct thorough assessments, listen to clients, and answer all of their questions and review information on treatment options.

Being inclusive and equitable means that staff composition is reflective of the diversity of the client populations they serve. It means minimally that all staff are adequately trained to recognize and address their own implicit and explicit biases so they can provide services that are affirming and inclusive of all identities and avoid racist, sexist, heterosexist, and trans-discriminatory practices that are invalidating, hurtful, and (re)traumatizing. Ideally, staff are trained in recognizing and dismantling structures, policies, and practices that are racist and discriminatory throughout the agency including holding each other accountable. For instance, they affirm the gender identities and sexual orientations of all clients in their messaging, forms, records, and practices. They share their pronouns and invite clients to share theirs as well. Their forms are in various languages and language interpretation services are available on site. Providers understand how implicit bias can influence clinical practice and how the experience of racism and discrimination over the course of a lifetime can lead to poor health. Providers are skilled and comfortable in having conversations with clients that explore their racial and cultural experiences and perspectives including their experiences of racism and discrimination in ways that are validating, constructive, and affirming and that lead to interventions that are culturally tailored and effective.

Inclusivity and equity also mean that all clients can easily access resources and services regardless of their personal circumstances. Equitable providers design their service environments with the needs of their most vulnerable, stressed, and disadvantaged clients first. It means that services are easily accessible and that the childcare, work or treatment schedules, transportation, and the ability of clients to get to services are acknowledged and addressed through responsive policies and procedures. Agency structures and procedures are also in place that regularly holds providers and leadership accountable to consistently provide services that are inclusive and equitable.

Organizations must be safe and trauma informed. Being trauma informed means that providers can sensitively and competently screen and assess for trauma and provide clients with support, education, and access to trauma services upon request. It means that practices and procedures are designed so they do not retraumatize clients. Intake and exam procedures are also conducted in ways that ensure safety and privacy. These are important ways to enhance rapport and engagement in treatment. Another important way to create safe environments that are welcoming, inclusive, safe, and equitable is the utilization of community health workers and/or peer providers or navigators. These individuals provide outreach and engagement services to clients by giving support, teaching coping skills, and helping them navigate the treatment environment. These individuals often share the same lived experiences as those of clients and can use those experiences to provide genuine and authentic support, hope, and guidance (Mancini 2018, 2019).

Showing Warmth, Respect, Patience, and Empathy
The ability of clinicians to convey a sense of warmth, respect, patience, and empathy to clients can lead to improved outcomes (Dowrick 2015; van Os et al. 2005; Jani et al. 2012). Supportive professionals have been found to be a key element of recovery for persons with serious mental health disorders (Mancini et al. 2005), and a strong therapeutic relationship is often viewed as an intervention in its own right (Dowrick 2015). Clinicians who build trust and rapport are able to convey a sense of warmth, affirmation, understanding, and support. This begins by engaging in active listening. Active listening involves a set of communication skills that convey to the client that they are respected, cared for, and heard. It also signals to clients that what they are experiencing is important and real. Hearing a client's words and their underlying concern while focusing directly on the client is an important initial step. This requires providers to face clients, give them their full attention, and avoid being distracted by computer screens, charts, and interruptions. This also involves allotting the necessary time to provide a competent consultation and avoid being rushed.

Clinicians can engage in active listening by doing the following: (1) make and maintain direct eye contact (if culturally appropriate); (2) sit facing the clients with an open stance; (3) ask open-ended questions designed to gather as much information from the client about their symptoms as possible; (4) listen intently to the client and patiently wait for the client to finish their story or encourage them to go on; and (5) be comfortable with silences and pauses and wait for the client to complete their thoughts. Clients with behavioral health concerns (e.g., depression, anxiety, trauma, and substance use) can often have difficulty concentrating, and can experience fatigue and shame. Reflecting back to the patient what you have heard them say is also a way to help the client know that they are understood and can encourage them to expand on their experiences. Writing down treatment instructions and reviewing them with clients can also improve treatment participation and follow-up.

Offering Hope and Optimism

After listening to clients, it is important to summarize what they say in order to assess accuracy. This practice can also be used to recognize strengths, share concerns, validate experiences, educate about alternatives, and provide the message that while what they are experiencing has implications of their health, they are not alone, and that help is available. Summarizing what has been said can help the provider and client develop a shared understanding of the problem. Thanking the client for sharing their concerns and complimenting them on the courage it took to come forward and ask for help are also important. In short, listen to people. Validate their experiences. Normalize what they are experiencing so they don't feel alone without minimizing the impact or seriousness of their distress. And drive home the message that while their behavioral health symptoms have health consequences, what they are experiencing is treatable, and their problems are solvable. Doing so can increase the chances a client continues in treatment, follows treatment protocols, and reports satisfaction with their treatment experience. It may also improve the sense of trust and respect necessary to encourage honest communication necessary for an accurate assessment (Dowrick 2015; van Os et al. 2005; Jani et al. 2012).

4.3 Assessing for Strengths and Resources

While developing a comprehensive and multidimensional understanding of client problems and concerns is the central feature of any assessment protocol, an understanding of client strengths is just as important. In a strength-based assessment approach, behavioral health providers create discursive space that explores how a person has coped with their issues and what special abilities, skills, and resources a person possesses. This type of assessment also identifies a person's hopes and dreams for the immediate and more distant future (Rapp and Goscha 2012). Understanding a client's strengths, hopes, and dreams can inform the treatment-planning process as it highlights the internal and external resources that can be redeployed to assist the person in coping with their problems. Strength-based assessment also helps continue to build rapport, increase motivation, and enhance self-efficacy in clients (Adams and Grieder 2014).

The strengths perspective values self-determination and views clients as experts in their own lives. Behavioral health providers invite clients to reflect upon their strengths and capacities in multiple domains and help them identify and (re)deploy those strengths to set goals and address behavioral and social problems. The approach also identifies areas in the client's life that need to be reinforced and strengthened. Problems are positioned as barriers to goals that can be overcome. As part of the assessment, the behavioral health provider takes on an approach that is conversational, engaging, encouraging, and affirming. Strength-based assessment is designed to help people acknowledge and utilize their abilities and resources to solve problems and to connect with natural resources and supports whenever possible (Rapp and Goscha 2012). Rapp and Goscha (2012) identify at least three main domain areas important for strength-based assessment that exist at the personal, interpersonal, and environmental levels: (1) personal skills and attributes; (2) interpersonal strengths and connections; and (3) environmental strengths and resources. When assessing personal, social, and environmental domains, it is important to first identify the things in the client's life that are going right, that can help them achieve their goals, what they have used in the past that they can use now, and what the client wants to accomplish in the future within these domains (2012).

Personal Skills, Character Traits, and Attributes

Clients are doing the best they can and are often doing better than they (or we) think. Why not identify and highlight those positive qualities and skills? The field of positive psychology has identified several broad character strengths and virtues that are constellations of persistent thoughts, perspectives, worldviews, behaviors, feelings, and tendencies that help define each person (Peterson and Seligman 2004). Peterson and Seligman (2004) have identified 24 character strengths and virtues that include integrity, love, kindness, gratitude, optimism, humor, bravery, self-control, leadership, forgiveness, teamwork, humility, curiosity, perseverance, and creativity to name several. Character strengths can be assessed and measured through the values in action (VIA) inventory of strengths (VIA-IS) (Peterson and Seligman 2004). It is important for clients (and providers) to know their character strengths so they can embrace and rely on them when needed. For instance, do clients have a good sense of humor? Are they humble, kind, generous, curious, brave, honest, or determined? Are they survivors? Are they protectors of their family? Knowing and embracing their positive traits help boost a client's sense of self-efficacy and guide them to rely on the parts of their selves that can be sources of strength and resilience.

It is also important to identify the skills and talents of an individual. What do they love to do and what do they know how to do well? What unique talents do they possess? What skills do they have that are important for achieving their goals? The beginning of the assessment process involves the identification of the strengths that people have used in the past to solve problems and the characteristics and attributes they currently have that they can use to work toward their goals. Identifying client skills and attributes can achieve three practice goals: (1) it frames the client more holistically and in positive terms rather than being problem focused; (2) it can help build rapport and treatment engagement; (3) it highlights areas that the client may have forgotten about and lead to increased motivation; and (4) it identifies resources that can be used to design and work toward identified goals (Rapp and Goscha 2012).

Interpersonal Strengths and Resources

A second domain of strength assessment focuses on interpersonal relationships and social support in the client's life such as helpful and supportive family, friends, coworkers, neighbors, and faith or community group members. These interpersonal resources can include people the person has relied on in the past, currently rely on, and could rely on in the future (Rapp and Goscha, 2012). It is important to assess if clients have people in their lives that can provide emotional and psychological support. Do they have someone they can confide in such as an intimate partner, child, parent, or close friend? Is there someone they can call upon to go for a walk, talk on the phone, have a cup of coffee, or go to the movies? In addition, it is important to explore if the person has people they can rely on to provide instrumental support such as transportation, childcare, or help with household chores. These organic forms of naturally occurring supports are far more reliable, holistic, efficient, and sustainable than support provided by professional sources (Rapp and Goscha 2012). Exploration of interpersonal relationships is also a form of culturally informed practice that validates worldviews that are more focused on interdependence rather than individualism. Clients from various cultural backgrounds place their interpersonal relationships at the center of their lives. When these relationships are stressed or fractured, it can lead to significant distress. Focusing explicitly on interpersonal health can help providers and clients collaboratively identify areas in the client's social network that are sources of strengths and areas that may require targeted interventions (Díaz et al. 2017).

Environmental Strengths and Resources
A third practice is to identify the positive assets and resources in each client's environment that have been and/or can be used to solve problems. This includes access to economic and basic resources such as income, transportation, safe housing, food, employment, education, and access to opportunities for recreation and meaningful activities. These resources can also include community or faith groups, schools, libraries, coffee shops or other businesses, or other neighborhood or community organizations that can provide access to needed resources. These resources can be highlighted to provide a more balanced picture of a client's ecology, which can often times be viewed as unnecessarily bleak or hopeless by the client. They can also be reorganized and redeployed to help solve client problems. Again, naturally available resources within the client's community or household are often more sustainable and efficient than professionally provided services (Rapp and Goscha 2012).

An assessment that only provides descriptions of barriers and problems lacks important information about how best to generate solutions that are organic to the person's lived reality. The strengths assessment can be a separate section of the assessment process, or it can be integrated throughout the process and act as an orienting perspective. For instance, assessment of personal strengths could be integrated into the assessment of behavioral health experiences, and assessment of interpersonal and environmental strengths could be a part of the assessment of social determinants of health discussed below. However documented, assessing for strengths helps the client (1) identify naturally occurring personal, social, and environmental resources they can rely on to help solve problems and (2) create a realistic sense of hope and optimism that can help motivate the person to work toward solutions to problems and build a sense of personal self-efficacy (Rapp and Goscha 2012).

4.4   Screening Areas for Common Behavioral Health Issues

Screening is an ongoing, formal process that begins when the client first presents for services and is used to identify the presence of symptoms, experiences, or problems that indicate the need for further assessment. Screening results are not a substitute for a full assessment and should not be used to make diagnoses. A positive screen does not confirm the presence of a disorder, but only indicates that symptoms of the disorder are present and that a full assessment is warranted. Assessment is a more detailed process to determine if a client meets the diagnostic criteria of a behavioral health disorder (e.g., major depressive disorder, post-traumatic stress disorder (PTSD), anxiety disorders, cognitive impairment, and substance use disorder) as identified by the American Psychiatric Association's fifth Edition of the Diagnostic and Statistical Manual of Mental Disorders (DSM-5) (APA 2013). It can also be used to confirm the presence of other issues that negatively impact behavioral health that requites exploration (e.g., interpersonal violence, poverty, discrimination, harmful drinking or other drug use, loneliness, suicidality, or housing instability). Screening results should be used to begin a conversation with the client about what the results mean for their health and to guide the assessment process. Figure 4.2 outlines the most common areas for behavioral health screening. Providers should universally screen for several common behavioral health problem areas in every new client as part of the intake process using brief, reliable, and valid instruments. Screening for psychiatric distress, trauma, stress, suicidal thinking, problem drinking, and drug use can be done in a remarkably efficient, sensitive, and reliable way with minimal questions.

4.4.1   Screening for Depression and Anxious Distress

Depressive and anxiety symptoms are prevalent, commonly comorbid with each other as well as other physical and behavioral health issues, and can lead to increased morbidity and early mortality. The two main symptoms of depression include a persistent pattern of low mood and lack of interest in all or almost all activities of daily living. This lack of interest and pleasure is sometimes called anhedonia. Depression also includes fatigue, disturbances in sleep, appetite, psychomotor activity, concentration, and persistent thoughts of worthlessness, guilt, and death. One of the most common screens for depression used in primary care and outpatient behavioral health settings is the Patient Health Questionnaire (PHQ-9) (Kroenke et al. 2001). The PHQ-9 is a publically available scale that screens for the presence of all nine depressive symptoms identified by the DSM-5. Five symptoms are required for a diagnosis with at least one being low mood or anhedonia (APA 2013). The PHQ-2 screens for the two main symptoms required for depression (e.g., low mood and anhedonia), and is also a reliable and valid screen for depression (Kroenke et al. 2003).

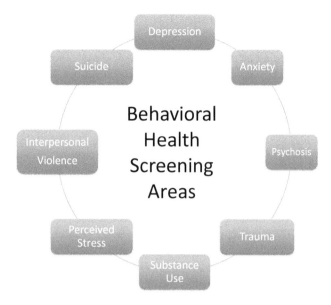

Fig. 4.2 Behavioral health screening areas

Anxiety is pathological worry or fear across a range of issues that is either excessive or experienced in the absence of perceived threats. This fear results in significant distress and avoidance behavior that can impair functioning. Symptoms include panic, nervousness, social anxiety, excessive worry, fear of a range of situations or objects (e.g., phobias), and obsessions and compulsions (APA 2013). One of the most common screens for anxiety is the Generalized Anxiety Disorder Scale (GAD-7) (Spitzer et al. 2006). The GAD-7 screens for seven prominent anxiety symptoms which include restlessness, excessive worry, uncontrollable worrying, inability to relax, being on edge, fear, and irritability.

A scale that combines depression and anxiety screening in four questions is the Patient Health Questionnaire 4 (PHQ-4) (Kroenke et al. 2009). Two questions focus on the two main depressive symptoms and the other two focuses on anxiety symptoms (nervousness and uncontrollable worry). Using the PHQ-4, providers ask clients how often over the last two weeks they have been bothered by the following problems: (1) feeling nervous, anxious, or on edge; (2) not being able to stop or control worrying; (3) experiencing little interest or pleasure in doing things; and (4) feeling down, depressed, or hopeless. The scale has four anchors (Not at all (0); Several days (1); More than half the days (2); and Nearly every day (3)). Scores for depression and anxiety can range from 0 to 6 point for each disorder. A score of 3 or greater indicates a positive screen for the presence of symptoms for that disorder (Löwe et al. 2010). These screens will be discussed further in Chap. 8.

4.4.2 Screening for Substance Use

Substance use including alcohol misuse can be quickly screened using a variety of scales including the CAGE-AID (*C*ut down, *A*nnoyed, *G*uilty, *E*ye-opener-*A*dapted to *I*nclude other *D*rugs) (Mayfield et al. 1974; Brown and Rounds 1995). Providers using this screen ask clients if: (1) they have ever felt they should *cut down* on their drinking or other drug use; (2) others have ever been *annoyed* with their drinking or drug use; (3) they had ever felt *guilty* by their drinking or drug use; (4) they have ever had to use drugs or alcohol in the morning as an *eye-opener* or to control withdrawal effects. A "yes" response to any two questions indicates a positive screen (Brown and Rounds 1995).

Other common screens include The Alcohol Use Disorders Identification Test (AUDIT)(Babor et al. 1989). This is a 10-item screen that is very popular in medical settings. The AUDIT screens for frequency and quantity of drinking as well as problem drinking, hazardous use, and alcohol use disorders (Babor et al. 1989, 2001). The Michigan Alcohol Screening Test (MAST) is a commonly used, reliable, and valid 28-item (yes/no) screen for alcohol use disorders (Selzer 1971). The screen assesses for lack of control over drinking behavior and whether the person has experienced a range of negative consequences related to drinking. There is a 24-item short-form geriatric version (SMAST-G) that is one of the first and most common screens for alcohol use disorders and problematic drinking behavior in older adults (Selzer 1971). A score of five or more positive responses indicates the presence of problem drinking (Blow et al. 1998). The 10-item Drug Abuse Screening Test (DAST-10) is a brief instrument that assesses for problematic and hazardous drug use and has been shown to have good reliability and validity (Skinner 1982; Gavin et al. 1989).

Prescreening questions can include asking clients if they drink or use drugs, how frequently they have drank or used drugs in the past two weeks, and how many drinks they have had in the past two weeks. The National Institute on Alcohol Abuse and Alcoholism (NIAAA) has set average daily and weekly drinking limits for men at no more than two drinks per day or 14 drinks per week. For persons who identify as female and persons over the age of 65, the daily limits are one drink per day and seven drinks per week. Hazardous drinking limits include five or more drinks within one day for men, and four or more drinks per day for women or persons over 65 years of age. Unfortunately, there are currently no specific guidelines for Trans Gender Non-Conforming (TGNC) persons. Persons who exceed the above drinking limits are at a higher risk of developing an alcohol use disorder and experiencing other health problems.

Providers can also ask two additional questions: (1) how many times in the past year have you had five or more drinks (four or more if client is over 65 years old or identifies as female)? An answer of more than one indicates the potential presence of hazardous drinking and (2) how many times have you used an illegal substance or misused a prescription medication in the past year? An answer greater than one indicates the potential presence of a substance use problem requiring further assessment (Smith et al. 2010). Screening instruments for substance use will be further covered in Chap. 10.

4.4.3   Adverse Childhood Events (ACEs) and Trauma

As reviewed in Chap. 2 and, later in Chap. 7, experiencing adverse childhood events and/or traumatic events can have a substantial, dose–response impact on a wide range of health and behavioral health domains including increased use of healthcare resources, comorbid medical conditions, depression, and substance use. Screening for ACEs and trauma can provide valuable information for providers that can inform treatment planning. Asking the question "Have you ever experienced or witnessed a situation where you thought your life was in danger?" can lead to important conversations about trauma and stress. Using an ACE questionnaire as routine part of intake can give providers an ACE score that can help them determine whether a more complete assessment for trauma is necessary and can give guidance on a proper course of treatment.

Two screens that provide important information regarding ACEs and trauma are the Revised Adverse Childhood Events Questionnaire (Finkelhor et al. 2013, 2015) and the Primary Care-Post Traumatic Stress Disorder Screen for DSM-5 (PC-PTSD-5) (Prins et al. 2003, 2015, 2016). Both are easy to administer and have been found to be useful and appropriate in primary care settings, outpatient and inpatient behavioral healthcare settings, emergency departments, and in integrated care settings. The Revised ACE questionnaire screens for most of the original ten ACEs as well as questions regarding peer bullying, peer rejection, and community violence exposure. The PC-PTSD-5 is a five-item scale that screens for probable PTSD symptoms in response to an identified traumatic event including intrusive thoughts or images (e.g., nightmares), dissociation (e.g., numbing), hyperarousal (e.g., being on guard), avoidance of reminders of the event, and experiencing guilt or self-blame regarding the event. A "yes" to any three questions suggest possible PTSD and warrants further assessment.

A valuable screen that combines items from the above instruments is the Patient Stress Questionnaire. This is a 26-item screen used in behavioral health and primary care settings that integrates items from the PHQ-9 (depression), GAD-7 (anxiety), PC-PTSD-5 (trauma), and AUDIT (alcohol use) to form a brief screen for the most common disorders listed above (SAMHSA 2020).

4.4.4   Perceived Stress

Like trauma, high perceived stress related to poverty, discrimination, violence, caregiving, occupation, and other stressors can lead to increased risks for depression, anxiety, and adverse health behaviors (e.g., smoking, drinking, poor diet, and sedentary lifestyle), resulting in higher rates of morbidity and premature mortality (Algren et al. 2018; Geronimus et al. 2006; Krueger and Chang 2008; Mancini and Farina 2019; Ng and Jeffery 2003). Given these clinical implications, identifying clients with high levels of perceived stress is an important component of any health assessment. Perceived stress can be effectively screened using the Perceived Stress Scale-4 (PSS-4) (Cohen et al. 1983). This four-item scale measures qualities of stress that include how overwhelming, negative, and persistent clients perceive their stress to be, and how much control the person thinks they have over their stress. Higher scores indicate more stress. This is a simple tool that can be used to quickly assess the stress burden of clients and indicate whether there is a need for intervention.

Perceived stress can also be assessed by simply asking people how stressed they feel. A reliable and valid single-item stress scale includes the question: "Stress refers to a situation where a person feels tense, restless, nervous, or anxious, or is unable to sleep at night because his/her mind is troubled all the time. Do you feel that kind of stress these days?" The anchors are Not at all (1); Only a little (2); To some extent (3); Rather much (4); and Very much (5). A score of 3 and above indicate intermediate to high stress levels (Elo et al. 2003).

Clients who score highly on stress can receive interventions designed to reduce stress that can include: (1) social support interventions (e.g., case management) designed to address and alleviate the burdens of poverty such as poor housing, income constraints, access to transportation and childcare, and other resources; (2) psychoeducation and stress reduction techniques such as mindfulness-based stress reduction (MBSR) interventions, which have been found effective in reducing stress (Janssen et al. 2018; Kabat-Zinn 1990); and/or (3) helping clients advocate for their rights if they are experiencing discrimination or other forms of unfair treatment at work, school, or other life domains that are causing stress.

4.4.5 Interpersonal Violence

Interpersonal violence is common and takes an enormous toll on the lives and health of millions of people (CDC 2020a, b). Two forms if interpersonal violence are intimate partner violence and community violence. Intimate partner violence (IPV) is defined as physical, sexual, or psychological violence, threats, intimidation, stalking, and other actions with the intent to control an intimate partner (Decker et al. 2018; CDC 2020a, b). Community violence is violence that is committed by strangers or acquaintances. This form of violence usually takes place outside of the home and can include fights, robberies, assaults, and homicides. Assessing for community violence involves asking clients if they have ever experienced physical violence in their community such as a violent attack, assault, being shot, stabbed, robbed, or beaten up. Assessment questions can also include asking about how safe a person feels in their community or neighborhood.

Screening for intimate partner violence can utilize a brief screening instrument that has been highly valid in a variety of settings. The HITS screening tool (Sherin et al. 1998; Rabin et al. 2009) is a four-item scale that asks clients if their partner has ever: physically **H**urt you, **I**nsulted or talked down to you, **T**hreatened you with harm, or **S**creamed or cursed at you. The scale uses the anchors (never, rarely, sometimes, fairly often, and frequently). Another question to ask people is simply whether or not they are afraid of their partner. When screening for IPV, providers should do so alone with the client in a confidential and private location and fully inform clients of the limits of confidentiality if they disclose whether they have experienced violence. Mandatory reporting laws vary by state in relation to IPV. Providers should know the laws of their respective geographic location and relay those constraints to the client before screening for IPV or other forms of violence. Professional language interpreters independent from the client's family or friends should be available to translate items on the scale or interview. Results should be discussed privately with the client in a calm and neutral tone. Providers should provide education and information about IPV regardless of disclosure. If a client screens positive for IPV, providers are encouraged to show concern, inform clients about the health implications, and ask clients if they would like to receive further assessment or other services. Services should be readily available and co-located at the setting. If services are not co-located on site, the provider should have formal referral relationships with outside community providers such as behavioral health providers, legal services, crisis teams, victim advocacy groups, and shelters so as to facilitate timely and effective referrals and following up (i.e., warm referrals) (Decker et al. 2018).

The information in the above screening areas can be used to guide the assessment process that will inform the development of the case conceptualization and subsequent person-centered care plan (Adams and Grieder 2014). In the next section, information regarding the psychiatric examination and social determinants of health will be reviewed. In each of these domains, it is important to identify past history and current difficulties for each area as well as the strengths, skills, and resources needed to address problems experienced in any domain area.

4.5   Behavioral Health Assessment Areas

Presenting Problems

Problem formulation guides and orients the assessment and treatment process. Problem formulation is a conceptualization of the presenting problems brought forth by the client. Problems are stated in clear, measurable, and solvable terms. Adequately exploring, describing, and defining the problem are vital steps toward proper assessment and treatment. What problems have brought the client to your agency? If part of a routine clinical exam or checkup—what pressing concerns or problems does the client have? What problems have they experienced in the past? The problems reviewed can include mental health symptoms (e.g., depression, anxiety, psychotic symptoms, and ADHD); substance use issues (e.g., problem drinking, substance misuses, and substance use disorders); experiencing stress, adverse events, interpersonal violence, or other traumas; suicidal behavior; social isolation; functional impairments; medical conditions; or social factors such as poverty, homelessness, or family-relational issues.

During this conversation, it can be helpful to clarify the problem from the client's point of view. Problem definition is not simply what the client says is the problem. While it is important to listen to the client and take their views into consideration, what the client perceives is the problem is not always accurate, complete, or stated in a way that is solvable. For instance, a client who is depressed and has negative core beliefs about themselves as helpless and unlovable often underestimate their ability to solve problems, take on too much responsibility for perceived problems, and overestimate the severity and future negative consequences of problems. This can lead to pessimism, hopelessness, and paralysis. In these situations, providers may need to help clients reframe problems so that they more accurately reflect the client's situation, their role and responsibilities in the problems, and the achievable solutions that can be undertaken by the client. This process can lead to relief, motivation, and action on the part of the client. This process relies on building trust and actively listening, reflecting, and exploring problems with clients during assessment.

Medical History

As reviewed in Chap. 2, behavioral health disorders are commonly comorbid with many chronic illnesses and that this relationship is often bidirectional. A medical history and evaluation can provide important information for behavioral health providers. For instance, several diseases such as diabetes, thyroid disease, delirium, Parkinson's disease, Huntington's disease, multiple sclerosis, asthma, arthritis, chronic pain, irritable bowel syndrome, cardiovascular and cerebrovascular disease, obesity, HIV/AIDS, hepatitis, lupus, fibromyalgia, and other diseases are either comorbid with behavioral health issues or have symptoms that mimic behavioral health symptoms such as depressed or labile mood, anxiety, hallucinations, attention problems, cognitive disorganization and deficits, and difficulty concentrating (APA 2013; Scott et al. 2016). While medical conditions can produce symptoms that mimic behavioral health disorders, it is also possible that behavioral health and medical conditions exist as separate comorbidities. As a result, it is paramount for behavioral health providers to know the degree to which behavioral health symptoms are a part of a medical condition and how medical and behavioral health symptoms impact each other. Other important medical information that behavioral health providers need to know are what medication the client is taking or has taken in the past, whether they have had any recent surgeries or procedures conducted in the past, and whether they are pregnant or nursing. Medical information can be collected as part of the routine physical examination, from medical records, or via an intake form or other self-report format.

Family History

Behavioral health issues often run in families, and conducting a careful review of family history for various behavioral health conditions can provide important information about the client system. Tools such as genograms and eco-maps can help providers understand past and current family structure, contexts, and dynamics that can inform assessment. A genogram (McGoldrick et al. 2020) provides a generational diagram of family structures that identify relationships within the client system that are supportive, stressful, or toxic. This diagram can outline who the client can rely on in their family, who relies on them, and relationships in the family that are negative and stressful due to mental illness, substance use, or violence. A genogram can also provide important information about positive or negative patterns that exist across generations. An eco-map (Hartman 1978) is rooted in the ecological framework and positions the client in the center of an expanding web of relationships with other systems such as household, immediate and extended family, friends, schools, neighborhood, community groups, work, service organizations and systems (e.g., criminal justice systems, health, or behavioral health systems), and faith communities. The eco-map identifies the quality of the relationships between the client and these other systems such as whether they are nurturing, helpful, stressful, or toxic (1978).

Functional Assessment

Functional assessment refers to the level to which a client can live independently and successfully complete daily activities and routines. Functional assessments are particularly important for persons with intellectual, developmental or physical disabilities, traumatic brain injury, dementia-related or cognitive impairments, and severe forms of mental illness who may need support living independently in the community (APA 2013). Some areas of a functional assessment include:

- Ability to effectively communicate and socialize with others and develop safe, positive relationships with others
- Safety or the ability to stay safe and avoid danger
- Occupational skills and abilities
- Physical mobility and ability to get around, such as walking or using assistive devices
- Sensory abilities such as seeing and hearing or the ability to use adaptive tools such as walking stick, braille, sign language, or assistive technologies
- Ability to complete activities of daily living (e.g., eating, using the toilet, bathing, and dressing) and instrumental activities of daily living (e.g., household chores, cooking, cleaning, laundry, and grocery shopping)
- Ability to budget, pay bills, and handle money
- Transportation—ability to drive a car or use of public transportation
- Literacy ability

Several scales can be used to assess functioning. A common scale that is part of the DSM-5 is the World Health Organization's Disability Assessment Scale (WHODAS 2.0) (APA 2013). The WHODAS 2.0 is a brief but comprehensive assessment scale that measures several functional domains including cognition, mobility, self-care, getting along with others, life activities, and community participation (Ustun et al. 2010).

Behavioral Health Symptoms

A behavioral health assessment includes an evaluation of a range of internalizing (e.g., depression and anxiety), externalizing (e.g., substance use, aggression, ADHD, mania, and disruptive disorders), and psychotic (e.g., hallucinations, delusions, and disorganized thinking) mental health symptoms that can assist in identification of behavioral health disorders and guide treatment planning and intervention selection. I will review specific information on diagnostic symptoms for depression, anxiety, PTSD, and substance use disorders in separate chapters in this book. Here, I will review some common behavioral health symptom areas that indicate the presence of a behavioral health disorder and how to assess for them. Table 4.1 outlines the most common behavioral health symptom domains and their relationship to behavioral health disorders. These symptom areas form the basis of the mental health status exam (MSE) discussed next.

The provider is best served by utilizing the screening information obtained in the early treatment meeting or intake process and the client's medical history to guide their assessment. This information can then be used to inform the mental status exam (MSE), which is a psychiatric exam that explores a range of symptoms areas and domains with the client. Providers should gather information regarding past and current use of psychiatric medications, psychiatric diagnoses, and psychiatric hospitalization or treatment history. The MSE relies on self-report of historical and current information from the client as well as observation of verbal and nonverbal behavior of the client by the service provider. Information from collateral contacts such as family or caregivers can also inform the MSE. Service providers should consider all observation within the context of their client giving consideration to culture, race, age, gender identity, ability, sexual orientation, religious preferences, and socioeconomic factors that may influence what the service provider is observing in their clients. The mental status exam can help service providers determine if mood, anxiety, psychotic, substance use, or other disorders such as delirium are present (Snyderman and Rovner 2009; Vergare et al. 2006). The following sections outline the specific components of the mental status exam that are displayed in Table 4.1.

Appearance The provider can initiate the MSE by observing the client's appearance upon arrival to the visit. Appearance can include grooming, dress, personal hygiene, and general demeanor such as eye contact, distinguishing features such as scars and tattoos, and attention to detail. A person with a disheveled or unkempt appearance, dirty clothing, poor hygiene, or inappropriate dress may indicate poverty, stress, or illness such as depression, addiction, or psychosis.

General Behavior General behavior includes the person's level of openness, politeness, calmness, and cooperation. Persons who are excessively guarded, nervous, suspicious, withdrawn, irritable, or resistant could be experiencing a range of issues such as depression, anxiety, substance use, psychosis, or mania. Persons experiencing intimate partner violence or abuse may also exhibit guarded or nervous behavior, especially if the abuser is present or nearby. The person may also be

Table 4.1 Common symptoms in mental health disorders

Symptom area	Depression	Anxiety	Mania	Psychosis	Delirium or intoxication
Appearance	Disheveled Poor grooming Poor hygiene	Disheveled Poor grooming Poor hygiene	Disheveled Poor grooming Poor hygiene, Inappropriate or provocative dress	Disheveled Poor grooming Poor hygiene	Disheveled Poor grooming Poor hygiene
General behavior	Irritable Withdrawn	Fearful Nervous Fidgety Guarded	Inappropriate Grandiose Irritable Aggressive Euphoric Interrupting Restless	Suspicious Distracted Irritable Guarded Resistant Withdrawn Fearful Aggressive	Disoriented Somnolent Hyperalert Disorganized Fluctuating alterations in consciousness Poor attention
Speech	Slow Low Soft Sad Monotone	Staccato Shaky or tremulous Fearful Nervous	Fast Loud Aggressive Angry Irritable Euphoric	Angry Paranoid Incoherent Disorganized Illogical Monotone Mutism	Slurred Incoherent Disorganized Shifting/labile tone
Motor	Bradykinesia	Agitated Restless Hand wringing Pacing Fidgety	Akathisia Inability to sit still Psychomotor agitation or restlessness Hyperactive	Parkinsonism (Rx) Akathisia (Rx) Catatonia Bradykinesia (Rx) Negativism Psychomotor agitation	Psychomotor agitation Bradykinesia Negativism Somnolence Lack of coordination
Affect	Sad Irritable Dysphoric Tearful Dysregulated	Fearful Irritable Nervous On edge	Euphoric Irritable Energized Dysregulation	Nervous/on edge irritable Fearful Dysregulated	Fluctuating between calm, euthymic, and irritated or dysphoric
Cognitions	Poor concentration Poor memory	Poor concentration Distracted	Distracted, Overly alert	Distracted Disorganized Poor memory Impulsive Lack of focus Impaired executive functioning Poor planning	Fluctuating consciousness ranging from alert to clouded, lethargic to somnolent and comatose

(continued)

Table 4.1 (continued)

Symptom area	Depression	Anxiety	Mania	Psychosis	Delirium or intoxication
Thought Content	Suicidal Self-blame Guilt Worthlessness	Obsessive Fearful Avoidant Preoccupied with feared stimuli Overestimate risks	Grandiose Delusions Flight of ideas Racing thoughts Incoherent Disorganized	Paranoid or bizarre delusions Disorganized Illogical Incoherent	Fluctuating Disorganized Labile Incoherent
Hallucinations	Auditory or visual hallucinations may be present during active mood syndrome	Not usually present	Auditory or visual hallucinations may be present during active mood syndrome	Evidence of internal stimuli in the form of auditory (e.g., voices) or visual hallucinations	
Insight Judgment	Insight and judgment can be impaired Impulsiveness a risk factor for suicide	Insight usually intact	Poor insight and judgment High impulsivity. High degree of risk behaviors and dangerousness when mania is present	Poor insight and judgment High impulsivity High degree of risk behaviors especially when using substances High victimization risk	Poor insight and judgment High impulsivity High degree of risk behaviors especially when using substances. High risk for victimization

Based on Snyderman and Rovner (2009) and Vergare et al. (2006)

having a bad day or may not like being asked personal questions. It is normative for clients to be a guarded or nervous in psychiatric interviews. Be sure to position the client's behavior within the context of the situation and other signs and symptoms.

Speech A client's speech can indicate a range of problems. Important factors to pay attention to speech include how much the person is talking (quantity), how fast they are talking (rate), how loud they are talking (volume), the tone of speech (e.g., angry or euphoric), and coherence of speech. For instance, persons speaking rapidly, loudly, and exhibiting grandiose flight of ideas may be experiencing a manic episode, ADHD, anxiety, or stimulant intoxication. Persons speaking very slowly, softly, and with an irritable or sad tone may be depressed. People speaking in ways that are illogical or incoherent may be experiencing disorganized thinking, which is commonly seen in clients experiencing delirium, psychosis, substance use, or cerebrovascular accident. Speech that is monotone or with a blunted effect may indicate psychosis or the side effects of psychiatric medication. Slurred speech could indicate the effects of overmedication, cerebrovascular accident stroke and transient ischemic attack (TIA's), or substance use, or it could also indicate a number of health disorders such as Bell's palsy, amyotrophic lateral sclerosis (ALS), multiple sclerosis (MS), or poorly fitting dentures or thought disorders.

Motor Movements This includes body movements, posture, and facial expressions. Some nervousness would be expected in an interview—but generally a person is expected to appear calm, relaxed, and animated. Signs of ill health would include overt restlessness (akathisia) or psychomotor agitation (e.g., the inability to sit still and excessive motor activity). These could indicate anxiety, ADHD, mania, psychosis, or addiction/withdrawal. These could also be side effects of neuroleptic/antipsychotic medication, which can also include tics, tremors, and involuntary fine motor movements (e.g., Tardive Dyskinesia or parkinsonism). Psychomotor retardation (bradykinesia), such as slowness of movement and physical/emotional reactions, can indicate depression, side effects of psychiatric medication (overmedication), or the negative symptoms of schizophrenia.

Affect/Mood It is important to screen for the presence of mood and anxiety disorders in patients, and this is usually done through patient self-report (Vergare et al. 2006). Ask people directly, "How would you describe your mood?", "Have you felt depressed, blue, sad, or discouraged lately?", "Have you felt angry or irritable lately?", "Have you felt euphoric, energized, and like you're out of control lately? (e.g., mania)," or "Have you felt nervous or on edge lately?" Any of these symptoms might indicate the presence of mood, anxiety, or a bipolar spectrum condition.

Thought Process and Content Thought processes include how clients express themselves in the visit, organize and communicate their ideas, and answer questions. Are statements logical and goal directed? Is the person able to answer questions appropriately? Do their answers make sense? For instance, clients who exhibit a flight of ideas or who express thoughts that are disorganized, incoherent, disconnected, obsessional, or delusional could indicate a number of conditions such as anxiety, depression, schizophrenia, substance use, or obsessive compulsive disorder. This can also be assessed via self-report or standardized instruments. Some questions to ask include: (1) Do you have intrusive thoughts or images that you can't control or shake that cause you anxiety? (2) Do you have an excessive fear of something? (3) Do you find yourself worrying about a lot of different things? (4) Do you think people are out to get you? (5) Do you think you have any special powers that other people don't have? (6) Do you feel guilty about things that happened a long time ago? (7) Do you think you're a bad person? The DSM-5 has a number of dimensional scales that can thoroughly assess for the above symptoms and point the provider in the direction of a potential diagnosis (APA 2013).

Suicidal/Homicidal Ideation Screening for suicidality and homicidality is important and should be a part of any intake and assessment process in integrated behavioral health settings. A detailed suicide assessment procedure is reviewed in Chap.

8. Basic questions to screen for suicidality include: Have you ever thought about hurting or killing yourself? If so, how often do you have these thoughts? How would you do it? Have you ever tried to kill yourself? Do you ever feel that life is not worth living? Questions to ask about homicidality include: Have you ever thought about killing or hurting other people to get even with them? If so, when was the last time you had those thoughts?

While there is little evidence supporting specific suicide screening instruments, a brief four-item screening instrument for suicide that can be used in a variety of settings is the Ask Suicide-Screening Questions questionnaire (ASQ) (Horowitz et al. 2012). In a 2012 study, a "yes" response to one or more of the four questions identified 97% of youth at risk for suicide (Horowitz et al. 2012). The screening questions include: In the past few weeks have you: (1) Wished you were dead? (2) Felt that you or your family would be better off dead? (3) Been having thoughts about killing yourself? (4) Have ever tried to kill yourself? (If yes, how?). A "yes" to any of the four questions requires the interviewer to ask a fifth question: Are you having thoughts of killing yourself right now? (If yes, please describe)

A positive screen for suicide is if the client answers "yes" to any of the first four questions. If they answer "yes" to the fifth question, the client is in imminent risk for suicide, requiring an emergency evaluation or risk assessment. Appropriate medical personnel or first responders should be notified. The client should not be left alone for any period of time. The client should not be out of sight of a professional and should be in a secure and safe environment until the full evaluation is complete. When a client answers "yes" to any of the first four questions, and "no" to question five, this is considered a nonacute positive screen requiring a suicide safety assessment to determine if a full mental health evaluation is needed. The client should not leave until evaluated for safety and a safety plan (see Chap. 8) is developed. Proper personnel responsible for client care should be alerted.

Hallucinations Hallucinations are perceptual experiences, sometimes referred to as internal stimuli, that occur in the mind of the client and are not perceptible to others. Common examples include hearing voices or other sounds that others do not hear, or seeing objects, images, distortions, or people that others do not see. In other words, people hear and see things that others do not. Hallucinations are common symptoms in persons with schizophrenia, bipolar spectrum disorders, major depression, delirium, dementia, intoxication, or withdrawal. In fact, most of us will experience a hallucination at some point in our lives. Exploratory questions to ask include: Do you see or hear things that upset you that others cannot? The provider should observe if the client is responding to any internal stimuli or auditory or visual hallucinations such as tracking eye movements, facial expression, body language, attention, or verbal responses.

Consciousness and Cognition Consciousness can be considered alert, clouded, somnolent, lethargic, and comatose. Cognition can include attention, concentration, and memory. Any disturbance or fluctuation of consciousness may indicate a delirium, which is a medical condition that must be immediately addressed (APA 2013).

Delirium is often misdiagnosed in older adults as dementia or cognitive impairment. This can be a lethal mistake. Delirium is often the result of a significant medical condition or event such as an infection (e.g., urinary tract infection and staph infection), stroke, drug overdose, intoxication, head trauma, nutritional deficit, or dehydration. Delirium is a confusional state that can share some symptoms and etiologies with dementia and depression. Delirium has several primary and secondary diagnostic features impacting a person's attention, memory, arousal, and awareness. Symptoms can be hyper- and hypoactive in nature. The primary diagnostic features for delirium are: (1) an acute disturbance in cognition (e.g., memory, language, orientation, and perception), awareness, and the ability to focus, sustain, and shift attention; (2) clinically significant symptoms develop rapidly (e.g., within hours), fluctuate over the course of a day, and result in a marked difference in baseline functioning; (3) disturbance is not part of a pre-existing neurocognitive condition and there is evidence (e.g., lab tests, examination, and medical history) symptoms are caused by a medical condition or substance (withdrawal, side effect, and intoxication); (4) fluctuating changes in psychomotor activity, mood and behavior that can include restlessness, agitation, euphoria, nervousness, aggressive behavior, paranoia, social withdrawal, confusion, disorganized speech, slurred words and incoherence, subdued motor activity, and limited arousal and attention (APA 2013).

These symptoms can often be misdiagnosed as fatigue, dementia, stroke, and psychiatric disorders including bipolar and schizophrenia spectrum disorders, and depressed or anxious mood. A particular challenge is the fact that hyper- and hypo-symptoms can fluctuate and cycle widely over the course of a delirium. This fluctuation and rapid onset are key indicators that a delirium may be present (Mandebvu and Kalman 2015; Kalish et al. 2014; APA 2013). Assessing for delirium can include using the Confusion Assessment Method (CAM), a brief screening instrument for delirium that assesses for the main diagnostic symptoms of depression including rapid onset, fluctuating course, and confusion and attention issues (Inouye et al. 1990; Wei et al. 2008).

Assessing for attention and concentration can also be done by asking a person to spell the word "W.O.R.L.D." backward and forward. You can ask them to do so with their name if they have trouble reading or spelling. You can also ask people to subtract serial 7's from a hundred (e.g. 100, 93, 86, 79…). Questions measuring cognition in an MSE must take into account a person's education and cultural background. Memory can also be assessed using a number of instruments including the Mini-Mental State Exam (MMSE) (Folstein et al. 1975) or the Mini-Cognitive Assessment Instrument (MINI-COG), which asks people to repeat and remember three words (e.g., dog, car, and tree). They are then asked to draw the hands on a clock that specifies a particular time (e.g., 3:35). Once this is complete, they are asked to recall and recite the three words they were given. The Mini-Cog is brief, sensitive, and easy to administer regardless of education level to detect cognitive impairment (Borson et al. 2003).

Insight and Judgment Insight is a person's awareness of illness, how it impacts their life and those around them, and their need for treatment. Persons with schizophrenia, bipolar disorder, and dementia may often lack insight into their illness and this (in schizophrenia) predicts poor treatment response (Lysaker and Buck 2007). Judgment is the level to which a client can appreciate and recognize the consequences of their actions. Persons with bipolar and schizophrenia spectrum disorders, dementia, and some personality disorders can sometimes struggle to exhibit sound judgment due to their symptoms. A common question used to assess judgment is: What would you do if you found a stamped envelope on the sidewalk? Persons who struggle to answer the question directly (e.g., put it in the nearest mailbox) may be having trouble with judgment that could indicate several disorders such as delirium, bipolar spectrum disorder, schizophrenia spectrum disorder, or dementia, among others.

4.6 Social Environmental Domains of Assessment

Racial health disparities are the result of health inequities in many social determinants of health (SDOH) related to income, health insurance access, access to transportation, childcare, food and other basic resources, adequate and stable housing, interpersonal safety, and environmental conditions among others (WHO 2010; Nuruzzaman et al. 2015; CSDH, 2008; Phelan et al. 2010). These differences in SDOH result from the creation and maintenance of racist policies and systems designed to benefit white populations at the expense of BIPOC communities. Health disparities can only be resolved through the dismantling of these racist systems and policies and the creation of new policies that seek to provide equitable access to the resources important to health (Kendi 2019). Health and behavioral health providers can play an important role in this work at multiple levels. The first step in addressing the social determinants of health is to routinely assess the social needs of all patients and provide them, either directly or through coordinated referrals, with the resources needed resolve unmet needs. Recent research in the field of family medicine suggests that many providers, particularly early career providers and those serving high need communities, are engaged in addressing SDOH at least in some form (NASEM, 2019; Nuruzzaman et al. 2015; Kovach et al. 2019). While addressing SDOH in clients is gaining ground and has shown to lead to care that is more holistic, effective, and efficient, barriers to effective implementation in clinical practice exist. These barriers include: (1) lack of provider training; (2) insufficient time in the clinical encounter; (3) lack of staffing and organizational capacity; (4) lack of community programming to address social needs outside of the clinic; and (5) lack of financial incentives and billing codes (Andermann 2018; Kovach et al. 2019). The need to change billing restrictions, provide training, enhance electronic health record prompts, and the routine deployment of community health workers and peer staff are just some areas that could enhance utilization of SDOH assessment and intervention (NASEM, 2019; Kovach et al. 2019). Figure 4.3 identifies the broad domains of the most common social determinants of health relevant for behavioral health assessment.

Several screening forms currently exist to guide efficient and effective SDOH assessment. For instance, the Protocol for Responding to and Assessing Patient Assets, Risks, and Experiences (PRAPARE Protocol) developed by the National Association of Community Health Centers (2016) asks a range of questions that address SDOH (NACHC 2019). The first section assesses demographic and language preferences for the patient. The form then assesses: (1) how many family members live in the home; (2) housing status; (3) money and resources including education level and employment situation, insurance status, and access to health care; (4) ability to pay for basic resources including utilities, food, childcare, and medicine; (5) access to transportation; (6) social and emotional health including social networks; (7) perceived stress; and (8) optional questions regarding refugee status, incarceration history, and safety/IPV. The protocol is a total of 21 questions and can be completed in a matter of minutes (NACHC 2019).

Another screening tool is the Center for Medicare and Medicaid Services and Center for Medicare and Medicaid Innovation (CMMI) Accountable Health Communities Health-Related Social Needs Screening Tool (Billioux et al. 2017). The tool screens for social needs that impact health such as homelessness, hunger, and interpersonal violence. This 26-item self-report tool is designed for healthcare providers to screen for the presence of health-related social needs in several areas. The five main areas of the screening form are: (1) housing instability; (2) need for utilities assistance; (3) access to food; (4) exposure to violence; and (5) transportation access. Several other questions were added to screen for mental health and substance use, financial stress, employment and education status, presence of family/community support, and disabilities. The tool is currently being tested at several Accountable Health Community (AHC) sites across the United States (Billioux et al. 2017). If it is not possible to implement the above tools into your practice setting, the following areas are relevant for social determinants of health and all or most should comprise a component of assessment.

Family and Community Support
Assess the quality of support the client has in their household and community. What important and positive relationships does the person currently have and what relationships were important in the past? What is the quality of their social support? Who is important to them and why? How do they get along with their neighbors? How would they rate the quality of their interpersonal relationships? Do they ever feel lonely or isolated?

Housing and Daily Living
In this section, the provider assesses the quality of the client's home life. What is the client's current housing situation? What do they enjoy about their home (what makes it "home")? What living skills do they have and what would be their ideal living situation? Also, what are the problems they encounter in their living situation (e.g., safety, homelessness, and lack of access to resources)? Is the housing safe and stable? Are there any health concerns such as mold, pests, fire hazards, lead paint, inadequate heating/cooling, plumbing, or appliances for cooking? Does the client feel safe in their community?

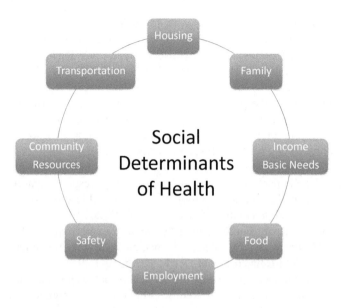

Fig. 4.3 Social determinants of health

Transportation
Access to safe, reliable, and affordable transportation is an important element in health and well-being. Having access to adequate transportation can enable the client to get to work or school, go shopping, and attend medical appointments. Assess clients' level of access to transportation to get them where they need to go. Do they have their own vehicle? Are they in a walkable or bikeable neighborhood? Are they on the train or bus line? How does the person get around? Do they lack access to affordable and accessible transportation that limits their ability to go to work or school, attend medical appointments, or complete daily living activities such as shopping?

Employment and Education
Stable employment and income are vital to health. Assess the employment status and education level of your client. What is the client's current work situation? What have they done in the past and what would they like to do now and in the future? How stable is their current employment? Are they looking for work or need help finding work? How satisfied are they with their job? How much stress does their job give them? What vocational skills does the person have? What do they aspire to do? What skills does the person have and what would they like to learn in the future?

Food Insecurity
Having regular access to healthy food is an important contributor to health. Does the person have access to healthy, affordable food? Has the person ever run out of food or not had money to buy food in the last 12 months? Does the person have easy

access to high quality, affordable grocery stores and markets? Has the person ever worried about running out of food in the last year?

Financial Resources and Basic Needs
Assess clients' ability to pay their bills and their level of financial strain. What are their sources of income and how well does their income meet their needs? What goals do they have regarding income and finances (e.g., savings, vacation, saving for home)? Has the person had or come close to having their utilities turned off or do they have trouble paying for utilities such as gas, heat, hot water, water, and electric? Do they have medical insurance and are they able to pay medical bills? How much money do they have leftover at the end of the month after paying monthly bills? How much do they worry about making ends meet?

Activity/Leisure/Recreation
What do they do for fun? How would they characterize their physical activity level? For instance, on average how many days a week do they exercise and how long is each activity? What are their hobbies and pursuits? What have they enjoyed in the past that they currently do not utilize? Do they have access to parks and other recreational activities? What low-cost recreational activities does the client have access to such as museums, science center, zoo, etc.?

Spirituality/Culture
Providers often feel uncomfortable assessing spirituality due to not being clear on the goal or the definition of spirituality (Starnino et al. 2014). Assessing spirituality means assessing anything that provides meaning, joy, and purpose to the person and helps them strive to be the best version of themselves that they can be. From this perspective, spirituality can go beyond religious descriptions and include hobbies, artistic endeavors, activities, activism, and other things that help people be whole and help the person feel a part of something bigger than themselves. These aspects of spirituality can then be used to help enhance people's recovery and well-being (Starnino et al. 2014). What gives a person a sense of accomplishment, meaning, and purpose? What activities initiate a sense of flow or engagement (see Chap. 3) or a sense of wholeness and well-being (Starnino et al. 2014)? These aspects can also be identity-forming activities such as cultural or religious traditions, rituals, foods, celebrations, beliefs, and values.

4.7   Common Components of the Behavioral Health Assessment

Assessment documentation formats vary across behavioral health settings. The following sections identify the most common and important areas that can comprise a behavioral health assessment. The information in these sections will be used to inform the case conceptualization and treatment planning process discussed in Chap. 5.

Demographic Information

Demographic information about the client includes age, sex, race, ethnic and/or cultural group, preferred gender identification (e.g., cis-gendered woman/man, trans woman/trans man, gender variant, intersex, two spirit) and preferred pronouns, sexual orientation, marital status, number of children, and roles within the household (parent, spouse, and adult caregiver). This section can also include relevant roles such as: are they a veteran or in the military, student, parent, adult caregiver, or retired?

Referral Information

How did the client come to the agency? Who or what agency referred the client to you? Is the client mandated or voluntary? Identify any other status information (e.g., inpatient and partial hospitalization) or where else the client receives services.

Presenting Problems

This section provides a description of the problem that brought the client to the agency and any relevant problems impacting treatment and behavioral health status of the client such as substance use, trauma, lack of support, life stressors, or grief. This can include other persons in the client's family or household that are impacted by, or are impacting, the problem. If the presenting problem is recurrent, describe how the client has experienced it and dealt with it in the past. Identify related difficulties that stem from the presenting problems and any personal, interpersonal, or environmental issues are exacerbating the presenting problem.

Client Strengths

This section includes strengths at the personal, interpersonal, and environmental level. It is important that client strengths be mentioned up front rather than anecdotally at the end of the assessment. The assessment is a narration of a client's life. It should leave the reader with an impression that, while the client has problems, they are balanced by several strengths and positive qualities. This section should outline personal strengths that include the following: (1) talents and abilities across a range of areas such as home, work, school, hobbies, recreation/sports, and other areas; (2) special abilities, attributes, and characteristics such as loving-kindness, friendship/camaraderie, courage, integrity, openness, conscientiousness, charisma, listening, gratitude, humor, grit/perseverance, and the ability to abide and survive disappointment; and (3) interests, aspirations, hopes, and dreams that drive and motivate the person to achieve. The strengths section should also identify supportive relationships and social networks in the client's life that they can lean on such as family, friends, faith, community, and work community, and any environmental strengths that exist such as stable housing, health insurance, or adequate income.

Current Living and Social Situation (SDOH)

This section includes information about the client's household and family situation including the number of people in the household, location, housing status (e.g., independent, residential, institutional, shelter, and homeless), and quality of housing (e.g., safe, affordable, in good repair, quality of plumbing, heat appliances, clean, number of bedrooms, and any problems with pests). It also includes information about the level of safety and environmental barriers such as lack of access to healthy food, transportation, recreation, or support, or the presence of environmental risks such as lead, pollution, crime, and violence. Financial resources are also discussed in this section and should include information on financial resources, basic needs, current occupational and income status, and benefits. Education and employment history can also be included in this section as well as the client's work skills, vocational training areas, or employment/education aspirations not included elsewhere.

Medical Problems

Provide a summary of the current health status of the client and any relevant health history such as current and past medical issues and ongoing or chronic medical needs, medication history and current medications and preferences, allergies, and any risk behaviors regarding alcohol use, diet/weight, smoking, drug use, sexual activity, and physical activity levels.

Behavioral Health Problems

Provide a summary of the current and historical behavioral health information. This includes psychiatric diagnosis and treatment history, current diagnoses and treatment, results of the most recent mental status exam, screening instruments, and assessments. This information also includes substance use history and current use patterns for alcohol, prescription and other drugs, caffeine, and nicotine.

Interpersonal Relationships

Summarize the quality of the most important interpersonal relationships in the client's life including intimate partners, family, and friends. It highlights important positive social supports and relationships as well as relationships that cause stress.

Safety and Trauma

For trauma, identify any history of interpersonal trauma (e.g., IPV, sexual abuse, and community violence) as a victim or perpetrator and report any childhood adverse events. Also note whether there is any family history of past or current psychiatric symptoms or diagnoses, addictions, suicide, or criminal behavior. For safety, identify any past or current threats to safety such as intimate partner violence, community violence, abuse and neglect, and the presence of any unsecure firearms in the home.

Functional Impairments

Summarize the level of functioning in the areas of psychological, behavioral, and living skills. Note any areas of impairment in daily or behavioral functioning such as developmental delay, intellectual functioning, problem solving, head trauma, or impairment in physical, language, or sensory functioning. Identify any problems in cognitive processes such as any cognitive deficits or impairments (e.g., traumatic brain injury (TBI), memory, mental, or language processing) and negative thinking patterns that may be related to negative automatic thoughts, cognitive distortions, or maladaptive schemas that can lead to negative emotions (e.g., depression, anger, and anxiety).

Legal Status
Note any history of or current legal difficulties (e.g., criminal charges, civil issues, and divorce/bankruptcy), incarceration, and criminal justice involvement including any criminal justice involvement of close family and friends.

4.8   Summary and Conclusion

Assessment is a process of gathering information from the client in order to inform the case conceptualization and treatment planning process. The assessment frames how problems and goals are conceptualized and delineates the range of strategies and interventions that will be selected to address identified problems and achieve goals. The assessment is the foundation of your work with the client. The process of assessment, since it is initiated at the beginning of the treatment relationship, also sets the stage for the developent of a trusting therapeutic alliance. The success of any particular treatment relationship is often determined during the assessment process. Assessment consists of engaging the client and introducing them to the therapeutic process while assessing for personal, social, and environmental strengths and capacities. It also involves screening for common health and behavioral health symptoms and the quality of several social, functional, and environmental domains. This information is combined with a careful analysis of family, medical, mental health, and substance use history. Providers then use this information to more fully assess for the presence of any symptoms that suggest the presence of a behavioral health disorder. This information is then organized and documented so as to inform the case conceptualization and treatment planning processes.

Case Study 4.1: Mr. Clarence Smith
Mr. Clarence Smith[1] is a 62-year-old cis-gendered Black man attending his primary care appointment with one of his daughters visiting him from out of town. She has been concerned for his physical and behavioral health for the last year. Clarence is kind, generous, hardworking, and enjoys cooking, working on old cars, fixing things around the house, and wood working. He likes to help friends and neighbors with home projects (he can do carpentry, plumbing, landscaping, and electrical) and enjoys talking about politics and world events with a close group of friends. Clarence lost his wife, Angela, of 40 years to a sudden and massive stroke approximately two years ago. They were in the kitchen making dinner one evening when Angela suddenly fell to the floor and was nonresponsive. Clarence called 911 and tried to resuscitate Angela, but the EMT said that she died almost instantly. Angela had just

---

[1] All names and other identifiers of this case have been changed to protect privacy and confidentiality.

retired from a large telecommunications company after 25 years of service. Clarence retired from the Postal Service two years earlier. Both had great retirement pensions and they had plans to travel, visit grandchildren, and work on the house.

Clarence didn't show much emotion at Angela's funeral. He has always been a stoic man. Clarence initially found comfort in his faith life and the close friends he spoke to each morning at a local coffee shop and played cards with once or twice a month. He and Angela have three grown children and four grandchildren. All live out of State, but kept in touch and visited relatively often. While he put on a strong public exterior after Angela's death, Clarence was devastated and continues to struggle with his grief. He blames himself for not being able to save Angela. He states, "It's my fault. I should have encouraged her to relax more. I should have done more to help her around the house. She should have retired when I did. I should have made her go to the doctor when she complained of those migraines. I should have done something! I was right there. I was an EMT in the army! I couldn't save her. My own wife and I couldn't save her."

He was also ashamed of himself for missing his wife so desperately even though it was two years after her death. He could not stop thinking about her and he could not shake his despair over Angela. He admits that he speaks to her often, apologizing for not being there enough and for past arguments. He reports having trouble sleeping at night because he thinks of Angela. He reports losing interest in cooking and taking care of the house, although he still accomplishes these tasks as if on autopilot. He reports feeling empty and alone. He started to avoid his friends because he did not want to talk about Angela and felt awkward. He is now isolated from family, friends, and his faith community due to restrictions from COVID-19. He states, "I stopped playing cards and going to church regularly for the past year, but I always went to breakfast with my friends and I looked forward to seeing my grandkids. Now that's gone too with this damn disease. I know if I get it, it might kill me. Sometimes I wonder if that wouldn't be such a bad thing. But I love my kids and grandkids. I wish I could see them more."

Clarence has a history of hypertension and Type 2 diabetes. He takes medication as prescribed for both conditions. Recently, Clarence has developed vision problems and an increase in painful neuropathy related to his diabetes. As a result, he has trouble walking long distances and he drives less. His house is a couple of miles away from the center of town. It is too far for him to walk. His children pay to have groceries delivered to his house once a week and have a neighbor call him and check on him each day. Clarence does not like relying on people for help and is reluctant to burden his friends or people at his church. This and the COVID-19 pandemic have resulted in Clarence spending most days staying home and watching TV. He feels tired all the time and has trouble concentrating and sleeping at night. He is often flooded with images of his wife collapsing and the confused and startled look on her face before she became unconscious, and the lifeless look on her face while he tried to revive her. He tries to avoid the kitchen as much as he can despite being an accomplished cook. As a result, the quality of his diet is declining. He reports frequent nightmares of the event and similar dreams where he is helpless to save the people he loves. Although never a person who drank much, he has begun to have two or three beers at night to help him fall asleep.

Overall, Clarence feels useless and stuck. When asked what he would like to be different about his life he pauses a long time and then states, "I'm not going to waste your time saying I want Angela back. She isn't coming back. I know that. I miss her. Sometimes I wish I could join her, but I'm not crazy and I don't want to die. I just wish I could miss her and remember her without thinking about how she died every damn minute of every damn day of my life. I try to forgive myself, but I can't. We had plans. It wasn't supposed to be this way. I guess I would like to still honor those plans in some way. I'm not interested in travelling the world, but I would like to feel useful and see my family and friends more. I miss them and I miss my friends. This conversation has made me realize how lonely I am. How closed in I feel. Unimportant. I guess I'd like that to change if it could."

Case Analysis
Clarence is a loving husband, father, and grandfather. He has cultivated a number of friends and is loved by many in his family. He is financially secure and has a safe and stable housing situation. He has many interests and talents. He also has access to basic resources and, while needing some help, currently has a good level of functioning. Despite these strengths, Clarence has suffered a significant loss with the death of his partner as well as other related losses of friends and purpose. He experiences a range of social stressors. He also exhibits several health and behavioral health symptoms and possesses several risk factors for increased morbidity and early mortality. Most importantly Clarence is experiencing significant grief due to the sudden, unexpected loss of his beloved wife, Angela. This would also constitute a traumatic event. Due to the circumstances of her death and his reported symptoms, Clarence also suffers from at least partial-PTSD. He witnessed Angela's death as he tried to resuscitate her. He reports intrusive thoughts (e.g., flashbacks and nightmares) and negative emotions and cognitions (e.g., self-blame, guilt, shame, numbing, and sadness), and avoidance (e.g., kitchen).

Clarence also reports depressive symptoms including low mood, loss of interest or pleasure in daily activities, persistent thoughts of guilt and worthlessness, fatigue, and sleep disturbances. He meets criteria for at least mild-to-moderate depression. Clarence also reports loneliness and social isolation from his family, friends, and faith community. While his isolation is exacerbated by the current pandemic, he also reported isolation beginning prior to the pandemic. He cannot attend gatherings with friends, go to church services, or complete daily errands due to concerns over contracting the virus. Clarence has a history of diabetes and hypertension. The symptoms from his diabetes appear to be worsening as evidenced by increased problems with vision and neuropathy. His diet is declining. Finally, Clarence reports drinking at least two or more beers nightly to help induce sleep. While this amount does not significantly exceed standardized daily drinking limits for alcohol, drinking alcohol may have negative health consequences given his age, depression, and comorbid health conditions.

Questions

What kind of help does Clarence need?

Based on the information in this case, what are three to five goals that would guide Clarence's treatment plan?

What interventions would be relevant given Clarence's current situation?

References

Adams, N., & Grieder, D. M. (2014). *Treatment planning for person-centered care: Shared decision making for whole health* (2nd ed.). Boston: Elsevier Press.

Algren, M. H., Ekholm, O., Nielsen, L., Ersbøll, A. K., Bak, C. K., & Andersen, P. T. (2018). Associations between perceived stress, socioeconomic status, and health-risk behaviour in deprived neighbourhoods in Denmark: A cross-sectional study. *BMC Public Health, 18*(1), 250. https://doi.org/10.1186/s12889-018-5170-x.

American Psychiatric Association. (2013). Diagnostic and Statistical Manual of Mental Disorders, Fifth Edition (DSM-5), American Psychiatric Association, Arlington, VA.

Andermann A. (2018). Screening for social determinants of health in clinical care: moving from the margins to the mainstream. Public health reviews, 39, 19. https://doi.org/10.1186/s40985-018-0094-7

Babor, T. F., De La Fuente, J. R., & Saunders, J. (1989). *AUDIT: Alcohol use disorders identification test: Guidelines for use in primary health care*. Geneva: World Health Organization.

Babor, T. F., Higgins-Biddle, J. C., Saunders, J. B., & Monteiro, M. G. (2001). *The alcohol use disorders identification test: Guidelines for use in primary care* (2nd ed.). World Health Organization. Retrieved March 27, 2020, at: https://www.who.int/publications-detail/audit-the-alcohol-use-disorders-identification-test-guidelines-for-use-in-primary-health-care

Billioux, A., Verlander, K., Anthony, S., & Alley, D. (2017). Standardized Screening for Health-Related Social Needs in Clinical Settings: The Accountable Health Communities Screening Tool. National Academy of Medicine Perspectives, 1-9. https://nam.edu/wpcontent/uploads/2017/05/Standardized-Screening-for-Health-Related-Social-Needs-in-Clinical-Settings.pdf.

Blow, F. C., Gillespie, B. W., Barry, K. L., Mudd, S. A., & Hill, E. M. (1998). Brief screening for alcohol problems in elderly populations using the Short Michigan Alcoholism Screening Test-Geriatric Version (SMAST-G). *Alcoholis: Clinical and Experimental Research, 22*(Suppl), 131A.

Borson, S., Scanlan, J. M., Chen, P., & Ganguli, M. (2003). The Mini-Cog as a screen for dementia: Validation in a population-based sample. *Journal of the American Geriatric Society, 51*(10), 1451–1454.

Bronfenbrenner, U. (1979). *The ecology of human development: Experiments by nature and design*. Cambridge, MA: Harvard University Press. ISBN: 0-674-22457-4.

Brown, R. L., & Rounds, L. A. (1995). Conjoint screening questionnaires for alcohol and other drug abuse: Criterion validity in a primary care practice. *Wisconsin Medical Journal, 94*(3), 135–140.

Center for Substance Abuse Treatment. (2006). *Screening, assessment, and treatment planning for persons with co-occurring disorders. COCE overview paper 2. DHHS publication no. (SMA) 06–4164*. Rockville: Substance Abuse and Mental Health Services Administration, and Center for Mental Health Services.

Centers for Disease Control and Prevention. (2020a). *Ten leading causes of death by age group, United States—2017*. 2020. WISQARS. https://www.cdc.gov/injury/wisqars/LeadingCauses.html. Retrieved March 12, 2020.

Centers for Disease Control and Prevention. (2020b). *Intimate partner violence.* https://www.cdc. gov/violenceprevention/intimatepartnerviolence/index.html. Retrieved March 12, 2020.

Cohen, S., Kamarck, T., & Mermelstein, R. (1983). A global measure of perceived stress. *Journal of Health and Social Behavior, 24,* 385–396.

Commission on Social Determinants of Health (CSDH). (2008). *Closing the gap in a genera- tion: Health equity through action on the social determinants of health* (Final report of the Commission on Social Determinants of Health). Geneva: World Health Organization.

Davidson, L., Tondora, J., Staeheli-Lawless, M., O'Connell, M. J., & Rowe, M. (2009). *A practi- cal guide to recovery-oriented practice: Tools for transforming mental health care.* New York: Oxford University Press.

De Ruysscher, C., Vandevelde, S., Vanderplasschen, W., De Maeyer, J., & Vanheule, S. (2017). The concept of recovery as experienced by persons with dual diagnosis: A systematic review of qualitative research from a first-person perspective. *Journal of Dual Diagnosis, 13*(4), 264–279.

Decker, M. R., Wilcox, H. C., Holliday, C. N., & Webster, D. W. (2018). An integrated public health approach to interpersonal violence and suicide prevention and response. *Public Health Reports, 133*(suppl. 1), 65s–79s.

Dell, N. A., Long, C., & Mancini, M. A. (In press). Models of recovery in mental illness: An over- view of systematic review. *Psychiatric Rehabilitation Journal.*

Díaz, E., Añez, L. M., Silva, M., Paris, M., & Davidson, L. (2017). Using the cultural formulation interview to build culturally sensitive services. *Psychiatric Services, 68*(2), 112–114. https:// doi.org/10.1176/appi.ps.201600440.

Dowrick, C. (2015). Therapeutic consultations for patients with depressive symptoms. *British Journal of General Practice, 65*(639), 550–551. https://doi.org/10.3399/bjgp15X687169.

Eaton, W. W., Muntaner, C., Smith, C., Tien, A., & Ybarra, M. (2004). Center for Epidemiologic Studies Depression Scale: Review and revision (CESD and CESD-R). In M. E. Maruish (Ed.), *The use of psychological testing for treatment planning and outcomes assessment* (3rd ed., pp. 363–377). Mahwah: Lawrence Erlbaum.

Elo, A. L., Leppänen, A., & Jahkola, A. (2003). Validity of a single-item measure of stress symp- toms. *Scandinavian Journal of Work, Environment, and Health, 29,* 444–451. https://doi. org/10.5271/sjweh.752.

Finkelhor, D., Shattuck, A., Turner, H., & Hamby, S. (2013). Improving the adverse childhood experiences study scale. *JAMA Pediatrics, 167*(1), 70–75.

Finkelhor, D., Shattuck, A., Turner, H., & Hamby, S. (2015). A revised inventory of adverse childhood experiences. *Child Abuse and Neglect, 48,* 13–21. https://doi.org/10.1016/j. chiabu.2015.07.011.

Folstein, M. F., Folstein, S. E., & McHugh, P. R. (1975). Mini-mental status. A practical method for grading the cognitive state of patients for the clinician. *Journal of Psychiatric Research, 12*(3), 189–198.

Gavin, D. R., Ross, H. E., & Skinner, H. A. (1989). Diagnostic validity of the DAST in the assess- ment of DSM-III drug disorders. *British Journal of Addiction, 84,* 301–307.

Germain, C. B., & Gitterman, A. (1980). *The life model of social work practice.* New York: Columbia University Press.

Germain, C. B., & Gitterman, A. (2008). *The life model of social work practice* (3rd ed.). New York: Columbia University Press.

Geronimus, A. T., Hicken, M., Keene, D., & Bound, J. (2006). "Weathering" and age patterns of allostatic load scores among blacks and whites in the United States. *American Journal of Public Health, 96,* 826–833.

Gottlieb, L. (2014). Strengths-based nursing: A holistic approach to care, grounded in eight core values. *American Journal of Nursing, 114,* 24–32.

Hartman, A. (1978). Diagrammatic assessment of family relationships. *Social Casework, 59,* 465–476.

Horowitz, L. M., Bridge, J. A., Teach, S. J., Ballard, E., Klima, J., Rosenstein, D. L., et al. (2012). Ask Suicide-Screening Questions (ASQ): A brief instrument for the pediatric emergency department. *Archives of Pediatrics & Adolescent Medicine, 166*(12), 1170–1176.

Inouye, S. K., van Dyck, C. H., Alessi, C. A., Balkin, S., Siegal, A. P., & Horwitz, R. I. (1990). Clarifying confusion: The confusion assessment method. A new method for detection of delirium. *Annals of Internal Medicine, 113*(12), 941–948.

Jani, B., Bikker, A. P., Higgins, M., Fitzpatrick, B., Little, P., Watt, G. C., & Mercer, S. W. (2012). Patient centeredness and the outcome of primary care consultations with patients with depression in areas of high and low socioeconomic deprivation. *British Journal General Practice, 62*(601), e576–e581. https://doi.org/10.3399/bjgp12X653633.

Janssen, M., Heerkens, Y., Kuijer, W., van der Heijden, B., & Engels, J. (2018). Effects of mindfulness-based stress reduction on employees' mental health: A systematic review. *PLoS One, 13*(1), e0191332. https://doi.org/10.1371/journal.pone.0191332.

Kabat-Zinn, J. (1990). *Full catastrophe living: Using the wisdom of your body and mind to face stress, pain and illness* (p. 1990). New York: Delacorte.

Kalish, V. B., Gillham, J. E., & Unwin, B. K. (2014). Delirium in older persons: Evaluation and management. *American Family Physician, 90*(3), 150–158.

Karls, J. M., & O'Keefe, M. (2008). *Person-in-environment system manual* (2nd ed.). Washington, DC: NASW Press.

Kendi, I. X. (2019). *How to be an antiracist*. New York: Random House.

Kovach, K. A., Reid, K., Grandmont, J., Jones, D., Wood, J., & School, B. (2019). How engaged are family physicians in addressing the social determinants of health? A survey supporting the American Academy of Family Physician's Health Equity Environmental Scan. *Health Equity, 3*(1). https://doi.org/10.1089/heq.2019.0022.

Kroenke, K., Spitzer, R. L., & Williams, J. B. W. (2001). The PHQ-9: Validity of a brief depression severity measure. *Journal of General Internal Medicine, 16*(9), 606–613.

Kroenke, K., Spitzer, R. L., & Williams, J. B. (2003). The patient health questionnaire-2: Validity of a two-item depression screener. *Medical Care, 41*(11), 1284–1292. https://doi.org/10.1097/01.MLR.0000093487.78664.3C.

Kroenke, K., Spitzer, R. L., Williams, J. B., & Löwe, B. (2009). An ultra-brief screening scale for anxiety and depression: The PHQ-4. *Psychosomatics, 50*(6), 613–621.

Krueger, P. M., & Chang, V. W. (2008). Being poor and coping with stress: Health behaviors and the risk of death. *American Journal of Public Health, 98*(5), 889–896. https://doi.org/10.2105/AJPH.2007.114454.

Lang, A. J., & Stein, M. B. (2005). An abbreviated PTSD checklist for use as a screening instrument in primary care. *Behaviour Research and Therapy, 43*, 585–594.

Lang, A. J., Wilkins, K., Roy-Byrne, P. P., Golinelli, D., Chavira, D., Sherbourne, C., Rose, R. D., Bystritsky, A., Sullivan, G., Craske, M. G., & Stein, M. B. (2012). Abbreviated PTSD checklist (PCL) as a guide to clinical response. *General Hospital Psychiatry, 34*, 332–338.

Leamy, M., Bird, V., Boutillier, L., Williams, J., & Slade, M. (2011). Conceptual framework for personal recovery in mental health: Systematic review and narrative synthesis. *British Journal of Psychiatry, 199*, 445–452. https://doi.org/10.1192/bjp.bp.110.083733.

Löwe, B., Wahl, I., Rose, M., Spitzer, C., Glaesmer, H., Wingenfeld, K., Schneider, A., & Brähler, E. (2010). A 4-item measure of depression and anxiety: Validation and standardization of the Patient Health Questionnaire-4 (PHQ-4) in the general population. *Journal of Affective Disorders, 122*(1–2), 86–95. https://doi.org/10.1016/j.jad.2009.06.019.

Lysaker, P. H., & Buck, K. D. (2007). Neurocognitive deficits as a barrier to psychosocial function in schizophrenia: Effects on learning, coping, & self-concept. *Journal of Psychosocial Nursing and Mental Health Services, 45*(7), 24–30. https://doi.org/10.3928/02793695-20070701-08.

Mancini, M. A. (2006). Consumer-providers theories of recovery from serious psychiatric disabilities. In J. Rosenberg (Ed.), *Community mental health: Challenges for the 21st Century* (pp. 15–24). New York: Brunner-Routledge.

Mancini, M. A. (2007). The role of self-efficacy in recovery from serious psychiatric disabilities: A qualitative study with fifteen psychiatric survivors. *Qualitative Social Work: Research and Practice, 6*, 49–74.

Mancini, M. A. (2018). An exploration of factors that effect the implementation of peer support services in community mental health settings. *Community Mental Health Journal, 54*(2), 127–137. https://doi.org/10.1007/s10597-017-0145-4/.

Mancini, M. A. (2019). Strategic storytelling: An exploration of the professional practices of mental health peer providers. *Qualitative Health Research., 29*(9), 1266–1276. https://doi.org/10.1177/1049732318821689.

Mancini, M. A., & Farina, A. S.J. (Epub ahead of print December 17, 2019). Co-morbid mental health issues in a clinical sample of Latinx adults: Implications for integrated behavioral health treatment. Journal of Ethnic & Cultural Diversity in Social Work, https://doi.org/10.1080/15313204.2019.1702132

Mancini, M. A., Hardiman, E. R., & Lawson, H. A. (2005). Making sense of it all: Consumer providers' theories about factors facilitating and impeding recovery from psychiatric disabilities. *Psychiatric Rehabilitation Journal, 29*(1), 48–55.

Mandebvu, F., & Kalman, M. (2015). The 3 Ds, and newly acquired cognitive impairment: Issues for the ICU nurse. *Critical Care Nursing Quarterly, 38*(3), 317–326. https://doi.org/10.1097/CNQ.0000000000000079.

Mayfield, D., McLeod, G., & Hall, P. (1974). The CAGE questionnaire: Validation of a new alcoholism screening instrument. *American Journal of Psychiatry, 131*, 1121–1123.

McCarthy-Jones, S., Marriott, M., Knowles, R., Rowse, G., & Thompson, A. (2013). What is psychosis? A meta-synthesis of inductive qualitative studies exploring the experience of psychosis. *Psychosis, 5*(1), 1–16.

McGoldrick, M., Gerson, R., & Petry, S. (2020). *Genograms: Assessment and intervention* (4th ed.). New York: W.W. Norton.

McKenzie-Smith, L. (2019). *Recovery experiences of forensic mental health service users.* Doctoral dissertation, Canterbury Christ Church University. http://create.canterbury.ac.uk/18413/1/Laura_McKenzie-Smith_MRP_2019.pdf

National Academies of Sciences, Engineering, and Medicine (NASEM). (2019). *Integrating social care into the delivery of health care: Moving upstream to improve the Nation's health.* Washington, DC: The National Academies Press. https://doi.org/10.17226/25467.

National Association of Community Health Centers (NACHC) (2019). Protocol for responding to and assessing patients' assets, risks and experiences (PRAPARE): Implementation and action toolkit. Downloaded at: https://www.nachc.org/wp-content/uploads/2020/08/NACHC_PRAPARE_ALL-Updated-8.24.20.pdf

Ng, D. M., & Jeffery, R. W. (2003). Relationships between perceived stress and health behaviors in a sample of working adults. *Health Psychology, 22*(6), 638–642. https://doi.org/10.1037/0278-6133.22.6.638.

Nuruzzaman, N., Broadwin, M., Kourouma, K., & Olson, D. P. (2015). Making the social determinants of health a routine part of medical care. *Journal of Health Care for the Poor and Underserved, 26*(2), 321–327. https://doi.org/10.1353/hpu.2015.0036.

Parker, D., Byng, R., Dickens, C., & McCabe, R. (2020). Every structure we're taught goes out the window: General practitioners' experiences of providing help for patients with emotional concerns. *Health and Social Care in the Community, 28*(1), 260–269. https://doi.org/10.1111/hsc.12860.

Peterson & Seligman. (2004). *Character strengths and virtues: A handbook and classification.* Washington, DC: APA Press.

Phelan, J. C., Link, B. G., & Tehranifar, P. (2010). Social conditions as fundamental causes of health inequalities: Theory, evidence, and policy implications. *Journal of Health and Social Behavior, 51*(Suppl), S28–S40. https://doi.org/10.1177/0022146510383498.

Prins, A., Ouimette, P., Kimerling, R., Cameron, R. P., Hugelshofer, D. S., Shaw-Hegwer, J., Thrailkill, A., Gusman, F.D., Sheikh, J. I. (2003). The Primary Care PTSD Screen (PC-PTSD):

Development and operating characteristics (PDF). Primary Care Psychiatry, 9, 9-14. doi: 10.1185/135525703125002360 PTSDpubs ID: 26676

Prins, A., Bovin, M. J., Kimerling, R., Kaloupek, D. G, Marx, B. P., Pless Kaiser, A., & Schnurr, P. P. (2015). *Primary Care PTSD Screen for DSM-5 (PC-PTSD-5)*. Downloaded on 5/28/20 at https://www.ptsd.va.gov/professional/assessment/screens/pc-ptsd.asp

Prins, A., Bovin, M. J., Smolenski, D. J., Marx, B. P., Kimerling, R., Jenkins-Guarnieri, M. A., Kaloupek, D. G., Schnurr, P. P., Kaiser, A. P., Leyva, Y. E., & Tiet, Q. Q. (2016). The Primary Care PTSD Screen for DSM-5 (PC-PTSD-5): Development and evaluation within a veteran primary care sample. *Journal of General Internal Medicine, 31*(10), 1206–1211. https://doi.org/10.1007/s11606-016-3703-5.

Prochaska, J. O., DiClemente, C. C., & Norcross, J. C. (1992). In search of how people change: Applications to addictive behaviors. *American Psychologist, 47*(9), 1102–1114. https://doi.org/10.1037//0003-066x.47.9.1102.

Rabin, R., Jennings, J. M., Campbell, J. C., & Bair-Merritt, M. H. (2009). Intimate partner violence screening tools: A systematic review. *American Journal of Preventive Medicine, 36*(5), 439–445. e4.

Rapp, C. A., & Goscha, R. J. (2012). *The strengths model: A recovery-oriented approach to mental health services*. New York: Oxford University Press.

Saleebey, D. (1996). The strengths perspective in social work practice: Extensions and cautions. *Social Work, 41*(3), 296–305.

SAMHSA. (2020). *Patient stress questionnaire*. Retrieved March 10, 2020, from: https://www.integration.samhsa.gov/clinical-practice/screening-tools

Scott, K. M., Lim, C., Al-Hamzawi, A., Alonso, J., Bruffaerts, R., Caldas-de-Almeida, J. M., Florescu, S., et al. (2016). Association of Mental Disorders with subsequent chronic physical conditions: World mental health surveys from 17 countries. *JAMA Psychiatry, 73*(2), 150–158. https://doi.org/10.1001/jamapsychiatry.2015.2688.

Peterson, C. & Seligman, M. (2004). *Character strengths and virtues: A handbook and classification*. New York: Oxford University Press.

Selzer, M. L. (1971). The Michigan alcohol screening test: The quest for a new diagnostic instrument. *American Journal of Psychiatry, 127*, 1653–1658.

Sherin, K., Sinacore, J. M., Li, X. Q., Zitter, R. E., & Shakil, A. (1998). HITS: A short domestic violence screening tool for use in a family practice setting. *Family Medicine, 30*(7), 508–512.

Skinner, H. A. (1982). Drug abuse screening test. *Addictive Behavior, 7*, 363–371.

Smith, P. C., Schmidt, S. M., Allensworth-Davies, D., & Saitz, R. (2010). A single question screening test for drug use in primary care. *Archives of Internal Medicine, 170*(13), 1155–1160. https://doi.org/10.1001/archinternmed.2010.140.

Snyderman, D., & Rovner, B. W. (2009). Mental status examination in primary care: A review. *American Family Physician, 80*(8), 809–814.

Spitzer, R. L., Kroenke, K., Williams, J. B., & Löwe, B. (2006). A brief measure for assessing generalized anxiety disorder: The GAD-7. *Archives of Internal Medicine, 166*(10), 1092–1097. https://doi.org/10.1001/archinte.166.10.1092.

Starnino, V. R., Gomi, S., & Canda, E. R. (2014). Spiritual strengths assessment in mental health practice. *British Journal of Social Work, 44*(4), 849–867.

Stewart, M., Belle-Brown, J., Donner, A., McWhinney, I. R., Oates, J., Weston, W. W., & Jordan, J. (2000). The impact of patient-centered care on outcomes. *Journal of Family Practice, 49*(9), 796–804.

Tondora, J., Miller, R., Slade, M., & Davidson, L. (2014). *Partnering for recovery in mental health: A practical guide to person-centered planning*. Hoboken: Wiley.

Ustun, T. B., Kostanjsek, N., & Rehm, S. C. (2010). *Measuring health and disability. Manual for the WHO Disability Assessment Schedule: WHODAS 2.0*. World Health Organization.

van Os, T. W., van den Brink, R. H., Tiemens, B. G., Jenner, J. A., van der Meer, K., & Ormel, J. (2005). Communicative skills of general practitioners augment the effectiveness of guideline-based depression treatment. *Journal of Affective Disorders, 84*(1), 43–51.

Vergare, M. J., Binder, R. L., Cook, I. A., Galanter, M., & Lu, F. G. (2006). *Practice guidelines for the psychiatric evaluation of adults* (2nd ed., pp. 23–25). Washington, DC: American Psychiatric Association.

Wei, L. A., Fearing, M. A., Sternberg, E. J., & Inouye, S. K. (2008). The confusion assessment method: A systematic review of current usage. *Journal of the American Geriatrics Society, 56*(5), 823–830. https://doi.org/10.1111/j.1532-5415.2008.01674.x.

World Health Organization. (2010). *A conceptual framework for action on the social determinants of health*. Geneva, Switzerland. www.who.int/sdhconference/resources/ConceptualframeworkforactiononSDH_eng.pdf. Accessed 30 May 2020.

Chapter 5
Person-Centered Treatment Planning

5.1   An Overview of Person-Centered Treatment Planning

Treatment planning can be a rich, collaborative process that produces a detailed plan of action designed to achieve a set of client goals that are specific, measurable, actionable, achievable, relevant, recovery-oriented, and time limited. Unfortunately, it is all too common that treatment plans are developed only to fulfill a bureaucratic requirement by providers with little or no client input. These plans are often placed in a drawer and never looked at again until it is time to review them as part of a mandated requirement. However, at their best, treatment plans are person-centered and strength-focused, and guide the therapeutic process (Adams and Grieder 2014; Tondora et al. 2014; Rapp and Goscha 2012). Treatment plans can function as a touchstone in times of confusion, frustration, or inertia. According to Rapp and Goscha (2012), the purpose of a treatment plan is to:

> "Create a mutual agenda for work between the person receiving services and their worker, which should be focused on achieving the goals that the person has set." (Rapp and Goscha 2012; pp. 130)

Part of effective integrated behavioral health practice is to use assessment data to develop coordinated care plans that help people achieve health and well-being. This is done through the provision of: (1) health and behavioral health treatments and interventions to reduce symptoms, improve functioning, and increase coping skills and (2) case management services to address violence, poverty, lack of basic resources, unemployment, inadequate housing, and other social determinants of health through advocacy and the acquisition of resources. These services can be provided as part of a collaborative care team or through structured and formal relationships with relevant outside providers.

A key component of the Patient Protection and Affordable Care Act (PPACA) is the promotion of person-centered care. Person-centered care is a perspective of care that considers the whole person. Providers using a person-centered approach to care

© Springer Nature Switzerland AG 2021   123
M. A. Mancini, *Integrated Behavioral Health Practice*,
https://doi.org/10.1007/978-3-030-59659-0_5

respect and value client perspectives, preferences, needs, and participation in treatment decisions (Mahoney 2011; Patient Protection and Affordable Care Act 2010; Stanhope & Ashenberg-Straussner 2018; Stanhope and Choy-Brown 2018). Person-centered treatment planning is the written action or service plan that directs all client care toward life goals identified by the client. These plans outline a time-limited course of action designed to help the client overcome barriers (e.g., health and behavioral health symptoms, lack of resources, skill deficits, social determinants of health) to achieving of their life goals (Adams and Grieder 2014; Rapp and Goscha 2012; Stanhope and Choy-Brown 2018; Tondora et al. 2014). Person-centered care planning is a core function of integrated behavioral health care and is defined as "providing care that is respectful of and responsive to individual patient preferences, needs, and values and ensuring that patient values guide all clinical decisions" (Institute of Medicine (IOM) 2001, pp. 40). Person-centered treatment plans are first and foremost collaborative and should be strength-based, accountable, focused on whole health, and utilize a shared decision-making (SDM) framework in the selection of treatment goals, objectives, and interventions (Berwick 2009; Stanhope & Ashenberg-Straussner 2018; Stanhope and Choy-Brown 2018).

Person-centered care orients services toward the goals identified by the client. Clients participate in clinical care decisions in collaboration with healthcare providers, toward holistic, recovery-oriented goals and objectives that move beyond symptom alleviation toward holistic well-being (Adams and Grieder 2014). The utilization of person-centered planning can increase the investment that people have in their care, motivating them to set and achieve goals that lead to health and positive treatment outcomes. For instance, person-centered planning has been found to significantly improve treatment engagement, participation, and medication usage rates in persons with serious mental illness (Stanhope et al. 2013).

In order for treatment planning to be person-centered, several process-related criteria need to be met. First, providers meet face-to-face with clients either in person or through telehealth visits to develop plans in *collaboration*. All aspects of the plan are agreed to by the client and shared with all relevant persons. The plan acts as a type of contract or covenant between the client and provider. Second, goals are in the clients' own words and all goals and interventions are *aligned* with the problems identified in the assessment and case conceptualization. For instance, in the client record, the assessment and treatment plan including the case conceptualization, problems, goals, and interventions should all reinforce each other and be in *alignment*. Long-term goals and treatment outcome goals should align with the assessment and case conceptualization. Objectives or smaller sub-goals should clearly lead to the achievement of larger life goals and treatment outcome goals. Interventions should realistically address each problem area or barrier to goal achievement. Case notes should document how interventions are being deployed to help the client and the progress being made toward achieving goals in the plan and so forth. Last, the provider has *fully informed* the client about the resources available and the benefits and potential risks or harms of any treatments, interventions, or services, including the benefits and harms associated with not taking action (e.g., watchful waiting). The client must also fully understand and endorse the plan and can readily recite all goals in the plan (Adams and Grieder 2014; Rapp and Goscha 2012; Stanhope and Choy-Brown 2018; Tondora et al. 2014).

Essentially, treatment planning consists of two components: (1) a case conceptualization that is comprised of a synthesis of the data collected during the assessment and a working hypothesis of the problems encountered by the client and (2) a treatment plan that consists of: (a) a recovery-statement that includes one to three *life goals*; (b) a series of *treatment outcome goals* and *objectives* that lead to the achievement of the larger, long-term life goal(s) identified in the recovery statement; and (c) selected interventions designed to achieve objectives and treatment outcome goals. Each of these aspects of the treatment plan will be reviewed in the sections that follow.

Collaborative Care Plans

Collaborative care planning occurs when teams of multidisciplinary professionals work together with clients to develop treatment plans that integrate health and behavioral health treatment in a coordinated and collaborative fashion. This approach has shown positive outcomes for both providers and clients (Collins 2010). Collaborative care plans can also promote health and behavioral health service integration because they include interventions designed to address health, mental health, and addiction issues, as well as social determinants of health. In short, collaborative care planning can integrate care in a way that addresses co-occurring needs. It is best that plans include interprofessional interventions that are integrated into the same team of professionals through a shared plan. Ideally, plans would be in a shared record and all providers would meet as a team to discuss each client, review progress toward goals, and adjust treatment approaches to accommodate progress (Stanhope and Choy-Brown 2018).

For care provided outside of the team, formal treatment relationships with outside providers are established in order to promote coordinated and effective referral, follow-up, and monitoring (e.g., so-called warm referral or hand-off). Cross-site communication and sharing of care plans is very important to coordinate and integrate care, particularly across disciplines and settings that use different practices, theories, and language to understand the problem. This can often be a barrier to high-quality care, but active communication and cross-site training can be an effective way to overcome these barriers. The Electronic Health Record (EHR) can also function as a barrier to person-centered care when the EHR is too rigid (e.g., fixed, strict drop-down menu options) and is not able to be customized to recognize individualized goals, objectives, and approaches to care. It is important for settings to be able to design their EHR systems in such a way as to meet their reporting requirements, while also being flexible enough to allow providers to design customized client care plans and for team members to share those plans with each other across the team and with clients (Stanhope and Choy-Brown 2018; Stanhope and Matthews 2019).

5.2   Formulating Case Conceptualizations and Treatment Plans

Treatment plans should be based on the information gathered through the assessment interview, medical records, family and other collateral contacts, and other relevant sources of information such as school, employment, and criminal justice records. Treatment plans begin with a "bridge" that summarizes, synthesizes, and integrates the information gathered from the assessment in such a way that clients and providers can make informed decisions about relevant treatment goals and the course of clinical treatment. In this chapter, I will refer to this bridge as the *case conceptualization* (Berman 2019; Wright et al. 2017). Case conceptualizations are also referred to as case or problem formulations (Lichner-Ingram 2012) and can be referred by other names. For instance, the Commission on Accreditation of Rehabilitation Facilities (CARF) refers to them as "interpretive summaries." They are also referred to as "integrative summaries" (Adams and Grieder 2014), or more generally as "summary and recommendations." Regardless of how they are termed, case conceptualizations follow similar developmental patterns. Adams and Grieder (2014) describe case conceptualizations (they use the term integrative summaries) as follows, "the written integrative summary documents the rationalization, and justification for the provider's recommendations and suggestions as well as promotes shared decisions about how best to proceed. It creates the platform from which the individual and the team/provider launch into creating the individual plan and charting a course for recovery and wellness." (Adams and Grieder 2014, pp. 78).

The provider develops case conceptualizations by synthesizing the subjective (e.g., client's story) and objective (e.g., case records, screening and test results) information collected during the assessment process to develop a working hypothesis of the client's problems and their potential solutions. This information is then used to develop a set of long-term and short-term goals that guide treatment decisions regarding the interventions, skills, and resources needed for the client to be successful. This process helps the client see their problems and potential solutions more clearly. For instance, the conceptualization should help clients recognize their resources, strengths, and capabilities; how the problem has developed and changed over time; the barriers that need to be overcome; and a path forward to recovery and wellness. The provider and client then use the case conceptualization to build their plan to address identified problems.

Case Conceptualization and Treatment Plan Components
Case conceptualizations: Case conceptualizations: (1) synthesize *subjective and objective data* of client's strengths and needs across biological, psychological, social, and environmental domains to formulate a set of relevant problems, and (2) use that data to develop *working hypotheses* as to the causes of those problems and their solutions. These components then drive the framing and development of a series of treatment planning goals.

Treatment plans: Treatment plans flow from the conceptualization and include three parts: (1) a recovery statement that lists one to three *long-term life goals*; (2) a set of three to five *treatment outcome goals* that guide treatment and lead to the

Case Conceptualization and Treatment Planning Process

(Based on: Adams & Grieder, 2014; Berman, 2019; Lichner-Ingram, 2012; Wright et al., 2017)

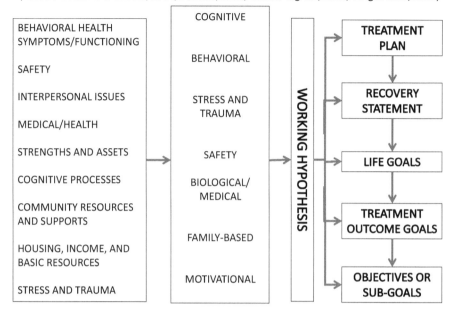

Fig. 5.1 Case conceptualization and treatment planning process. (Based on: Adams and Grieder 2014; Berman 2019; Lichner-Ingram 2012; Wright et al. 2017)

achievement of life goals; and (3) a series of specific, concrete, actionable *objectives* (sometimes referred to as sub-goals) whose completion will ultimately lead to achievement of each treatment outcome goal. Figure 5.1 provides a description of the components of the case conceptualization and treatment planning process.

5.2.1   The Case Conceptualization

Summarization of Client Assessment Data

Case conceptualizations begin with a summary of assessment data about the client's health and behavioral health needs that include presenting symptoms, diagnoses, screening, and testing results and client health and behavioral health history. This section should also identify client insight into problems and their motivation and commitment to address identified issues (e.g., stage of change). The data that should inform the case conceptualization includes a summary and synthesis of at least some of the following areas covered in Chap. 4: (1) strengths and assets; (2) presenting symptoms or problems; (3) summary of current and historical physical and behavioral health conditions, functioning, and diagnoses; (4) substance use history; (5) trauma history; (6) interpersonal relationships and social network; and (7) relevant social determinants of health related to safety, housing, income, and access to basic resources (e.g., food, utilities, medicine, transportation, clothing). Case conceptualization may not include all of this information—but this is the main information from which conceptualizations are often developed (Adams and Grieder 2014; Tondora et al. 2014).

The data from the above areas are used to create a problem list. The *problem list* should be a comprehensive list of clear, solvable targets that are relevant to client recovery or well-being. These targets should also align with client preferences and values. The problem list will naturally lead with the presenting problems identified by the client supplemented by results of screening and diagnostic tests and relevant information from the biopsychosocial assessment. Possible domains of functioning where problems emerge include: (1) physical health concerns and illnesses; (2) psychiatric symptoms such as negative thinking patterns, anxiety, stress, depression, psychosis, or trauma symptoms; (3) addictive behaviors; (4) unhealthy relationships; (5) education and occupational functioning; (6) legal and financial concerns; (7) environmental concerns (e.g., housing and neighborhood safety, lack of basic resources, and other SDOH); and (8) a lack of coping skills (e.g., assertiveness, problem solving, social skills, anger management, illness management). Identifying the most important problem areas is vital. Parsimony is also important, as you don't want to overwhelm the person. The problem list should be limited to three to five priority areas that will lead to the design of specific goals and interventions (Berman 2019; Lichner-Ingram 2012).

Hypothesis Formulation

In the case conceptualization, the provider synthesizes client subjective self-reports and objective data from the assessment about specific areas from the problem list (e.g., problem statement) into working hypotheses regarding the origins of the problems or how and why the problems have emerged (e.g., adverse childhood events and negative formative experiences, hypercritical parenting, trauma, psychiatric symptoms, negative thinking patterns, substance use, interpersonal conflict, lack of coping skills). Providers ground their working hypotheses within a particular theoretical orientation that is most appropriate and best suited to solving the problem. There are several theories that can be relied upon to solve the problem. Usually, these are limited by the training and orientation of the provider; however, providers should strive to utilize the theories and approaches that have been found to be most effective in solving their client's problems. Below is a list of some of the most common theories and approaches and their application (Berman 2019; Lichner-Ingram 2012).

1. Cognitive theory: These approaches are used when problems can be best explained by cognitive processes that include the development of maladaptive schemas, negative thinking patterns, and self-talk that lead to depression, anxiety, aggressive behavior, social withdrawal, substance use, self-harm, or avoidance. Interventions can include cognitive reframing and cognitive processing therapy.

2. Behavioral theory: Behavioral approaches are used to conceptualize how learned behaviors and thinking patterns are positively and negatively reinforced. These

approaches also focus on developing coping skills to address problematic behaviors. Do client problems stem from conditioned responses (e.g., avoidance) to antecedents in the environment that lead to negative consequences? Is the client so overwhelmed that they feel paralyzed or stuck? Is the client suffering from intrusive memories and hyper-arousal symptoms due to trauma? Does the client lack a particular skill to cope effectively with problems (e.g., anger management, problem solving)? Interventions designed to reduce anxious feelings, indecision, paralysis, and problem behaviors include behavioral activation, relaxation, and mindfulness-based interventions; coping skill development (e.g., problem-solving skills, assertiveness training, anger management, illness self-management); and exposure-based therapies such as prolonged exposure, EMDR, and trauma-informed CBT.

3. Stage-based approaches: These approaches are used to conceptualize interventions that complement a person's stage of change (e.g., precontemplation, contemplation, preparation, action, and maintenance). Persons in precontemplation, contemplation, and early preparation stages of change may benefit from harm reduction and motivational enhancement approaches. Persons in late preparation, action, and maintenance stages may benefit from more cognitive-behavioral approaches that focus on directly confronting problems, developing health life-styles, and preventing relapse such as cognitive behavioral therapy, exposure-based therapies, and abstinence-based substance use treatments and approaches.

4. Biological-based approaches: Can genetics, organic processes, family history, or medical illnesses (e.g., diabetes, hyper/hypothyroidism, cancer, cerebrovascular or cardiovascular disease) explain behavioral health symptoms such as severe melancholic depression, psychosis, mania, and severe anxiety? For these sources, approaches that use medications, nutritional, rehabilitative, and other medical interventions to reduce or eliminate symptoms may be relevant. This may include the use of psychiatric medications or electroconvulsive therapy (ECT) to reduce intense psychiatric symptoms as part of a stepped approach to care that also includes application of psychotherapeutic approaches.

5. Family-based approaches: Family-based approaches rely on family systems theory to address relational problems within the couple or family system to improve communication and understanding, resolve conflict, clarify roles, and increase functionality. These approaches may include interpersonal therapy (IPT), brief strategic family therapy, and family psychoeducation.

6. Safety approaches: Safety approaches are used to address immediate safety concerns related to interpersonal violence (e.g., intimate partner violence, community violence), homelessness, non-suicidal self-injury (NSSI), suicidality, homicidality, severe substance abuse or dependence, or severe psychotic or manic symptoms. This will include a range of approaches such as crisis housing, medical or psychiatric hospitalization, legal advocacy, safety planning, and harm reduction (e.g., opioid replacement, needle exchange/safe injection sites, emergency contraception, detoxification services) (Mancini et al. 2008, 2010; Mancini and Wyrick Waugh 2013). They may also include fulfilling mandated reporting requirements, mandated treatment, and involvement of law enforcement.

7. Stress and trauma: Approaches in this domain focus on addressing issues related to the experience of high stress, life crisis, violence, stressful transitions, traumatic events, and the experience of bereavement and grief due to a significant loss. The experience of adverse childhood events, traumatic experiences, and high levels of chronic perceived stress can lead to a range of physical and behavioral health problems. The continuous experience of discrimination, violence, and inequitable access to resources commonly experienced by Black, Indigenous, and People of Color (BIPOC) persons, people in poverty, and members of the LBGTQ community are sources of high morbidity and early mortality. This domain includes a range of approaches and perspectives including (but not limited to): (1) affirming therapeutic practices in the domains of gender, sexual orientation, race, and culture; (2) approaches that help people process grief and loss; (3) accessing resources to address the impacts of violence (e.g., shelter, victim advocacy, childcare, employment); (4) trauma-informed practices; and (5) mindfulness-based relaxation approaches and wellness strategies to reduce stress and anxiety.

Working hypotheses are used to explain client problems and utilize a range of perspectives. Working hypotheses should begin with a clear problem statement that provides a distillation of the client and provider's perspective of the problem(s), including the main issues(s) that will be addressed in treatment. This should align with the list of problem areas identified by the provider and client. The working hypothesis is the central thread of the conceptualization. These hypotheses can then be used to design goals, service plans, and interventions for clients. The case conceptualization concludes with a set of recommendations about how to solve those problems that are in line with the theories and hypotheses identified previously. Recommendations usually imply what needs to happen to solve the problem (e.g., learning problem-solving skills, cognitive reframing, relaxation techniques, increased social activity). Recommendations then lead to treatment goals and objectives, which then ultimately lead to specific interventions and techniques (Berman 2019; Lichner-Ingram 2012). These areas will be discussed next.

5.2.2 The Treatment Plan

Treatment plans consist of three components. The first is the recovery statement that is comprised of a client's goal(s) for a happy life (e.g., life goals). These goals are big, broad, long-term goals the client identifies as most important. These goals may include things like "Find a job," "Go to school," "Move into my own place," "Get discharged or graduate," "Achieve sobriety," or "Feel more confident in myself." The second is the identification of specific and measurable treatment outcome goals with appropriate responsibility and timeline for completion. What does the client want to have accomplished by the end of treatment? This may include resolving the perceived barriers to treatment. Treatment outcome goal(s) should be succinct, recovery-oriented, and written in plain language. Treatment outcome goals guide treatment decisions and are the main goals that are achieved through the specific application of treatment approaches. For instance, if the life goal is "Get a job," then treatment outcome goals may center on areas like reducing alcohol or substance use, entering and completing vocational rehabilitation or an employment training program, applying for a job, completing resume and developing interviewing skills, and learning a specific vocational or employment skill. Treatment outcome goals are the main, end-point goals related to treatment. These should ultimately contribute to the life goal(s). The third area of the plan is the identification of concrete, specific objectives that lead to the achievement of treatment outcome goals. This will include interventions performed by the provider or provider team as well as referrals to outside service agencies. Objectives (sometimes referred to as "sub goals") are very specific and include things like, "completing a wellness plan," "using problem-solving skills to solve a particular problem," "applying for benefits," "completing thought change records each week," and "completing weekly exposure-exercises." Objectives are the intervention techniques and strategies that lead to the achievement of treatment outcome goals (Adams and Grieder 2014; Rapp and Goscha 2012; Tondora et al. 2014).

Types of Goals and Goal Development
Goal development is a process of identifying large, meaningful goals; breaking them down into manageable segments; and then identifying strategies designed to achieve those smaller parts. One of the most challenging practice areas in behavioral health is working with clients on setting meaningful, measurable, and achievable goals. At worst, care plans consist of goals set by the provider with minimal input or buy-in from the client. These recycled, meaningless goals are rarely reviewed or achieved. This is unethical practice and a waste of valuable time and energy that could be used to actually achieve something. Another problematic practice issue are goals set by the client that are unrealistic, vague, or confusing. These goals are also unlikely to be achieved. At their best, care plans include a series of collaboratively developed goals that are not only relevant, clear, crisp, measurable, and challenging but also achievable. These goals have the best chance of being accomplished and leading to positive outcomes. And so, as a provider, it is important to listen intently on what the client wants and then help them shape those goals into a framework that will lead to success. In the sections that follow, I outline a process and structure of goal development. Figure 5.1 provides a description of how life goals, treatment outcome goals, and objectives align with each other. As can be seen, objectives support treatment goals and treatment goals support achievement of the larger life goals of the client (Adams and Grieder 2014).

The Recovery Statement
The recovery statement is the ultimate purpose of treatment. It guides all goal development and treatment activities. This statement is grounded in the presenting problem list and assessment information and is mainly comprised of one to three "Happy Life Goals" in a concise statement that drives the client and orients treatment. It is the lodestar of the treatment process and acts as an orienting guide when things get confusing. Recovery statements are inherently person-centered and should come

from the client and be in their primary interest. The life goals that comprise these statements should be clear, succinct, positive, and measurable. It should be apparent when the life goals in the statement are accomplished. The recovery statement is a set of responses or solutions to identified problems and should be of primary interest to the client. Recovery statements are written in complete narrative sentences using the client's own words and should reflect client preferences and desires.

The recovery statement is a means to build trust, enhance collaboration, and set the general course for treatment. While at times the life goals contained in the statement can seem unrealistic to providers, the goals reflect the hopes and dreams of clients and can build motivation to work toward well-being and recovery. Goals that are important to the provider should not replace client goals, nor should client goals be changed, watered down, or otherwise altered to be more reflective of provider preferences. These are the goals that are important to the client and should guide treatment. However, the provider can help give advice regarding goal selection, wording, prioritization, and sequencing to maximize success. When disagreements arise, it may be helpful to prioritize goals according to Maslow's hierarchy of needs by first prioritizing urgent medical or safety needs and then prioritizing needs related to belonging and love, followed by self-esteem and self-actualization needs.

Sample List of Life Goal Statements
A sample of happy life goals include:

- I want to get a job.
- I want my own apartment or living space.
- I want to move to a better neighborhood where my family and I feel safe.
- I want to increase my income.
- I want to have more independence.
- I want to get an associate's degree in culinary arts so that I can be a chef.
- I want to be safe.
- I want to get my diabetes under control.
- I want to learn how to better manage my symptoms so that I can … feel better … argue less with my partner … be less fearful … go out more … enjoy life more, etc.
- I want to learn how to assert myself so that I can more effectively get my needs met.
- I want to meet a romantic partner and have more friends.
- I want to stop drinking and get along better with my family.
- I want to learn how to be a better parent and partner.

Treatment Outcome Goals
Treatment outcome goals are in service to broader life goals contained in the recovery statement. Each life goal should have one to five treatment outcome goals that address problems and barriers that interfere with achievement of life goals. Treatment outcome goals are the main goals that are worked on as part of treatment and address problems in various domains of functioning. Treatment outcome goals should be S.M.A.A.R.R.T or *S*pecific, *M*easurable, *A*ctionable, *A*chievable, *R*elevant, *R*ecovery-oriented and *T*ime-limited. For instance, treatment outcome

goals should be *specific and measurable*. They should identify an increase in something positive (e.g., skills, number of positive thoughts in a day, number of fruits and vegetables eaten in a day or week, increase in the number of social contacts), a decrease in something negative (e.g., depressive or anxious symptoms, cholesterol levels, number of drinks per day, HbA1c levels, change in weight or BMI levels, nicotine or drug use, negative thoughts), or the achievement of something (e.g., employment, sobriety, an academic or training degree/certificate, discharge from hospital). The client and provider should be able to easily measure progress and know when the goal has been achieved. Treatment outcome goals should also be something that is *actionable and achievable*; that is, something the client can actively work toward that is *relevant to them* and contributes to their overall *recovery* and can be *achieved* in a *reasonable amount of time*. These goals can sometimes overlap with a life goal. For instance, if the life goal is "I want a job," then clearly one of the goals may be focused on searching, applying, and interviewing for a job. However, other treatment outcome goals may address areas related to that life goal, but are not specifically listed in the recovery statement or identified as a life goal (e.g., reducing substance use, using medication) (Adams and Grieder 2014; Rapp and Goscha 2012; Tondora et al. 2014) (Fig. 5.2).

For instance, a treatment outcome goal may address an area that is a barrier to achieving a life goal such as symptoms related to health or mental health disorders, substance use, or a resource deficit. Using the employment example (e.g., "I want a job), a set of treatment outcome goals may address barriers to employment such as reducing drug or alcohol use, increasing coping skills, gaining access to transportation or basic resources, or identifying work preferences or skill areas. Resolving these areas might then be included as treatment outcome goals along with the goal

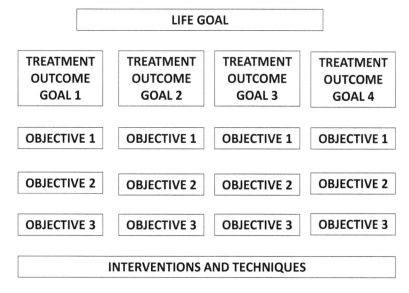

Fig. 5.2 Life goals, treatment outcome goals, and objectives

Domain	Definition	Good Examples	Poor Examples
Specific	The goals are clear, concise, and describe what will be accomplished and who will do what.	Khalid will reduce the number of daily drinks by 50% within the next 30 days.	Khalid will stop drinking.
Measurable	You know when it is achieved. It can be counted or measured in some way.	Clarisse will be able to identify 3 cognitive distortions she typically engages in by next week.	Clarisse will complete psychoeducation about her negative thinking patterns.
Actionable and Achievable	Person has the power to accomplish the goal in a reasonable time frame.	George will submit applications to two local community colleges within the next month.	George will get an associate's degree.
Relevant and Recovery-Oriented	Goal aligns with recovery and what the client wants.	Peter will complete his wellness recovery action plan within the next 30 days and speak to his doctor about lowering his Rx dosage	Peter will take his medication as prescribed.
Time-Limited	Date of completion is specified.	Victoria will experience a reduction in depressive symptoms by 50% within the next 30 days.	Victoria will reduce her depressive symptoms.

Fig. 5.3 Creating S.M.A.A.R.R.T. goals. (Based on Adams and Grieder 2014)

of employment because they are in service to the employment goal. Other examples may include: achieve sobriety, get my diabetes under control, secure child care, reduce negative thinking, use medication, buy a car, move closer to transportation lines, apply for a bus pass, or access to social services). It is often the case that providers identify a treatment approach or strategy designed to achieve the outcome goal such as medication, psychotherapy, coping skill development, or case management. This process of strategizing and problem solving, if done collaboratively, teaches clients how to break large goals down into smaller, more achievable parts and is an intervention in and of itself. Figure 5.3 defines each component of the S.M.A.A.R.R.T goals format and offers some good and not-so-good examples of SMAARRT goals.

Collaborating with Clients to Develop Outcome Goals

Collaboration, education, and communication are the keys to developing goals that are efficient, relevant, and likely to succeed. Client motivation is a vital component in determining goal achievement. If clients aren't motivated, they are unlikely to pursue goals. Motivation is enhanced through collaboration and education. Sometimes, providers must discuss goals that clients may be less motivated to pursue. It is important to ask permission to discuss these goals. When permission is granted, work together to outline the benefits and drawbacks of a particular goal and be sure to always tie it back to the recovery statement or life goals. Be flexible in how you might address treatment outcome goals, and assess the client's motivation to select and structure goals and the interventions needed to achieve them. If clients outright refuse to work on a goal you find important, move on. It is their choice. It is not worth damaging the relationship to insist on working on goals that have little chance of being accomplished. Ask if it is OK to revisit the goal at another time.

Objectives or Sub-Goals

Objectives or "sub-goals" are the smaller action steps to achieving the treatment outcome goals described above. Each treatment outcome goal should include a list of smaller objectives (Adams and Grieder 2014). Objectives are accomplished through services and interventions. They are smaller, more detailed, and more specific than treatment outcome goals. They include interventions techniques, tasks, and micro-practices. Objective completion should naturally lead to achievement of one or more treatment outcome goals. Objectives keep clients on track for achieving larger treatment outcome goals. While treatment outcome goals will often identify a treatment strategy or approach such as CBT, objectives will go one step further and identify a more specific technique linked to the strategy such as identifying negative thinking patterns through the use of thought change records or developing problem-solving skills through the completion of a problem-solving exercise or skills group.

For instance, a client with negative thinking patterns that lead to depressive mood may have a treatment outcome goal that reads: "Reduce severity of depressive symptoms as measured through a standardized depression symptoms inventory by 50% through CBT." A set of objectives linked to this goal might look something like this: (1) understand and identify two to three relevant cognitive distortions through psychoeducation by March 31, 2021 and (2) reframe negative thinking patterns related to perfectionistic thinking by identifying two to three alternative thoughts using thought change records and the "examining the evidence" approach by April 30, 2021 (see Chap. 9 for more information on these methods). These are very specific objectives, but you can see how accomplishing these smaller objectives can lead to a reduction of depressive symptoms. Note that the use of CBT methods here is not random. The use of these methods is rooted in the hypothesis that depressive symptoms are at least partly caused by negative thinking patterns. This hypothesis develops from the assessment and case conceptualization. If the case conceptualization identified biological or medical causes of depressive symptoms, then the client, while maintaining the original outcome goal of reduced depressive symptoms, may have additional objectives focused on selecting and using medication as part of a stepped approach (medication + psychotherapy). If the depressed mood was seen as part of trauma or family conflict, then exposure-based therapy or family-focused approaches would be selected as interventions, respectively.

Like treatment outcome goals, objectives should also be S.M.A.A.R.R.T. (e.g., specific/simple, measurable, actionable, achievable, relevant, recovery-oriented, and time-limited). Objectives should be *specific* and clearly identify an activity in clear and easy-to-understand language. Objectives should also be *measurable* and any change should be easily recognizable and observable by others. Change can be measured by self-report, standardized instrument, or behavioral observation, completion of a task, or counting something. Objectives should be collaboratively developed and be relevant to the client's recovery. Furthermore, there should be a reasonable time frame depending on the goal with a completion date. Time frames should be specific to the circumstances of the person, not the reporting requirements of the agency. Time frames can motivate people, but they can also overwhelm people. Be sure they are balanced. An objective statement should identify an outcome, an activity, and a measurement (Adams and Grieder 2014). Table 5.1 provides examples of life goals, treatment outcome goals, objectives, and interventions for several brief vignettes.

Examples of Objectives
1. Jeff will report an 80% reduction in drinking within the next 30 days as measured by the number of standard drinks consumed per week. Jeff will also report 0 binge-drinking episodes defined as four or more drinks per day during this time.
2. Alexis will demonstrate a reduction in depressive symptoms by 50% as evidenced by lower scores on the CES-D depression scale in the next six weeks.
3. Nora will use the activity scheduling form to schedule and carry out three pleasurable activities during times of low mood in the next week.
4. Jake will use the examining the evidence exercise to explore and evaluate two negative automatic thoughts identified through the thought record this week.
5. Claire will engage in brief relaxation exercises daily for the next weeks and rate her anxiety level before and after the exercises.
6. Michelle will attend three yoga sessions with her friend Jasmine at the YMCA and rate her anxiety level before and after each session.
7. Michael will use the "what went well" exercise nightly for the next 2 weeks and rate his mood before and after each exercise.

Objectives should also be appropriate and relevant to the treatment setting and reflect what is actually happening at the team level. For instance, objectives should be reasonable in regard to number, type, complexity, and time frame given the constraints and realities presented by the setting and the capacities of the individual (e.g., developmental level, age, psychiatric history, skill/functioning level, culture, and stage of change). They should be clearly worded, understandable, and challenging, but not overwhelming. Objectives should identify the *actions* that people will do. Objectives that seek to help people "gain insight" or "understanding" are too vague and not observable. How will people demonstrate they have gained insight? How will they show you they have benefitted from psychoeducation? Objectives should be in *alignment* with the assessment, conceptualization, outcome goals, and ultimately the life goals of the client. A thread should connect all of these elements, and they should all exist in harmony with each other (Adams and Grieder 2014).

Provider Traps and Pitfalls When Creating Treatment Plan Goals
Developing goals collaboratively with clients can be challenging, especially when providers and clients disagree on the problem and how goals should be sequenced and prioritized. Here are some ways to prevent or navigate these issues.

Table 5.1 Examples of life goals, treatment outcome goals, and objectives

Client description[a]	Recovery statement	Life goal	Treatment outcome goals	Objectives	Interventions
Johnette, 32, receives case management services from a community mental health center. She currently lives in a group home with other persons with serious mental illness.	I want to have a life!	I want to work.	Client will be employed at least part-time within the next 3 months.	Client will complete resume in 2 weeks.	Supported employment
				Client will complete job search and identify 1–3 positions in 1 month.	
				Client will apply for 1 to 3 jobs in 2 months.	
		I want my own place.	Client will live in own apartment in the next 6 months.	Client will collaborate with case worker to apply for supported housing placement within the next month.	Supported housing
				Client will collaborate with peer provider to complete wellness recovery action plan in the 45 days.	Case management
				Client will attend independent living skills group with peer counselor twice a week while waiting for placement.	Peer support
				Client will complete financial education class within the next 2 months offered at local education collaborative.	Wellness recovery action planning
		I want to make some friends.	Client will develop friendships with 1–2 new friends in the next 3 months.	Client will demonstrate skills on how to develop safe relationships after attending peer led socialization group.	Socialization skill development
				Client will introduce herself to 3 new people at social club in the next 60 days.	Peer support
				Client will go on 2 to 3 social activities (e.g., dinner, outing) in the next 45 days.	

(continued)

Table 5.1 (continued)

Client description[a]	Recovery statement	Life goal	Treatment outcome goals	Objectives	Interventions
Brody, 40, is an IT specialist. Since his divorce 5 years ago he has experienced depression and hypertension. He engages in harmful drinking (3–4 beers after work per day). He is currently overweight by 30 pounds and is pre-diabetic. He expresses loneliness and chronic thoughts of worthlessness and anxiety.	I want to feel healthy, strong, and loved.	I want to lose weight and gain muscle.	Client will lose 20 pounds and reduce glucose level by 20% in the next 6 months.	Client will attend nutritional consultation to get dietary recommendation (i.e., diet) to improve weight and diabetic symptoms.	Behavioral activation
				Client will attend beginner power yoga classes 2–3 times a week.	Relaxation
				Client will join walking group at work and walk 3+ times a week in nearby park.	
		I want to be less depressed and nervous.	Client will experience a 50% reduction in depression scores in 2 months.	Client will complete activity log to identify times during day they are most depressed.	Behavioral activation
				Client will structure activities to target times when most likely to be depressed.	Cognitive reframing
				Client will identify 2 cognitive distortions and rational replacement thoughts using thought change records.	
				Client will demonstrate relaxation skills in-session and practice at home several times a week and as needed	Relaxation training

Client description[a]	Recovery statement	Life goal	Treatment outcome goals	Objectives	Interventions
		I want to meet a romantic partner.	Client will go on 1–2 social activities in the next 2 months	Client will complete online dating profile.	Socialization
				Client will complete 2–4 new social activities (e.g., classes, outings, events) per month.	
				Client will re-engage with 1–2 friends and increase social activities with friends 1–2 times a month.	
Jess, 29, is a full-time hair stylist and part-time bartender. They have experienced PTSD symptoms (e.g., nightmares, arousal, avoidance) after a recent incident of violence in which they were verbally threatened and assaulted by a patron at work while closing the bar. The patron pushed them and threatened them and their partner with violence before other co-workers intervened.	I want to feel safe, and I want to move on from this experience so it doesn't control my life anymore.	I want to be free from these nightmares.	Client will report 75% reduction in intrusion and arousal symptoms.	Client will demonstrate understanding of the CBT model of PTSD in the next 21 days.	Exposure-based therapy
				Client will identify specific elements of event that were problematic.	Safety planning
				Client will engage in 5–10 sessions of imaginal exposure (EMDR) and report declining subjective distress.	Advocacy
				Client will identify external symptom cues in the next week.	
				Client will engage in 5–10 weeks of in vivo exposure to identified symptom cues (safety permitting).	

(continued)

Table 5.1 (continued)

Client description[a]	Recovery statement	Life goal	Treatment outcome goals	Objectives	Interventions
		I want to go back to work without being afraid.	Client will go to work each shift and report 75% reduction in subjective distress.	Client will develop personal safety plan to ensure safety in home life.	
				Client will collaborate with counselor to develop safety plan for re-engaging with work in the next 15 days.	
				Client will work with employer to advocate for implementation of safety plan to ensure safe work environment (e.g., different shift, safety protocols for closing) in the next 15 days.	
				Client will develop response plan (e.g., legal action, alternative employment) if employer will not comply with safety plan.	
		I want to feel calm and less on edge and angry.	Client will report 50% reduction in arousal symptoms	Client will demonstrate competence in practicing mindfulness-based relaxation techniques in the next 30 days.	Relaxation training
				Client will seek out peer support such as joining trans support group and/or advocacy opportunities for trans rights and protections in the next 60 days.	Self-help
					Advocacy

All names and other identifiers of clients have been changed to protect privacy and confidentiality

1. **Do not substitute your preferences for the clients'** under the guise of what is "realistic" or "appropriate." Remember, "achievable" is not the same as "realistic." For instance, if you do not think a client's goal is "realistic" and you try to steer them away from their goal toward something you think is more "appropriate," then you are just substituting your goal for the clients'. That's not being realistic. That's being paternalistic. Good luck trying to motivate the client to achieve that goal. Why would they? It isn't their goal. It's yours. Paternalism has no place in person-centered treatment planning. It is understandable when providers want to protect clients from getting too stressed out and having a relapse. However, this can sometimes result in overprotection of clients. Clients have the right to take calculated risks that can lead to success *or* failure. It is important to support clients no matter what—win or lose. If they succeed—cheer them on. Failure is also an opportunity to learn something. If they fail, help them get back up and problem solve solutions for what went wrong so they can be successful in the future.

2. **Keep goals measurable**. Goals that are too vague and abstract do not get accomplished. The goal, "I want to be happy," is a good goal to have, but it is not measurable. Help clients break "happy" down into measurable goals that, if achieved, would lead to happiness. These goals might include: I want my depressive symptoms to be reduced; I want to think more positive thoughts about myself; I want to make new friends; I want my own place; I want to lose weight; I want to stop drinking so much. Goals should always be recovery-oriented, grounded in the needs of the individual, and have a positive impact on the person's life—that is, when they are achieved, the person is healthier, happier, more fulfilled, and more secure. But more importantly, we need to know when they are achieved. When goals are specific, measurable, and time-limited, we have a better chance of knowing if we are on the right track.

3. **Keep it simple**. When goals and objectives are too detailed, they can become overwhelming and confusing. Goals and objectives should be written with parsimony in mind. Be sure to match the level of detail with the capacities and abilities of your client. Goals should be challenging and exciting, but not overwhelming. If clients have multiple morbidities, goals and objectives can get complex. Helping clients prioritize goals related to basic needs and safety first can be a good way to help clients work toward goals in such a way as to build success. Objectives should also be written in clear language so the client knows exactly what they have to do between sessions for homework. Objectives should be easy to remember, include all the necessary steps, and sequenced in such a way so that they lead to goal achievement. Clients with behavioral health issues often have trouble concentrating and remembering things. Clients who have sequenced tasks and instructions in writing or on a digital device can stay on track and be successful. Conducting check-ins with clients between sessions to see how they are progressing and to give encouragement and feedback is also a good practice.

4. **Keep it concise**. Similar to having too many details, having too many goals can lead clients to feel stuck and demoralized, which then leads to resistance and

eventually loss to follow-up. Stick to three to five treatment outcome goals that are relevant and important to the client. Encourage clients to start with goals that are "low hanging fruit" and can be accomplished quickly. That way they can build momentum and gain some success. Break bigger goals down into achievable steps that can be celebrated as they are achieved.

5. **Keep life goals, treatment outcome goals, and objectives in alignment.** This will make your supervisor and auditors happy. Remember: (1) life goals are the ultimate endpoint for the client; (2) treatment outcome goals are more specific, but still broad and are what is achieved at the end of treatment and lead to the achievement of life goals; (3) treatment outcome goals should be clear, global, and lead to well-being; and (4) objectives are the specific action steps necessary to achieve the treatment outcome goals. They identify who will do what by a certain date.

6. **Pacing is important.** If you're moving too fast, clients can get overwhelmed and give up. If you are moving too slow, clients can get bored and lose focus and motivation. Providers need to repeatedly check in with clients to make sure that the pacing of change is challenging, but not overwhelming. It is best to start slow and then speed up as needed. If you find that the client becomes overwhelmed and did not complete their between-session tasks, explore with them why they weren't able to complete the assignment. This usually takes place at the start of each session when you review assignments and set the agenda. Be honest about pacing and be flexible enough to speed up or slow things down as needed. In addition to monitoring assignment completion, check progress on outcome goals through symptom measures or other measurements (e.g., self-report, observation, collateral contacts, records). Is there improvement? Has the client shown any successes or progress? Intermediate success energizes the process and keeps clients motivated as they see their progress. Use these measures as gauges to see if the pacing of intervention is appropriate. Inviting clients to discuss these issues directly is also important.

7. **Avoid "dead person," "process," or "participation" goals.** Will your client achieve all of their goals if they just drop dead one day? Then you have dead person goals. A goal list that says the person will stop drinking, stop smoking, avoid sweets, stop being depressed, stop gambling, and not be angry, are unlikely to be successful. While "stop and avoid" goals are inevitable, it is important to mix in "improve, get, develop, and learn goals." People need something positive to work toward such as employment, independent housing, recreation, making friends, getting stronger. Make goals positive, meaningful, and recovery-oriented (Adams and Grieder 2014).

Also avoid using "process" or "participation" goals as treatment outcome goals or objectives. These goals focus on participation or adherence in some treatment or therapy program. Although they may be related or supportive to a treatment outcome goal or objective, they should not replace them. Treatment outcome goals and objectives accomplish something. Participation goals identify a type of strategy to achieve an objective. You may be required to have participation or process goals such as "the client will attend therapy sessions three times a week," "the client will take medications as prescribed 80% of the time," or "the client will complete a six-week anger management program" as part of your plan—but position them as "sub-objectives". Do not confuse these with treatment outcome goals or objectives. A treatment plan with only participation goals will not be effective. Think about it this way—imagine that you have a client that wants to feel less depressed and angry, and all of their goals and objectives are related to participating in groups, taking medications, and attending therapy sessions. What if after six months of doing all of these things, they still experience the same symptoms, problems, and issues they did when they started despite participating in treatment? Maybe they have even gotten worse. Yet, all goals would have been achieved. Success! But that's not success from the client's perspective since they would be no better off. That's a great way for clients to become demoralized and pessimistic about future help-seeking. *Outcome goals lead to change* (e.g., reduced symptoms, increased skills). *Objectives accomplish something* (e.g., identify cognitive distortions, complete a job application, demonstrate a coping skill). Participation in treatment identifies a means to achieve those goals and objectives—but they are not the goals or objectives themselves.

8. **Respond to setbacks in a positive way**. Setbacks are the expectation, not the exception. Prepare your client for relapse and setbacks since this is a part of the therapy process. Do not react with dismay or disappointment when setbacks happen. Be sincere and supportive, but stay balanced. The task after a setback is to identify what went wrong, adjust the plan, and move ahead.

5.3 Selecting Interventions

Interventions are the treatments, services, and resources necessary for a client to overcome barriers, solve problems, and accomplish their goals (Adams and Grieder 2014). When selecting interventions, the provider should have *a complete understanding of the best and most effective range of interventions* designed to address clients' identified problems and goals. Providers should also have a *complete understanding of the different resources that exist in the community* that the client can access either on their own or through referral. Providers should have formal relationships with the most important outside resources to facilitate the referral and follow-up processes, including organizations that address physical and behavioral health, violence and safety, and social determinants of health. And providers should have a *complete understanding of their client's* preferences, capacities, and stage of change for a particular problem in order to select interventions that are in alignment with those elements. For instance, when selecting a substance use intervention for a client in the contemplation stage of change, motivational approaches would be more appropriate than an intervention designed for the action stage of change such as substance abuse counseling or Alcoholics Anonymous. Clients should have a menu of relevant treatment options to choose from to ensure they select interventions that are effective and compatible with their goals and preferences.

Key elements in intervention selection include: (1) the *modality* (e.g., cognitive behavioral therapy) including the specific *techniques* that will be used such as psychoeducation, evaluating negative thinking patterns, or exposure; (2) *who* will provide the intervention (e.g., discipline, setting, agency, person); (3) *when* the intervention will be provided and the *frequency* (e.g., how many sessions and how many times a week or month) including if clients are expected to do assignments or tasks between sessions; (4) *intensity* (e.g., 30 minutes, one hour), *duration* (e.g., how many days, weeks, months, or sessions will the treatment last in total); (5) *where* the intervention will take place (e.g., agency, setting—home, school, work, hospital, clinic, store, center); and (6) *the rationale* for why the intervention was chosen (e.g., the purpose of the intervention, why was it selected, what problem is it designed to solve, and what goal it serves). The rationale for the intervention should logically match the problem and goal. For instance, how will CBT help a person's depressive symptoms and how will it help the person meet a particular objective or goal? (Adams and Grieder 2014; Rapp and Goscha 2012; Tondora et al. 2014).

Shared Decision-Making
When conducting person-centered treatment planning, interventions in the plan should be selected by clients who are fully informed about the range of options available including the risks and benefits associated with each service. When selecting interventions, providers should rely on a *shared decision-making (SDM)* approach. Shared decision-making is a process of collaborative decision-making between providers and clients that involves consideration of all available information and options and then supporting and respecting the client's choices regarding treatment (Charles et al. 1997; Deegan and Drake 2006; Drake and Deegan 2009; Elwyn et al. 2012; Stanhope and Choy-Brown 2018). Like person-centered care, SDM is associated with greater patient participation in treatment and satisfaction with treatment decisions (Glass et al. 2012; Loh et al. 2007). Implementing shared decision-making perspectives, like other recovery-oriented practices, takes intentionality, organizational support, and collaborative learning within practice communities (Macdonald-Wilson et al. 2017; Mancini and Miner 2013). Providers who use a shared decision-making approach are guided by a perspective that prioritizes client self-determination and a strong, supportive therapeutic relationship. Clients are not just coldly given the options for treatment and left to decide for themselves. Providers help clients become aware and informed of the options and choices that exist and give them decision support that is thorough and understandable. They help clients figure out what is most important to them so that they can develop personal preferences that are informed by awareness of the given risks and benefits of all available options, including doing nothing. In this way, clients and providers work in partnership to identify the best options for treatment given according to client preferences and goals (Elwyn et al. 2012).

All aspects of available interventions, including evidence of effectiveness, benefits, and potential adverse effects, should be explained to the person in clear, easy-to-understand language. They should also know the full range of benefits and adverse effects of any treatment, as well as the risk and benefits of not engaging in a particular approach (e.g., doing nothing, watchful waiting). Providers should use all available evidence including empirical evidence, clinical expertise (e.g., practice wisdom), and personal experiences when informing clients. Iatrogenic effects such as side effects from medication, distress from exposure-based treatments, and experiencing rejection from the taking of social risks can lead to real negative effects. Clients should be fully informed and supported in their decisions. For instance, the adverse effects of psychiatric medications include metabolic problems, weight gain, sexual side effects, dry mouth, drooling, tremors, restlessness, and an increased risk for suicide among other serious adverse effects. These effects should be clearly explained to the client and a plan for monitoring and addressing them should be developed if the client agrees to use them. For instance, if a client decided to take antipsychotic medications because the adverse effects are less problematic than doing nothing, the provider and the client can discuss ways to minimize the adverse effects such as lower dosing, complementary medications, monitoring and planning, and the use of wellness strategies to either replace or supplement medications and reduce adverse or unintended effects of the drug.

Providers should thoroughly explore all areas of concern and ask for feedback and questions that clients may have regarding any intervention. For instance, if employment is a goal for clients on disability, they will need to know the changes that may occur to their entitlement benefits if they gain employment such as a reduction in assistance or changes to their medical coverage. Providers and clients can then collaborate to figure out how to best move forward, considering the given client preferences, needs, and available solutions (Stanhope and Choy-Brown 2018; Tondora et al. 2014).

During sessions, it is important for providers to create a warm, empathic environment in which the client has as much time and encouragement as needed to explore concerns and solutions. Providers should also have a range of information available for clients to take home and review on their own. Practicing from this perspective also requires providers to be culturally competent and responsive. Language interpretation services should be easily accessible. Providers should be representative of the community they serve, and a diverse array of service options that are responsive to the cultural practices and preferences of the client are vital. Community health workers or peer specialists should be utilized to help the clients gain a more authentic understanding based on personal experiences from someone who has undergone the treatment first-hand (Mancini 2018, 2019). Honesty, frankness, and transparency are key attributes for providers as are the skills of active, empathic listening and reflection.

Sometimes clients may make decisions that conflict with your professional opinion. This may include not pursuing an intervention (e.g., watchful waiting) or preference for an alternative approach with limited evidence of effectiveness. In these instances, providers should be honest and clear about interventions they think are ineffective or pose unnecessary risks and work to help the client or family find a solution to their problem. While it is important to be flexible, one cannot endorse interventions that are ineffective or may pose a significant risk or threat to the client. Providers should be transparent about this upfront (Adams and Grieder 2014).

The Importance of Stages of Change

Providers should help clients select goals, objectives, and interventions aligned with a person's stage of change. For instance, education, harm reduction, and motivational interventions are good for persons in pre-contemplation and contemplation. Motivation and action-related interventions are more appropriate for preparation and action stages. Relapse prevention strategies are ideal for persons in the maintenance stage. Stage assessment is ongoing and should be updated as treatment progresses (Adams and Grieder 2014).

Different Types of Interventions

- Medications and biological interventions
- Psychotherapeutic interventions such as cognitive behavioral therapy, problem-solving therapy, and interpersonal psychotherapy
- Psychoeducation/bibliotherapy
- Skill development: social, assertiveness, anger management, wellness, problem solving
- Trauma-informed interventions
- Brief family therapy approaches
- Psychiatric rehabilitation approaches
- Intensive case management
- Peer support
- Self-help
- Natural occurring resources and events in the community

Mobilizing Supports and Resources

The provider should have a clear understanding of the community resources available to address a range of health, mental health, and social problems. Person-centered planning helps clients access outside resources to address problems. The provider should prioritize the use of existing natural supports within the client's household and family and then work outward to extended family and friends, neighborhood, and local community resources to help clients get their needs met and address social determinants of health (Rapp and Goscha 2012). Providers should routinely ask: What sources of help exist in the person's social network that can provide needed resources such as transportation, socialization, basic needs, and other help? Natural supports are the individuals, relationships, organizations, and communities that can help the person achieve well-being. The benefit of natural supports is that they are often low cost, culturally tailored, enduring because they are integrated within the community, and bidirectional, providing benefit both to the client and the supporter (Rapp and Goscha 2012).

For resources that require assistance from outside the person's natural support network, providers should have close, formal relationships with several important community agencies and resources. These community resources can include different types of health and behavioral health organizations, social service organizations, victim advocacy groups, child care organizations, shelters, housing and employment organizations, community groups, faith groups, self-help resources (e.g., Alcoholics Anonymous or Narcotics Anonymous), mentoring programs, and programs that provide help with basic resources. Having formal relationships with outside providers can lead to a smooth transition of services and increase the likelihood that clients will successfully engage with services (e.g., warm referral). It also helps enhance the ability of the provider to coordinate services and follow up on progress.

5.4 Documenting Progress

It is important for providers to consistently document the progress clients are making toward their goals in detailed and frequent progress notes. Progress notes should align with the plan for services including the assessment, case conceptualization, and treatment plan. For instance, if you used a cognitive behavioral-based framework in your hypothesis to explain a client's depressed and anxious symptoms, then your progress notes should document your use of cognitive behavioral interventions to achieve cognitive behavioral-oriented outcome goals and objectives. In short, providers should use progress notes to evaluate and document client progress on activities that are in service to stated goals and the notes should align with the broader plan for services. There are certainly times when new problems arise that require attention. These should be documented, and any problems and new interventions should be linked back to the original goal by describing how the new issues impact the identified goals so as to justify a response. Treatment plans should then be updated accordingly to accommodate the new information. New problems can also signal the need for the creation of new goals and objectives if it is deemed necessary to address to ensure successful achievement of life goals.

Progress notes have several functions. First, they communicate to others the specific interventions and activities of treatment and the progress people make toward the goals identified in the plan. Second, they outline the work of the provider and client toward those goals, and they provide documentation of the things that have been successful and unsuccessful. Third, they hold treatment providers and clients accountable to the plan by evaluating progress and tracking where people are on the recovery journey. This is important for insurance payers and auditors who want to know how the provider is benefiting the client in an efficient and effective manner. Progress notes are essential in the communication, coordination, and evaluation of services and are vital in the continuous quality improvement process.

Several formats for progress notes exist. They all have similar characteristics. First, progress notes always identify progress clients are making toward specific goals. Second, they identify the interventions that are being used to achieve the goals and objectives identified by the client. Third, they assess and evaluate the response to those interventions. And fourth, they identify a future plan of action to address the results of the evaluation. Progress note formats often depend on the setting. For instance, some settings do not have a specific format, but rely on more unstructured narratives. If this is the case, the four areas mentioned above should be included in each and every note. Notes should be taken for every interaction with

SOAP	DAP	PIE
Subjective Data: Information that comes from the client in their own words and self-report..	Data: Combination of subjective and objective data	Problems: Objective and subjective data, regarding social, behavioral, and physical health symptoms and problems
Objective: Results of professional observations, tests, medical history, and measures		
Assessment/Impact: Initially this includes diagnoses. Later progress notes include an evaluation of the impact of interventions and results of any subsequent measures or observations. (i.e., "What went well and what didn't?")	Assessment: Same as SOAP	Interventions: Description of the interventions for each target problem
Plan: Next steps in the treatment process based on the results of the assessment/impact section	Same as SOAP	Evaluation: Evaluation of the impact of interventions

Fig. 5.4 Progress note formats. (Based on: Adams and Grieder 2014)

the client or family as well as for any new information that comes to the attention of the worker from outside the client or client system (e.g., reports or conversations with probation officers, other providers, teachers, employers, or medical personnel).

Progress Note Formats

The most common progress note formats are the SOAP and DAP formats. The SOAP format stands for *S*ubjective, *O*bjective, *A*ssessment, and *P*lan. The DAP format stands for *D*ata, *A*ssessment, and *P*lan. These approaches contain the same information. Another format is the PIE format, which stands for *P*roblem, *I*ntervention and *E*valuation. Figure 5.4 outlines the components of each of the above progress note formats.

Data In the SOAP format, subjective and objective data are the comments, observations, and perspectives regarding the problems, goals/objectives, and interventions of the client (subjective), and provider observations and results from tests and measures (objective), respectively. The DAP format combines the subjective and objective data into the Data section. In the PIE format, the *P*lan section includes the objective and subjective data, observations, and perspectives of the client and provider regarding social, behavioral, and physical health symptoms and problems (Adams and Grieder 2014).

Assessment of Impact of Interventions The second domain of the progress note is a description of interventions used by the provider, the target problem that the intervention was designed to address, and the perceived impact of the interventions on the target problem. This assessment can be described through self-report, observations, or through results of standardized tests, assessments, or measures. Assessment of interventions should also include the client and provider's perspective on the quality and value of the intervention and what could have been improved upon. In other words, what went well and what didn't? This data is reported in the *assessment* section of the SOA*P* and DA*P* formats. Description of the interventions on target problems corresponds to the *intervention* section of the P*I*E format. Evaluation of intervention impact corresponds to the *evaluation* section of the PI*E* format (Adams and Grieder 2014).

Plan The *plan* section of the DA*P* and SOA*P* format describes the next steps in the treatment process based on the results of the assessment/impact section. This section also corresponds to the *evaluation* section in the PI*E* format. The plan should include documentation that the intervention will continue as planned if the goal or problem areas are still being addressed. If the problem has been solved or the goal achieved, then success should be noted and the next steps in the treatment process outlined. If the intervention was deemed insufficient, then the plan moving forward should be described. This may mean increasing intensity of services, adding or discontinuing services, or extending the intervention for a longer period (Adams and Grieder 2014).

The purpose of the progress note is to offer an easily deciphered description of the work (problem/goal, intervention, response, next steps) between the client and the provider, and the progress made (or not). Continuous documentation of progress ensures that the provider and the client are aware of what is happening in the relationship and what needs to change (if anything). If progress is shown, it can strengthen the relationship and signal when services can end. If progress is not shown, it provides a feedback loop that can signal the need to change approaches or strategies in order to better solve problems. In short, progress notes hold the client and provider accountable to progress.

Progress notes can also be collaborative between the client and the provider. For instance, concurrent or collaborative documentation is an important strategy that involves sharing and reviewing notes with clients and giving clients the opportunity to add input or revisions. This approach increases accountability, transparency, engagement, and accuracy. Progress notes are not a secret. People should be included in the documentation of their lives, and people have a right to read and have input in what is written about them. This can increase client satisfaction in the process and can increase positive outcomes and treatment adherence (Stanhope et al. 2013).

Collaboration can also be across team members, so that if team members are working on various problems, a shared progress note can capture the data, assessment, and plan from each team member to create a more integrated documentation system. Having separate progress notes across areas and in separate records dealing with addictions, mental health, physical health, and social areas can lead to fragmented, disorganized care. Having a shared note in one place organized across problems, goals, and intervention can lead to better communication and collaboration across team members, enhancing coordination of care.

Treatment Planning Review

Treatment plans should be reviewed on a routine basis, and care settings often have requirements for when treatment plans are reviewed. For instance, community mental health centers are often required to review initial treatment plans after 30 days and then subsequent plans are reviewed quarterly or semi-annually. In general, it is good practice to view the treatment plan as a living document that is continually reviewed, revised, and updated. Reviewing progress toward goals and evaluating the result of specific interventions is good behavioral health practice. This helps hold the provider and client accountable and keep both working toward shared and agreed upon goals. Reviewing the treatment plan on a routine basis can also lead to more efficient treatment because new problems or barriers to treatment can be identified sooner. This can lead to creative and collaborative problem-solving between the client and provider to keep treatment on track.

5.5   Summary and Conclusion

Person-centered treatment planning is a collaborative process that synthesizes the information gathered in the psychosocial assessment to develop a detailed case conceptualization of client problem areas. This information is then used to identify goals and develop a documented action plan to achieve those goals in a set time frame. Person-centered treatment planning is a partnership between the provider and the client who work together to set goals and select the best interventions to achieve those goals based on client preferences and informed choices. Treatment plans guide the service relationship and provide a roadmap for problem-solving and goal achievement. When done well, treatment planning can be a form of intervention that models for the client how to work collaboratively with others, solve problems, set and achieve goals, monitor progress, and can also build client self-efficacy. Treatment planning also offers a way to assess and monitor progress for continuous quality improvement.

Case Study 5.1: The Case of Clarence Smith (Continued)
(See Case Study 4.1 from Chap. 4)
Case Review

Mr. Clarence Smith[1] is a 62-year-old Black man who lost his wife, Angela, suddenly to a stroke 2 years ago. He reports sadness, loss of interest in daily activities, trouble sleeping, and fatigue. He blames himself for not being able to help his wife and reports drinking 2 or more beers a night to help him sleep. He has also experienced a traumatic event in that he witnessed his wife's death and could not resuscitate her.

---

[1]All names and other identifiers of this case have been changed to protect privacy and confidentiality.

He experiences persistent and intrusive thoughts and nightmares, negative cognitions (e.g., self-blame), and emotions (e.g., sadness, anxiety) related to the event. He also avoids the place where the event happened. He has a history of co-morbid diabetes and hypertension. While both conditions are currently controlled with medication, he is experiencing increased vision and neuropathy symptoms. Mr. Smith is a retired postal worker, father of three, and grandfather of four. He has a loving relationship with his family, but they live out of state. He reports a rich social network that includes several friends and a faith community. However, he reports he is not able to socialize with friends and family due to the restrictions related to COVID-19. He reports feeling lonely, sad, and worthless, and he blames himself for his wife's death. When asked what Mr. Smith would like to improve in his life, he reported that he would like to: (1) feel more useful; (2) see his family and friends more; and (3) reduce ruminative thoughts regarding Angela's death.

Case Conceptualization

Clarence is struggling with symptoms of PTSD, depression, and grief. His symptoms are complicated by his social isolation and ruminative thoughts about his wife's death. He has also begun to drink in order to sleep. The combination of depression, loneliness, diabetes, hypertension, drinking, and grief can lead to significant health consequences and early mortality if not addressed. Based on conversations with Clarence about the above symptoms and situation, the following recommendations were collaboratively developed: (1) reduce his depressive symptoms through psychotherapy to accept the loss of Angela and develop healthier thinking patterns around her death (e.g., reduce self-blame and guilt) and behavioral activation to schedule activities during the day; (2) reduce his trauma symptoms by prolonged exposure, EMDR, or cognitive processing therapy in order to reduce intrusive thoughts and negative cognitions and mood; (3) increase his socialization with others through re-connecting him safely with friends, family, and faith community in person through safe outside events like conversing in a park with masks and social distancing and virtually connecting with his faith community and family online or on the phone; (4) get more exercise through daily activity scheduling of walks or through home equipment such as a stationary bike, and completing daily errands; (5) advise him to reduce or eliminate his drinking, particularly before bed, as this can exacerbate depressive symptoms and reduce sleep; (6) explore antidepressant medication as a supplement to psychotherapy to reduce depressive symptoms if needed; and (7) address his diabetes through improved meal planning, a review of his medication, and exploring the use of orthotics, rehabilitative exercises, and other means to reduce pain in his feet.

Questions

What are five SMAARRT treatment outcome goals and relevant objectives that could help Clarence achieve his life goals?

What specific intervention approaches and techniques could be used to help Clarence? What natural supports could be incorporated in the plan?

What strengths does Clarence have that could be used to help him achieve his goals?

References

Adams, N., & Grieder, D. M. (2014). *Treatment planning for person-centered care: Shared decision making for whole health* (2nd ed.). Boston, MA: Elsevier Press.

Berman, P. S. (2019). *Case conceptualization and treatment planning: Integrating theory with clinical practice* (4th ed.). Los Angeles: Sage.

Berwick, D. (2009). What "patient-centered" should mean: Confessions of an extremist. *Health Affairs, 28*(4), w555–w565. https://doi.org/10.1377/hlthaff.28.4.w555.

Charles, C., Gafni, A., & Whelan, T. (1997). Shared decision-making in the medical encounter: What does it mean? (or it takes two to tango). *Social Science and Medicine, 44*(5), 681–692.

Collins, C. (2010). *Evolving models of behavioral health integration in primary care.* New York: Milbank Memorial Fund.

Deegan, P. E., & Drake, R. E. (2006). Shared decision making and medication management in the recovery process. *Psychiatric Services, 57*(11), 1636–1639. https://doi.org/10.1176/ps.2006.57.11.1636.

Drake, R. E., & Deegan, P. E. (2009). Shared decision making is an ethical imperative. *Psychiatric Services, 60*(8), 1007. https://doi.org/10.1176/ps.2009.60.8.1007.

Elwyn, G., Frosch, D., Thomson, R., Joseph-Williams, N., Lloyd, A., Kinnersley, P., et al. (2012). Shared decision making: A model for clinical practice. *Journal of General Internal Medicine, 27*(10), 1361–1367.

Glass, K. E., Wills, C. E., Holloman, C., Olson, J., Hechmer, C., Miller, C. K., & Duchemin, A. M. (2012). Shared decision-making and other variables as correlates of satisfaction in health care decisions in a United States National Survey. *Patient Education and Counseling, 88*(1), 100–105.

Institute of Medicine (IOM). (2001). *Crossing the quality chasm: A new health system for the 21st century.* Washington, DC: National Academy Press.

Lichner-Ingram, B. (2012). *Clinical case formulations: Matching the integrative treatment plan to the client* (2nd ed.). Hoboken: Wiley.

Loh, A., Simon, D., Wills, C. E., Kriston, L., Niebling, W., & Harter, M. (2007). The effects of a shared decision-making intervention in primary care of depression: A cluster-randomized controlled trial. *Patient Education and Counseling, 67*, 324–332.

Macdonald-Wilson, K., Hutchison, S. L., Karpov, I., Wittman, P., & Deegan, P. E. (2017). A successful implementation strategy to support adoption of decision making in mental health services. *Community Mental Health Journal, 53*(3), 251–256. https://doi.org/10.1007/s10597-016-0027-1.

Mahoney, K. (2011). Person-centered planning and participant decision making. *Health and Social Work, 36*(3), 233–235.

Mancini, M. A. (2018). An exploration of factors that effect the implementation of peer support services in community mental health settings. *Community Mental Health Journal, 54*(2), 127–137. https://doi.org/10.1007/s10597-017-0145-4/.

Mancini, M. A. (2019). Strategic storytelling: An exploration of the professional practices of mental health peer providers. *Qualitative Health Research, 29*(9), 1266–1276. https://doi.org/10.1177/1049732318821689.

Mancini, M. A., & Linhorst, D. M. (2010). Harm reduction in community mental health settings. *Journal of Social Work in Disability & Rehabilitation, 9*, 130–147.

Mancini, M. A., & Miner, C. S. (2013). Learning and change in a community mental health setting. *Journal of Evidence Based Social Work, 10*(5), 494–504.

Mancini, M. A., & Wyrick-Waugh, W. (2013). Consumer and practitioner perceptions of the harm reduction approach in a community mental health setting. *Community Mental Health Journal, 49*(1), 14–24.

Mancini, M. A., Hardiman, E. R., & Lawson, H. A. (2005). Making sense of it all: Consumer providers' theories about factors facilitating and impeding recovery from psychiatric disabilities. *Psychiatric Rehabilitation Journal, 29*(1), 48–55.

Patient Protection and Affordable Care Act. (2010). P.L. 111-148, 124 Stat. 1025; 2010.

Rapp, C. A., & Goscha, R. J. (2012). *The strengths model: A recovery-oriented approach to mental health services*. New York: Oxford University Press.

Stanhope, V., & Ashenberg-Straussner, S. L. (Eds.). (2018). *Social work and integrated health care: From policy to practice and back*. New York: Oxford University Press.

Stanhope, V., & Choy-Brown, M. (2018). Chapter 10: Person-centered care. In V. Stanhope & S. L. Ashenberg-Straussner (Eds.), *Social work and integrated health care: From policy to practice and back* (pp. 148–165). New York: Oxford University Press.

Stanhope, V., & Matthews, E. B. (2019). Delivering person-centered care with an electronic health record. *BMC Medical Informatics and Decision Making, 19*(1), 168. https://doi.org/10.1186/s12911-019-0897-6.

Stanhope, V., Ignolia, C., Schmelter, B., & Marcus, S. (2013). Impact of person-centered planning and collaborative documentation on treatment adherence. *Psychiatric Services, 64*, 76–79.

Tondora, J., Miller, R., Slade, M., & Davidson, L. (2014). *Partnering for recovery in mental health: A practical guide to person-centered planning*. Hoboken: Wiley.

Wright, J. H., Brown, G. K., Thase, M. E., Ramirez Basco, M., & Gabbard, G. O. (2017). *Learning cognitive behavioral therapy: An illustrated guide* (Core competencies in psychotherapy) (2nd ed.). Arlington, VA: American Psychiatric Publishing.

Chapter 6
Integrated Behavioral Health Approaches to Interpersonal Violence

6.1 An Overview of Violence and Health

Interpersonal violence is a multidimensional phenomenon that has an enormous impact on society. Intimate partner violence (IPV) is a form of interpersonal violence perpetrated by a current or former partner or spouse that includes physical and sexual assault, verbal insults and threats, manipulative behaviors, economic abuse, psychological/emotional abuse, and stalking (CDC 2018; Decker et al. 2018). Perpetrators of IPV use one or more of these forms of violence systematically to establish and maintain power and control over a current or former partner/spouse. *Community violence* is another form of interpersonal violence that is experienced in settings outside of the home (e.g., playgrounds, schools, residences outside the person's home, cars, the street) by persons who are not immediate family members (e.g., strangers, acquaintances, rivals, friends, classmates). Community violence includes fights, physical assaults, and firearm-related violence (Decker et al. 2018).

Primary care settings represent a key site for screening and intervention for violence due to the high prevalence of violence in the population and the high number of injuries seen in medical settings that result from violence. Survivors of violence experience a range of comorbid health, behavioral health, and social problems and are at a higher risk for re-injury and re-experiencing violence in the future. Furthermore, different types of violence are often comorbid and intertwined with each other and share common risk and protective factors resulting in a survivor or perpetrator of one form of violence being at a much higher risk for experiencing or engaging in other forms of violence (Finkelhor et al. 2011; Hamby and Grych 2013; Wilson et al. 2014). Public health prevention strategies for various forms of violence are available and can occur at the individual, family, and community level, making the integration of screening, assessment, and intervention practices for various forms of violence in medical settings possible and imperative. In this chapter, I will explore several best practices with regard to screening and intervention for interpersonal violence in integrated behavioral health settings. Approaches that specifically address intimate partner violence (IPV) and community violence will be reviewed.

© Springer Nature Switzerland AG 2021
M. A. Mancini, *Integrated Behavioral Health Practice*,
https://doi.org/10.1007/978-3-030-59659-0_6

6.2 Epidemiological Impact of Violence on the Population

Data from the National Crime Victimization Survey indicated that violence victimization, after years of decline, has risen 20% from 2015 to 2018, mainly due to increases in rape and sexual and physical assaults. In 2018, there were six million violent incidents. This is a 13% rise (800,000 incidents) from 2017. The rate of rape or sexual assaults per 1,000 persons over the age of 12 almost doubled from 1.4 victimization/1,000 to 2.7/1,000 in 2018 (Morgan and Oudekerk 2019). In 2017, over 19,500 people or 6/100,000 people died from homicide and of that number, over 14,500 (4.5/100,000) were due to firearms (Kochanek et al. 2019). Violence and homicide disproportionally impact communities of color and younger persons (Sumner et al. 2015). Homicides are among the top-five leading causes of death for persons under the age of 45 and the third leading cause of death of persons between the ages of 15 and 34. For Black and Latinx persons in that age range, it is the leading and second leading cause of death, respectively (Heron 2019). Even more tragically, homicide is the second leading cause of death for Black children in the United States under the age of 10 (Heron 2019).

Men are more likely to engage in homicidal behavior (Curtin et al. 2016; Cooper and Smith 2011; Kann et al. 2018) and almost four times more likely to be victims of homicide than women (Cooper and Smith 2011). However, homicide is one of the leading causes of death for women (Heron 2019), with IPV accounting for half of all female homicides (Petrosky et al. 2017; Stöckl et al. 2013). Homicide disproportionately impacts women of color as it is the second leading cause of death for black women under the age of 20 and fourth leading cause of death for black women between the ages of 20 and 44, and it is the fifth leading cause of death for Latinx women under the age of 45 and is the sixth leading cause of death for white women between the ages of 20 and 44 (Heron 2019). Violence against the transgender and gender nonconforming (TGNC) community is increasing. Since 2013, nearly 200 TGNC persons have been murdered in the United States, the vast majority (80–90%) of whom are black transgender women (HRC 2020). In 2019, at least 27 TGNC persons were murdered. In the first half of 2020, at least 21 TGNC persons have been murdered (HRC 2020). The murder rates of TGNC persons are likely severe undercounts.

6.2.1 Ecological Factors that Impact Violence

There are several inter-related social and ecological factors that impact violence across individual, interpersonal, community, and societal levels (Decker et al. 2018; Sumner et al. 2015). Table 6.1 outlines the risk and protective factors for violence victimization and perpetration at the individual, interpersonal, and community levels. At the individual level, the experience of trauma, poverty, unemployment, substance use, and poor mental health are key factors that can increase the risk of experiencing violence (Capaldi et al. 2012; Decker et al. 2018; Sumner et al. 2015).

Table 6.1 Risk and protective factors for experiencing violence

Level	Risk factors	Protective factors
Individual	**Victimization:** Trauma Poverty Unemployment Substance use Poor mental health Difficult temperament **Perpetration:** Unemployment Conduct disorder or antisocial personality disorders (ASPD) History of violence Young age Depression Substance use High anger and hostility Witnessing or experiencing IPV as a child Unplanned pregnancy Negative affectivity Emotional dysregulation Low cognitive problem-solving/ cognitive inflexibility	**Perpetration and victimization** Problem-solving ability Cognitive flexibility Flexible temperament Emotional regulation Prosocial behaviors and emotional competence High self-efficacy Positive affectivity
Interpersonal	**Victimization:** Relationships marked by high conflict and tension Perceived isolation and loneliness Financial stress **Perpetration:** Criminal behavior, association with violent or aggressive peers Substance use and mental illness in the home Intergenerational violence transmission through witnessing or experiencing violence Adversity as a child Having parents with less than a high school education	**Both perpetration and victimization** Positive peers Social connectedness with positive nurturing adults Positive marriages Social support
Community	Schools with poor safety cohesion and efficacy High drug and gun trafficking Chronic poverty High alcohol availability Low social cohesion High male incarceration rates	**Both perpetration and victimization** Access to healthy schools Neighborhood cohesion Access to a range of comprehensive and coordinated community resources and services

Based on CDC (2019)

Risk factors identified by the Centers for Disease Control and Prevention (CDC) for violence perpetration include low income and unemployment, conduct disorder or antisocial personality disorders (ASPD), history of violence, young age, depression, substance use, high anger and hostility, witnessing or experiencing IPV as a child, and unplanned pregnancy (CDC 2019; Yakubovich et al. 2018). At the interpersonal level, the most common risk factors for interpersonal violence include relationships marked by high conflict and tension, perceived isolation and loneliness, financial stress, criminal behavior, association with violent or aggressive peers, substance use and mental illness in the home, intergenerational violence transmission through witnessing or experiencing violence and adversity as a child, and having parents with less than a high school education (CDC 2019; Decker et al. 2018; Capaldi et al. 2012; Sumner et al. 2015; Yakubovich et al. 2018). At the community level, risk factors for violence include schools with poor safety, cohesion, and efficacy; high drug and gun trafficking in communities; chronic poverty; high alcohol availability; low social cohesion; and high male incarceration rates (CDC 2019; Capaldi et al. 2012; Decker et al. 2018; Sumner et al. 2015; Yakubovich et al. 2018). Racist social policies play a large role in the development of these risk factors. Policies that result in housing discrimination, lack of universal health care, lack of political power due to voter suppression and discrimination, over-incarceration, racial profiling, and police violence can lead to racial inequities, concentrated economic disadvantages, segregation, and ultimately higher rates of community violence (Sumner et al. 2015).

Effectively addressing community violence is not a mystery. We know what works. While chronic toxic stress and concentrated economic disadvantage are some of the most pronounced risk factors for violence, protective factors include social connectedness with positive, nurturing adults; positive marriages; older age; social support; access to healthy schools and positive peers; neighborhood cohesion and efficacy; and access to a range of comprehensive and coordinated community resources and services. Given these protective factors, community violence can be effectively reduced or eliminated through the development of policies that reduce economic inequality through increased access to employment, good schools, affordable and safe housing, and health care (CDC 2016, 2019; Niolon et al. 2017).

6.2.2   Impact of Violence on Health

Exposure to violence can lead to a range of negative health and mental health outcomes. For instance, exposure to violence in childhood can lead to higher rates of psychopathology such as depression, post-traumatic stress disorder (PTSD), personality disorders such as antisocial and borderline personality disorder, conduct disorders, anxiety disorders, substance use disorders, and suicide (Sumner et al. 2015). Violence exposure can lead to higher rates of risk behaviors such as high-risk sexual behaviors leading to sexually transmitted infections (STIs) and sedentary lifestyle leading to obesity (Sumner et al. 2015). Violence exposure can also lead to later problems with employment, income, housing, and family relationships, and is also associated with various diseases that include cancer, cardiovascular and cerebrovascular disease, and diabetes (Norman et al. 2012; Hillis et al. 2004; García-Moreno and Riecher-Rössler 2013; Felitti et al. 1998). To summarize, violence exposure is one of the most important risk factors for a range of physical health, mental health, and social outcomes, making routine screening and intervention for violence a necessary part of health and behavioral health professional practice.

6.3 Integrated Behavioral Health Practices to Address Violence

Given the multidimensional impact violence has on health and well-being, a variety of approaches to preventing and treating the impact of violence at the individual, family, community, and societal level are needed.

6.3.1 Universal Prevention Programs

Universal prevention programs that can reduce the risk of IPV include bystander-training programs in schools and universities designed to help bystanders spot and interrupt the perpetration of violence. These programs reduce violence and violence acceptance (Coker et al. 2016, 2019). In addition, providing rape awareness and resistance training in schools can help reduce the risk of IPV and sexual violence (Senn et al. 2015). For prevention of community violence, school climates that hold students to high expectations and provide safe and healthy environments for students to learn are crucial (Niolon et al. 2017). Universal prevention approaches in elementary schools that promote safety and community, such as the "Good Behavior Game," a classroom management strategy that teaches and reinforces emotional competence, problem-solving skills, and prosocial behaviors, can reduce aggressive behaviors (Petras et al. 2008).

6.3.2 Trauma-Informed Care Approaches

Trauma-informed approaches provide comprehensive, responsive care to persons who have experienced violence and trauma while increasing safety and access to resources. These approaches can reduce re-traumatization in health settings and re-victimization (SAMHSA 2014; Sumner et al. 2015). Screening, brief interventions, and treatment referrals in healthcare settings have shown good outcomes in reducing violence, and identifying and responding to IPV and child abuse and neglect in clients (Dubowitz et al. 2009, 2011; Feder et al. 2011; Sumner et al. 2015; Nelson et al. 2012; Strong et al. 2016). Trauma-focused cognitive behavioral therapy (CBT) approaches to reduce the symptoms of PTSD and depression can reduce the risk for future IPV victimization (Iverson et al. 2011). For instance, school-based approaches that use CBT and somatic approaches to help children and adolescents exposed to violence develop coping skills have been shown to be effective in reducing depression and PTSD symptoms in school children (Stein et al. 2003; Mancini 2020). CBT can also help people learn effective anger management, communication, and problem-solving skills to reduce violence perpetration and re-victimization (Lipsey et al. 2007). Family-focused interventions most effective in reducing the impact of violence include child and family counseling, multi-systemic therapy, parenting education, training, and home visitation programs. Parent training and home visitation programs have been shown to be particularly effective in reducing violence in the home (Bilukha et al. 2005; Kaminski et al. 2008, pp. 62, 63).

6.3.3   Hospital-Based Violence Intervention Programs (HVIP)

Hospital-based violence intervention programs (discussed in more detail later) provide free, longitudinal access to advocacy, case management, and counseling to survivors of community and intimate partner violence. These programs can reduce re-injury rates and are cost effective (Cooper et al. 2006). Collaborative care approaches that offer stepped care including motivational approaches, CBT, medications, and case management targeting depression, PTSD, substance use, and violence risk behavior in injured adolescents presenting to the ER showed significant positive outcomes (Zatzick et al. 2014).

Multi-tiered approaches that provide universal trauma-informed care, screening, and brief motivational interventions and longer-term, targeted case management and wraparound services that help people access resources, skills, and safe environments are important ways that hospitals and medical settings can interrupt the cycle of violence (Health Research and Educational Trust 2015). Developing collaborations with legal and justice advocacy organizations, behavioral health providers, and community-based agencies that serve survivors of violence are important ways that primary care settings can ensure that clients experiencing violence gain access to advocacy and legal services (restraining orders, protective orders), safe housing, food, medical care, and child care (Sumner et al. 2015).

6.3.4   Law Enforcement Strategies

At the community level, enactment of laws that restrict firearm possession and purchase for persons with restraining orders, mental health issues, and perpetrators of domestic violence and enactment of safe storage laws and programs can save lives and lead to reductions in violence, homicide, and suicide. Reducing the availability of alcohol in communities and universities can also reduce violence perpetration (Decker et al. 2018). Policing strategies that reduce drug and gun trafficking in communities such as *In the Crossfire*, and programs such as *Cure Violence*, that use trained community members who have experienced violence to interrupt violent altercations and retribution before violence can spread can be very effective in reducing community violence and homicides (Webster et al. 2013; Henry et al. 2014; Butts et al. 2015; Koper and Mayo-Wilson 2006; Delgado et al. 2017).

6.4 Assessment and Interventions for Intimate Partner Violence

6.4.1 Overview of Intimate Partner Violence

Intimate partner violence (IPV) occurs when a relationship partner engages in a pattern of behavior with the intention to establish and maintain power and control over another person. The behaviors used to maintain power and control include physical violence such as hitting, pushing, strangling, biting or inflicting injury through the use of a weapon. IPV also includes sexual violence including rape and sexual assault. IPV also include a range of controlling behaviors and tactics. Persons who engage in IPV also rely on a combination of intimidation and threats of violence to the partner or other family members including children, stalking, using mental health biases (i.e., "no one will believe you because you're crazy"), emotional abuse (i.e., put downs, contempt), social isolation (i.e., restricting or monitoring access to friends and family), jealousy, and restricting access to resources such as social status, money, important documents, and other resources as a means to control another person (CDC 2018; Decker et al. 2018; Black et al. 2011). For persons in the immigrant and refugee community, including victims of human trafficking, tactics can include using language privilege or restricting the learning of the dominate language in a community, threatening immigration status or deportation, or preventing access to important documents such as passports, birth certificates, IDs, licenses, or green cards.

6.4.1.1 Epidemiology of Intimate Partner Violence

One in four women will experience and report being impacted by intimate partner violence (IPV) in their lifetime and one in five will experience rape (Smith et al. 2018; Black et al. 2011). Nearly 45% of all women and one in five men will report lifetime sexual victimization other than rape. Over half of all reported rapes are by an intimate partner (Black et al. 2011; Smith et al. 2018). Nearly 1 in 10 women in the United States have been raped by an intimate partner and almost a quarter have experienced physical assault by an intimate partner (Black et al. 2011). One in seven men report experiencing physical violence by an intimate partner, one in seventy-one men report being raped, and one in nineteen men report being stalked in their lifetime (Black et al. 2011). Black, Indigenous, and Persons of Color (BIPOC) experience IPV at higher rates than persons who identify as white (Breiding et al. 2014).

Approximately one in five black and non-Hispanic white women, one in seven Latinx women, and one quarter of women who identify as American Indian or Alaskan Native will experience rape in their lifetime (Black et al. 2011). IPV is also very prevalent in the LGBTQ+ communities. Approximately 60% of bisexual women and 37% of bisexual men reported lifetime experience of sexual assault, physical violence, and stalking (Walters et al. 2013). Lesbian women (44%) and gay men (26%) reported high lifetime prevalence rates for sexual assault, physical violence, and stalking (Walters et al. 2013). Rates of IPV for persons who identify as transgender are higher than in persons who identify as cisgender (Langenderfer-Magruder et al. 2016). Over half of transgender persons report experiencing IPV in their lifetime (James et al. 2016). The lifetime prevalence of physical and sexual violence for transgender persons is 35% and 47%, respectively (Landers and Gilsanz 2009; James et al. 2016).

For adolescents, approximately 12% of women and 4.5% of men reported sexual coercion, while 25% of adolescents reported emotional abuse by their partner (CDC 2012). Nearly 80% female survivors of rape experienced their first rape before age 25 and approximately 42% experienced their first rape before the age of 18.

6.4.1.2   The Impact of Intimate Partner Violence on Health and Well-Being

Assessing for IPV in healthcare settings is important because experiencing IPV places a person at a significant risk for a multitude of health problems. Injuries from assaults include bruises, broken bones, knife and gunshot wounds, burns, lacerations, and spinal cord injuries. Physical violence also results in traumatic brain injury (TBI) in over 70% of women experiencing IPV (Arias and Corso 2005; Chrisler and Ferguson 2006). More than two-thirds of persons experiencing IPV experienced strangulation at least once. Of that number, the average number of times they report strangulation is over five. Death from a strangulation incident can occur days afterward due to delayed swelling of breathing pathways injured during the event (Barker et al. 2019; Chrisler and Ferguson 2006; Coker et al. 2002; Messing et al. 2018).

Persons experiencing IPV are also at risk for a range of other serious health problems due to experiencing chronic stress. These can include chronic disease conditions such as high blood pressure, heart disease, asthma, irritable bowel syndrome, migraine headaches, joint conditions, and chronic pain (Black 2011; Coker et al. 2002). The stress of IPV can also place a person at risk for several behavioral health conditions such as suicidality, unipolar and post-partum depression, antisocial behavior, anxiety, substance use (including opioid abuse), full and partial post-traumatic stress disorder (PTSD), and smoking (Ackard and Neumark-Sztainer

2002; Beydoun et al. 2012; Coker et al. 2002; Ludermir et al. 2010; Kim-Godwin et al. 2009). Experiencing IPV also has implications for maternal and sexual health. Mothers experiencing IPV have higher rates of both miscarriages and unwanted pregnancies. They are also more likely to give birth prematurely and have low-birth-weight babies due to stress and engaging in maladaptive coping behaviors such as smoking, drinking, and drug use. Women are also more likely to have sexually transmitted infections (STIs) and urinary tract infections (UTIs) because their partners may refuse to wear protection or it is unsafe to insist on protection (Miller et al. 2010; Sarkar 2008). Over half (55%) of women with HIV have experienced IPV in their lifetimes compared to 36% of non-HIV infected women (Machtinger et al. 2012; Black 2011).

6.4.2 Implementing Approaches to Address IPV in Integrated Behavioral Healthcare Settings

IPV has a broad impact on health and well-being indicating the need for clear policies and procedures to address IPV that are trauma-informed, safe, and effective. The US Department of Health and Human Services has identified routine and universal screening and intervention as a covered preventative service. This policy was based on the 2011 recommendation by the Institute of Medicine's Consensus report on Clinical Preventative Services for Women that universal IPV screening and counseling be provided in healthcare settings. A systematic review found screening and brief interventions at primary care sites that involved empathic listening, support, education, and referral to IPV services can lead to reduced violence, improved safety behaviors, and greater utilization of IPV resources in the community (Bair-Merritt et al. 2014). IPV interventions can also reduce risks for reproductive coercion in family planning and reproductive health sites. IPV interventions at family planning sites to address reproductive coercion that involve screening, education, empathic listening, and providing access to birth control, emergency contraception, and referrals to IPV services led to lower rates of pregnancy coercion and higher rates of patients ending abusive relationships (Miller et al. 2010, 2011).

Despite their effectiveness, implementation of universal screening and brief interventions in routine healthcare settings have proven to be a challenge (Decker et al. 2012). Effective translation requires creating a clinical environment that is supportive of addressing IPV such as: (1) having leadership and champions promoting the importance of IPV services across the organization; (2) having information pamphlets and posters in the waiting room about the effect of IPV on health and information on IPV services in the community; (3) the presence of clinical and non-clinical staff that are trained in trauma-informed practices; (4) providing routine screening procedures for IPV and brief interventions for IPV that involve universal education on healthy relationships; and (5) information/access to victim advocacy and service organizations either on-site or through warm referrals (Decker et al. 2012; IOM 2011a, b; McCaw 2011; Miller et al. 2015b).

It should be noted that the goal is not for clients and patients to disclose IPV or to leave the relationship, both of which can jeopardize the safety of the patient. Persons experiencing IPV face an increased risk of being killed when in the process of leaving a relationship (Bachman and Salzman 2000). Responding to IPV from a trauma-informed perspective means moving from disclosure and detection as the main goal, to initiating a conversation about violence that ensures patient safety and confidentiality, while also providing education, service access, and support (Miller et al. 2015a).

The common barriers to effectively initiating a conversation about IPV include low provider comfort and skill levels with discussing IPV, not having enough time or privacy in the clinical encounter to discuss IPV, and providers not knowing what to do if there is a positive disclosure due to lack of effective response procedures or IPV services available either on-site or through referral, and lack of follow-up care and monitoring. Simply screening for IPV without providing effective service provision or linkage for survivors provides little benefit and may even be harmful (Klevens et al. 2012; Wathen and MacMillan 2012). When providers have clear guidelines and skills on how to effectively respond to IPV disclosures and serve persons who screen positive for IPV, they are more comfortable with discussing IPV and more effective in their clinical encounters (McCaw et al. 2001).

Addressing these issues involves several important initiatives. First, it is important to deploy ongoing staff training on how to embed IPV screening, universal education, and information about available community resources into clinical encounters. This also includes providing safety cards to all clients in order to engage them in a conversation about universal education. Providers need to be made aware of and understand that the goal of IPV conversations is not to get clients to disclose, but to provide information and education regardless of disclosure. Training should also include opportunities for providers to discuss their concerns and experiences and give providers opportunities to practice through scripts and role-plays.

Second, it is vital to have in place a trauma-informed and integrated system of care that is responsive to health and safety of persons experiencing IPV and has clear, concrete policies regarding the provision of services to patients who disclose IPV. Provider discomfort with IPV screening and education often stems from not having clear response guidelines for when a client discloses IPV. Confusion around mandatory reporting requirements, lack of awareness of community resources, and a lack of system integration and partnership with IPV organizations, complicate this matter. The best way to ensure that providers are effective and comfortable is to have clear guidelines on what to do when someone identifies as an IPV survivor. Provision of integrated, on-site services is the best way for clients to gain access to services (Decker et al. 2012).

If services cannot be co-located on site, then warm referrals defined by clear protocols and guidelines to community IPV service organizations that provide legal advocacy and services, child care, safe housing/shelter, and food access are best. A warm referral process means having in place bi-directional partnerships with community-based IPV service organizations that include billing and referral procedures through an official Memorandum of Understanding (MOU) with outside IPV organizations that guide the referral process. During training, it is best for health and behavioral health providers to meet and have contact with IPV providers in the community in order to establish rapport and facilitate referral processes. Ongoing cross-training between health care and IPV partners can strengthen the relationships between these service entities, increase integration of services, and reduce fragmentation. Strong community partnerships need to be established and maintained to ensure adequate referral to services. These protocols should be tested before screening commences. This ensures an active referral process or "warm hand-off" that goes beyond just giving clients a business card and phone number. Organizations, such as Futures without Violence.org and IPVHealth.org, have evidence-based training toolkits, webinars, and resources addressing the intersection of health and violence in healthcare settings, including multilingual safety cards for multiple communities and settings (Miller et al. 2015a; Decker et al. 2012).

Third, it is vital for settings to have champions for IPV screening and intervention throughout the organization and that IPV services are integrated throughout all organizational processes, policies, and procedures. This includes having visible posters, brochures, and information about IPV in waiting rooms and restrooms. Prompts for IPV screening and brief interventions should be integrated in electronic management systems that can prompt and guide providers through the screening process. IPV procedures should also be integrated into clinical checklists, progress notes, and medical records forms and databases. Follow-up and tracking of client outcomes is important to ensure they received appropriate services and are being adequately served. IPV-related clinical goals and objectives should be integrated into all strategic planning, policy manuals, hiring guidelines, trainings, and continuous quality improvement processes (Decker et al. 2012).

6.4.2.1   Mandated Reporting of IPV

Mandatory reporting laws require certain persons and professionals (e.g., healthcare workers, social workers, counselors, teachers) to report to state or federal authorities suspected or actual abuse of vulnerable persons (Jordan and Pritchard 2018). These laws vary by state, but reportable offenses typically involve: (1) victims of violence that involve a weapon (e.g., firearm injuries); (2) child abuse, neglect, or trafficking; (3) adult/elder abuse, neglect, or trafficking; and (4) domestic violence or sexual assault (Jordan and Pritchard 2018). While reporting laws vary, most states compel social workers, nurses, physicians, and other healthcare professionals to report offenses to state authorities (e.g., law enforcement, child or adult protective services) despite the wishes of the survivor (Durborow et al. 2013). Mandatory reporting laws for domestic violence can have significant negative consequences for victims of IPV (Lippy et al. 2020).

Many states also designate workers in domestic violence shelters as mandated reporters, which can lead to negative psychological consequences to IPV survivors parenting in these shelters (Fauci and Goodman 2020). Persons experiencing IPV may experience mandatory reporting laws if they disclose their experiences to a healthcare worker directly, if they experience an IPV-related injury from a weapon, or they may be reported if they have children in the home exposed to domestic violence, which is often seen as a form of child harm. In 18 states, anyone over the age of 18 is mandated to report IPV, which may also include members of the survivor's social network. Mandated reporting laws, as they pertain to IPV, have been found to have several negative consequences including lack of disclosure to medical care providers and delay of medical care for fear that a report will be filed resulting in law enforcement and social service involvement, court exposure, arrest, and removal of children from the home (Durborow et al. 2013; Jordan and Pritchard 2018; Lippy et al. 2020). BIPOC mothers who experience IPV are particularly at risk as they have been found to be more likely have their cases referred to child protective services compared to white mothers who are more likely to be referred to shelters or behavioral health services (Dosanjh et al. 2008). Lippy et al. (2020) found that fear of being reported can prevent IPV survivors from seeking support from formal and informal networks. They also found that transgender and gender nonconforming (TGNC) survivors were reluctant to disclose IPV because they were afraid law enforcement would arrest them noting the long history of police misconduct and brutality toward the TGNC population (Lippy et al. 2020); Stotzer 2014). Women were more likely to be concerned about losing their children and immigrant survivors were often concerned about being deported (Lippy et al. 2020). The experiences of persons who have been reported indicated that the experience made their situation worse due to involvement in the criminal justice and child welfare systems and subsequent loss of stability in the domains of housing, finances, and family. The experience of persons of color differed from white women. The abusers of women of color who were reported were less likely to be arrested than those who abused white women. BIPOC mothers were also more likely to lose their children after being reported (Lippy et al. 2020).

For persons experiencing IPV, help-seeking is important and potentially life-saving. Unfortunately, evidence is emerging that suggests that the presence of mandatory reporting laws contribute to inequitable access to health care and services. Informing clients in advance that their abuse could be reported may lessen the likelihood that women will disclose abuse to healthcare providers (Jordan and Pritchard 2018). Further, mandated reporters often only need reasonable suspicion that violence has occurred in order to report an offense. A compendium is available through the Futures without Violence website that identifies mandated reporting laws for each state and the US Territory (Lizdas et al. 2019).

6.4.3   Common Screening and Assessment Practice for Intimate Partner Violence

Two factors have led to a rise in routine screening for IPV in primary care settings: (1) the decision by the Department of Health and Human Service to make IPV screening a covered preventative service; and (2) Affordable Care Act's mandated prohibition of the discriminatory practice by insurance companies of making the experience of IPV a pre-existing condition (Decker et al. 2012; IOM 2011a, b;

Lippy et al. 2020; Lizdas et al. 2019). While screening for violence should be a universal and routine part of care, screening is not enough. It is equally important to provide both universal education to clients about IPV and health, and easy access to needed services for persons who need them.

Screening for IPV should always be done in a private setting and when the client and provider are alone. The CDC has a list of effective and easy-to-administer scales for IPV (Basile et al. 2007). A brief IPV screening instrument that has been used in a variety of settings and can be deployed as a written form or as part of a clinical interview, is the Extended Hurt, Insult, Threaten, Scream screening tool (E-HITS) (Iverson et al. 2015). This tool is an extension of the well-known Hurt, Insult, Threaten, Scream (HITS) tool for IPV (Rabin et al. 2009; Shakil et al. 2014; Sherin et al. 1998). The E-HITS tool is a five-item scale that asks clients over the last 12 months how often their partner has: (1) physically *H*urt you; (2) *I*nsulted or talked down to you; (3) *T*hreatened you with harm; (4) *S*creamed or cursed at you; or (5) forced you to have *Sexual* activities. The scale anchors and scores are: never = 1, rarely = 2, sometimes = 3, fairly often = 4, and frequently = 5. Scores range from 5 to 25. A score of 7 or more indicates a positive screen for IPV.

Another common tool is the Partner Violence Screen (PVS) (Feldhaus et al. 1997). The PVS is a three-item "Yes" and "No" screen that asks clients: (1) Have you ever been hit, kicked, punched, or otherwise hurt by someone within the past year (if so, by whom?); (2) Do you feel safe in your current relationship?; and (3) Is there a partner from a previous relationship who is making you feel unsafe now? Any "yes" answer and recognition that the violence is from a current or past partner is a positive screen for IPV. It is also important and useful to ask clients if they have ever experienced reproductive coercion. This is particularly important in settings that provide reproductive health services.

6.4.4   Brief Interventions for IPV in Integrated Behavioral Health Settings

Providers should routinely engage in brief interventions for IPV after screening regardless of whether or not a person discloses IPV. Brief interventions usually involve providing universal education about IPV and its connection with health in a supportive and conversational manner. This often includes handing out brochures and safety cards. Practitioners also provide access to IPV services to clients either on-site or through warm referrals with trusted IPV providers in the community. Two overlapping models for brief IPV intervention will be discussed next: The CUES Approach and the Systems Approach to IPV intervention. Futures without Violence is a nonprofit organization that has promoted the CUES approach to screening and brief intervention for intimate partner violence (See: Futures without Violence.org). The CUES approach to IPV intervention has three facets: (1) Discussing **C**onfidentiality; (2) Providing **U**niversal Education and **E**mpowerment; and (3) **S**upporting Clients through a warm referral (Miller and Anderson 2018; Miller et al. 2011, 2015a, b, 2017). Table 6.2 outlines each of the components of the CUES

Table 6.2 CUES approach to addressing intimate partner violence in health settings

Domain	Definition	Script
Confidentiality	Make patients aware of the limits of confidentiality (e.g., mandatory reporting laws) when discussing violence as early in the clinical encounter as possible through direct conversations, signage, and intake forms Use sensitive and caring language that recognizes the difficulty in talking about IPV, and detail situations that would require them to report violence to law enforcement To ensure client safety and privacy, providers should never ask about IPV or human trafficking with other people in the room If a language interpreter is used, it should be a professional that is affiliated with the setting, and not a family member or friend **Do not:** Signal that IPV-related screening questions are perfunctory and not important Violating confidentiality rules by asking about IPV with family or partners present	"Before we begin, I need to inform you that this is a safe place and that what you tell me is confidential. That means I will not share what you tell me with anyone outside of this room except if you tell me [include any limits on disclosure relevant to your state or jurisdiction]" "In my experience, clients (or patients) are sometimes going through things that may have a negative impact on their health and safety, but that they are not comfortable telling me because they are afraid for their safety or the safety of someone they love. No matter what you decide to tell me, the information and resources I share with you today can be used by you or someone else important to you"

(continued)

Domain	Definition	Script
Universal education and empowerment	Provide universal education about healthy and unhealthy relationships and how relationships can impact health *Disclosure is not the goal.* The goal is initiating conversations about healthy and unhealthy relationships and educating the client about the impacts of unhealthy relationships *Normalize the conversation.* Sit facing your client and start the conversation by letting the client know that you are interested in making sure that all of your clients are healthy and part of that is by educating clients about healthy and unhealthy relationships *Educate* clients by introducing safety cards focused on characteristics of healthy and unhealthy relationships Give your client a tour of the safety card by reviewing the signs of healthy and unhealthy relationships Highlight that unhealthy or unsafe relationships do not always include physical or sexual abuse, but can also be defined by other abusive practices such as restricting contact with others, stalking, use of put-downs, threats, controlling money and resources, or using jealously to control behavior Review safety information on the back of the card (e.g., safety plans, organizations, hotlines, text-lines and other resources) Review resources provided by your agency on-site or through referral **Do not:** Jeopardize safety of the client by suggesting upon disclosure that the client should leave the relationship or call law enforcement	"I'm going to give you two of these cards—one is for you in case you ever need it because relationships are complex and can change, and the other is for someone you care about who may be in an unhealthy relationship that you want to help" "On the back of the card there is information in case you or someone you care about ever needs help. There is a safety plan as well as hotlines and text-lines that are staffed 24-hours-a-day by people that understand unhealthy or complicated relationships and are ready to help"

(continued)

Domain	Definition	Script
Supporting clients	Be ready to help. Following a disclosure, be prepared to respond to clients in an effective, safe, and compassionate way *Validate* the client by expressing: (1) you are sorry to hear this is happening; (2) it is not their fault; (3) they are not alone; and (4) what they are experiencing is unacceptable Indicate that what you are hearing makes you *concerned* for their overall safety, health, and well-being *Reduce harm* by asking the client how you can be helpful and offering help in regard to safety plans, medication adherence (i.e., for partners who control access to medications), access to birth control and other forms of pregnancy prevention such as emergency contraception, and developing plans for adequate exercise, nutrition, and sleep can be very useful to the client Provide a menu of service options either on-site or through warm referrals to outside resources designed to support survivors of IPV such as a shelter, advocacy, counseling programs, support groups, and social service agencies Offer the client the option of making the phone call in your office on your phone in situations where the client's phone is controlled by their partner Know the advocate you are calling and have a pre-arranged referral plan and organizational partnership to ensure a successful referral **Do not:** Engaging in victim blaming by asking: "Why do you stay?" "Why not just leave him?" "Think about your kids?" Re-traumatizing or triggering the client by interrogating or probing for all the sensitive details of the abuse	"I have a range of options for you to choose from that I am happy to tell you about. These include learning about some options and resources we offer here and by our partners in the community. Some clients/patients find talking to an advocate or counselor helpful. I can connect you with a colleague that I know and who has helped many of our clients. She has lots of information about how to seek help. Would you like me to connect you to my colleague? You can call right here in the office and we can use my phone"

Based on Miller and Anderson (2018) and (Miller et al. 2011, 2015a, b, 2017) approach with helpful practice suggestions and scripts. The table also identifies practices to avoid that can be harmful to clients.

6.4.4.1 Confidentiality

Initiating conversations about violence should be a universal practice in integrated care settings. Disclosure can happen at any point in a clinical encounter. As a result, providers of the CUES approach are directed to make patients aware of the limits of confidentiality when discussing violence as early as possible. This can be communicated in signage and on intake forms. Providers should also inform clients directly about the limits of confidentiality through sensitive and caring conversations that recognize the difficulty in talking about IPV, and detail situations that would require them to report violence to law enforcement. Clients need to know the limits of confidentiality before direct or indirect questions are asked about IPV. To ensure client safety and privacy, providers should never ask about IPV or human trafficking with other people in the room. If a language interpreter is used, it should be a professional that is affiliated with the setting, and not a family member or friend.

Mandatory reporting requirements vary by state. Every state has mandatory reporting requirements for providers in the case of child or elder abuse. Several states also have reporting requirements for bodily injury due to weapons or interpersonal or self-inflicted violence. Therefore, it is imperative that providers know the limits of confidentiality and reporting requirements in their jurisdiction around disclosure of IPV and clearly describe those limits to their client before any questions are asked about IPV. A script that can be helpful includes:

> Before we begin, I need to inform you that this is a safe place and that what you tell me is confidential. That means I will not share what you tell me with anyone outside of this room except if you tell me [include any limits on disclosure relevant to your State or jurisdiction].
>
> In my experience, clients (or patients) are sometimes going through things that may have a negative impact on their health and safety, but that they are not comfortable telling me because they are afraid for their safety or the safety of someone they love. No matter what you decide to tell me, the information and resources I share with you today can be used by you or someone else important to you.

Mandatory disclosure warnings are a complex issue. Issuing these warnings can often reduce the likelihood for disclosure due to fear of the consequences of being reported. These consequences can be severe, particularly for BIPOC and TGNC persons, and include criminal justice and child protective services involvement, arrest, jeopardized safety, and loss of familial and economic well-being (Lippy et al. 2020). Further research is needed on policies and procedures that allow survivors of IPV to disclose their experiences without automatically triggering a report, since mandated reporting can result in harm due to exposure to unjust systems with histories of racism and violence toward the poor, BIPOC, and TGNC communities.

6.4.4.2   Providing Universal Education About Healthy Relationships and Empowering Clients

Providing universal education to clients about healthy and unhealthy relationships and the impact of violence on health is a form of primary prevention for violence. This approach can also be a form of secondary prevention for clients with histories of IPV who are at risk for further violence, and a form of tertiary (harm reduction) prevention for those actively in relationships marked by IPV. Providers should begin by normalizing universal education about violence and how relationships can impact health in positive and negative ways. Universal education about violence should be positioned as a way of ensuring the optimal health of clients (Miller and Anderson 2018; Miller et al. 2011, 2015a, b, 2017).

The most effective way to have these conversations is by introducing safety cards focused on characteristics of healthy and unhealthy relationships. These small, discreet cards have information about the different forms of IPV, characteristics of healthy and unhealthy relationships, the negative health effects of violence, and a list of resources for those who wish to seek help. A good practice is to give two cards to clients, so they can give the card to someone they care about who may be in an unhealthy relationship. This can empower clients to help others and may also lead them to evaluate their own relationship. An example of what to say includes:

> I'm going to give you two of these cards – one is for you in case you ever need it because relationships are complex and can change, and the other is for someone you care about who may be in an unhealthy relationship that you want to help.

Providers should ensure they use plain and simple language and use an agency-based interpreter when necessary. There are several common principles for initiating these conversations. First is that *disclosure is not the goal*. The goal is initiating conversations about healthy and unhealthy relationships and educating the client about the impacts of unhealthy relationships. The second is *normalization*. Sit facing your client and start the conversation by letting the client know that you are interested in making sure that all of your clients are healthy and part of that is by educating clients about healthy and unhealthy relationships. The third principle is *education*. Introduce the safety card by explaining that the card is designed to provide information about the characteristics of relationships that are unsafe and can lead to health problems. Continue the conversation by giving your client a tour of the safety card, reviewing the signs of healthy and unhealthy relationships. Be sure to highlight that unhealthy or unsafe relationships do not always include physical or sexual abuse, but can also be defined by other abusive practices such as restricting contact with others; stalking; use of put-downs; threats; controlling access to family, money, children, and resources; or using jealousy to control behavior. After educating clients about healthy and unhealthy relationships, professionals should review helpful safety information on the back of the card (Miller and Anderson 2018). This information includes safety plans, organizations, hotlines, text-lines, and other resources for the client. Professionals should try these lines themselves so that they can better inform clients about what they can expect when they use these resources. A common script to guide the conversation includes:

On the back of the card there is information in case you or someone you care about ever needs help. There is a safety plan as well as hotlines and text-lines that are staffed 24-hours-a-day by people that understand unhealthy or complicated relationships and are ready to help.

6.4.4.3 Supporting Clients: Be Ready to Help

Professionals should have open and honest conversations about violence one-on-one with clients. During these conversations, disclosures can happen. Providers need to be prepared to respond sensitively and effectively when they do. Clients report preferring IPV assessment practices that focus on improving health and safety and are done in a private, one-on-one manner. Clients who talk with health-care providers about IPV experiences are four times more likely to seek help and over 2.5 times more likely to leave the relationship (McCloskey et al. 2006). It should be noted that the risk of homicide increases substantially when victims are in the process of leaving a relationship, particularly when a firearm is in the home, indicating the need for a coordinated referral process that can ensure that clients receive the support, information, advocacy, and protection they need to safely leave an abusive relationship (Bachman and Salzman 2000).

Therefore, professionals need to be prepared to respond to clients in an effective, safe, and compassionate way. It is not the time to explore traumatic details of the relationship or to encourage clients to leave the relationship or call the police, as this may not be the safest option for the client at the time. Professionals should also avoid describing the relationship using alienating terms such as "violent," "rape," or "abusive," and use terms like "complicated," "unsafe," or "unhealthy." The primary responsibility of the provider in these encounters is to validate the client by showing concern, reduce harm, and provide education and resources to the client. *Validating* the experience means expressing to the client that: (1) you are sorry to hear this is happening; (2) it is not their fault; (3) they are not alone; and (4) what they are experiencing is unacceptable. Showing *concern* means expressing to the client that what you are hearing makes you concerned for their overall safety, health, and well-being. *Reducing harm* means asking the client how you can be helpful. Offering help in regard to safety plans, medication adherence (i.e., for partners who control access to medications), access to birth control and other forms of pregnancy prevention such as emergency contraception, and developing plans for adequate exercise, nutrition, and sleep can be very useful to the client. Finally, it is important for behavioral health professionals to be prepared to provide services either on-site or through referrals to outside resources designed to support survivors of IPV such as a shelter, advocacy, counseling programs, support groups, and social service agencies. Providing a warm referral to clients and a follow-up visit are the best ways to ensure that clients get the help they need and increase the likelihood of a successful referral. This will require organizational relationships and training. Warm referrals are those in which providers are able to connect the client with a professional resource they know either by phone or face-to-face. Offering the client the option of making the phone call in the provider's office on the provider's phone is important in situations where the client's phone is controlled by their partner. Knowing the advocate that the provider is calling and having a pre-arranged referral plan and organizational partnership will be essential to ensuring a successful referral (Miller and Anderson 2018; Miller et al. 2011, 2015a, b, 2017).

Offering a menu of options can be helpful in encouraging clients to choose an option that is appropriate for them. Some sample scripts to assist clients in deciding about resources include:

> I have a range of options for you to choose from that I am happy to tell you about. These include learning about some options and resources we offer here and by our partners in the community. Some clients/patients find talking to an advocate or counselor helpful? I can connect you with a colleague that I know and who has helped many of our clients. She has lots of information about how to seek help. Would you like me to connect you to my colleague? You or I can call right here in the office and we can use my phone.

If services are available on-site, providers can arrange to walk the person over to the person providing IPV services. Asking clients, "How else can I be helpful to you?", is also important to give clients an opportunity to identify ways you can help that are tailored to the specific needs of the client.

Unfortunately, providers who are untrained, unsupported, or lack comfort in IPV assessment can say and do things that are counter-productive and even dangerous. There are some practices and statements that are not helpful and can jeopardize the safety of clients. *Here are some practices to avoid:*

- Signaling that IPV-related screening questions are perfunctory and not important such as asking IPV screening questions in a rote manner with your back to the client, not asking the questions at all, or just listing them on an intake form and not following up.
- Violating confidentiality rules by asking about IPV with family or partners present.
- Jeopardizing safety of the client by suggesting upon disclosure that the client should leave the relationship or call law enforcement.
- Engaging in victim blaming by asking, "Why do you stay?" "Why not just leave him?" "Think about your kids?"
- Re-traumatizing or triggering the client by interrogating or probing for all the sensitive details of the abuse.

As reviewed above, IPV assessment that is empowering and effective requires active, empathic listening that involves adequate time, privacy, focus, eye contact, and concern. Documentation of IPV includes indicating if the person was assessed for IPV or the reason IPV screening and assessment did not occur. The client's screening and assessment responses should be recorded as well as any observed health impacts if IPV is disclosed. The provider should also thoroughly document their responses regarding the provision of education, support, resources, and referrals.

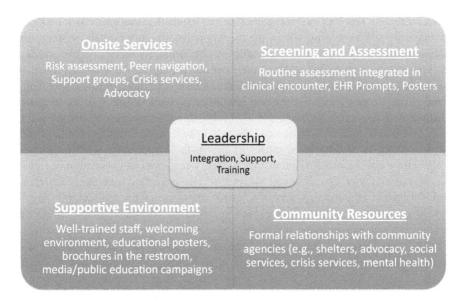

Fig. 6.1 Systems approach to IPV. (Based on Decker et al. 2012; Miller et al. 2015a)

6.4.4.4   A Systems Approach to IPV

A closely related approach to the CUES intervention is the Kaiser Permanente's Systems approach to assessing and addressing IPV in health settings (Miller et al. 2015b; Decker et al. 2012; IOM 2011a, b; McCaw 2011). This approach incorporates the practices outlined in the CUES intervention above, but also includes other factors relevant for adequate implementation of IPV assessment in healthcare settings. Figure 6.1 outlines the main components to the systems approach to IPV intervention. A key component of the systems approach is for clients to access IPV services at any point in the healthcare system including primary care and ambulatory care sites, reproductive health settings, emergency settings, and hospital-based settings. The systems approach integrates IPV universal assessment and treatment services throughout the entire healthcare environment. The approach can dramatically increase the rates of IPV treatment access (Miller et al. 2015a).

The systems approach has four inter-related components. First, leadership and support of the approach throughout the system is required. Leadership support ensures that the approach can be thoroughly implemented into all aspects of patient care and sustained in the organization. Brief, ongoing training of all staff on IPV screening, assessment, education, intervention, and referral is required to ensure adequate uptake and dissemination of the approach. Second, screening and assessment procedures are integrated and supported throughout the system. Clinicians are trained to inquire directly about IPV and know how to respond to disclosure in a trauma-informed and effective manner to ensure safety and support of the client. An important aspect of the systems approach is that IPV screening, assessment, resources, and services are integrated in the clinical encounter. This includes prompts for IPV screening within the electronic health record (EHR) system, the availability of IPV resources to the patient (e.g., community services, safety cards), and posters in exam rooms and waiting areas that prompt IPV discussion. Third, a supportive environment is established that includes trauma-informed and well-trained staff, educational posters, and brochures available in the waiting area and restrooms, and community education about IPV through newspapers, social media, radio, billboard, and online resources. Fourth, linkage to community resources and cross-training is an important aspect of the systems approach. Healthcare sites should have active, formal relationships with IPV resources in the community such as legal advocacy groups, domestic violence service providers, emergency and transitional housing, childcare services, crisis response teams, behavioral health resources, support groups, and employment programs. Formal relationships ensure warm referrals and increase the likelihood of follow-up. Further, cross-training opportunities between healthcare and community agencies increase knowledge and skill transfer within the service environment. Lastly, IPV service are provided onsite. This can include risk and safety assessments, support groups, advocacy services, peer navigators, and triage services for behavioral health. These five areas ensure that IPV services are uniformly and universally integrated within the service system landscape and increase access to health, advocacy, behavioral health, and social services for IPV survivors (Decker et al. 2012; Miller et al. 2015a).

6.5   Hospital-Based Violence Intervention Programs for Community-Based Violence

The experience of community-based violence is increasingly being recognized as a disease process requiring a set of secondary and tertiary public health interventions designed to intervene and prevent continued morbidity and early mortality. Morbidity and mortality due to firearm-related and other violent injuries are a public health epidemic in many US cities. In the United States, there are 67,000 firearm injuries and nearly 40,000 firearm deaths annually costing billions of dollars (CDC Wonder Database 2020). In 2017, almost 15,000 persons were murdered with firearms. Homicide is one of the top-five leading causes of death for persons under 45 years of age. Homicide is the third leading cause of death for people between the ages of 15 and 34. It is also the leading cause of death for Black Americans and the second leading cause of death for Latinx persons in that age range (Heron 2019). For Black children between the ages of 1 and 9, homicide was the second leading cause of death in the United States. (Heron 2019). The rise in youth who experience violence in the United States has emerged as a public health crisis requiring transdisciplinary approaches to prevention and intervention (Cunningham et al. 2009). Recent epidemiological data indicate that physical assault of children and youth are common. Over half of youth under the age of 18 report experiencing a physical assault, and nearly two-thirds of youth between the ages of 14 and 17 have experienced an assault. Approximately 10% of youth under the age of 18 report experiencing an injury from a physical assault in the last year (Finkelhor et al. 2015).

Experiencing an assault-related injury places a person at a higher risk of future re-injury. Youth who come to the ED with an assault injury are 40% more likely to experience gun violence within two years than youth who come to the ED without an assault injury. For youth with co-occurring PTSD and substance use disorders, re-injury rates were found to be substantially higher. Survivors who also have access to firearms and held positive views of retaliation were particularly at risk for re-injury and death (Carter et al. 2015; Copeland-Linder et al. 2012: Cunningham et al. 2014). Other risk factors for assault re-injury include previous fights, being injured by a weapon, and seeing someone else get shot with a firearm (Cheng et al. 2003). Experiencing a firearm-related (or other penetrating trauma) injury can increase the risk for retaliatory violence, weapon carrying, and future injuries (Kubrin and Weitzer 2003; Brooke et al. 2006; Wiebe et al. 2011). Firearm-related re-injury rates range from 25% to 44% over five years with an average of 2.6 injuries (Sims et al. 1989; McCoy et al. 2013). For a person experiencing two or more firearm-related injuries, the re-injury rate can be as high as 77%, with each subsequent injury associated with an increased risk for death (Brooke et al. 2006). Assault-injured youth who come to the emergency room are more likely to have behavioral health issues, to have experienced adverse childhood events, PTSD, and substance use (Corbin et al. 2013; Cunningham et al. 2014). Firearm-related injuries are also enormously expensive to treat. The cost for firearm-related injuries requiring admission to the ER in 2010 was estimated at more than $420,000 per patient, and the cost for patients discharged from the ER was $120,000 (Lee et al. 2014).

In addition to experiencing behavioral health conditions, other important risk factors for violence can largely be categorized as social determinants of health including socioeconomic (e.g., poverty), poor education, high unemployment, environment degradation, and low-quality housing (Dicker 2016). These rates have made reducing and preventing violence re-injury through addressing social determinants of health a priority for hospital-based violence prevention networks across the country. Retaliatory violence often occurs within six months of an ER visit (Wiebe et al. 2011). This suggests that the initial time during and after an ER visit is a critical time for intervention to prevent re-injury and possibly death through engagement in services (Cunningham et al. 2014; Carter et al. 2018; Copeland-Linder et al. 2012).

Hospital emergency departments are a common point of contact for persons who experience violent injuries and represent important sites for violence prevention and intervention. Hospital-based violence intervention programs (HVIPs) provide health, behavioral health, and social services to persons who have experienced injuries due to community violence such as penetrating injuries (e.g., firearm-related injuries, stabbings) and blunt force injuries (i.e., fists, club) from assaults. Providers from these programs provide outreach to assault-injured youth and their families. HVIP providers seek to engage patients while in the hospital and provide wraparound follow-up care after discharge. There is a growing body of evidence that shows these programs are cost-effective, improve employment and educational outcomes, and interrupt the transmission of violence by reducing re-injury rates, criminal justice involvement, and weapon carrying (Cunningham et al. 2009, 2015; Chong et al. 2015; Cooper et al. 2006; Juillard et al. 2015; Purtle et al. 2015; Smith et al. 2013; Zatzick et al. 2014).

Providers within hospital-based violence intervention programs seek to engage clients and their families in services quickly while they are in the hospital (i.e., bedside engagement). Offering services in close temporal proximity to injury can increase the likelihood survivors will engage in service because they may be more motivated and open to change. Once enrolled, service clients gain access to free, comprehensive, longitudinal, wraparound services designed to address health, behavioral health, interpersonal, and social service needs (Cheng et al. 2008a, b). For instance, many programs provide free case management services for 6 months to a year following injury. Case managers provide counseling, advocacy, mentoring, system navigation and care coordination, access to transportation and basic resources, and assistance accessing health, behavioral health, and social services in the community. Clients can also receive educational support, employment training, and job placement services (Aboutanos et al. 2011; Juillard et al. 2015, 2016; Cheng et al. 2008a, b; Lumba-Brown et al. 2017; Martin-Mollard and Becker 2009; Purtle et al. 2013; Smith et al. 2013).

Successful implementation of HVIPs may require coordination, leveraging, and integration of resources from multiple domains and levels (Bell et al. 2018; Health Research and Educational Trust 2015). Patients who experience gun and other forms of community violence are already vulnerable and face a devastating range of consequences following their injury (Juillard et al. 2016; Richardson et al. 2016). Hospital-Based Violence Intervention programs have the potential to save lives, reduce costs, and interrupt cycles of violence *and* the poverty that perpetuates it (Bell et al. 2018; Health Research and Educational Trust 2015). Effective implementation requires extensive coordination, a committed network of champions consisting of transdisciplinary professionals, and institutional partnerships with hospitals, universities, community providers, and funders (Bell et al. 2018; Health Research and Educational Trust 2015).

6.6   Summary and Conclusions

Interpersonal violence, particularly violence involving firearms, is an epidemic in the United States impacting health, home, and community. Given the prevalence of interpersonal violence in the community and its negative and generational impact on a range of health indicators, violence assessment and intervention in health and behavioral health settings must be a priority. Assessing for intimate partner violence requires health systems to create safe, welcoming spaces that promote compassionate and courageous conversations about healthy and unhealthy relationships. Survivors of IPV need to know they are in control of their story and must have easy access to effective, comprehensive, and affordable interventions to address the broad range of health impacts resulting from violence.

Community violence, especially involving firearm-related injuries in youth, must be addressed through a broad range of policy and practice interventions. Hospitals represent important settings in which to intervene to prevent re-injury and retaliation in assault-injured youth. Homicide represents the leading cause of death for Black Americans under 40. This is directly the result of decades of racist social policies designed to segregate Black and Brown communities and limit their access to wealth and health through discrimination in the domains of housing, employment, health, and education leading to unemployment, unsafe neighborhoods, under-resourced schools, and profound poverty. Policy reforms that seek to eliminate racial wealth inequality and poverty and guarantee equitable access to employment, health care, and quality education, are the only way to reduce this epidemic of violence. Further, reducing access to unsecure firearms represents an effective means to reducing gun violence across America. Currently, rise in calls for racial justice and police reform and the realities of systemic health inequities exposed by the COVID-19 pandemic provide a unique opportunity to forge new policy priorities focused on equity and justice, both of which are vital to physical and behavioral health.

Case Study 6.1: Jessica Sanders

Jessica Sanders[1] is a 31-year-old cisgendered, white woman attending her first annual physical exam at her new primary care doctor's office. Jessica notices that the office has many wall posters that bring awareness to depression, drinking, substance use, and violence prevention. She also notices brochures in the restroom that discuss healthy and unhealthy relationships, intimate partner violence, and resources for persons who are survivors of violence and human trafficking. She also noticed on the intake form questions about her depression, anxiety, stress, and drinking levels. Jessica is married and has two children. She works in the human resources department at a medium-sized financial management company. Jessica's doctor, Cynthia Johnson, walks in to the exam room. After the nurse leaves, Dr. Johnson begins her exam with a brief, private conversation with Jessica. She sits directly across from Jessica. She first informs Jessica about the limits of confidentiality.

> Dr. Johnson: I may ask you some questions about your health and mental health, including your drinking and drug use, stress levels, and your relationships. These are routine questions I ask all my patients because they are all areas that impact health. Before we begin, I need to inform you that this is a safe place and that what you tell me is confidential. That means I will not share what you tell me with anyone outside of this room except if you tell me your children are in danger of abuse or neglect. In that situation I am a mandated reporter and must report this to State authorities. Know that your safety and the safety of your children are my priority. In my experience, patients are sometimes going through things that may have a negative impact on their health and safety, but that they are not comfortable telling me because they are afraid for their safety or the safety of someone they

---

[1]All names and other identifiers of this case have been changed to protect privacy and confidentiality.

love. No matter what you decide to tell me, the information and resources I share with you today can be used by you or someone else important to you.

Dr. Johnson begins by reviewing Jessica's intake form and going over any significant information. Jessica's intake form indicates that her levels of stress and anxiety are high and her depressive scores are approaching the clinical cut off for a positive score. Jessica reports that she has never abused alcohol or substances of any kind. She reports she occasionally has a beer when out with friends and has never used illegal drugs. She has no prior history of mental health or medical problems or disorders and she has no previous suicide attempts or ideation. Dr. Johnson asks Jessica open-ended questions about her stress and anxiety levels and if there are any issues at home or at work.

> Dr. Johnson: Your stress levels seem pretty high and your depression levels are approaching significance. Stress can have a negative impact on health. Do you mind if we have talk about your stress?
> Jessica: I guess so.
> Dr. Johnson: Good. What kind of stress are you experiencing at home or at work?

Jessica discloses that has been married to Steven for 10 years. They were 'high school sweethearts'. They have two children. Jimmy who is 7 and Matthew who is 9. They live in a single-family home in a working class neighborhood about 30 minutes from Jessica's work. Steven works as a salesman for a local auto-parts retailer. He is on the road often and works long hours. Jessica often has to shoulder the load in terms of the children when Steven is on the road. Jessica used to be able to rely on her mother to watch Matthew and Jimmy and to help her with things around the house. Unfortunately, Jessica's mother has Parkinson's and suffered a recent stroke about six months ago that has exacerbated her symptoms. She is in a rehabilitation center. She will probably have to go into a nursing home after she leaves the hospital. This leaves Jessica with a tremendous burden both financially and socially. Jessica becomes tearful at this point in the interview.

> Jessica: I just feel so alone and isolated with having to care for the children and my mom. I'm losing my friends and I miss my mom. You know, she is slipping away from me. Jessica also indicates that she is becoming increasingly overwhelmed at work and caring for her family. She feels lonely and isolated.
> Dr. Johnson: I'm so sorry this is happening to you. You're not alone and there is help. I'm concerned that this is having a negative impact on your health. We have resources right here at the clinic that you may find helpful. Would you like to hear about them?

Jessica indicates that she would like to learn more and Dr. Johnson tell Jessica that she is going to refer her to the social worker who works on the team who can help her get access to some help and maybe sign her up for a caregiver support group. Dr. Johnson also makes a referral for Jessica to the clinics health and wellness program to assist Jessica in learning some relaxation skills. There is also a yoga program and meditation hours each morning. Dr. Johnson then asks Jessica to describe her relationship with Steven.

> Jessica: Steven helps around the house when he can but he is always on the road. He works long hours and tries to do what he can, but when he comes home he is exhausted. He tries, he really does, and he helps with my mom, but we just can't do it all alone.

> Dr. Johnson: Sounds like a very stressful situation. I am going to ask you some questions about your safety. Unhealthy relationships can have a negative impact on health. Have you ever been afraid of Steven or feared for your safety? Do you experience any abuse from Steven? For instance, has Steven ever hit you or physically tried to harm you in any way? Does he insult you, threaten you or scream at you? Has he ever forced you to have sex or get pregnant?
>
> Jessica (in a monotone): No. We love each other and he does the best he can. I think he wishes he could do more, but his job is very stressful.
>
> Dr. Johnson: Are there any unsecured firearms in the home?
>
> Jessica: Steve does have a pistol for protection. It is in a locked safe. I don't like having it around the house with the boys. We keep it locked up at all times.

Dr. Johnson then reviews the safety card that describes the characteristics of healthy and unhealthy relationships and their impact on health. She also reviews the information on the card about how to stay safe and the resources available in the community for persons who experience intimate partner violence. Dr. Johnson also states that there are resources at the clinic for persons experiencing IPV.

> Dr. Johnson: "We have social workers on staff that can link you with resources directly in the community. We have a relationship with several organizations in the community that can provide a safe place to live, legal advocacy and child care. We can connect people to those resources right here in the office. I know these are difficult conversations. I'm going to give you two of these cards – one is for you in case you ever need it because relationships are complex and can change, and the other is for someone you care about who may be in an unhealthy relationship that you want to help. On the back of the card there is information in case you or someone you care about ever needs help. There is a safety plan as well as hotlines and text-lines that are staffed 24-hours-a-day by people that understand unhealthy or complicated relationships and are ready to help. After the exam, lets go down and talk to Diane, our social worker, who can tell you about some of our resources that can help with taking care of your mom and to help reduce your stress. I'd like to see you in a few weeks just to check in and see how you're doing. Is that OK?

One Month Later

Jessica arrives for her appointment and Dr. Johnson reviews with Jessica what has been happening. Jessica was able to secure some additional resources for her mom with the help of the social workers. She also was able to get some respite childcare help so she could visit her mom more. She has been attending the caregiver support groups and, while skeptical at first, has really found them to be helpful.

Jessica hesitates and then states that she has been thinking a lot about the resources she was given at the last meeting regarding IPV. She has reflected a lot on her relationship with Steven and how unhealthy it has been. She thinks that a lot of her stress has to do with Steven, rather than her mom. Jessica indicates that although always jealous, Steven has become increasingly suspicious of Jessica over the last five years of their marriage. He always thinks that she is having an affair. Two years ago he made her quit her previous job and forced her to work at her current job where he had a friend in the building that could 'keep an eye' on her. Steven became concerned about what Jessica did with her co-workers at lunch and after work and so forbade her to go out and forced her to come home every night right after work. He also forbade her to leave the house without his permission while he was away saying that he had someone watching the house. Steven said that if she disobeyed him or ever did anything to betray him he would take the kids and she would never see them again. In the past year Steven has also increased his drinking to the point that it is interfering with his work. He has become increasingly erratic and Jessica fears for her safety and that of her children. Jessica states that she is not necessarily ready to leave Steven because she is afraid of what he may do, but she is willing to have a more detailed conversation about what options are available.

> Jessica: Our conversation made me realize how messed up everything is. How mean and paranoid he is. Honestly, he's never hit me or the kids, but he says terrible things to me, especially when he's drunk and his jealousy has really isolated me and made be really stressed. I really can't stand it anymore. And now his drinking? Who knows what he's capable of. I'd like to know what my options are to keep me and my kids safe.

Dr. Johnson and Jessica call in the social worker and they get to work on developing a menu of options so Jessica can choose the right one for her and her family.

Epilogue

Eventually Jessica leaves Steven and stayed for a while in a temporary shelter with her children. She also got a restraining order and gained full custody. She is now living on her own home with her children and doing well. Her mother is recuperating and making strides. Her anxiety and panic have subsided and she found a new position at another company. She recently received a promotion. Steven eventually went to treatment for alcoholism.

Questions

What elements in the above case were important in helping Jessica improve her health?

What provider and setting characteristic were helpful?

How could the above case been different if mandatory reporting laws required Dr. Johnson to report IPV?

What if Dr. Johnson never asked about IPV in the first place or provided resources – how could the outcome have been different?

What other services were important in helping Jessica get help?

References

Aboutanos, M. B., Jordan, A., Cohen, R., Foster, R. L., Goodman, K., Halfond, R. W., Poindexter, R., Charles, R., Smith, S. C., Wolfe, L. G., Hogue, B., & Ivatury, R. R. (2011). Brief violence interventions with community case management services are effective for high-risk trauma patients. *The Journal of Trauma, 71*(1), 228–237. https://doi.org/10.1097/TA.0b013e31821e0c86.

Ackard, D. M., & Neumark-Sztainer, D. (2002). Date violence and date rape among adolescents: Associations with disordered eating behaviors and psychological health. *Child Abuse & Neglect, 26*(5), 455–473. https://doi.org/10.1016/s0145-2134(02)00322-8.

Arias, I., & Corso, P. (2005). Average cost per person victimized by an intimate partner of the opposite gender: A comparison of men and women. *Violence and Victims, 20*(4), 379–391.

Bachman, R., & Salzman, L. (2000). *Violence against women: Estimates from redesigned survey.* Washington, DC: U.S. Bureau of Justice Statistics.

Bair-Merritt, M. H., Lewis-O'Connor, A., Goel, S., Amato, P., Ismailji, T., Jelley, M., Lenahan, P., & Cronholm, P. (2014). Primary care-based interventions for intimate partner violence:

A systematic review. *American Journal of Preventive Medicine, 46*(2), 188–194. https://doi.org/10.1016/j.amepre.2013.10.001.

Barker, L. C., Stewart, D. E., & Vigod, S. N. (2019). Intimate partner sexual violence: An often overlooked problem. *Journal of Women's Health, 28*(3), 363–374. https://doi.org/10.1089/jwh.2017.6811.

Basile, K. C., Hertz, M. F., & Back, S. E. (2007). *Intimate partner violence and sexual violence victimization assessment instruments for use in healthcare settings: Version 1.* Atlanta: Centers for Disease Control and Prevention, National Center for Injury Prevention and Control. https://www.cdc.gov/violenceprevention/pdf/ipv/ipvandsvscreening.pdf. Accessed 4 May 2020.

Bell, T. M., Gilyan, D., Moore, B. A., Martin, J., Ogbemudia, B., McLaughlin, B. E., Moore, R., Simons, C. J., & Zarzaur, B. L. (2018). Long-term evaluation of a hospital-based violence intervention program using a regional health information exchange. *Journal of Trauma and Acute Care Surgery, 84*(1), 175–182.

Beydoun, H. A., Beydoun, M. A., Kaufman, J. S., Lo, B., & Zonderman, A. B. (2012). Intimate partner violence against adult women and its association with major depressive disorder, depressive symptoms and postpartum depression: A systematic review and meta-analysis. *Social Science & Medicine, 75*(6), 959–975. https://doi.org/10.1016/j.socscimed.2012.04.025.

Bilukha, O., Hahn, R. A., Crosby, A., Fullilove, M. T., Liberman, A., Moscicki, E., Snyder, S., Tuma, F., Corso, P., Schofield, A., Briss, P. A., & Task Force on Community Preventive Services. (2005). The effectiveness of early childhood home visitation in preventing violence: A systematic review. *American Journal of Preventive Medicine, 28*(2 Suppl 1), 11–39. https://doi.org/10.1016/j.amepre.2004.10.004.

Black, M. C., Basile, K. C., Breiding, M. J., Smith, S. G., Walters, M. L., Merrick, M. T., Chen, J., & Stevens, M. R. (2011). *The National Intimate Partner and Sexual Violence Survey (NISVS): 2010 summary report.* Atlanta: National Center for Injury Prevention and Control, Centers for Disease Control and Prevention.

Breiding, M. J., Chen, J., & Black, M. C. (2014). *Intimate partner violence in the United States – 2010.* Atlanta: National Center for Injury Prevention and Control, Centers for Disease Control and Prevention.

Brooke, B. S., Efron, D. T., Chang, D. C., Haut, E. R., & Cornwell, E. E., 3rd. (2006). Patterns and outcomes among penetrating trauma recidivists: It only gets worse. *The Journal of Trauma, 61*(1), 16–20. https://doi.org/10.1097/01.ta.0000224143.15498.bb.

Butts, J. A., Roman, C. G., Bostwick, L., & Porter, J. R. (2015). Cure violence: A public health model to reduce gun violence. *Annual Review of Public Health, 36*, 39–53. https://doi.org/10.1146/annurev-publhealth-031914-122509.

Capaldi, D. M., Knoble, N. B., Shortt, J. W., & Kim, H. K. (2012). A systematic review of risk factors for intimate partner violence. *Partner Abuse, 3*(2), 231–280. https://doi.org/10.1891/1946-6560.3.2.231.

Carter, P. M., Dora-Laskey, A. D., Goldstick, J. E., Heinze, J. E., Walton, M. A., Zimmerman, M. A., Roche, J. S., & Cunningham, R. M. (2018). Arrests among high-risk youth following emergency department treatment for an assault injury. *American Journal of Preventative Medicine, 55*(6), 812–821.

Carter, P. M., Walton, M. A., Roehler, D. R., Goldstick, J., Zimmerman, M. A., Blow, F. C., & Cunningham, R. M. (2015). Firearm violence among high-risk emergency department youth after an assault injury. Pediatrics, 135(5), 805–815. https://doi.org/10.1542/peds.2014-3572

Centers for Disease Control and Prevention. (2016). *Preventing multiple forms of violence: A strategic vision for connecting the dots.* Atlanta: Division of Violence Prevention, National Center for Injury Prevention and Control, Centers for Disease Control and Prevention.

Centers for Disease Control and Prevention. (2018). *Intimate partner violence.* Updated June 2018. https://www.cdc.gov/violenceprevention/intimatepartnerviolence/index.html. Accessed 30 Apr 2020.

Centers for Disease Control and Prevention. (2019). National Center for Injury Prevention and Control. Intimate Partner Violence: Risk and protective factors for violence perpetration.

https://www.cdc.gov/violenceprevention/intimatepartnerviolence/riskprotectivefactors.html. Accessed 1 May 2020.

Centers for Disease Control and Prevention. (2020). National Center for Injury Prevention and Control. Web-based Injury Statistics Query and Reporting System, 2018. http://www.cdc.gov/injury/wisqars. Accessed 30 Apr 2020.

Cheng, T. L., Schwarz, D., Brenner, R. A., Wright, J. L., Fields, C. B., O'Donnell, R., Rhee, P., & Scheidt, P. C. (2003). Adolescent assault injury: Risk and protective factors and locations of contact for intervention. *Pediatrics, 112*(4), 931–938. https://doi.org/10.1542/peds.112.4.931.

Cheng, T. L., Haynie, D., Brenner, R., Wright, J. L., Chung, S. E., & Simons-Morton, B. (2008a). Effectiveness of a mentor implemented violence prevention intervention for assault-injured youths presenting to the emergency department: Results of a randomized trial. *Pediatrics, 122*, 938–946.

Cheng, T. L., Wright, J. L., Markakis, D., Copeland-Linder, N., & Menvielle, E. (2008b). Randomized trial of a case management program for assault-injured youth: Impact on service utilization and risk for re-injury. *Pediatric Emergency Care, 24*, 130–136.

Chong, V. E., Smith, R., Garcia, A., Lee, W. S., Ashley, L., Marks, A., Liu, T. H., & Victorino, G. P. (2015). Hospital-centered violence intervention programs: A cost-effectiveness analysis. *American Journal of Surgery, 209*(4), 597–603. https://doi.org/10.1016/j.amjsurg.2014.11.003.

Chrisler, J. C., & Ferguson, S. (2006). Violence against women as a public health issue. *Annals of the New York Academy of Sciences, 1087*, 235–249. https://doi.org/10.1196/annals.1385.009.

Coker, A. L., Davis, K. E., Arias, I., Desai, S., Sanderson, M., Brandt, H. M., & Smith, P. H. (2002). Physical and mental health effects of intimate partner violence for men and women. *American Journal of Preventive Medicine, 23*(4), 260–268. https://doi.org/10.1016/s0749-3797(02)00514-7.

Coker, A. L., Bush, H. M., Fisher, B. S., Swan, S. C., Williams, C. M., Clear, E. R., & DeGue, S. (2016). Multi-college bystander intervention evaluation for violence prevention. *American Journal of Preventive Medicine, 50*(3), 295–302. https://doi.org/10.1016/j.amepre.2015.08.034.

Coker, A. L., Bush, H. M., Brancato, C. J., Clear, E. R., & Recktenwald, E. A. (2019). Bystander program effectiveness to reduce violence acceptance: RCT in high schools. *Journal of Family Violence, 34*(3), 153–164. https://doi.org/10.1007/s10896-018-9961-8.

Cooper, A. D., & Smith, E. L. (2011). *Homicide trends in the United States, 1980–2008*. Washington, DC: Bureau of Justice Statistics.

Cooper, C., Eslinger, D. M., & Stolley, P. D. (2006). Hospital-based violence intervention programs work. *Journal of Trauma, 61*(3), 534–540.

Copeland-Linder, N., Johnson, S. B., Haynie, D. L., Chung, S. E., & Cheng, T. L. (2012). Retaliatory attitudes and violent behaviors among assault-injured youth. *Journal of Adolescent Health, 50*(3), 215–220. https://doi.org/10.1016/j.jadohealth.2011.04.005.

Corbin, T. J., Purtle, J., Rich, L. J., Rich, J. A., Adams, E. J., Yee, G., & Bloom, S. L. (2013). The prevalence of trauma and childhood adversity in an urban, hospital-based violence intervention program. *Journal of Health Care for the Poor and Underserved, 24*(3), 1021–1030. https://doi.org/10.1353/hpu.2013.0120.

Cunningham, R., Knox, L., Fein, J., Harrison, S., Walton, M., Dicker, R., Calhoun, D., Becker, M., & Hargarten, S. W. (2009). Before and after the trauma bay: The prevention of violent injury among youth. *Annals of Emergency Medicine, 53*(4), 490–500.

Cunningham, R. M., Ranney, M., Newton, M., Woodhull, W., Zimmerman, M., & Walton, M. A. (2014). Characteristics of youth seeking emergency care for assault injuries. *Pediatrics, 133*(1), e96–e105. https://doi.org/10.1542/peds.2013-1864.

Cunningham, R. M., Carter, P. M., Ranney, M., Zimmerman, M. A., Blow, F. C., Booth, B. M., Goldstick, J., & Walton, M. A. (2015). Violent reinjury and mortality among youth seeking emergency department care for assault-related injury. *JAMA Pediatrics, 169*(1), 63. https://doi.org/10.1001/jamapediatrics.2014.1900.

Curtin, S. C., Warner, M., & Hedegaard, H. (2016). Increase in suicide in the United States, 1999–2014. *NCHS Data Brief, 241*, 1–8.

Durborow, M. A., Lizdas, K. C., O'Flaherty, A., Marjavi, A. (2013). Compendium of state and U.S. territory statutes and policies on domestic violence and health care. San Francisco, CA: Futures Without Violence.

Decker, M. R., Frattaroli, S., McCaw, B., Coker, A. L., Miller, E., Sharps, P., Lane, W. G., Mandal, M., Hirsch, K., Strobino, D. M., Bennett, W. L., Campbell, J., & Gielen, A. (2012). Transforming the healthcare response to intimate partner violence and taking best practices to scale. *Journal of Women's Health, 21*(12), 1222–1229. https://doi.org/10.1089/jwh.2012.4058.

Decker, M. R., Wilcox, H. C., Holliday, C. N., & Webster, D. W. (2018). An integrated public health approach to interpersonal violence and suicide prevention and response. *Public Health Reports, 133*(suppl. 1), 65s–79s.

Delgado, S. A., Alsabahi, L., Wolffe, K., Alexander, N., Cobar, P., & Butts, J. A. (2017). *The effects of cure violence in the South Bronx and East New York, Brooklyn.* https://johnjayrec.nyc/2017/10/02/cvinsobronxeastny. Accessed 8 Sept 2018.

Dicker, R. A. (2016). Hospital-based violence intervention: An emerging practice based on public health principles. *Trauma Surgery & Acute Care, 1*(1), e000050. https://doi.org/10.1136/tsaco-2016-000050.

Dosanjh, S., Lewis, G., Mathews, D., & Bhandari, M. (2008). Child protection involvement and victims of intimate partner violence: Is there a bias? *Violence Against Women, 14*(7), 833–843. https://doi.org/10.1177/1077801208320247.

Dubowitz, H., Feigelman, S., Lane, W., & Kim, J. (2009). Pediatric primary care to help prevent child maltreatment: The Safe Environment for Every Kid (SEEK) Model. *Pediatrics, 123*(3), 858–864. https://doi.org/10.1542/peds.2008-1376.

Dubowitz, H., Lane, W. G., Semiatin, J. N., Magder, L. S., Venepally, M., & Jans, M. (2011). The safe environment for every kid model: Impact on pediatric primary care professionals. *Pediatrics, 127*(4), e962–e970. https://doi.org/10.1542/peds.2010-1845.

Fauci, J. E., & Goodman, L. A. (2020). "You don't need nobody else knocking you down": Survivor-mothers' experiences of surveillance in domestic violence shelters. *Journal of Family Violence, 35*, 241–254. https://doi.org/10.1007/s10896-019-00090-y.

Feder, G., Davies, R. A., Baird, K., Dunne, D., Eldridge, S., Griffiths, C., Gregory, A., Howell, A., Johnson, M., Ramsay, J., Rutterford, C., & Sharp, D. (2011). Identification and Referral to Improve Safety (IRIS) of women experiencing domestic violence with a primary care training and support programme: A cluster randomised controlled trial. *Lancet, 378*(9805), 1788–1795. https://doi.org/10.1016/S0140-6736(11)61179-3.

Felitti, V. J., Anda, R. F., Nordenberg, D., Williamson, D. F., Spitz, A. M., Edwards, V., Koss, M. P., & Marks, J. S. (1998). Relationship of childhood abuse and household dysfunction to many of the leading causes of death in adults. The Adverse Childhood Experiences (ACE) study. *American Journal of Preventive Medicine, 14*(4), 245–258. https://doi.org/10.1016/s0749-3797(98)00017-8.

Finkelhor, D., Turner, H., Hamby, S., & Ormrod, R. (2011). *Polyvictimization: children's exposure to multiple types of violence, crime and abuse.* Office of Juvenile Justice and Delinquency Prevention and Centers for Disease Control and Prevention, Juvenile Justice Bulletin, National Survey of Children's Exposure to Violence. NCJ 235504. https://www.ncjrs.gov/pdffiles1/ojjdp/235504.pdf. Accessed 1 Apr 2020.

Finkelhor, D., Turner, H. A., Shattuck, A., & Hamby, S. L. (2015). Prevalence of childhood exposure to violence, crime, and abuse: Results from the National Survey of Children's Exposure to Violence. *JAMA Pediatrics, 169*(8), 746–754. https://doi.org/10.1001/jamapediatrics.2015.0676.

Feldhaus, K. M., Koziol-McLain, J., Amsbury, H. L., Norton, I. M., Lowenstein, S. R., & Abbott, J. T. (1997). Accuracy of 3 brief screening questions for detecting partner violence in the emergency department. JAMA, 277(17), 1357–1361.

García-Moreno, C., & Riecher-Rössler, A. (2013). *Violence against women and mental health.* Basel: Karger.

Hamby, S., & Grych, J. (2013). *The web of violence: Exploring connections among different forms of interpersonal violence and abuse.* New York: Springer Briefs in Sociology.

Health Research & Educational Trust. (2015, March). *Hospital approaches to interrupt the cycle of violence*. Chicago, IL: Health Research & Educational Trust. Accessed at www.hpoe.org

Henry, D. B., Knoblauch, S., & Sigurvinsdottir, R. (2014). *The effect of intensive CeaseFire intervention on crime in four Chicago police beats: Quantitative assessment*. Chicago: University of Chicago.

Heron M. (2019). Deaths: Leading causes for 2017. National vital statistics reports: from the Centers for Disease Control and Prevention, National Center for Health Statistics, National Vital Statistics System, 68(6), 1–77. Cooper AD, Smith EL. Homicide Trends in the United States, 1980–2008. Washington, DC.

Hillis, S. D., Anda, R. F., Dube, S. R., Felitti, V. J., Marchbanks, P. A., & Marks, J. S. (2004). The association between adverse childhood experiences and adolescent pregnancy, long-term psychosocial consequences, and fetal death. *Pediatrics, 113*(2), 320–327. https://doi.org/10.1542/peds.113.2.320.

Human Rights Campaign. (2020). *Violence against the transgender and gender non-conforming community in 2020*. https://www.hrc.org/resources/violence-against-the-trans-and-gender-non-conforming-community-in-2020. Accessed 7 July 2020.

Institute of Medicine (IOM). (2011a). *Preventing violence against women and children: Workshop summary*. Washington, DC: The National Academies Press.

Institute of Medicine (IOM). (2011b). *Clinical preventive services for women: Closing the gaps*. Washington, DC: The National Academies Press.

Iverson, K. M., Gradus, J. L., Resick, P. A., Suvak, M. K., Smith, K. F., & Monson, C. M. (2011). Cognitive-behavioral therapy for PTSD and depression symptoms reduces risk for future intimate partner violence among interpersonal trauma survivors. *Journal of Consulting and Clinical Psychology, 79*(2), 193–202. https://doi.org/10.1037/a0022512.

Iverson, K. M., King, M. W., Gerber, M. R., Resick, P. A., Kimerling, R., Street, A. E., & Vogt, D. (2015). Accuracy of an intimate partner violence screening tool for female VHA patients: A replication and extension. *Journal of Traumatic Stress, 28*(1), 79–82. https://doi.org/10.1002/jts.21985.

Jordan, C. E., & Pritchard, A. J. (2018). Mandatory reporting of domestic violence: What do abuse survivors think and what variables influence those opinions? *Journal of Interpersonal Violence*, 886260518787206. Advance online publication. https://doi.org/10.1177/0886260518787206.

Juillard, C., Smith, R., Anaya, N., Garcia, A., Kahn, J. G., & Dicker, R. A. (2015). Saving lives and saving money: Hospital-based violence intervention is cost-effective. *Journal of Trauma, 78*(2), 252–258.

Juillard, C., Cooperman, L., Allen, I., Pirracchio, R., Henderson, T., Marquez, R., Orellana, J., Texada, M., & Dicker, R. A. (2016). A decade of hospital-based violence intervention: Benefits and shortcomings. *Journal of Trauma, 81*(6), 1156–1161.

James, S. E., Herman, J. L., Rankin, S., Keisling, M., Mottet, L., & Anafi, M. (2016). The Report of the 2015 U.S. Transgender Survey. Washington, DC: National Center for Transgender Equality.

Kann, L., McManus, M.S., Harris, W.A., Shanklin, S.L., Flint, K.H., Queen, B,… Ethier, K.A. (2018). Youth risk behavior surveillance – United States, 2017. Morbidity and Mortality Weekly Review (MMWR), 67(8), 1–114.

Kaminski, J. W., Valle, L. A., Filene, J. H., & Boyle, C. L. (2008). A meta-analytic review of components associated with parent training program effectiveness. *Journal of Abnormal Child Psychology, 36*(4), 567–589. https://doi.org/10.1007/s10802-007-9201-9.

Kim-Godwin, Y. S., Clements, C., McCuiston, A. M., & Fox, J. A. (2009). Dating violence among high school students in southeastern North Carolina. *The Journal of School Nursing, 25*(2), 141–151. https://doi.org/10.1177/1059840508330679.

Klevens, J., Kee, R., Trick, W., Garcia, D., Angulo, F. R., Jones, R., & Sadowski, L. S. (2012). Effect of screening for partner violence on women's quality of life: A randomized controlled trial. *JAMA, 308*(7), 681–689.

Kochanek, K. D., Murphy, S. L., Xu, J. Q., & Arias E. (2019). Deaths: Final data for 2017. *National Vital statistics reports, 68(9)*. Hyattsville, MD: National Center for Health Statistics. https://www.cdc.gov/nchs/data/nvsr/nvsr68/nvsr68_09-508.pdf?utm_source=link_newsv9&utm_campaign=item_268094&utm_medium=copy. Accessed 1 June 2020.

Koper, C. S., & Mayo-Wilson, E. (2006). Police crackdowns on illegal gun carrying: A systematic review of their impact on gun crime. *Journal of Experimental Criminology, 2*(2), 227–261.

Kubrin, C. E., & Weitzer, R. (2003). Retaliatory homicide: Concentrated disadvantage and neighborhood culture. *Social Problems, 50*, 157–180.

Landers, S., Gilsanz, P. (2009). The health of lesbian, gay, bisexual, and transgender (LGBT) persons in Massachusetts. Massachusetts Department of Public Health. Retrieved from http://www.mass.gov/eohhs/docs/dph/commissioner/lgbt-health-report.pdf

Langenderfer-Magruder, L., Whitfield, D. L., Walls, N. E., Kattari, S. K., & Ramos, D. (2016). Experiences of intimate partner violence and subsequent police reporting among LGBTQ adults in Colorado: Comparing rates of cisgender and transgender victimization. *Journal of Interpersonal Violence, 31*(5), 855–871. https://doi.org/10.1177/0886260514556767.

Lee, J., Quraishi, S. A., Bhatnagar, S., Zafonte, R. D., & Masiakos, P. T. (2014). The economic cost of firearm-related injuries in the United States from 2006 to 2010. *Surgery, 155*(5), 894–898. https://doi.org/10.1016/j.surg.2014.02.011.

Lippy, C., Jumarali, S. N., Nnawulezi, N. A., Peyton-Williams, E., & Burk, C. (2020). The impact of mandatory reporting laws on survivors of intimate partner violence: Intersectionality, help-seeking and the need for change. *Journal of Family Violence, 35*, 255–267. https://doi.org/10.1007/s10896-019-00103-w

Lipsey, M. W., Landenberger, N. A., & Wilson, S. J. (2007). Effects of cognitive-behavioral programs for criminal offenders. *Campbell Systematic Reviews.* https://doi.org/10.4073/csr.2007.6.

Lizdas, K. C., O'Flaherty, A., Durborow, N., & Marjavi, A. (2019). *Compendium of state and U.S. territory statutes and policies on domestic violence and health care* (4th ed.). Futures Without Violence. http://fvpf.convio.net/site/EcommerceDownload/Compendium%204th%20Edition%202019%20Final-1793.pdf?dnl=111966-1793-Wl1qlxwQAk8UYXM4. Accessed 4 May 2020.

Ludermir, A. B., Lewis, G., Valongueiro, S. A., de Araújo, T. V., & Araya, R. (2010). Violence against women by their intimate partner during pregnancy and postnatal depression: A prospective cohort study. *Lancet, 376*(9744), 903–910. https://doi.org/10.1016/S0140-6736(10)60887-2.

Lumba-Brown, A., Batek, M., Choi, P., Keller, M., & Kennedy, R. (2017). Mentoring pediatric victims of interpersonal violence reduces recidivism. *Journal of Interpersonal Violence,* 886260517705662. Advance online publication. https://doi.org/10.1177/0886260517705662.

Machtinger, E. L., Wilson, T. C., Haberer, J. E., & Weiss, D. S. (2012). Psychological trauma and PTSD in HIV-positive women: A meta-analysis. *AIDS and Behavior, 16*(8), 2091–2100. https://doi.org/10.1007/s10461-011-0127-4.

Mancini, M. A. (2020). A pilot study evaluating a school-based, trauma-focused intervention for immigrant and refugee youth. *Children and Adolescent Social Work Journal, 37*, 287–300. https://doi.org/10.1007/s10560-019-00641-8.

Martin-Mollard, M., & Becker, M. (2009). *Key components of hospital-based violence intervention programs.* http://nnhvip.org/wp-content/uploads/2010/09/key.pdf. Accessed 1 June 2020.

McCaw, B. (2011). Using a systems-model approach to improving IPV services in a large health care organization. In *The Institute of Medicine (IOM) preventing violence against women and children: Workshop summary* (pp. 169–184). Washington, DC: The National Academies Press.

McCaw, B., Berman, W. H., Syme, S. L., & Hunkeler, E. F. (2001). Beyond screening for domestic violence: A systems model approach in a managed care setting. *American Journal of Preventative Medicine, 21*(3), 170–176.

McCloskey, L. A., Lichter, E., Williams, C., Gerber, M., Wittenberg, E., & Ganz, M. (2006). Assessing intimate partner violence in health care settings leads to women's receipt of interventions and improved health. *Public Health Reports, 121*(4), 435–444. https://doi.org/10.1177/003335490612100412.

McCoy, A. M., Como, J. J., Greene, G., Laskey, S. L., & Claridge, J. A. (2013). A novel prospective approach to evaluate trauma recidivism: The concept of past trauma history. *The Journal of Trauma and Acute Care Surgery, 75*, 116–121.

Messing, J. T., Patch, M., Wilson, J. S., Kelen, G. D., & Campbell, J. (2018). Differentiating among attempted, completed, and multiple nonfatal strangulation in women experiencing intimate partner violence. *Women's Health Issues, 28*(1), 104–111. https://doi.org/10.1016/j.whi.2017.10.002.

Miller, E. & Anderson, J. (2018). *The "CUES" approach to Address IPV/Human Trafficking and intersections with HIV in Primary Care: what's the evidence?*. Webinar sponsored by Futures without Violence. Downloaded at: https://www.futureswithoutviolence.org/wp-content/uploads/Demo-Site-Webinar-3-Final.pdf

Miller, E., Decker, M. R., McCauley, H. L., Tancredi, D. J., Levenson, R. R., Waldman, J., Schoenwald, P., & Silverman, J. G. (2011). A family planning clinic partner violence intervention to reduce risk associated with reproductive coercion. *Contraception, 83*(3), 274–280. https://doi.org/10.1016/j.contraception.2010.07.013.

Miller, E., Goldstein, S., McCauley, H. L., Jones, K. A., Dick, R. N., Jetton, J., et al. (2015a). A school health center intervention for abusive adolescent relationships: A cluster RCT. *Pediatrics, 135*, 76–85. https://doi.org/10.1542/peds.2014-2471.

Miller, E., McCaw, B., Humphreys, B. L., & Mitchell, C. (2015b). Integrating intimate partner violence assessment and intervention into healthcare in the United States: A systems approach. *Journal of Women's Health, 24*(1), 92–99. https://doi.org/10.1089/jwh.2014.4870.

Miller, E., McCauley, H. L., Decker, M. R., Levenson, R., Zelazny, S., Jones, K. A., Anderson, H., & Silverman, J. G. (2017). Implementation of a family planning clinic-based partner violence and reproductive coercion intervention: Provider and patient perspectives. *Perspectives on Sexual and Reproductive Health, 49*(2), 85–93. https://doi.org/10.1363/psrh.12021.

Miller, E., Decker, M. R., McCauley, H. L., Tancredi, D. J., Levenson, R. R., Waldman, J., Schoenwald, P., & Silverman, J. G. (2010). Pregnancy coercion, intimate partner violence and unintended pregnancy. Contraception, 81(4), 316–322. https://doi.org/10.1016/j.contraception.2009.12.004

Morgan, R. E. & Oudekerk, B. A. (2019, September). Criminal *victimizations, 2018*. Washington, DC: Bureau of Justice Statistics, U.S. Department of Justice. https://www.bjs.gov/content/pub/pdf/cv18.pdf. Accessed 4 May 2020.

Nelşon, H. D., Bougatsos, C., & Blazina, I. (2012). Screening women for intimate partner violence: A systematic review to update the U.S. Preventive Services Task Force recommendation. *Annals of Internal Medicine, 156*(11), 796–282. https://doi.org/10.7326/0003-4819-156-11-201206050-00447.

Niolon, P. H., Kearns, M., Dills, J., Rambo, K., Irving, S., Armstead, T., & Gilbert, L. (2017). *Preventing intimate partner violence across the lifespan: A technical package of programs, policies, and practices*. Atlanta: National Center for Injury Prevention and Control, Centers for Disease Control and Prevention.

Norman, R. E., Byambaa, M., De, R., Butchart, A., Scott, J., & Vos, T. (2012). The long-term health consequences of child physical abuse, emotional abuse, and neglect: A systematic review and meta-analysis. *PLoS Medicine, 9*(11), e1001349. https://doi.org/10.1371/journal.pmed.1001349.

Petras, H., Kellam, S. G., Brown, C. H., Muthén, B. O., Ialongo, N. S., & Poduska, J. M. (2008). Developmental epidemiological courses leading to antisocial personality disorder and violent and criminal behavior: Effects by young adulthood of a universal preventive intervention in first- and second-grade classrooms. *Drug and Alcohol Dependence, 95*(Suppl 1), S45–S59. https://doi.org/10.1016/j.drugalcdep.2007.10.015.

Petrosky, E., Blair, J. M., Betz, C. J., Fowler, K. A., Jack, S., & Lyons, B. H. (2017). Racial and ethnic differences in homicides of adult women and the role of intimate partner violence – United States, 2003-2014. *MMWR. Morbidity and Mortality Weekly Report, 66*(28), 741–746. https://doi.org/10.15585/mmwr.mm6628a1.

Purtle, J., Rich, L. J., Bloom, S. L., Rich, J. A., & Corbin, T. J. (2015). Cost-benefit analysis simulation of a hospital-based violence intervention program. American journal of preventive medicine, 48(2), 162–169. https://doi.org/10.1016/j.amepre.2014.08.030

Purtle, J., Dicker, R., Cooper, C., Corbin, T., Greene, M. B., Marks, A., Creaser, D., Topp, D., & Moreland, D. (2013). Hospital-based violence intervention programs save lives and money. *Journal of Trauma, 75*(2), 331–333.

Rabin, R. F., Jennings, J. M., Campbell, J. C., & Bair-Merritt, M. H. (2009). Intimate partner violence screening tools: A systematic review. *American Journal of Preventive Medicine, 36*(5), 439–445.e4. https://doi.org/10.1016/j.amepre.2009.01.024.

Richardson, J. B., St. Vil, C., Sharpe, T., Wagner, M., & Cooper, C. (2016). Risk factors for recurrent violent injury among black men. *Journal of Surgical Research, 204*, 261–266.

Sarkar, N. N. (2008). The impact of intimate partner violence on women's reproductive health and pregnancy outcome. *Journal of Obstetrics and Gynaecology, 28*(3), 266–271. https://doi.org/10.1080/01443610802042415.

Senn, C. Y., Eliasziw, M., Barata, P. C., Thurston, W. E., Newby-Clark, I. R., Radtke, H. L., & Hobden, K. L. (2015). Efficacy of a sexual assault resistance program for university women. *The New England Journal of Medicine, 372*(24), 2326–2335. https://doi.org/10.1056/NEJMsa1411131.

Shakil, A., Bardwell, J., Sherin, K., Sinacore, J. M., Zitter, R., & Kindratt, T. B. (2014). Development of verbal HITS for intimate partner violence screening in family medicine. *Family Medicine, 46*(3), 180–185.

Sherin, K. M., Sinacore, J. M., Li, X. Q., Zitter, R. E., & Shakil, A. (1998). HITS: A short domestic violence screening tool for use in a family practice setting. *Family Medicine, 30*(7), 508–512.

Sims, D. W., Bivins, B. A., Obeid, F. N., Horst, H. M., Sorensen, V. J., & Fath, J. J. (1989). Urban trauma: A chronic recurrent disease. *The Journal of Trauma, 29*, 940–947.

Smith, R., Dobbins, S., Evans, A., Balhotra, K., & Dicker, R. A. (2013). Hospital-based violence intervention: Risk reduction resources that are essential for success. *The Journal of Trauma and Acute Care Surgery, 74*, 976–982.

Smith, S. G., Zhang, X., Basile, K. C., Merrick, M. T., Wang, J., Kresnow, M., & Chen, J. (2018). *The National Intimate Partner and Sexual Violence Survey (NISVS): 2015 data brief – Updated release.* Atlanta: National Center for Injury Prevention and Control, Centers for Disease Control and Prevention.

Stein, B. D., Jaycox, L. H., Kataoka, S. H., Wong, M., Tu, W., Elliott, M. N., & Fink, A. (2003). A mental health intervention for schoolchildren exposed to violence: A randomized controlled trial. *JAMA, 290*(5), 603–611. https://doi.org/10.1001/jama.290.5.603.

Stöckl, H., Devries, K., Rotstein, A., Abrahams, N., Campbell, J., Watts, C., & Moreno, C. G. (2013). The global prevalence of intimate partner homicide: A systematic review. *Lancet, 382*(9895), 859–865. https://doi.org/10.1016/S0140-6736(13)61030-2.

Stotzer, R. L. (2014). Law enforcement and criminal justice personnel interactions with transgender people in the United States: A literature review. *Aggression and Violence Behavior, 19*(3), 263–277. https://doi.org/10.1016/j.avb.2014.04.012.

Strong, B. L., Shipper, A. G., Downton, K. D., & Lane, W. G. (2016). The effects of health care-based violence intervention programs on injury recidivism and costs: A systematic review. *The Journal of Trauma and Acute Care Surgery, 81*(5), 961–970. https://doi.org/10.1097/TA.0000000000001222.

Substance Abuse and Mental Health Services Administration (SAMHSA). (2014). *Trauma-informed care in behavioral health services.* Rockville: Substance Abuse and Mental Health Services Administration.

Sumner, S. A., Mercy, J. A., Dahlberg, L. L., Hillis, S. D., Klevens, J., & Houry, D. (2015). Violence in the United States: Status, challenges, and opportunities. *JAMA, 314*(5), 478–488.

Walters, M. L., Chen, J., & Breiding, M. J. (2013). *The national intimate partner and sexual violence survey (NISVS): 2010 findings on victimization by sexual orientation.* Atlanta: National Center for Injury Prevention and Control, CDC.

Wathen, C. N., & MacMillan, H. L. (2012). Health care's response to women exposed to partner violence: Moving beyond universal screening. *JAMA, 308*(7), 712–713.

Webster, D. W., Whitehill, J. M., Vernick, J. S., & Curriero, F. C. (2013). Effects of Baltimore's Safe Streets Program on gun violence: A replication of Chicago's CeaseFire Program. *Journal of Urban Health: Bulletin of the New York Academy of Medicine, 90*(1), 27–40. https://doi.org/10.1007/s11524-012-9731-5.

Wiebe, D. J., Blackstone, M. M., Mollen, C. J., Culyba, A. J., & Fein, J. A. (2011). Self-reported violence-related outcomes for adolescents within eight weeks of emergency department treatment for assault injury. *The Journal of Adolescent Health, 49*(4), 440–442. https://doi.org/10.1016/j.jadohealth.2011.01.009.

Wilson, N., Tsao, B., Hertz, M., Davis, R., & Klevens, J. (2014). *Connecting the dots: An overview of the links among multiple forms of violence.* Oakland: National Center for Injury Prevention and Control, Centers for Disease Control and Prevention (Atlanta, GA) and Prevention Institute.

Yakubovich, A. R., Stöckl, H., Murray, J., Melendez-Torres, G. J., Steinert, J. I., Glavin, C., & Humphreys, D. K. (2018). Risk and protective factors for intimate partner violence against women: Systematic review and meta-analyses of prospective-longitudinal studies. *American Journal of Public Health, 108*(7), e1–e11. https://doi.org/10.2105/AJPH.2018.304428.

Zatzick, D., Russo, J., Lord, S. P., Varley, C., Wang, J., Jurkovich, G., et al. (2014). Collaborative care intervention targeting violence risk behaviors, substance use, and post-traumatic stress and depressive symptoms in injured adolescents: A randomize clinical trial. *JAMA Pediatrics, 168*(6), 532–539. https://doi.org/10.1001/jamapediatrics.2013.4784.

Chapter 7
Trauma-Informed Behavioral Health Practice

7.1 Chapter Overview

The last 30 years of scientific inquiry has firmly established the profound impact toxic stress and traumatic events have on the mind and body. Experiencing early adverse events, toxic stress, and/or traumatic events can alter the physiology of the body and make people more susceptible to a range of chronic diseases, depressive and anxiety disorders, addiction, violence, and suicide (Burke-Harris 2018; CDC 2020; Felitti and Anda 2010; Perry and Szalavitz 2017; Van der Kolk, 2015). The impact of the COVID-19 pandemic will resonate in health and behavioral health treatment systems for years to come by increasing the number of persons coping with trauma in the population much like the events of 9-11 and the wars in Vietnam, Afghanistan, and Iraq. COVID-19 will impact rates of trauma and toxic stress exposure in the population in a number of ways. First, lockdowns will result in an increase in the experience and intensity of intimate partner violence as families are trapped at home with abusive partners in high-stress situations with no means for escape. This will increase rates of exposure to violence, leading to higher rates of post-traumatic stress disorder (PTSD) and placing survivors at risk for health and mental health problems that may last for years. The lockdown will also lead to backlog of cases resulting in a disruption in detection and identification of IPV in the community as health and behavioral health appointments are cancelled. It will also disrupt the ability of victims to access services and resources such as shelters, health care, legal advocacy, and childcare. The increase in toxic stress exposure to children that result from these disruptions will have lifelong impacts on their health and well-being.

Second, survivors of COVID-19, particularly those in intensive care units (ICUs) and who were placed on ventilators, are already reporting an increase in PTSD and depressive symptoms. The experience of being in an ICU and on a ventilator is known to produce trauma symptoms, particularly nightmares and flashbacks. The increase in persons in ICUs and on ventilators will likely result in a corresponding increase in PTSD prevalence in the population. Likewise, PTSD seen in the health-care workforce is likely to increase. The experiences of healthcare workers and first responders experiencing the constant fear of infection due to a lack of personal protective equipment (PPE), and their exposure to vast numbers of patient deaths will increase the likelihood of PTSD and other behavioral health issues in this population. Third, family members who lost loved ones to the virus and were unable to say goodbye and process their grief may also experience increased rates of PTSD, depression, anxiety, and substance use. Last, the stress experienced by tens of millions of people, particularly in Black and Brown communities, due to the health and economic impact of this pandemic may have behavioral health implications for years to come.

These are just some of the implications of this still unfolding crisis. But the COVID-19 pandemic exists within a network of other intersecting epidemics that have roiled the United States for generations and magnify the impact of COVID-19. The epidemic of police violence perpetrated on Black Americans and the inequities in health, education, and wealth experienced by generations of Black families due to racist policies and practices are two interrelated examples. The epidemic of community violence as a result of the poverty generated by these same inequities that has resulted in generations of stressed and traumatized youth and adults is another. A fourth example is the increases in substance use and suicide, particularly by firearms, that have impacted all communities across the United States. The sheer magnitude of these challenges can be overwhelming. Indeed, the current US healthcare system is not equipped currently to deal with it effectively. Addressing trauma in the community from a behavioral health practice standpoint requires an approach to practice that is trauma-informed and universally integrated across healthcare settings. In this chapter, I will review the impact of trauma on the mind and body and how to screen, assess, and treat trauma in a way that is sensitive, compassionate, and effective.

7.1.1   Trauma-Related Definitions and Terms

7.1.1.1   Traumatic Events

An event is considered *traumatic* if it is perceived to be potentially life-threatening and overwhelms our ability to cope. The Diagnostic and Statistical Manual of Mental Disorders (DSM-5) defines trauma as "Exposure to actual or threatened death, serious injury, or sexual violence." (APA 2013; p. 271). Exposure is defined as directly experiencing trauma, witnessing trauma happening to someone else, learning that a traumatic event has happened to someone close to you (e.g., parent, child, spouse, sibling, close friend, or relative), or repeatedly experiencing extreme details or the effects of traumatic events such as seeing or collecting remains, providing first aid or medical care to persons experiencing life-threatening events, or responding to the scene of disasters, wars, violent acts, or fires (APA 2013).

Table 7.1 Traumatic events impacting behavioral health

Domains	Events
Accidents, illness, and disasters	Natural disaster (e.g., flood, hurricane, earthquake, tornado)
	Fire
	Transportation accident (e.g., car, boat)
	Other serious accident
	Exposure to environmental toxic substance
Interpersonal violence	Sexual assault
	Any unwanted/uncomfortable sexual experience
	Physical assault (e.g., being punched, slapped, kicked, threatened with a weapon)
	Captivity (e.g., being held/detained, held hostage, kidnapped)
War, community violence, poverty	Experiencing war or combat exposure (military or civilian)
	Witnessing or experiencing severe human suffering (e.g., war, famine, extreme poverty)
Death and injury	Sudden, unexpected death of someone close
	Life-threatening illness or injury
	Serious injury, harm, or death you caused to someone else
	Sudden, violent death such as suicide or homicide (witnessing or learning about it happening to someone)

Based on: Blake et al. (1995), Weathers et al. (2013a)

Table 7.1 lists examples of traumatic events that impact health within several major domains. Examples of traumatic events are numerous and include experiencing war, famine and disease, interpersonal violence (e.g., physical abuse, rape, sexual abuse, extreme neglect, robbery, assault, kidnapping), accidents (e.g., motor vehicle, falls, heavy machinery), fire and explosions, and natural disasters (e.g., flood, earthquakes, hurricanes, tornados).

While the DSM-5 requires traumatic events to be potentially life-threatening, events such as experiencing discrimination, learning that your spouse has been having an affair or wants a divorce, getting fired, loss of one's home, loss of an ability (e.g., eyesight, paralysis), or learning one has a chronic disease can be so life-shattering and unexpected that they overwhelm our ability to cope. These events, too, can lead to significant trauma symptoms. Experiencing forms of interpersonal violence are more likely to lead to post-traumatic effects. For instance, complex traumatic stress is experiencing repeated, long-term interpersonal violence. Complex trauma is most often associated with the childhood experience of sexual or physical abuse and neglect in the home or in homes where there is intimate partner violence (NCTSN 2020).

The effects of traumatic experiences can be diverse and long-lasting. First and foremost, trauma, particularly interpersonal violence, disrupts the ability to form and maintain healthy relationships with other people. Trauma can lead to negative beliefs about the self, others, and the world that lead to a sense of personal helplessness, shame and worthlessness, fear and mistrust for others, and a sense of hopelessness for the future. Experiencing trauma can also lead to emotional dysregulation, dissociation, negative effects on memory and concentration, and a reduction in the ability to cope with future stress and adversity. These effects can lead to depressed mood, anxiety, hypervigilance, and avoidant behaviors such as substance use and social withdrawal (SAMHSA 2014a, b).

7.1.1.2   Adverse Childhood Events

Adverse childhood events (ACEs) are defined as the experience of one or more negative or toxic life stressors that have been found to have long-ranging effects on health. Table 7.2 lists examples of ACEs that impact health within several major domains. These experiences include physical, sexual, or emotional abuse; physical or emotional neglect; living in a household with a person who has a mental illness, substance use disorder, or who is in prison; parental divorce; and death of a care-giver, among other events. Some of these experiences are not considered life-threatening as defined by the DSM-5; however, they exert a long-term negative impact on emotional and physical health (Burke-Harris 2018; Felitti and Anda 2010).

Table 7.2 Adverse childhood events impacting behavioral health

Domains	Events
Child maltreatment	Emotional abuse
	Sexual abuse
	Physical abuse
	Physical neglect
	Emotional neglect
Toxic family stress	Household mental illness or substance abuse
	Someone close had a bad accident or illness
	Parents always arguing
	Mother treated violently
	Parental divorce
	Household member incarcerated
	No good friends (at time of interview)
Peer, school, and community-based toxic stress	Property victimization (non-sibling)
	Peer victimization (non-sibling)
	Community violence exposure
	Socioeconomic status
	Below-average grades
Other domains needing further study	Death of a parent
	Lack of access to food
	Experiencing discrimination

Based on Finkelhor et al. (2015)

7.1.1.3 Post-Traumatic Stress Disorder

Post-traumatic stress disorder (PTSD) is the experience of a range of debilitating and distressing symptoms at least one month after exposure to a traumatic event that causes significant distress and functional impairment. These symptoms occur across four different clusters and include symptoms related to intrusive memories of the event, continued hyperarousal and vigilance following the event, negative mood (e.g., sadness, anger, fearfulness) and cognitive symptoms (e.g., dissociation, hope-lessness, helplessness, shame, guilt), and avoidance of trauma cues or reminders of the event (e.g., people, places, objects) that can include substance use and social withdrawal.

7.1.1.4 Trauma-Informed Care

The experience of trauma and untreated symptoms related to full, or partial, PTSD can increase the risk for comorbid health and behavioral health issues and hinder recovery from these conditions (Pietrzak et al. 2011; Schnurr 2015). Trauma-informed practice environments prioritize the safety of clients and promote trust, collaboration, healing, empowerment, and recovery from the effects of trauma. Providers or organizations that operate from a trauma-informed care (TIC) lens: (1) recognize the impact of trauma on health and behavioral health and integrate trauma awareness into all practices, policies, and procedures; (2) understand the strategies that lead to recovery; (3) routinely screen and assess for the signs and symptoms of trauma; (4) eliminate practices that have the potential to be re-traumatizing to cli-ents; and (4) deploy practices that are responsive to those who may have experi-enced trauma and that create a practice environment that promotes safety, empowerment, and healing (SAMHSA 2014a, b).

7.1.2 The Epidemiology of Trauma

7.1.2.1 PTSD and Health

Trauma activates the natural stress response system that prepares the body to fight an adversary, run away from danger, or freeze in the face of danger. These responses are rooted in our limbic system and brain stem—areas that control emotion (e.g., anger, disgust, fear) and autonomic responses (e.g., heart rate, breathing, blood pressure, consciousness). Traumatic stress is often sensory in that it activates our sense of sight, sound, smell, taste, and touch, and records signals from those senses in our memory. These memories can lead to somatic reactions to reminders or cues of the event such as emotional dysregulation (e.g., fear, anxiousness, hypervigi-lance, anger), intrusive and sometimes dissociative thoughts (e.g., flashbacks, numbing), and behavioral reactions (e.g., avoidance, aggression, withdrawal, freezing, substance use). Trauma memories serve a survival function and are designed to prevent a recurrence of trauma or death through increased vigilance, arousal, and avoidance. However, when these memories are triggered by cues in the environment and lead to distress when no danger exists or that is out of proportion to any potential danger, they can impair functioning and lead to the development of PTSD (APA 2013; Burke-Harris 2018; Van der Kolk 2015). Traumatic events involving interpersonal violence, especially sexual violence, intimate partner violence, and community violence, are the most likely events to lead to PTSD and can have a long-term impact on the health and well-being of many of our clients (Goldstein et al. 2016).

For instance, PTSD is associated with higher rates of chronic diseases such as cardiovascular and cerebrovascular disease, cancer, hypertension, metabolic disease, and autoimmune diseases (Gradus et al. 2015; Howard et al. 2018; Husarewycz et al. 2014; Kessler et al. 1995; Remch et al. 2018; Song et al. 2018; Spitzer et al. 2009). Violence can also lead to higher rates of visible and invisible injuries such as traumatic brain injury (Halbauer et al. 2009). All of these factors can compromise health and impact the ability of people to take care of themselves, engage in preventative care, and adhere to treatment resulting in persistent morbidity, disability, and early mortality (Burke-Harris 2018; Felitti and Anda 2010; CDC 2020; Leeies et al. 2010; Perry and Szalavitz 2017; Van der Kolk 2015).

7.1.2.2 Prevalence of Trauma and PTSD

The majority of people who experience a traumatic event do not develop PTSD. However, PTSD is a highly prevalent behavioral health condition in the community that is often comorbid with other behavioral health conditions (Goldstein et al. 2016). In the United States, nearly 70% of people experience a lifetime traumatic event. Lifetime prevalence rates of PTSD range from 6% to 8% nationally and 12-month rates for PTSD are nearly 5% (Goldstein et al. 2016; Kilpatrick et al. 2013). Women experience higher PTSD prevalence rates than men and the potential of experiencing PTSD increases with increased exposure to traumatic events (Kilpatrick et al. 2013). Over half of the general population (53%) will experience some form of interpersonal violence (58.6% of women and 47.1% of men). Almost a third of the general population (30%) and over 40% of women will experience a sexual assault. Over 40% of people and 45% of women will experience physical assault. Approximately half will experience a disaster, accident, or fire (Kilpatrick et al. 2013).

PTSD increases the odds of experiencing other behavioral health disorders including all anxiety disorders, major depressive disorders, substance use disorders, antisocial and borderline personality disorders. Persons with PTSD are 3 times more likely to have a co-occurring mood disorder, over 2.5 times more likely to have anxiety disorder, and 1.5 times more likely to have a substance use disorder (Goldstein et al. 2016). Despite the prevalence of PTSD, only 60% of persons with the condition receive treatment with a 4.5-year delay, on average, between onset and treatment (Goldstein et al. 2016).

7.1.2.3 Adverse Childhood Experiences and Health

Adverse childhood events (ACEs) are childhood experiences that are considered toxic or traumatic and can have a drastic impact on health (Felitti et al. 1998). The negative impact on health can develop regardless of whether a person develops full or even partial PTSD. These events are often silenced and buried in people's lives, but nonetheless have important health effects later in life. The ACE study, a large longitudinal study of over 17,000 middle-class, employed, college-educated people with good health insurance, found that experiencing any of the ten adverse childhood events mentioned below can have important health consequences later in life (Anda et al. 2006; Felitti et al. 1998; Whitfield et al. 2003). Examples of these events include growing up in a household where the person experienced: (1) emotional abuse; (2) physical abuse; (3) sexual abuse; (4) emotional neglect; (5) physical neglect; (6) parental separation or divorces; (7) domestic violence; (8) a person with a substance use disorder or problem drinking; (9) a depressed, mentally ill, or suicidal family member; and (10) someone in the house that had gone to prison. ACEs were found to be very common with about two-thirds of the sample having experienced at least one ACE (and 87% of those had more than one), and one in eleven people having experienced six or more ACEs (Felitti and Anda 2010). The impact of trauma on the brain and body can place people at risk for a range of negative behavioral, social, and physical health problems later in life (Anda et al. 2006; Whitfield et al. 2003).

For instance, childhood exposure to interpersonal violence led to increased rates of depression, substance use, and experiencing or perpetrating interpersonal violence in adulthood (Edwards et al. 2003; Whitfield et al. 2003). A higher number of ACEs were also linked to higher rates of cancer (Brown et al. 2013), COPD (Anda et al. 2008), heart disease (Dong et al. 2004), diabetes (Deschenes et al. 2018), and autoimmune diseases such as rheumatoid arthritis (Dube et al. 2009).

It is also important to note that the impact of ACEs on health occurs in a dose-response relationship. Figure 7.1 lists the dose response impact of ACEs on several health outcomes. For instance, four or more ACEs increased the risk for chronic obstructive pulmonary disease (COPD) by 390%, hepatitis by 240%, depression by 460%, and attempted suicide by an ominous 1220%. A person with an ACE score of 6 was 4600% more likely to be an IV drug user and 3100% (31-fold) to 5000% (50-fold) more likely to attempt suicide than a person with 0 ACEs (Dube et al. 2001). For every increase in ACE score, the risk for suicide attempts increased 60%. Experiencing any one of the ten identified ACEs increased suicide attempts 200–500% (2–5 fold) (Dube et al. 2001). Experiencing any six ACEs shortened life expectancy by 20 years.

Adverse childhood experiences disrupt neurological development through chronic activation of the stress response systems. This overactivation can lead to bio-psychosocial problems such as emotional dysregulation, hypervigilance, aggressive behavior, and low impulse control. These problems, in turn, can result in impairment in the ability to connect with other people and to the adoption of high-risk behaviors that can cause chronic comorbidity and early death (Burke-Harris

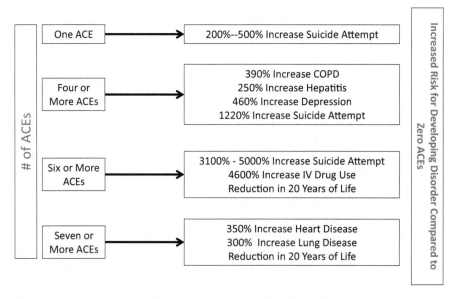

Fig. 7.1 Post-traumatic stress disorder symptoms (Based on APA 2013)

2018; Felitti et al. 1998; Van der Kolk 2015; Perry and Szalavitz 2017). For instance, it was found that higher ACE scores were associated with a higher prevalence of unhealthy coping behaviors such as smoking (Anda et al. 1999), alcohol and drug use (Dube et al. 2003; Strine et al. 2012), and obesity (Williamson et al. 2002). However, when controlling for these behaviors, the impact of ACEs was still profound. This is due to the impact of chronic stress on the brain and nervous system. Major chronic unrelieved stress leads to overactivation of the hypothalamic pituitary adrenal axis (HPA axis), the release of pro-inflammatory chemicals, and the suppression of immune system functioning that can lead to many of these health and behavioral health problems. This means that the experience of ACEs can change the body and brain via the stress response system in such a profound way that the experience of these events *by themselves* can lead to high morbidity and mortality if left untreated (Burke-Harris 2018).

7.2   Trauma-Informed Care

Trauma-informed approaches are heavily influenced by the ecological systems framework discussed in Chap. 2, which views human development and behavior as the result of the dynamic relationships that exist between an individual and their environment (Bronfenbrenner 1979, 2009; Bronfenbrenner and Morris 2007). Well-being is impacted by the fit between the biopsychosocial needs of the individual, and the resources and conditions available to them in their physical and social environments. Assessment and treatment should, therefore, focus on helping establish a good fit between individual characteristics (e.g., age, gender, culture, health and mental health, temperament and traits, education, and socioeconomic status, interpersonal relationships (e.g., social support, safety), and various social determinants of health (e.g., housing, income, neighborhood/community, and access to basic resources including health care). The Substance Abuse and Mental Health Services Administration (SAMHSA) has identified four assumptions and six principles of trauma-informed care (TIC) (2014). These will be reviewed next.

7.2.1   Trauma-Informed Care Definition and Assumptions

Trauma-informed care (TIC) is an approach to service delivery that fully recognizes the short-term and long-term impact of trauma on the health and well-being of service recipients, and responds with practices that promote safety, collaboration, trust, and empowerment (Elliott et al. 2005; Niolon et al. 2017; SAMHSA 2014a, b). SAMHSA has identified four assumptions that define trauma-informed care for organizations and providers. Table 7.3 lists the principles and practices of each of those assumptions. First, providers and organizations *realize* that trauma is prevalent in the lives of clients and that experiencing trauma exerts an impact on the health and well-being of client systems. Trauma sensitivity and awareness are integrated into all aspects of care, including screening and assessment, treatment, and follow-up care. A practice at the heart of trauma-informed care is asking the question *What happened? What happened* to this person? *What happened* to this family? *What happened* to this school? *What happened* to this community? Trauma awareness means positioning the behaviors of clients, families, organizations, and communities as reactions and attempts to adapt to the impact of traumatic stress. In other words, when providers practice TIC, they assume that trauma, experienced individually or collectively, and not traits inherent to the person or group, is the driving force behind behaviors that lead to negative health consequences. Framing behaviors in this way can diffuse judgmental feelings and responses by providers, reducing the risk of re-traumatization of the client (SAMHSA 2014a, b).

Second, being aware and sensitive to the prevalence and impact of trauma requires providers and organizations to be able to *recognize* trauma in those they serve. This is accomplished through the routine deployment of trauma-informed screening and assessment procedures designed to identify the presence of PTSD or other health effects related to stress and trauma (SAMHSA 2014a, b). Third, trauma-informed programs, organizations, and systems *respond* to trauma by integrating trauma-informed services across all levels of care. Health and behavioral health settings that are trauma-informed have in place trained staff, policies, procedures, and practices designed to create a safe, welcoming environment and provide clients with access to effective treatments and services that address the multidimensional impact of trauma on individual, social, and environmental levels (SAMHSA 2014a, b).

Table 7.3 The four Rs of trauma-informed care

Domain	Principle	Practices
Realize	Providers *realize* that trauma is common and has a drastic impact on health.	View symptoms, behaviors, and problems through a trauma lens. Ask: What may have happened to this person? How might trauma influence what I am seeing?
Recognize	Providers are trained to *recognize* trauma in clients.	Providers understand the signs and symptoms of trauma/PTSD and how trauma impacts the mind and body. Providers are trained to deploy routine and universal screening and assessment procedures and measures in a sensitive manner that ensures privacy and confidentiality.
Respond	Providers and programs effectively *respond* to trauma through training, policies, practices, and procedures.	Trauma awareness is integrated throughout the setting. Programs strive to create trust by ensuring an environment that is welcoming, transparent, safe, and kind, and begins when the client walks through the door or calls to schedule an appointment. The program provides trauma services either on-site or through direct, formal partnerships with community providers.
Resist	Providers and programs *resist* practices that could be re-traumatizing to clients.	Through systematic procedures, providers routinely (re)-assess their practices, policies, and procedures to ensure they are trauma-sensitive in this regard.

Based on SAMHSA (2014a)

Lastly, trauma-informed providers, organizations, and systems *resist* practices that are toxic and re-traumatizing to clients *and* staff by creating practice environments that are safe, nurturing, and conducive to the development of well-being (SAMHSA 2014a, b). These four assumptions represent the basic foundation underlying trauma-informed care. Trauma-informed care is also guided by several practice principles that I will review in the next section.

7.2.2 Principles of Trauma-Informed Care

Trauma-informed care is guided by six overarching practice principles that are infused into all levels of care. First, TIC organizations are dedicated to the promotion of physical, emotional, psychological, and interpersonal *safety* of clients served by the organization and the staff providing those services. Second, TIC organizations ensure that all clinical and organizational decisions prioritize *transparency and trust* with providers and clients. Third, trauma-informed organizations rely on *peer providers* with lived experience of trauma to use their stories to engage clients in treatment, build trust and hope, and promote healing and recovery. Fourth, trauma-informed care is person-centered and prioritizes *collaboration and mutuality* with clients. This means that service relationships are partnerships where power is shared.

Fifth, TIC organizations place an emphasis on *empowerment and choice*. This means that services are designed to promote recovery, health, and healing, and that clients can choose from a range of options that are aligned with their preferences and needs. Providers rely on shared decision-making models during care planning and treatment to ensure that clients are able to make informed decisions about the course of their care every step of the way. Sixth, trauma-informed programs provide *culturally-tailored services* that are sensitive and responsive to multiple intersecting identities such as race, ethnicity, culture, language, gender identity, and sexual orientation. Providers are trained to recognize and address bias, and care is provided with recognition of historical trauma caused by racist, heterosexist, sexist, and patriarchal policies and practices. TIC organizations eliminate practices and policies that reinforce stereotypes and lead to biased care, and implement policies, practices, procedures, and structures designed to ensure care that is responsive, affirming, and inclusive to the needs of service recipients with multiple identities (SAMHSA 2014a, b).

7.2.3   Implementation of Trauma-Informed Care Practice and Policies

Trauma-informed organizations ensure that trauma-informed care practices are fully integrated into the systems, structures, policies, and procedures of the program (Mancini and Miner 2013). Areas in which trauma-informed practices are integrated include intake procedures, staff training and professional development, screening and assessment procedures, policies regarding how to ensure safety and confidentiality of clients, hiring and retention policies of staff, physical space, monitoring and addressing compassion fatigue and burnout among staff, referral procedures, and continuous quality improvement initiatives. Programs also assess and address policies and practices that can be re-traumatizing such as the use of seclusion and restraints, power dynamics of provider-client relationships, lack of inclusive forms, lack of power over decision-making, being rushed through clinical appointments, physical touching and being placed in vulnerable positions, forced removal of clothing and invasive procedures, lack of privacy, and overly-personal questions. Trauma-informed practices utilize welcoming environments that are calm, affirming, and soothing. Providers take a holistic view of the client and engage in screening and assessment procedures for trauma in a safe, slow, and private manner. Providers utilize a collaborative approach offering clients choices among a range of holistic treatment options (e.g., group or individual counseling, yoga, nutrition, peer support, acupuncture, and meditation) offered on-site or through a warm referral process.

The implementation of trauma-informed care covers a number of domains identified by the Substance Abuse and Mental Health Services Administration (SAMHSA 2014a, b). First, trauma-informed care should be embraced by the highest levels of *leadership*. Peers with lived experience in trauma should be included in organizational decision-making processes, staff training, and the delivery and evaluation of services. Empowered champions for trauma-informed care should be positioned throughout the organization to increase acceptance and adoption of TIC practices. Second, TIC approaches should be part of the operations of the organization written specifically into all policy and procedure manuals and be a part of the organization's mission and vision. Third, the physical environment of the organization should be safe, welcoming, and collaborative. Fourth, TIC approaches should guide all decisions regarding organizational partnerships and collaborations. Referrals to outside services should only be to trauma-informed agencies and service sectors. Fifth, all providers receive continuous training in screening, assessment, and treatment services that are trauma-sensitive and culturally responsive. Sixth, trauma sensitivity is a consideration in hiring, supervision, and evaluation of all staff and leadership. Seventh, procedures are in place to ensure that staff have adequate access to self-care strategies and resources. Last, trauma-informed care is integrated into records, billing, and monitoring systems (Mancini and Miner 2013; SAMHSA 2014a, b).

7.3　Post-Traumatic Stress Disorder (PTSD) Diagnostic Criteria

A diagnosis of PTSD requires the persistent experience of symptoms related to the experience of a traumatic event for at least one month. There are four main clusters of PTSD symptoms: (1) intrusion/re-experiencing; (2) arousal/hypervigilance; (3) negative alternations in cognition and mood; and (4) avoidance. Figure 7.2 lists the main symptoms for PTSD within each of these four clusters. Symptoms should be severe enough to cause significant distress and impairment in functioning (i.e., interpersonal relationships, employment, daily activities). The DSM-5 has a modified set of diagnostic criteria for children under the age of seven. For adults, adolescents, and children over the age of 6, the following criteria are required for a diagnosis of PTSD. Table 7.4 lists the major diagnostic criteria for post-traumatic stress disorder.

7.3.1　Criteria A: Exposure to a Traumatic Event

A traumatic event is defined as actual or threatened exposure to death, injury, or violence and can include direct experience, witnessing first-hand traumatic events experienced by others, being made aware of traumatic events that have happened to close persons, or being repeatedly exposed to the details of traumatic events

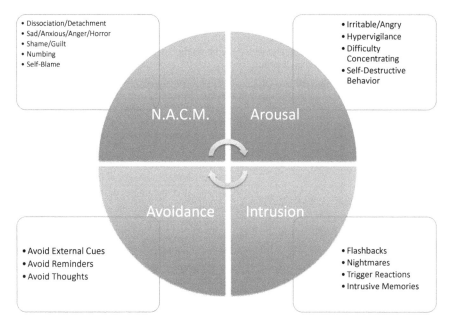

- Dissociation/Detachment
- Sad/Anxious/Anger/Horror
- Shame/Guilt
- Numbing
- Self-Blame

- Irritable/Angry
- Hypervigilance
- Difficulty Concentrating
- Self-Destructive Behavior

N.A.C.M.   Arousal

Avoidance   Intrusion

- Avoid External Cues
- Avoid Reminders
- Avoid Thoughts

- Flashbacks
- Nightmares
- Trigger Reactions
- Intrusive Memories

Fig. 7.2 Dose-response impact of ACEs (Based on: Anda et al. 2008; Dube et al. 2001; Dong et al. 2004)

experienced by others (APA 2013). Examples of traumatic events include: experiencing or witnessing interpersonal and community violence such as sexual assault, physical assault, assault with a weapon, combat or exposure to war, kidnapping or being detained, natural disasters, fire and explosions, serious accidents, life-threatening illness or injury, witnessing sudden violent death or serious injury, and witnessing intense human suffering (APA 2013; Blake et al. 1995).

The two most profound clusters of traumatic events that have the highest probability of leading to PTSD are experiencing sexual trauma and when traumatic events happen to close loved ones such as spouses, children, and parents. Experiencing sexual violence holds the highest likelihood of developing PTSD, with 33% of persons experiencing this form of violence developing PTSD. Thirty percent of persons who experience the sudden loss of a loved one or whose loved one experiences a life-threatening injury, illness, or trauma will go on to develop PTSD symptoms. Approximately 11–12% of persons experiencing or witnessing interpersonal and community-based violence or war may go on to develop PTSD (Kessler et al. 2014).

7.3.2   Criteria B: At Least One Intrusion or Re-experiencing Symptom

One of the hallmarks of PTSD is the presence of intrusive thoughts and re-experiencing of the traumatic event. For a PTSD diagnosis, a person must experience at least one symptom from this cluster following a traumatic event (APA 2013).

Table 7.4 Post-traumatic stress disorder diagnostic criteria

Symptoms should be present for at least one month following the event and cause significant impairment in functioning. Symptoms should not be solely the result of medical condition, substance use, or another mental disorder.

Criteria A: Exposure to traumatic event(s)	Actual or threatened exposure to death, injury, or violence Exposure can include direct experience, witnessing, learning about traumatic events happening to close persons, or repeated exposure to the details of trauma
Criteria B: One or more intrusion symptoms	Recurrent, involuntary, unwanted, distressing memories, thoughts, images of the event
	Repeated, vivid nightmares of the event
	Dissociative flashbacks or re-experiencing the event as if it is re-occurring
	Experiencing cognitive, emotional, or physiological reactions to reminders/cues of the event
Criteria C: Evidence of avoidance of reminders of the event	Repeated attempts to avoid internal reminders of the event (e.g., thoughts, feelings, images) through substance use, self-harm, high-risk behaviors
	Repeated attempts to avoid external reminders of the event such as people, places, situations, or objects through isolation, social withdrawal, relocation, or other means of strategic avoidance
Criteria D: Two or more symptoms of negative alterations in cognitions and mood	Inability to remember an important aspect of the traumatic event(s)
	Negative beliefs about the self, others, or world
	Persistent, distorted cognitions about the cause or consequences of the traumatic event(s) (e.g., it's all my fault or I am forever damaged)
	Lack of interest or pleasure in activities
	A persistent negative emotional state: sadness, anxiety, anger, guilt/shame
	Emotional numbness or the inability to experience positive emotions such as joy or satisfaction
	Dissociation or feeling detached or estranged from other people
Criteria E: Two or more symptoms of heightened arousal and reactivity	Problems sleeping
	Exaggerated startle response
	Persistent hypervigilance for danger or feeling "on guard"
	Recklessness
	Feeling on edge or persistently irritable

Based on APA (2013)

Intrusion symptoms can include prolonged, frequent, and vivid nightmares about the event; dissociative flashbacks where the person re-experiences the elements of the event as if it were happening again; and constant intrusive thoughts and memories of the event (e.g., can't stop thinking about it). Another important element of intrusion symptoms is cognitive, affective, or physiological reactions to cues or reminders of the event. For instance, a person who has experienced rape may have a psychological or physiological stress response if they smell the same or similar cologne as their attacker, leading to flashbacks, hypervigilance or nervousness, nausea, fear, sadness, or irritability that can interfere with functioning. It should be noted that the person may not be aware of what is happening or that this particular cue is significant, despite experiencing these emotional or physiological reactions (APA, 2013).

7.3.3 Criteria C: Persistent Avoidance of Reminders Related to the Event

Memories and reminders of the traumatic event are persistently distressing to persons with PTSD over time. A sign of PTSD is engaging in repeated efforts to avoid internal (e.g., distressing memories or feelings) or external reminders or cues associated with the event (e.g., places, people, or situations). This avoidance can result in maladaptive coping behaviors that can include alcohol and substance use, social withdrawal, and isolation. Avoidance behaviors can include *either* attempts to avoid unwanted memories of the event, or external triggers of the event such as people, place, things, and situations (APA, 2013).

7.3.4 Criteria D: At Least Two Negative Alterations in Cognitions and Mood Symptoms

This cluster of symptoms was newly introduced to DSM-5 to capture the psychological distress and dysphoria that is a key feature of the trauma experience and PTSD. Persons with PTSD may experience a range of negative thoughts, feelings, and beliefs about the traumatic event. This cluster includes a wide range of symptoms associated with the traumatic event such as experiencing: (1) dissociative amnesia regarding the details of the event; (2) feelings of guilt, self-blame, shame, and negative self-concept due to the event; (3) negative emotions such as anhedonia, depressed mood, anxiety, and fear; and (4) detachment and feelings of numbness or the inability to experience positive emotions (APA, 2013).

7.3.5   Criteria E: At Least Two Alterations in Reactivity and Arousal Symptoms

Persons with PTSD often experience a prolonged activation of the stress response system that can lead to high rates of health problems. Signs and symptoms of hyperarousal include irritability and anger, sleep disturbances, behavior that is reckless to self or others, increased vigilance for danger, and an exaggerated startle response (APA 2013).

7.4   Screening and Assessment for Traumatic Stress and PTSD

Universal screening and assessment for traumatic stress and PTSD in health and behavioral health settings is a key part of trauma-informed care. Effective screening and assessment for traumatic stress are rooted in safety, trust, respect, and compassion. Clients need to feel that they are in a safe place to disclose traumatic experiences and that their stories will be heard and validated. Clients also need to trust that their responses are confidential and must be made fully aware of any limitations to confidentiality or reporting requirements before being asked about trauma. Providers need to ensure that they ask about trauma in a private setting, utilize active listening skills, and show respect and compassion. Language interpreters should be independent professionals, rather than family or friends of the client. Persons who disclose trauma need to feel like it was a good idea to tell their story. Trauma assessment should also be ongoing as the relationship between provider and client develops over time. Initial screening for trauma should be in a sensitive way, and conversations about the impact of stress and trauma on health can signal to reluctant clients that they are in a safe place to discuss their trauma. Providers should provide education to clients about the role of trauma in health regardless of whether they disclose experiencing trauma. If they do disclose, providers should normalize the symptoms that often are associated with traumatic events. Positive screenings should lead to further assessment and access to trauma services provided onsite or a referral to outside behavioral health settings that specialize in trauma-focused care. Screening and assessment should include assessing for ACEs, traumatic events, and symptoms of PTSD. Table 7.5 lists information about several common screening and assessment instruments for PTSD. Each of these instruments will be discussed in more detail in the sections that follow.

Table 7.5 Screening and assessment instruments for PTSD

Scale name	Description	References
Life events checklist	Screens for exposure for 17 common traumatic events including natural disasters, various forms of violence, illness, accidents, and war	Weathers et al. (2013a)
Primary care PTSD screen for DSM-5 (PC-PTSD-5)	Brief, 5-item screen for possible PTSD. Uses "yes" and "no" items that screen for intrusive thoughts, avoidance, hypervigilance, numbness or detachment, and guilt or self-blame. A "yes" to any three items indicates a positive screen.	Prins et al. (2016)
The PTSD checklist for DSM-5 (PCL-5)	The PCL-5 is a 20-item self-report assessment checklist that corresponds to the 20 symptoms of the DSM-5 across four diagnostic symptom clusters: intrusion/re-experiencing, hyperarousal, negative alteration in cognition and mood, and avoidance. The PCL-5 scores can be summed and compared to a clinical cut-off to assess severity, or the scale can be used as a diagnostic instrument. Preliminary severity cut scores range from 28 to 37 depending on the population and setting.	Weathers et al. (2013)
Clinician-administered PTSD scale for DSM-5 (CAPS-5)	The CAPS-5 is a 20-item semi-structured clinical interview that measures PTSD diagnosis and also offers a severity score. It is considered the gold standard for research and clinical assessment of PTSD. The symptoms correspond to the 20 main PTSD symptoms in the DSM-5 across four clusters (intrusion, avoidance, arousal, and negative alterations in cognition and mood). Symptom frequency and severity are measured using a 5-point scale (0 = absent; 1 = mild/sub-threshold; 2 = moderate/threshold; 3 = severe/markedly elevated; and 4 = extreme/incapacitated). In order to indicate the presence of clinical symptoms, a score of '2' or higher is required.	Weathers et al. (2013b)
Posttraumatic stress disorder symptoms scale interview for DSM-5 (PSSI-5)	The PSSI-5 is a 24-item semi-structured interview schedule that assesses the presence of a traumatic event and measures the 20 DSM-5 symptoms for PTSD. Symptoms are assessed on a 5-point scale that measures frequency and severity ranging from 0 (not at all) to 4 (6 or more times a week/severe). Scores of 1 or higher indicate the presence of symptoms. Scores can range from 0 to 80. The clinical cut-off score for a probable diagnosis of PTSD is 23.	Foa et al. (2016a)
Post-traumatic diagnostic scale for DSM-5 (PDS-5)	The PDS-5 is a 24-item self-report measure that assesses the presence of a traumatic event and measures the 20 DSM-5 symptoms for trauma. This measure is the self-report version of the PSSI-5 interview schedule. The clinical cut-off score for a probable diagnosis of PTSD is 28.	Foa et al. (2016b)

7.4.1 Adverse Childhood Experiences

The experience of adverse childhood events and traumatic events has been linked to a range of health issues. The experience of four or more adverse childhood events (ACEs) has been associated with higher rates of cancer, behavioral health issues such as depression, heart disease, diabetes, and suicide, controlling for negative health behaviors and socioeconomic issues (Felitti et al. 1998). The original ACE questionnaire uses "yes" and "no" questions to assess whether clients have ever experienced any of the original ten ACEs, which included the experiences of intimate partner violence, emotional and physical abuse and neglect, sexual assault, divorce, having a person in the household who has been in jail, used alcohol or drugs, or had a mental illness. The concept of ACEs has been expanding to include items measuring peer victimization, peer rejection or isolation, and community violence (Cronholm et al. 2015). This has led to the revised inventory of adverse childhood events (Finkelhor et al. 2015). The addition of these items has increased the sensitivity of the original measure to predicting mental health issues. The addition of low SES has also increased predictive ability of the measure for health issues (Finkelhor et al. 2015). Both versions of the scale can be found online and at the Centers for Disease Control and Prevention (CDC) website.

7.4.2   Traumatic Events

A common screen for DSM-5 traumatic events is the Life Events Checklist (LEC-5) (Weathers et al. 2013a). This checklist is part of two well-validated screening and assessment instruments: The PTSD Checklist for DSM-5 (PCL-5) (Weathers et al. 2013) and the Clinician-Administered PTSD Scale for DSM-5 (CAPS-5) (Blake et al. 1995). The LEC was originally developed as part of the CAPS. The LEC-5 screens for 17 common traumatic experiences including: experiencing various forms of interpersonal violence (e.g., physical and sexual assault, kidnapping, war, being threatened), natural disasters, fire, accidents, and life-threatening medical conditions. The purpose of the LEC is to identify the experience of a potentially traumatic event and as a result, it does not have a specific score or scoring procedure.

7.4.3   Post-Traumatic Stress Disorder

Primary Care Post-Traumatic Stress Disorder Screen for DSM-5 One of the most common screening tools in health settings for PTSD is the Primary Care-Post Traumatic Stress Disorder Screen for DSM-5 (PC-PTSD-5) (Prins et al. 2016). This is a five-item "yes" and "no" screen that assesses whether a client has experienced significant symptoms associated with a traumatic event(s) in the past month. The symptoms assessed by the scale are: (1) experienced nightmares about the event(s) or unwanted thoughts about the event; (2) engaged in attempts to avoid situations or thoughts that serve as reminders of the event or had to try hard not to think about the event; (3) experienced hypervigilance such as being "on guard," watchful, or easily startled; (4) experienced a sense of being numb or detached from activities or environment; and (5) experienced a sense of guilt or was unable to stop blaming themselves or others for what happened or the effects of what happened. A positive screen is a "yes" to any three items and indicates the need for further assessment for PTSD. This instrument has shown excellent psychometric properties in primary care settings and good sensitivity (score of 3) and specificity with a cut score of 4 for maximum efficiency. The screen has shown good diagnostic accuracy and is very effective in routine settings (Prins et al. 2016). The scale is in the public domain and can be accessed at the National Center for PTSD in the US Department of Veterans Affairs.

This screening instrument and others can lead to important clarifying conversations about trauma in the client's life. First, be sure to clarify whether the client experienced a traumatic event by asking the client to identify the event they feel has led to their symptoms. Be sure that the event is life-threatening. Experiencing troubling or stressful events that are not necessarily traumatic, but lead to depressed or anxious symptoms may be better classified as an adjustment disorder (APA, 2013). It is also important to ask how symptoms have interfered with work or interpersonal functioning. Lastly, it is important to assess whether any traumatic events the client identified are continuing to happen such as ongoing violence. Clients who disclose ongoing violence should be provided resources and referrals to legal and advocacy services, social services, behavioral health counseling and crisis response services, shelters, childcare services, and hotlines if safe to do so. If it is not safe to give the client brochures, providers should give them to the client verbally and offer the client the option to use the provider's office phone to make contact with referrals. Trauma-informed practice requires health settings that screen for trauma to offer services to survivors of violence on-site or through an active warm referral process. If the incident requires mandated reporting, consult with the client on how best to file the report in such a way that their safety is enhanced rather than diminished.

The PTSD Checklist for DSM-5 (PCL-5) The PCL-5 is a 20-item checklist that corresponds to the 20 symptoms of the DSM-5 across four diagnostic symptom clusters: intrusion/re-experiencing, hyperarousal, negative alteration in cognition and mood, and avoidance (Weathers et al. 2013). This measure uses the Life Events Checklist (LEC-5) to identify traumatic events. It is a self-report measure in which respondents identify how much distress each symptom has caused them in the past month on a 5-point scale that ranges from (0) not at all to (4) extremely. The PCL is easy to administer and score and has shown solid psychometric properties and diagnostic utility (Blevins et al. 2015; Bovin et al. 2016; Wortmann et al. 2016). Like the PC-PTSD-5, this measure is in the public domain and can be accessed at the National Center for PTSD in the US Department of Veterans Affairs.

The PCL-5 scores can be summed and compared to a clinical cut-off to assess severity or the scale can be used as a diagnostic instrument. Diagnosis of PTSD may be made if scores of 2 (Moderately) or higher are indicated on at least one intrusion symptom (Cluster B); one avoidance symptom (Cluster C); two arousal symptoms (Cluster D); and two negative alterations in cognition and mood symptoms (Cluster E). Preliminary Severity cut-off scores range from 28 to 37 depending on the population (military vs civilian), setting (medical clinic vs. VA), and reason for assessment. (Blevins et al. 2015).

Clinician Administered PTSD Scale for DSM-5 (CAPS-5) The CAPS-5 is a 20-item semi-structured clinical interview that measures PTSD diagnosis and also offers a severity score (Weathers et al. 2018). It is considered the gold standard for research and clinical assessment of PTSD. The symptoms correspond to the 20 main PTSD symptoms in the DSM-5 across four clusters (i.e., intrusion, avoidance, arousal, and negative alterations in cognition and mood). Symptom frequency and severity are measured using a 5-point scale (0 = absent; 1 = mild/sub-threshold; 2 = moderate/threshold; 3 = severe/markedly elevated; and 4 = extreme/incapacitated). In order to indicate the presence of clinical symptoms, a score of '2' or higher is required. Scoring for the CAPS-5 has been streamlined to combine frequency and intensity symptoms, and clinicians have a frequency and severity guideline that instruct them on how to score the scale. For instance, a score of 2 requires a minimum frequency of twice a month and a minimum intensity of "clearly present." A score of 3 requires a minimum frequency of twice a week and a minimum intensity of "pronounced." The CAPS-5 has shown good psychometric properties. It has good test-retest reliability (r = 0.78) and good internal consistency (0.88) for the severity score and showed good convergent validity with the PCL-5 (Weathers et al. 2013a, b). The CAPS is more time-consuming and is a more complicated measure to implement and score than other self-reports measures. Clinical training is required to utilize the scale effectively. The CAPS can be obtained from the National Center for PTSD in the US Department of Veterans Affairs. It is not available in the public domain.

Post-Traumatic Stress Disorder Symptoms Scale Interview for DSM-5 (PSSI-5) The PSSI-5 is a 24-item semi-structured interview schedule that assesses the presence of a traumatic event and measures the 20 DSM-5 symptoms for PTSD (Foa et al. 2016a). Symptoms measured are for the index traumatic event or the event that produces the most severe self-reported symptoms if multiple traumatic events have been experienced. The 20 symptoms correspond to the four DSM-5 symptoms clusters. Symptoms are assessed on a 5-point scale that measures frequency and severity ranging from 0 (not at all) to 4 (6 or more times a week/Severe). Scores of 1 or higher indicate the presence of symptoms. Scores can range from 0 to 80. Two items measure distress and interference with functioning, and a score of 2 or higher on either item is positive for clinical distress or interference in functioning. Two other items indicate duration of symptoms and delayed onset. Similar to DSM-5, a positive assessment requires the presence of one intrusion symptom, one avoidance symptom, two symptoms of negative cognition and mood, and two symptoms of arousal experienced for one or more months. The clinical cut-off score for a probable diagnosis of PTSD is 23, and the scale has shown excellent psychometric properties as a reliable and valid scale of PTSD. The sensitivity of the PSSI-5 is 0.82 and specificity is 0.71. The PSSI-5 showed good internal consistency (0.89) and test-retest reliability (r = 0.87) and showed good convergent validity with other measures of PTSD (Foa et al. 2016a). However, as compared to the CAPS-5, the 29% false positive rate of the PSSI-5 might be due to a lower scoring threshold leading to the propensity for an increased risk of false positives (Weathers et al. 2013b). This scale is not in the public domain and must be requested by the authors.

Post-Traumatic Diagnostic Scale for DSM-5 (PDS-5)   The PDS-5 is a 24-item self-report measure that assesses the presence of a traumatic event and measures the 20 DSM-5 symptoms for trauma. This measure is the self-report version of the PSSI-5 interview schedule. The items measuring symptoms are the same as the PSSI-5 and utilize the same scoring anchors and thresholds. The clinical cut-off score for a probable diagnosis of PTSD is 28, and the scale has shown excellent psychometric properties with an internal consistency score of 0.95 and a test-retest reliability score of 0.90. The scale showed good convergent validity with the PSSI ($r = 0.85$) and the PCL-S ($r = 0.90$). The PDS-5 showed a 78% agreement with the PSSI and is a valid self-report scale of PTSD (Foa et al. 2016b). This scale is not in the public domain and must be requested by the authors.

7.5   Treatment Guidelines for PTSD (NICE Guidelines 2005)

Treatment guidelines for PTSD for behavioral health providers include a range of treatment and practices that have shown to be effective in addressing the impacts of trauma and PTSD in the population. Routine health and behavioral health settings are key places where PTSD intervention can occur. As mentioned previously, many people with PTSD do not receive treatment or deal with the symptoms of PTSD for many years before receiving treatment. Table 7.6 lists the recommended guidelines for PTSD treatment drawn largely from the National Institute for Clinical Excellence (NICE). Specific guidelines to consider for treatment include the following:

Conduct Universal Screening and Education for Trauma and IPV for All Clients   These are important integrated treatment strategies to identify and address PTSD in routine health settings to help people avoid years of needless suffering. Trauma and IPV should be a part of normal and routine patient education. The role of trauma and health should be provided to all patients regardless of disclosure. Trauma-informed practices should be followed, which include assessing clients (especially children) separately from partners and caregivers. Primary care providers should ask clients about trauma symptoms and traumatic events in a sensitive and person-centered manner. Clients who screen positive for trauma should automatically have further assessment. For assessed clients who have PTSD or partial PTSD symptoms, care should be coordinated either within the team or through warm referral processes with trusted outside providers that specialize in trauma treatment for which there exist a formal referral arrangement. Providers should also consider the needs of families and caregivers, and assess and address practical and social support issues as they arise.

Table 7.6 Practice guidelines for PTSD

Guideline	Description
Universal screening and education	Providers screen and assess for trauma and intimate partner violence for all clients. Screening and assessment are done in a private setting alone with the client. Providers utilize empathic, active listening practices during assessment. Providers provide universal education to clients about healthy and unhealthy relationships, the impact of trauma and IPV on health. Providers give clients informational brochures (e.g., safety cards) about safe relationships and where to get help if services are needed.
Watchful waiting after a traumatic event	For clients who have experienced a traumatic event: (1) closely monitor for the emergence of symptoms for several weeks; and (2) encourage proper sleep, healthy diet, regular meals, exercise, preferred activities or hobbies, and utilization of social support system. For survivors of IPV: (1) conduct safety assessment; (2) show concern and empathy; (3) provide access to IPV services (e.g., counseling, housing/shelter, legal advocacy, social services, child care); (4) provide harm reduction with follow up for those unable or unwilling to utilize services (e.g., emergency contraception, hotline numbers, and safety cards).
Avoid critical incident stress debriefing (CISD)	Single-session CISD after a traumatic event is ineffective in preventing PTSD symptoms and may be harmful, and is therefore not recommended. Watchful waiting with follow-up is the preferred method.
Provide access to evidence-based treatment services	For clients who experience full or partial PTSD symptoms, encourage social support and provide access to evidence-based treatments for PTSD including: (1) prolonged exposure (PE); cognitive processing therapy (CPT); trauma-focused cognitive behavioral therapy (TF-CBT); eye movement desensitization and reprocessing therapy (EMDR); and cognitive behavioral interventions for trauma in schools (C-BITS).
PTSD comorbidity	For PTSD and mild-to-moderate depression, consider treating PTSD first. For PTSD and severe depression, treat depression first if depressive symptoms interfere with PTSD treatment. For PTSD and suicidality, treat suicidality first. For PTSD and substance use disorders, treat substance use first or simultaneously.

Based on NICE (2005)

Watchful Waiting For clients who have recently experienced a traumatic event, *watchful waiting* is the preferred method. This involves close monitoring of symptom emergence and follow-up of clients over several weeks or months. Encourage proper sleep, healthy diet, regular meals, exercise, preferred activities or hobbies, and utilization of social support. Screening for PTSD symptoms and then treating with evidence-based interventions once symptoms appear is the preferred approach (Rose et al. 2002).

For situations involving IPV, providers should conduct a safety assessment, show concern, and provide access to IPV services including counseling, legal advocacy, childcare, and social services (housing/shelter, income support, food access) on-site or through warm referral process. For clients who prefer not to engage in services due to safety concerns or other reasons, providers should offer harm reduction services such as emergency contraception and safety cards with hotline numbers and community resources. Providers should follow-up with the client at the next visit and extend an offer to refer for services as needed.

Avoid Critical Incident Stress Debriefing (CISD)   CISD is often provided to survivors in the aftermath of a life-threatening incident. Examples of persons receiving CISD can include survivors of a mass shooting or violent encounter, students after a school suicide, or bank employees following an armed robbery. In CISD, trained specialists meet with survivors soon after the event to assess its impact on survivors and their sense of safety, provide an opportunity for survivors to discuss the event and share their feelings and thoughts, provide survivors with information about trauma reactions and what to expect in the coming days, and assist in re-entry into the setting. There is no evidence that CISD after a traumatic event is effective in preventing PTSD symptoms and there is some evidence that the approach can be harmful. Therefore, single session CISD with persons who experience a traumatic event is not recommended. *Watchful waiting* with follow-up is the preferred method.

Offer Access to Evidence-Based Treatments and Increase Social Support   After detection, there are a range of effective treatments that help people reduce and cope with the symptoms of PTSD (APA, 2017). It is also important to increase social support networks as increased social support has been found to enhance the positive effect of treatment (Price et al. 2018). Some of the most proven effective and evidence-based treatments for PTSD are: (1) prolonged exposure (Foa et al. 2007); (2) eye movement and desensitization and reprocessing therapy (EMDR) (Bisson and Andrew 2007; Shapiro 2017); trauma-focused cognitive behavioral therapy (Mannarino et al. 2012); cognitive processing therapy (Resnick et al. 2016); and school-based cognitive behavioral approaches for children (Difede et al. 2014; Jaycox et al. 2012; Jonas et al. 2013). Non-directive or supportive therapy shows no evidence of alleviating PTSD symptoms (Bisson et al. 2013).

Medications for sleep (hypnotics) should be considered on a short-term basis. Currently, no pharmacological treatments have been approved specifically for PTSD. Antidepressants can be used with clients who experience significant comorbid depression, significant hyperarousal that interferes with treatment, or who have not responded to psychological PTSD symptoms or are not interested in psychological treatment for PTSD (NICE Guidelines 2005). For comorbid depression and PTSD, providers should consider treating PTSD first as this can result in a resolution of depression symptoms. For clients with very severe depressive symptoms that make PTSD treatment difficult, treating depression first is best. For PTSD and suicidality, suicidality should be addressed first. For those with comorbid PTSD and substance use issues that may interfere with PTSD treatment, providers should treat substance use issues first or simultaneously. Recognition of traumatic grief and PTSD treatment can exist side by side.

7.6   Treatment Approaches for Post-Traumatic Stress Disorder

7.6.1   Theoretical Orientation

Several psychotherapies have been identified that are strongly recommended in the treatment of PTSD. The four most commonly identified psychotherapies are: (1) prolonged exposure (PE) (Foa et al. 2007); (2) eye movement and desensitization and reprocessing therapy (EMDR) (Bisson and Andrew 2007; Bisson et al. 2013; Shapiro 2017); (3) trauma-focused cognitive behavioral therapy (TF-CBT) (Mannarino et al. 2012); and (4) cognitive processing therapy (CPT) (Resnick et al. 2016). All of the above treatments are rooted in cognitive behavioral therapy (CBT) and are usually delivered in 10–15 sessions. The core theory of CBT approaches is that thoughts, emotions, and behaviors are connected and distorted thinking patterns about the self, others, and the world lead to negative emotions and maladaptive behaviors. The key to more positive emotions and more healthy behaviors is to identify and challenge distorted or negative thinking patterns.

Two main theories help to explain PTSD in persons who experience traumatic events and underlie each of the above approaches. The social cognitive theory of PTSD suggests that people try to integrate and make sense of their trauma with previously held beliefs about the self, others, and world. A person's perceived self-efficacy or the beliefs in one's ability to effectively cope with traumatic stress and loss mediates how well a person copes with stress and whether a person experiences post-traumatic stress reactions (Benight and Bandura 2004). When self-efficacy beliefs around control, trust, and safety are unrealistic, the person can develop a distorted and maladaptive understanding of their experience. This can then lead to the emergence and maintenance of negative cognitions and emotions associated with PTSD such as shame, anger, self-loathing, fear, guilt, and self-blame which then lead to maladaptive coping behaviors such as avoidance, withdrawal, substance use, and aggression. The experience of the physiological experiences of trauma such as flashbacks, hyperarousal, and numbing or dissociation can reinforce these maladaptive coping behaviors (Benight and Bandura 2004). For instance, beliefs about control, safety, and trust in others can be shattered by trauma, leading to confusion and self-blame. Similarly, trauma can confirm previously held unrealistic beliefs about the self, others, and world such as, "I am worthless/unlovable," "People are dangerous or out for themselves," or "bad things happen to bad people," or "I am helpless." This can lead to anger, depression, self-blame (e.g., I deserved it), substance use, fear, and social withdrawal. Identifying and challenging these unrealistic beliefs leads to a reduction in feelings of helplessness, worthlessness, brokenness, and unlovability and a subsequent reduction in anxiety, depression, and substance use symptoms and behaviors commonly comorbid with PTSD (Benight and Bandura 2004).

Low perceived self-efficacy for coping with the effects of the traumatic event can lead to avoidance, rumination, and stress. High perceived coping self-efficacy is a key mediator for recovery from traumatic experiences. Persons who believe that they can overcome the effects of trauma, particularly those with social support, have better recovery outcomes and are less likely to experience prolonged PTSD. Persons with low perceived coping self-efficacy, either due to their previous beliefs being shattered or confirmed by the traumatic event, struggle to recover. Providers can enhance the perceived self-efficacy of their clients and a sense of control through the development of mastery experiences related to coping behaviors. Helping people develop effective coping skills through mastery experiences can challenge negatively held perceptions regarding their ability to cope with stress and trauma, and increase their perceived coping self-efficacy by providing evidence that they can manage their fears, control symptoms, and improve psychosocial functioning. This can be done through graduated imaginal and in vivo exposure to fear stimuli where stress responses to fear stimuli are neutralized and people develop a sense of mastery over their lives, while developing more realistic understandings about their experiences and ability to cope. The focus of treatment then is to help people develop a sense of control and agency through enhancing their perceived self-efficacy by providing clients with guided mastery experiences (Benight and Bandura 2004).

Emotional processing theory is the second theory that positions PTSD as the result of the development of a fear structure residing in one's memory consisting of a network of associations, feelings, physiological responses, and thoughts related to the traumatic event (Foa and Kozak 1986; Rauch and Foa 2006). This structure is activated when a person comes into contact with reminders of the traumatic event. Once activated, the underlying fear structure produces PTSD intrusion symptoms such as unwanted thoughts, feelings, and images that lead to anxiety, hyperarousal, and avoidance behaviors such as a social withdrawal, substance use, and avoidance of objects, situations, and places. Desensitization to the stimuli through systematic, repeated, and prolonged imaginary and in vivo exposure, and processing of traumatic memories in a safe space dismantles this fear structure. New, competing meanings and perceptions of the event (e.g., thoughts, meanings, feelings, and behaviors related to traumatic stimuli) are thought to emerge through repeated imaginary and in vivo exposure (Foa et al. 2006). The next sections will expand on five leading psychotherapies for the treatment of PTSD: prolonged exposure, cognitive processing therapy, EMDR, trauma-informed CBT, and Cognitive Behavioral Intervention for Trauma in Schools (C-BITS). Table 7.7 lists descriptions of several effective approaches to PTSD. Each of these approaches will be discussed more specifically in the sections that follow.

7.6.2 Prolonged Exposure

Prolonged exposure therapy for PTSD (PE) is one of the most effective frontline treatments for PTSD across a range of populations (Foa et al. 2007; Foa et al. 2009; IOM 2008; Rauch et al. 2012; Powers et al. 2010). PE has been effectively implemented in primary care settings (Cigrang et al. 2011) and has been shown to reduce comorbid depression, anxiety, and PTSD symptoms in persons with co-occurring substance use disorders (Rothbaum et al. 2005; Sannibale et al. 2013; Foa et al. 2013; Mills et al. 2012; Coffey et al. 2016). Foa and Kozak (1986) first proposed that PTSD symptoms are rooted in a fear structure maintained and reinforced through avoidance behaviors. Prolonged exposure addresses this fear structure through three mechanisms: (1) psychoeducation about trauma, symptoms, and treatment; (2) in vivo and imaginal exposure; and (3) emotional processing.

People who suffer from PTSD often have cognitive distortions about the self, others, and world related to the event. One example is a belief that they possess low perceived coping self-efficacy and see themselves as completely incompetent and incapable of handling or managing the impact of the traumatic event (Benight and Bandura 2004). Trauma survivors may also see their symptoms as evidence of insanity, brokenness, or weakness. Another unrealistic belief is an overestimation of danger and a view of the world and other people as completely dangerous or untrustworthy (Foa and Riggs 1995). The combinations of these maladaptive thoughts can lead to incapacitating symptoms of PTSD such as avoidance of people, places, and things; using drugs and alcohol to cope with symptoms; and chronic feelings of depression, shame, guilt, and fear (Foa and Kozak 1986; Rauch and Foa 2006).

PE therapists seek to modify fear structures and cognitive distortions by exposing the person to the feared stimuli or memory and challenging their typical avoidant coping responses. The effectiveness of PE is predicted on the processes of habituation and emotional processing that lead to a reduction in symptom severity and avoidance behaviors. Activation of the fear structure through repeated and prolonged exposure of the client to trauma stimuli within a safe and supportive environment leads to habituation or a decrease in emotional reactivity and intensity of the emotional and physiological symptoms. As exposure to traumatic stimuli begins to be associated with less physiological reactivity and pain, clients develop more realistic information into their beliefs about self and others in relation to the traumatic event. In other words, they begin to "get used" to the content as it becomes less and less physiologically triggering and reactive (Rauch and Foa 2006). As people become more habituated, they develop a sense of self-efficacy and mastery and are less likely to believe that they are incompetent, broken, or damaged or that the world and other people are completely dangerous (Benight and Bandura 2004). As clients' perceived self-efficacy increases, they engage in less avoidance behaviors. As clients' beliefs in their own competence gets stronger and their reactivity to trauma cues is further reduced, they are more likely to competently manage thoughts and emotions when they come across reminders of the trauma in real-life situations. The reduction of these negative beliefs then leads to improvement in other trauma-related symptoms such as depression and anxiety (Foa and Rauch 2004).

Table 7.7 Evidence-based treatments for post-traumatic stress disorder

Intervention	Description	References
Prolonged exposure	Addresses fear structure and cognitive distortions through three mechanisms: (1) psychoeducation about trauma, symptoms, and treatment; (2) repeated in vivo and imaginal exposure exercises; and (3) emotional processing. Reduces PTSD intrusion, avoidance, and arousal symptoms through repeated exposure exercises. Imaginal exposure involves verbally recounting the details of the event and processing the thoughts and emotions that emerge. In vivo exposure is conducted in between sessions to cues related to the trauma. Reduces negative alterations in cognitions and mood and increases self-efficacy through cognitive reframing and emotional processing. Effective for a range of populations including adults, veterans, survivors of interpersonal violence, and persons with comorbid substance use issues. Can be used in inpatient, outpatient, and primary care settings.	Foa EB, Hembree E, Rothbaum BO. Prolonged Exposure Therapy for PTSD: Emotional Processing of Traumatic Experiences, Therapist Guide, Oxford University Press, New York 2007
Cognitive processing therapy	Changes maladaptive thinking patterns about the trauma in relation to self, others, and the world to more realistic beliefs that can lead to less emotional reactivity (e.g., fear, anger, and depression) through cognitive reframing and development of more adaptive coping behaviors. Cognitive processing therapy has five focus areas: (1) safety, (2) trust, (3) control, (4) self-esteem, and (5) intimacy. CPT relies on: (1) psychoeducation, (2) imaginal exposure through writing about the trauma (optional), and (3) in-session and home-based activities using thought change records to identify and challenge maladaptive thinking patterns in the five focus areas and replace them with more realistic thoughts that are grounded in facts, evidence, and reality. CPT improves self-efficacy/mastery, coping skills, and the survivor's ability to form healthy relationships while reducing PTSD symptoms (e.g., intrusion, avoidance, negative alterations in cognitions and mood, hyperarousal), depression, and anxiety. Effective for adults and veterans, and appropriate for a range of inpatient and outpatient clinical settings.	Resnick et al. (2016). Cognitive processing therapy for PTSD: A comprehensive manual. New York, NY: Guilford Press
Trauma-focused CBT	TF-CBT incorporates elements of cognitive processing therapy, relaxation, and imaginal exposure and coping skill development. TF-CBT improves ability to enhance safety and manage symptoms and behaviors through: (1) psychoeducation about the cognitive model; (2) development of coping skills including relaxation/deep breathing, assertiveness, forming healthy relationships, and establishing a safety plan; (3) the use of imaginal exposure through the cognitive and emotional processing of a written trauma narrative; (4) parallel family counseling sessions that help caregivers process grief, improve communication around the trauma with their child, and reinforce the work that goes on in therapy. Effective in reducing PTSD, anxiety, depressive symptoms, and behavioral issues. Effective for children and adolescents who have experienced physical and sexual abuse. Approach can be used in inpatient, residential, and outpatient therapy settings.	Mannarino et al. (2012). Trauma-focused cognitive-behavioral therapy for children: Sustained impact of treatment 6 and 12 months later. Child maltreatment, 17(3), 231–241. Doi: https://doi. org/10.1177/1077559512451787

(continued)

Table 7.7 (continued)

Intervention	Description	References
EMDR	Uses a combination of (1) imaginal exposure; (2) emotional and cognitive processing; (3) bi-lateral eye movements where clients visually track an object (e.g., pen, fingers) that the therapist moves slowly, laterally, across their visual field during exposure exercises; and (4) in vivo exposure that focuses on desensitization of external cues for PTSD symptoms between sessions. During imaginal exposure, clients are asked to repeatedly revisit intense moments of the traumatic event in their mind and narrate the thoughts they experienced during the event and the thoughts they currently hold about the event while they simultaneously track an object that the therapist slowly moves across their visual spectrum. The theory of EMDR is the bilateral movement helps clients reduce emotional reactivity related to the trauma, process and resolve traumatic memories, and reframe negative, maladaptive thoughts related to the event such as mistrust of others, self-blame, incompetence, guilt, shame, taking too much responsibility for the event, or lack of control over one's life. Effective for a range of populations including children, adults, and veterans. A brief approach that can be used in inpatient and outpatient settings.	Shapiro (2017). Eye movement desensitization and reprocessing: Basic protocols, principles, (3rd Ed.) Guilford, New York.
C-BITS	C-BITS is a brief, 10–12 session, school-based intervention that provides structured sessions with youth between 9 and 18 years of age who have suffered from trauma. Group sessions consist of: (1) psychoeducation about trauma and how it impacts the mind and body; (2) identifying and reframing maladaptive thoughts related to safety, control, and self-blame (3) teaches coping skills related to problem-solving, emotional regulation, and relaxation; and (4) addresses trauma symptoms through construction and analysis of a trauma narrative that is done one-on-one with a therapist. Therapists also teach psychoeducation and behavior management skills to parents and teachers in parallel sessions. Effective for school-aged children and adolescents.	Jaycox et al. (2012). Cognitive behavioral intervention for trauma in schools. Journal of Applied School Psychology, 28, 239–255.

7.6.3   Psychoeducation

During a course of therapy, information about the cognitive, emotional, and behavioral aspects of trauma and how PE works to mitigate these effects are explained to the client in the first few sessions and reinforced throughout therapy. For instance, during psychoeducation providers explain how fear structures are reinforced through avoidance and how exposure to traumatic memories can challenge this avoidance directly in a safe space and lead to a reduction in symptoms and the creation and integration of a healthier and more realistic counter-narrative to the trauma.

7.6.4   Exposure

Exposure takes two forms. In vivo *exposure* is when clients refrain from avoiding traumatic external stimuli such as places, objects, sounds, and smells associated with the trauma. Clients are asked to routinely and slowly expose themselves to these feared stimuli gradually and in a safe manner. Clients may develop a hierarchy of feared stimuli that they rate from a scale of 1 (low fear) to 100 (high or extreme fear). Clients then work their way up from low fear-producing stimuli to high fear-producing stimuli. Exposure should *never* place the client at risk for re-traumatization or re-victimization. A second type of exposure is *imaginal exposure*. When using imaginal exposure, the therapist asks the client to relive the trauma memory by reimagining the traumatic event and narrating the details of what happened, what they were thinking, and how they felt. Clients are asked to engage with the emotional content of the trauma, and as they recite the memory, they will be asked to describe how they felt at particular moments of the traumatic event (Rauch and Foa 2006). The client will narrate each episode of the trauma from beginning to end using present tense language and highlight parts of the trauma narrative that were particularly intense and distressing. During the narration, the therapist will ask the client to "rate" their distress using a subjective unit of distress scale (SUDS), which is a simple scale of 1–100 with lower scores indicating less distress and higher scores indicating more distress. A SUDS rating is taken at baseline, during distressing elements of the trauma, and then at the end.

7.6.5   Emotional Processing

During and after exposure, therapists work with clients to process emotions related to the trauma through a discussion of how the trauma has impacted their lives and the thoughts and feelings they experience in relation to the trauma. Effective emotional processing of beliefs about the trauma and subjective distress after exposure sessions have been associated with increased improvement in symptoms (Cox et al.

2020). Therapists ask clients to talk about how their beliefs about themselves and others in regard to safety, control, self-efficacy, and relationships have changed since the trauma and then how these views have shifted since the start of therapy. Therapists encourage two to three exposure exercises during each therapy session and also encourage clients to engage in in vivo exposure in between sessions if it is safe to do so. Repeated exposure over time usually results in habituation and a reduction in intensity and intrusiveness of symptoms in 10–12 sessions. Therapists will also teach clients grounding techniques to combat dissociation and numbing that may be associated with trauma as well as relaxation techniques and the use of coping cards in order to help client manage hyperarousal symptoms during and between sessions (Rauch et al. 2012).

7.6.6 Eye Movement Desensitization and Reprocessing (EMDR)

EMDR is highly effective in reducing PTSD, anxiety, dissociation, and depressive symptoms with results similar to PE (Bisson and Andrew 2007; IOM 2008; Rothbaum et al. 2005). EMDR involves the combination of cognitive processing and imaginal exposure and is designed to open up new opportunities to re-process past traumatic events and make more adaptive associations between events and thoughts. The approach also focuses on desensitization of external cues for PTSD symptoms (Shapiro 2017). EMDR can take from 8 to 12 sessions depending on the number of traumatic events. Single traumatic events can be addressed in about 6 sessions. More complex or multiple traumas may take longer to address. EMDR providers take a thorough client history of trauma experiences and identify specific traumatic events and thoughts. Clients also receive psychoeducation on how trauma impacts the mind and body, the EMDR approach, and skills to manage distressing symptoms both at home and during sessions. These skills can include progressive relaxation or mindfulness-based approaches to managing distress.

EMDR is designed to help clients reduce emotional reactivity related to the trauma, process and resolve traumatic memories, and reframe negative, maladaptive thoughts related to the event. The client is asked to engage in an imaginal exposure exercise where they revisit the traumatic event in their mind and narrate the thoughts they experienced during the event and the thoughts they currently hold about the event. These thoughts may include themes such as mistrust of others, self-blame, incompetence, guilt, shame, taking too much responsibility for the event, or lack of control over one's life. They are also asked to identify bodily, physical, and emotional sensations related to the distress. Clients are asked to identify a more positive belief they would like to hold about the event and themselves in relation to the traumatic event. They are asked to rate the level of their belief in the positive thought on a scale of 1–10, with 1 being no belief and 10 being complete belief in the thought.

As the client focuses on the thoughts, anxiety and heightened physical hyper-arousal from the event, they are simultaneously asked to focus their attention on visually tracking an object (e.g., pen, fingers) that the therapist slowly moves later-ally across their visual field. The client is asked to just notice their bodily sensations and thoughts as they focus on the event and track the object. The provider and client may engage in these stimulation sessions for various lengths. At the end, the pro-vider asks the client to just let go of all of their thoughts, take deep breaths, and then just notice and report what feelings, thoughts, images, or sensations come into their minds. This process occurs until habituation, or the reduction in arousal, is achieved. The client and therapist may engage in repeated sets during one session. Once the anxiety has been reduced, the client is asked to name a maladaptive thought experi-enced during the trauma and replace it with a more adaptive thought. For instance, "It's all my fault," is replaced with "I did the best I could with the knowledge I had at the time,", or "It was an accident – I am not responsible for what happened." The maladaptive thought of "bad things happen to bad people" may be replaced with "bad things can happen to anyone," or "something bad happened to me, but it does not define who I am." The thought "I was weak and powerless" can be replaced with "I have survived something terrible. It has not broken me and it is in the past." When the anxiety or distress has been reduced for the target memory, the provider will ask the client to re-rate their level of belief in the positive thought they identified and then use that thought to focus on additional distressing memories.

The theory behind EMDR is that the bilateral movement helps to both distract the client and reduce emotional tension, while helping the client to access the trau-matic memory. Accessing the memory provides the client with an opportunity to make associations between the memory and more adaptive thoughts or information. The taking in of new information and making new, more adaptive associations leads to resolution or a more complete and accurate understanding of the events. This resolution can then lead to a sense of relief and a reduction in distress, arousal, and avoidance behaviors (Shapiro 2017).

7.6.7 Cognitive Processing Therapy (CPT)

Experiencing traumatic events can impact how you view yourself (e.g., competent vs incompetent), others (e.g., trustworthy vs untrustworthy), and the world (e.g., safe vs dangerous). Cognitive processing therapy focuses on scrutinizing and chal-lenging maladaptive thoughts related to the trauma that can lead to negative emo-tions and problematic, unhealthy avoidance behaviors (Resnick et al. 2016). Maladaptive beliefs about the self, others, and world that exist prior to the trauma can be either confirmed or shattered by the event, leading to maladaptive thinking and coping patterns. For instance, the goal of CPT is to change maladaptive thinking patterns about the trauma to more realistic beliefs that can lead to less emotional reactivity (e.g., fear, anger, depression) and teach more adaptive coping behaviors. The approach uses psychoeducation, imaginal exposure through writing about the trauma, and a series of in-session and home-based activities using thought-change records and other worksheets and assignments designed to identify and challenge maladaptive thinking patterns and replace them with more realistic thoughts that are grounded in facts, evidence, and reality. The approach is designed to improve self-efficacy, safety, coping skills, and the survivor's ability to form healthy, trusting relationships while also reducing avoidance, depression, and anxiety symptoms (Resnick et al. 2014, 2016).

Treatment begins with a careful history of traumatic events and psychoeducation about how trauma and maladaptive thinking patterns impact the self and relationships with others based in emotional processing and social cognitive learning theory. The therapy quickly moves to the development of an impact statement written by the client that outlines their views of why the trauma happened and how the trauma has changed their lives in relation to self-esteem, functioning, relationships, emotions, thoughts, and behaviors. The client is then asked to write a full account of the traumatic event that includes sensory details such as sights, sounds, smells, as well as thoughts and emotions experienced during the event. The client is asked to read the account every day, and they are encouraged to experience the feelings they have without avoiding them. The client also revises the account as new details and information emerges. The provider then collaborates with the client to identify maladaptive thinking patterns and cognitive distortions. Cognitive distortions include all-or-nothing thinking, overgeneralizing, negative filtering, or thinking that is biased toward overemphasis on negative information and ignoring evidence of positive traits, accomplishments, or developments.

Cognitive processing therapy has five focus areas: (1) safety, (2) trust, (3) control, (4) self-esteem, and (5) intimacy. The first focus area, safety, includes many common maladaptive thoughts about safety in relation to self and others. In this focus area, providers and clients identify and challenge unrealistic beliefs about safety so that they are more balanced. These beliefs can include irrational expectations about personal vulnerability, the perceived ability to control one's safety, and the overestimation of the dangerousness of other people and the outer world. These irrational beliefs can lead to anxiety, social withdrawal, and impairment of interpersonal functioning (Resnick et al. 2016).

The second focus area deals with the trust of one's own judgment and the intent of other people. Trauma can lead to maladaptive beliefs around trust such as, "I must exercise perfect judgment all the time," "I cannot trust myself to make any decisions," and "I cannot trust others intentions because people are only out for themselves." These thoughts can cause problems in interpersonal functioning and lead to self-doubt, anger, fear of being left behind, anxiety, and suspiciousness (Resnick et al. 2014, 2016).

The third focus area identifies and challenges maladaptive thoughts around power and control. These usually deal with beliefs about over-control (e.g., I need to have perfect control at all times over all situations), or helplessness (I have no control over anything that happens to me). Symptoms associated with these beliefs can include numbing, problems with boundaries, avoidance, or feelings of anger, passivity, submissiveness/lack of assertiveness, self-destructive behaviors, and anger. In this section, people learn balance and how to know what they can and cannot control, how to share power and set limits with others to improve functioning in relationships (Resnick et al. 2014, 2016).

The fourth area focuses on identifying and challenging unrealistic and negative beliefs about the self, such as beliefs of worthlessness and unlovability that can lead to shame, guilt, anxiety, depression, self-destructive behavior, fear of being alone, panic, dependency in relationships, and avoidance through drugs or alcohol. Trauma can shatter positive beliefs about the self, or it can radically (and unrealistically) ratify previously held negative views of the self. Maladaptive beliefs can include "bad things happen to bad people so I am bad because this happened to me," or "what happened is all my fault and I deserved it." Corrective thoughts can include "bad things happen to good people," "My trauma doesn't make me a bad person or undeserving of happiness," "People make mistakes, they aren't defined by them and no one deserves to be harmed," and "Bad things happen and sometimes there is no explanation." Self-esteem is also related to a person's perceived ability to cope with the effects of trauma. This module focuses on identifying and challenging unrealistic views of the self and building self-soothing skills (Resnick et al. 2014, 2016).

The fifth area focuses on repairing the ability to connect with the self and others that involve both feeling comfortable with oneself and developing healthy intimate relationships with others. Trauma disrupts the ability to form relationships and connections with oneself and other people leading to loneliness, alienation, emptiness, and social isolation. This increases the risk of self-destructive behaviors, including substance use and suicide as well as anger, aggression, and emotional numbing. Healthy intimate relationships involve taking risks and being vulnerable, which are areas that are impacted by trauma. This area challenges unrealistic thoughts about intimate relationships (e.g., "My problems are all my fault") and helps people develop the communication skills needed to nurture intimate relationships (Resnick et al. 2014, 2016).

In each of the above areas, clients learn how to identify and challenge maladaptive thinking patterns. After learning about common cognitive distortions that keep people stuck, clients learn skills in identifying and challenging these distortions when they happen in real time. Through the repeated deployment of thought change records and Socratic questioning as homework, clients identify, challenge, and reframe distorted thinking patterns in real-life situations and then discuss these events in session. Questions used to challenge problematic beliefs and thinking patterns include: What is the evidence for and against your beliefs? Does your belief include all of the facts and information or does it focus on only one part of the story? Are there other ways of thinking about this? What cognitive distortions might be operating here? Is there evidence of extreme beliefs (e.g., always, perfect, never)? Is this belief more rooted in facts or feelings/habits? What would be an alternative way of thinking about this situation in a more balanced way that includes all of the facts? These questions are used to loosen associations between maladaptive thoughts and emotional reactions and invites the client to substitute and try out an alternative thought that is more fact-based and balanced, leading to a reduction in negative emotions, reactivity, and avoidance (Resnick et al. 2014, 2016).

7.6.8   Trauma-Focused Cognitive Behavioral Therapy (TF-CBT)

TF-CBT is a very well-established cognitive behavioral therapy and is a top-tier evidence-based practice for treating trauma in children and youth (Bisson and Andrew 2007; Silverman et al. 2008). TF-CBT has been found to reduce PTSD-related symptoms such as abuse-related distress, behavioral issues, anxiety, and depression (Mannarino et al. 2012). It incorporates elements of cognitive processing therapy, relaxation, and imaginal exposure. In TF-CBT, clients are first provided psychoeducation about trauma symptoms, health, and the cognitive behavioral model of PTSD. They are then taught several coping skills designed to improve their ability to enhance safety and manage symptoms and behaviors such as relaxation, deep breathing, assertiveness, forming healthy relationships, and establishing a safety plan. Once children have a firm grasp of trauma's effect on the mind and body and have practices and learned coping behaviors, they are asked write a narrative (e.g., story, picture book, poem, lyrics) about their trauma that identifies all of the different parts of the memory including sensory information, thoughts, behaviors, and feelings. The client is asked to then revise the narrative again and again as the therapist and child work together to reframe negative thoughts about the event regarding safety, trust, responsibility, healthy relationships, and self-esteem. At the end of the story, the child re-writes the future in positive terms in order to integrate the event as something that is only one part of the child's life. The child reads the story repeatedly with the therapist one-on-one. The child will also read the story to caregivers at the end of therapy when appropriate. Parents are given family counseling sessions that help them talk about the event with their child and reinforce the work that goes on in therapy (Cohen et al. 2006, 2012; Deblinger et al. 2011; Mannarino et al. 2012).

TF-CBT occurs in three general phases. In phase one, providers focus on developing coping skills with clients. During this phase the client and provider build trust and develop a supportive, therapeutic working relationship. Usually, the first component of this phase is psychoeducation about trauma, the cognitive model of trauma and identifying the cues that can trigger traumatic responses (Cohen et al. 2006). During psychoeducation providers and clients work together to identify key themes about the trauma or themes that cut across multiple traumas. These themes will be addressed throughout therapy and guide treatment choices. For instance, themes about lack of safety and being able to trust others, or themes of self-blame may be important areas of exploration throughout therapy. Providers also offer parallel skills sessions with non-offending caregivers, offering them psychoeducation about trauma, parenting skills designed to create safe and supportive environments and to correct maladaptive thinking patterns toward themselves (e.g., "I should have protected him better," This is my fault") and the youth (e.g., "He's using the trauma as an excuse"), and to utilize effective methods for managing behavioral issues and emotional dysregulation.

Clients are also taught relaxation skills and coping skills to manage negative thinking patterns and emotional dysregulation. Relaxation skills can include breathing exercises, progressive muscle relaxation, yoga, and mindfulness approaches and imagery work. Affective coping skills are taught and modeled to teach youth how to appropriately express positive and negative emotions. This may include teaching youth how to identify emotions and express them appropriately through role-plays and modeling. To increase the ability to tolerate distressing emotions and manage affective dysregulation, providers teach youth distraction strategies (e.g., exercise, playing games, contacting friends), mindfulness strategies (e.g., identifying feelings or sensations and viewing them without judgment), strategies to identify emotions in other people, and cognitive coping strategies that help youth identify negative thoughts and replace them with a more accurate and positive thoughts or interpretations. These coping skills are also reviewed with caregivers in parallel sessions so that they can utilize and reinforce them in the home.

This phase concludes with a focus on enhancing safety and developing safety plans. Safety plans include: (1) understanding how to protect one's self and avoid danger through personal safety skills; (2) accessing external resources for assistance with needs (i.e., how to ask for help); (3) addressing self-harm and reckless behaviors; (4) educating caregivers about triggers; (5) appropriate behavioral responses to dysregulation that can lead to an enhanced sense of safety and security; (6) identifying and developing nurturing relationships with trusting and safe adults in the community; and (7) developing a repertoire of activities that enhance well-being and help to develop healthy interpersonal relationships. For clients with complex trauma and ongoing threats such as being in a residential care facility, enhancing safety and developing a safety plan may be covered in the first part of phase one (Cohen et al. 2012).

Phase two involves developing and processing the trauma narrative (TN). The skills in phase one are implemented in order to prepare youth to successfully navigate the stress and emotional content of processing trauma memories. Youth can begin phase 2 when they have a good ability to self-regulate emotions. This phase is not always provided in TF-CBT. Studies have found that providing TF-CBT without this phase has been associated with better behavioral management and fewer externalizing behaviors in the home. This may be due to the overemphasis in parenting behaviors. However, inclusion of the TN has been associated with less anxiety, fear, and abuse-specific distress (Deblinger et al. 2011).

The trauma narrative can be written as a storybook, play, poem, or song or other written form of narrative depending on the age of the child. Single event traumas focus on the sensory, emotional, and cognitive aspects of the event itself, while complex trauma can involve themes that have been identified by the client that cut across multiple traumas. Development of the trauma narrative occurs as a collaboration over several sessions between provider and client. The provider also shares elements of the narrative development process with the caregiver in parallel sessions. This is done to prepare the caregiver to hear the narrative in a conjoint session with the client and to educate and inform the caregiver about how the trauma was experienced by the youth. Silence and avoidance are often a part of trauma, and caregivers may not understand the nuances of how the client has experienced the events. The purpose of developing the trauma narrative is for the youth to develop new meaning and understanding of the trauma as well as become habituated to the event through repeated imaginal exposure while the narrative is written. Like prolonged exposure, this phase may also involve the creation of a fear hierarchy and gradual in-vivo exposure exercises to external elements related to the trauma that are subjects of avoidance by the client such as situations (e.g., being alone, the dark), places (e.g., school, playground), or people.

Phase three includes consolidation and closure exercises. In this phase the client shares their trauma narrative with their caregiver in a conjoint session. The purpose of sharing the narrative with a caregiver is to transfer trust built with the therapist to the caregiver and for the youth to trust that the caregiver can handle the trauma and respond supportively. The therapist continues to meet with the youth as they implement what was learned in session and to troubleshoot any setbacks or problems that may arise. Grief work may also be implemented in this phase to help the youth cope with losses they have experienced that they have not been able to adequately process due to their trauma.

EMDR and TF-CBT have both been found to significantly improve clinical symptoms and may be associated with positive improvements in brain connectivity and functioning (Diehle et al. 2015; Santarnecchi et al. 2019). One benefit of each approach is the "distance" that they create between the client and the trauma. For instance, TF-CBT creates distance through writing of the trauma narrative vs speaking it. While EMDR's exposure has the client speak about the event, the client is asked only to relay the most distressing part of the trauma in short, staccato bursts while being distracted with the bilateral visual tracking.

7.6.9 Cognitive Behavioral Intervention for Trauma in Schools (C-BITS)

Accessing treatment for trauma in children can be difficult, especially for low-income and underserved youth who have experienced stress and trauma and often lack access to behavioral health services. As a result, there has been a rise in school-based programs designed to offer free, brief, culturally tailored treatment in school settings. Schools represent a stable environment where youth can access highly competent mental health services during school hours that can improve symptoms and behavior without burdening caregivers with extra costs related to treatment fees, child and elder care, transportation, and taking unpaid sick time. School-based treatments are inexpensive, effective, and accessible. Providing mental health services in schools can provide youth with access to mental health services to address educational and behavioral health problems they would not otherwise be able to access (Alegria et al. 2015; Atkins et al. 2006; Pfeiffer and Goldbeck 2017). These early intervention opportunities can reduce health disparities in children of color and can lead to educational and socioeconomic benefits (Alegria et al. 2015; Sawhill and Karpilow 2014).

One such approach is the Cognitive Behavioral Intervention for Trauma in Schools (C-BITS) (Allison and Ferreira 2017; Jaycox et al. 2012; Kataoka et al. 2003; Stein et al. 2003). C-BITS has been found to improve psychosocial and academic functioning and reduce symptoms of trauma and depression in youth and has also been found to be effective in immigrant and refugee populations (Allison and Ferreira 2017; Jaycox et al. 2012; Kataoka et al. 2003; Stein et al. 2003). C-BITS is a brief, 10–12 session, school-based intervention that provides structured sessions with youth between 9 and 18 years of age. Group sessions consist of: (1) psychoeducation about trauma and how it impacts the mind and body; (2) identifying and reframing maladaptive thoughts related to safety, control, and self-blame (3) teaching coping skills related to problem-solving, emotional regulation, and relaxation; and (4) addressing trauma symptoms through construction and analysis of a trauma narrative that is done one-on-one with a therapist. Therapists also teach psychoeducation and behavior management skills to parents and teachers in parallel sessions. The approach is very effective in reducing symptoms, increasing psychosocial functioning, and has an excellent retention rate (Allison and Ferreira 2017; Jaycox et al. 2010).

Other school-based options for children can include the use of somatic approaches. Trauma can lead to increase in physiological arousal (e.g., elevated heart rate, racing thoughts, anxiety, aggression, freezing or numbing, and dissociation) (Ogden and Minton 2000). This arousal can endure long after the event has taken place, disrupting a child's ability to function and regulate emotions, leading to problem behaviors, learning difficulties, depression, and anxiety (Buckner et al. 2009; Warner et al. 2013). This dysregulation can also interfere with a child's ability to successfully engage with language-based cognitive behavioral trauma interventions because they require a high degree of emotional and physical regulation (Perry 2009; Raio et al. 2013). Interventions that rely primarily on physical and somatic activities such as grounding exercises (e.g., lightly tapping on extremities and putting feet firmly on the floor), stretching and movements exercises (e.g., yoga, martial arts), and relaxation and mindfulness exercises (e.g., deep breathing, muscle relaxation), can help children learn coping skills that can help them regulate their emotions and prepare them for language-based interventions (Corrigan et al. 2011; Mancini 2020; Farina and Mancini 2017; Perry 2009; van der Kolk 2015; Warner et al. 2014).

7.7 Summary and Conclusions

The experience of trauma and adverse events in childhood represent one of the most significant social predictors of negative health outcomes. Trauma can lead to a range of physical and behavioral health problems including depression, anxiety, PTSD, addiction, diabetes, cancer, and heart disease. These poor health outcomes combined with higher rates of suicide, substance use, smoking, sedentary life style, and unhealthy eating lead to significant rates of morbidity and early mortality. The experience of ACEs significantly increases the risk of illness and early death. Fortunately, several cognitive behavioral-based interventions have been shown to decrease the symptomatic effects of traumatic stress including prolonged exposure, trauma-focused CBT, cognitive processing therapy, EMDR, and C-BITS. Unfortunately, like many other behavioral health disorders, accessing effective treatment has been a problem for people who suffer the consequences of trauma. Trauma-informed care approaches in health and school-based settings that include creating safe care environments that routinely utilize screening and assessment approaches can identify people in need of treatment. Once identified, helping people access treatment on-site or through coordinated referrals can lower the risk of illness and premature mortality in clients who suffer from partial and full PTSD. Trauma prevention includes investment in programs that promote healthy parenting, prenatal and postnatal care, access to child care and early childhood education, and the creation of healthy, resourced schools where children and youth can easily access trauma-informed approaches to care that represent efficacious and cost-effective ways to reduce the impact of trauma on children and families and promote healthy communities.

Case Study 7.1: Dr. Tracey Williams
Dr. Tracey Williams[1] is a 35-year-old black transgender & gender nonconforming (TGNC) person referred to an outpatient behavioral health counseling agency from the victims' advocacy bureau for behavioral health symptoms related to a recent traumatic event. Tracey identifies as gender non-binary and uses the pronouns they/them/their. Tracey is a peer counselor and instructor in the human services department of a large community college system. Tracey is also a certified yoga instructor. Tracey is an advocate for young, transgender youth. They also lead a yoga class exclusively for transgender persons. They enjoy biking, working out, cooking, painting, and teaching. They say that their teaching is the most important act they do as a human being. It is their passion and their life's work. Tracey and their partner were both assaulted by a group of four, white cis-gendered men in their twenties while walking home from a restaurant one evening. The men passed them on the opposite side of the street and then followed them for several blocks yelling racist slurs and anti-TGNC insults. They eventually surrounded Tracey and their partner and told them they were going to "get what they deserve." Two of the men held Tracey while the other two punched and kicked their partner who suffered facial lacerations, a fractured left orbital, and several bruised ribs. Tracey was also slapped and punched several times in the face and kicked while they were on the ground, suffering lacerations, bruises, a mild concussion, and a cracked tooth. The assault

---

[1] All names and other identifiers of this case have been changed to protect privacy and confidentiality.

was interrupted when a passing car stopped and the men scattered. The passengers called 911. The police have not found the assailants.

At intake, Tracey states: "I was sure I was going to die and I am quite convinced that if that car did not stop when it did they would have raped one or both of us first, before killing us. That's what they told us they were going to do. I do not doubt their intent. I remember bits and pieces of the actual assault. The fear I felt when they were following us. Their words were vile, but quite frankly, I've heard it all before. It was the edge in their voice. It was…determined, drunk and angry. I have learned to recognize that edge from the more routine hate that I receive. I knew then they weren't going away. I remember the smell of the awful, cheap cologne the one who held my arms was wearing. I remember watching them beat my partner. I remember when they punched them in the face, the sound of it, and the way their head snapped back. I thought they were dead at that moment and I remember wishing right then and there that they would just kill me, too. The police came. More white men with their smirks and lack of compassion. As a black trans person – the police are not my friends. Hospital staff. Same. You would expect a bit of sensitivity given that this was an attempted lynching. Some acknowledgement of the horror we just experienced as a couple. Nothing. Robots. I may expect it – but it still shocks me – the lack of compassion I experience - the *depth* of it. I've learned through past therapy that it says more about them than me. But I still feel rage. What happened to us was a hate crime and it didn't even make the local paper. A hate crime and they have no leads even though they have a description from four witnesses. I think about what happened all day. Every day and every night I wait for them to come back to finish the job. I see them everywhere I go - grocery store, gym, running in the park. I stopped going out. I don't want to go out any more. I feel like my body is a target more than usual. I feel like they are still out there because *they are* and that they could just come up on me one day and say, "hey, remember us?" And not just *them*, but anyone. If it happened once, why not again with a new set of psychos? I feel like anyone can do anything to me and get away with it. I am on guard all day long. I'm irritable and exhausted. I have nightmares every night. I think they are going to be one of my students or I will see one of them on campus. They were about that age. Maybe I will hear their laughter – I still hear it every day. I do know that when one of my students walks in with that same nasty cologne on I am going to lose it, I just know it. The daily experience of being black and trans is something I have weathered my whole life, but now I just can't cope with it. I don't go out anymore. I work from home as much as I can. My partner and I fight all the time because their "over it" and I want to talk about it and they don't. They aren't over it, by the way. Their nightmares are worse than mine. They're in denial. But that is how they deal with things. They have a gun now that they carry and they say it makes them feel safer. Part of me is a little jealous – I wish it were that easy for me. It has been over two months of this. I am exhausted. When will it end?"

The counselor asks Tracey what they want to accomplish as part of their therapy. Tracey does not mix their words.

Tracey: I have been in counseling my whole life. I know what is possible. I want to feel safe. I want to sleep. I want the thoughts and the ruminations to stop. I do not want to take psychiatric medication. I want to be able to concentrate and work and write. I want to go about my business without fear. I want to stop being angry and afraid at people who are not worth it. I want to breathe deep. I want to smile and laugh and talk to my partner about what has happened to us and to talk to our friends about what happened to us. I am frozen in time. I want to thaw. Can you help me do that, please? I like the symbols you have around here that tell me that this is supposedly a safe space for someone like me, but I have learned that the mental health profession struggles helping people with identities like mine. If you cannot help me, please tell me now so I can find someone who can. I do not have time to waste.

Case Analysis and Guiding Questions

What does trauma-informed care look like for Tracey?

What specific symptoms is Tracey currently experiencing?

Do their symptoms meet criteria for one or more behavioral health disorders and, if so, which one(s)?

What are specific treatment outcome goals and objectives that would be relevant for Tracey given the information provided in this case?

What symptoms will you specifically target?

What interventions will you utilize that were covered in this chapter to address those symptoms?

What strengths and resources will you rely on when working with Tracey?

How will you ensure that Tracey receives care that is affirming, sensitive, and responsive to their multiple identities?

What obstacles exist for providers who are cis-gendered in forming a therapeutic and affirming relationship with Tracey?

References

Alegria, M., Greif-Green, J., McLaughlin, K. A., & Loder, S. (2015). *Disparities in child and adolescent mental health and mental health services in the U.S.* New York: The William T Grant Foundation.

Allison, A. C., & Ferreira, R. J. (2017). Implementing cognitive behavioral intervention for trauma in schools (CBITS) with Latino youth. *Child and Adolescent Social Work Journal, 34,* 181–189.

American Psychiatric Association. (2013). *Diagnostic and statistical manual of mental disorders, fifth edition (DSM-5).* Arlington: American Psychiatric Association.

American Psychological Association. (2017). Clinical practice guideline for the treatment of post-traumatic stress disorder (PTSD) in adults. Retrieved from https://www.apa.org/ptsd-guideline/ptsd.pdf

Anda, R. F., Croft, J. B., Felitti, V. J., Nordenberg, D., Giles, W. H., Williamson, D. F., & Giovino, G. A. (1999). Adverse childhood experiences and smoking during adolescence and adulthood. *JAMA, 282,* 1652–1658.

Anda, R. F., Felitti, V. J., Bremner, J. D., Walker, J. D., Whitfield, C., Perry, B. D…Giles, W. H. et al. (2006). The enduring effects of abuse and related adverse experiences in childhood: A convergence of evidence from neurobiology and epidemiology. European Archives of Psychiatry and Clinical Neuroscience, 256(3), 174–186. doi:https://doi.org/10.1007/s00406-005-0624-4.

Anda, R. F., Brown, D. W., Dube, S. R., Bremner, J. D., Felitti, V. J., & Giles, W. H. (2008). Adverse childhood experiences and chronic obstructive pulmonary disease in adults. *American Journal of Preventative Medicine, 34*(5), 396–403.

Atkins, M. S., Frazier, S. L., Birman, D., Abdul Adil, J., Jackson, M., Gracyk, P. A., et al. (2006). School-based mental health services for children living in high poverty urban communities. *Administration and Policy in Mental Health and Mental Health Services Research, 33*(2), 146–159.

Benight, C. C., & Bandura, A. (2004). Social cognitive theory of post-traumatic recovery: The role of perceived self-efficacy. *Behavior Research and Therapy, 42,* 1129–1148.

Bisson, J. I., Roberts, N. P., Andrew, M., Cooper, R., & Lewis, C. (2013). Psychological therapies for chronic post-traumatic stress disorder (PTSD) in adults. *Cochrane Database of Systematic Reviews, 2013(12),* Art. No.: CD003388. https://doi.org/10.1002/14651858.CD003388.pub4.

Bisson, J., & Andrew, M. (2007). Psychological treatment of post-traumatic stress disorder (PTSD). The Cochrane database of systematic reviews, (3), CD003388. https://doi.org/10.1002/14651858.CD003388.pub3

Blake, D. D., Weathers, F. W., Nagy, L. M., Kaloupek, D. G., Gusman, F. D., Charney, D. S., & Keane, T. M. (1995). The development of a clinician-administered PTSD scale. *Journal of Traumatic Stress, 8*(1), 75–90. https://doi.org/10.1007/BF02105408.

Blevins, C. A., Weathers, F. W., Davis, M. T., Witte, T. K., & Domino, J. L. (2015). The posttraumatic stress disorder checklist for DSM-5 (PCL-5): Development and initial psychometric evaluation. *Journal of Traumatic Stress, 28*, 489–498. http://dx.doi.org.ezp.slu.edu/10.1002/jts.22059.

Bovin, M. J., Marx, B. P., Weathers, F. W., Gallagher, M. W., Rodriguez, P., Schnurr, P. P., & Keane, T. M. (2016). Psychometric properties of the PTSD checklist for diagnostic and statistical manual of mental disorders-fifth edition (PCL-5) in veterans. *Psychological Assessment, 28*, 1379–1391. http://dx.doi.org.ezp.slu.edu/10.1037/pas0000254.

Bronfebrenner, U., & Morris, P. A. (2007). The bioecological model of human development. *Handbook of Child Psychology.* https://doi.org/10.1002/9780470147658.chpsy0114.

Bronfenbrenner, U. (1979). *The ecology of human development: Experiments by nature and design.* Cambridge, MA: Harvard University Press.

Bronfenbrenner, U. (2009). *The ecology of human development: Experiments by nature and design.* Cambridge, MA: Harvard University Press.

Brown, M. J., Thacker, L. R., & Cohen, S. A. (2013). Association between adverse childhood experiences and diagnosis of cancer. *PLoS One, 8*(6), e65524. https://doi.org/10.1371/journal.pone.0065524.

Buckner, J. C., Mezacappa, E., & Beardslee, W. R. (2009). Self-regulation and its relations to adaptive functioning in low income youths. *American Journal of Orthopsychiatry, 79*(1), 19–30. https://doi.org/10.1037/a0014796.

Burke-Harris, N. (2018). *The deepest well: Healing the long-term effects of childhood adversity.* New York: Houghton Mifflin Harcourt.

Cigrang, J. A., Rauch, S. A., Avila, L. L., Bryan, C. J., Goodie, J. L., Hryshko-Mullen, A., & Peterson, A. L. (2011). Treatment of active-duty military with PTSD in primary care: Early findings. *Psychological Services, 8*(2), 104–113. https://doi.org/10.1037/a0022740.

Coffey, S. F., Schumacher, J. A., Nosen, E., Littlefield, A. K., Henslee, A. M., Lappen, A., & Stasiewicz, P. R. (2016). Trauma-focused exposure therapy for chronic posttraumatic stress disorder in alcohol and drug dependent patients: A randomized controlled trial. *Psychology of addictive behaviors: Journal of the Society of Psychologists in Addictive Behaviors, 30*(7), 778–790. https://doi.org/10.1037/adb0000201.

Cohen, J. A., Mannarino, A. P., & Deblinger, E. (2006). *Treating trauma and traumatic grief in children and adolescents.* New York: The Guilford Press.

Cohen, J. A., Mannatino, A. P., Kliethermes, M., & Murray, L. A. (2012). Trauma-focused CBT for youth with complex trauma. *Child Abuse and Neglect, 36*(6), 528–541.

Corrigan, F. M., Fisher, J. J., & Nutt, D. J. (2011). Autonomic dysregulation and the window of tolerance model of the effects of complex emotional trauma. *Journal of Psychopharmacology, 25*(1), 17–25. https://doi.org/10.1177/0269881109354930.

Cox, K. S., Wangelin, B. C., Keller, S. M., Lozano, B. E., Murphy, M. M., Maher, E. K., et al. (2020). Emotional processing of imaginal exposures predicts symptom improvement: Therapist ratings can assess trajectory in prolonged exposure for posttraumatic stress disorder. *Journal of Traumatic Stress.* https://doi.org/10.1002/jts.22493. [Epub ahead of print].

Cronholm, P. F., Forke, C. M., Wade, R., et al. (2015). Adverse childhood experiences: Expanding the concept of adversity. *American Journal of Prevention Medicine, 49*, 354–361.

Deblinger, E., Mannarino, A. P., Cohen, J. A., Runyon, M. K., & Steer, R. A. (2011). Trauma-focused cognitive behavioral therapy for children: Impact of the trauma narrative and treatment length. *Depression and Anxiety, 28*(1), 67–75. https://doi.org/10.1002/da.20744.

Deschenes, S. S., Graham, E., Kivimaki, M., & Schmitz, N. (2018). Averse childhood experiences and the risk of diabetes: Examining the roles of depressive symptoms and cardiometabolic dysregulations in the Whitehall II cohort study. *Diabetes Care, 41*(10), 2120–2126.

Diehle, J., Opmeer, B. C., Boer, F., Mannarino, A. P., & Lindaur, R. J. L. (2015). Trauma-focused cognitive behavioral therapy or eye movement desensitization and reprocessing: What works in children with posttraumatic stress symptoms? A randomized controlled trial. *European Child and Adolescent Psychiatry, 24*, 227–236.

Difede, J., Olden, M., & Cukor, J. (2014). Evidence-based treatment of post-traumatic stress disorder. *Annual Review of Medicine, 65*, 319–332. https://doi.org/10.1146/annurev-med-051812-145438.

Dong, M., Giles, W. H., Felitti, V. J., Dube, S. R., Williams, J. E., Chapman, D. P., & Anda, R. F. (2004). Insights into causal pathways for ischemic heart disease: Adverse childhood experiences study. *Circulation, 110*, 1761–1766.

Dube, S. R., Anda, R. F., Felitti, V. J., Chapman, D. P., Williamson, D. F., & Giles, W. H. (2001). Childhood abuse, household dysfunction, and the risk of attempted suicide throughout the life span: Findings from the adverse childhood experiences study. *JAMA, 286*(24), 3089–3096. https://doi.org/10.1001/jama.286.24.3089.

Dube, S. R., Felitti, V. J., Dong, M., Chapman, D. P., Giles, W. H., & Anda, R. F. (2003). Childhood abuse, neglect and household dysfunction and the risk of illicit drug use: The adverse childhood experience study. *Pediatrics, 111*(3), 564–572.

Dube, S. R., Fairweather, D., Pearson, W. S., Felitti, V. J., Anda, R. F., & Croft, J. B. (2009). Cumulative childhood stress and autoimmune disease. *Psychosomatic Medicine, 71*, 243–250.

Edwards, V. J., Holden, G. W., Felitti, V. J., & Anda, R. F. (2003). Relationship between multiple forms of childhood maltreatment and adult mental health in community respondents: Results from the adverse childhood experiences study. *American Journal of Psychiatry, 160*(8), 1453–1460.

Elliott, D. E., Bjelajac, P., Fallot, R. D., Markoff, L. S., & Reed, B. G. (2005). Trauma-informed or trauma-denied: Principles and implementation of trauma-informed services for women. *Journal of Community Psychology, 33*(4), 461–477.

Farina, A., & Mancini, M. A. (2017). Evaluation of a multi-phase trauma-focused intervention with Latino youth. *Advances in Social Work, 18*(1), 270–283. https://doi.org/10.18060/21296.

Felitti, V. J., & Anda, R. F. (2010). The relationship of adverse childhood experiences to adult health, well being, social function and health care. (Chapter 8 pp. 77–87). In R. A. Lanius, E. Vermetten, & C. Pain (Eds.), *The impact of early life trauma on health and disease: The hidden epidemic*. Cambridge: Cambridge University Press.

Felitti, G., Anda, R., Nordenberg, D., et al. (1998). Relationship of child abuse and household dysfunction to many of the leading cause of death in adults: The adverse childhood experiences study. *American Journal of Preventive Medicine, 14*, 245–258.

Finkelhor, D., Shattuck, A., Turner, H., & Hamby, S. (2015). A revised inventory of adverse childhood experiences. *Child Abuse & Neglect, 48*, 13–21. https://doi.org/10.1016/j.chiabu.2015.07.011.

Foa, E. B., & Kozak, M. J. (1986). Emotional processing of fear: Exposure to corrective information. *Psychological Bulletin, 99*(1), 20–35. https://doi.org/10.1037/0033-2909.99.1.20.

Foa, E. B., & Riggs, D. S. (1995). Posttraumatic stress disorder following assault: Theoretical considerations and empirical findings. *Current Directions in Psychological Science, 4*(2), 61–65. https://doi.org/10.1111/1467-8721.ep10771786.

Foa, E. B., Huppert, J. D., & Cahill, S. P. (2006). Emotional processing theory: An update. In B. O. Rothbaum (Ed.), *Pathological anxiety: Emotional processing in etiology and treatment* (pp. 3–24). New York: The Guilford Press.

Foa, E. B., Hembree, E., & Rothbaum, B. O. (2007). *Prolonged exposure therapy for PTSD: Emotional processing of traumatic experiences: A therapist guide*. New York: Oxford University Press.

Foa, E. B., Yusko, D. A., McLean, C. P., Suvak, M. K., Bux, D. A., Oslin, D., et al. (2013). Concurrent naltrexone and prolonged exposure therapy for patients with comorbid alcohol dependence and PTSD: A randomized clinical trial. *JAMA, 310*(5), 488–495.

Foa, E. B., McLean, C. P., Zang, Y., Zhong, J., Powers, M. B., Kauffman, B. Y., Rauch, S., Porter, K., & Knowles, K. (2016a). Psychometric properties of the posttraumatic diagnostic symptom scale interview for DSM–5 (PSSI–5). *Psychological Assessment, 28*(10), 1159–1165. https://doi.org/10.1037/pas0000259.

Foa, E. B., McLean, C. P., Zang, Y., Zhong, J., Powers, M. B., Kauffman, B. Y., Rauch, S., Porter, K., & Knowles, K. (2016b). Psychometric properties of the posttraumatic diagnostic scale for DSM–5 (PDS–5). *Psychological Assessment, 28*(10), 1166–1171. https://doi.org/10.1037/pas0000258.

Foa, E. B., Keane, T. M., Friedman, M. J., & Cohen, J. A. (Eds.). (2009). Effective treatments for PTSD: Practice guidelines from the International Society for Traumatic Stress Studies (2nd ed.). The Guilford Press.

Foa, E. B., & Rauch, S. A. (2004). Cognitive changes during prolonged exposure versus prolonged exposure plus cognitive restructuring in female assault survivors with posttraumatic stress disorder. Journal of consulting and clinical psychology, 72(5), 879–884. https://doi.org/10.1037/0022-006X.72.5.879

Goldstein, R. B., Smith, S. M., Chou, S. P., Saha, T. D., Jung, J., Zhang, H., Pickering, R. P., Ruan, W. J., Huang, B., & Grant, B. F. (2016). The epidemiology of DSM-5 posttraumatic stress disorder in the United States: Results from the National Epidemiologic Survey on Alcohol and Related Conditions-III. *Social Psychiatry and Psychiatric Epidemiology, 51*(8), 1137–1148. https://doi.org/10.1007/s00127-016-1208-5.

Gradus, J. L., Farkas, D. K., Svensson, E., Ehrenstein, V., Lash, T. L., Milstein, A., Adler, N., & Sørensen, H. T. (2015). Posttraumatic stress disorder and cancer risk: A nationwide cohort study. *European Journal of Epidemiology, 30*(7), 563–568. https://doi.org/10.1007/s10654-015-0032-7.

Halbauer, J. D., Ashford, J. W., Zeitzer, J. M., Adamson, M. M., Lew, H. L., & Yesavage, J. A. (2009). Neuropsychiatric diagnosis and management of chronic sequelae of war-related mild to moderate traumatic brain injury. *Journal of Rehabilitation Research and Development, 46*(6), 757–796. https://doi.org/10.1682/jrrd.2008.08.0119.

Howard, J. T., Sosnov, J. A., Janak, J. C., Gundlapalli, A. V., Pettey, W. B., Walker, L. E., & Stewart, I. J. (2018). Associations of initial injury severity and posttraumatic stress disorder diagnoses with long-term hypertension risk after combat injury. *Hypertension, 71*(5), 824–832. https://doi.org/10.1161/HYPERTENSIONAHA.117.10496.

Husarewycz, M. N., El-Gabalawy, R., Logsetty, S., & Sareen, J. (2014). The association between number and type of traumatic life experiences and physical conditions in a nationally representative sample. *General Hospital Psychiatry, 36*(1), 26–32. https://doi.org/10.1016/j.genhosppsych.2013.06.003.

Institutes of Medicine (IOM). (2008). *Treatment of posttraumatic stress disorder: An assessment of the evidence*. Washington, DC: National Academies Press.

Jaycox, L. H., Cohen, J. A., Mannarino, A. P., Walker, D. W., Langley, A. K., Gegenheimer, K. L., & Schonlau, M. (2010). Children's mental health care following Hurricane Katrina: A field trial of trauma focused psychotherapies. *Journal of Traumatic Stress, 23*, 223–231.

Jaycox, L. H., Kataoka, S. H., Stein, B. D., Langley, A. K., & Wong, M. (2012). Cognitive behavioral intervention for trauma in schools. *Journal of Applied School Psychology, 28*, 239–255.

Jonas, D.E., Cusack, K., Forneris, C.A., Wilkins, T.M., Sonis, J., Middleton, J.C., Feltner, C., Meredith, D., Cavanaugh, J., Brownley, K.A., Olmsted, K.R., Greenblatt, A., Weil, A., Gaynes, B.N. (2013). Comparative Effectiveness Review No. 92. Agency for Healthcare Research and Quality; Rockville, MD. Psychological and pharmacological treatments for adults with posttraumatic stress disorder (PTSD) (AHRQ Publication No. 13-EHC011-EF). http://www.effectivehealthcare.ahrq.gov/reports/final.cfm. Accessed 21 Oct 2015.

Kataoka, S. H., Stein, B. D., Jaycox, L. H., Wong, M., Escudero, P., Tu, W., & Fink, A. (2003). A school-based mental health program for traumatized Latino immigrant children. *Journal of American Academy of Child and Adolescent Psychiatry, 42*, 311–318.

Kessler, R. C., Sonnega, A., Bromet, E., Hughes, M., & Nelson, C. B. (1995). Posttraumatic stress disorder in the National Comorbidity Survey. *Archives of General Psychiatry, 52*(12), 1048–1060. https://doi.org/10.1001/archpsyc.1995.03950240066012.

Kessler, R. C., Rose, S., Koenen, K. C., Karam, E. G., Stang, P. E., Stein, D. J., Heeringa, S. G., Hill, E. D., Liberzon, I., McLaughlin, K. A., McLean, S. A., Pennell, B. E., Petukhova, M., Rosellini, A. J., Ruscio, A. M., Shahly, V., Shalev, A. Y., Silove, D., Zaslavsky, A. M., Angermeyer, M. C., et al. (2014). How well can post-traumatic stress disorder be predicted from pre-trauma risk factors? An exploratory study in the WHO World Mental Health Surveys. *World Psychiatry: Official Journal of the World Psychiatric Association (WPA), 13*(3), 265–274. https://doi.org/10.1002/wps.20150.

Kilpatrick, D. G., Resnick, H. S., Milanak, M. E., Miller, M. W., Keyes, K. M., & Friedman, M. J. (2013). National estimates of exposure to traumatic events and PTSD prevalence using DSM-IV and DSM-5 criteria. *Journal of Traumatic Stress, 26*(5), 537–547. https://doi.org/10.1002/jts.21848.

Leeies, M., Pagura, J., Sareen, J., & Bolton, J. M. (2010). The use of alcohol and drugs to self-medicate symptoms of posttraumatic stress disorder. *Depression and Anxiety, 27*(8), 731–736. https://doi.org/10.1002/da.20677.

Mancini, M. A. (2020). A pilot study evaluating a school-based, trauma-focused intervention for immigrant and refugee youth. *Child and Adolescent Social Work Journal, 37*, 287–300. https://doi.org/10.1007/s10560-019-00641-8.

Mancini, M.A. & Miner, C.S. (2013). Learning and change in a community mental health setting. Journal of Evidence Based Social Work. 10(5), 494–504

Mannarino, A. P., Cohen, J. A., Deblinger, E., Runyon, M. K., & Steer, R. A. (2012). Trauma-focused cognitive-behavioral therapy for children: Sustained impact of treatment 6 and 12 months later. *Child Maltreatment, 17*(3), 231–241. https://doi.org/10.1177/1077559512451787.

Mills, K.L., Teesson, M., Back, S.E., Brady, K.T., Baker, A.L., Hopwood, S....Ewer, P.L. (2012). Integrated exposure-based therapy for co-occurring posttraumatic stress disorder and substance dependence: A randomized controlled trial. JAMA, 308(7), 690–699.

National Child Traumatic Stress Network. (2020). Complex trauma. Retrieved 26 Mar 2020 at: https://www.nctsn.org/what-is-child-trauma/trauma-types/complex-trauma

National Institute for Clinical Excellence. (2005). *Post traumatic stress disorder: The management of PTSD in children and adults in primary and secondary care.* London: The Royal College of Psychiatrists and British Psychological Society.

Niolon, P. H., Kearns, M., Dills, J., Rambo, K., Irving, S., Armstead, T., & Gilbert, L. (2017). *Preventing intimate partner violence across the lifespan: A technical package of programs, policies, and practices.* Atlanta: National Center for Injury Prevention and Control, Centers for Disease Control and Prevention.

Ogden, P., & Minton, K. (2000). Sensorimotor psychotherapy: One method for processing traumatic memory. *Traumatology, 6*(3), 149–173. https://doi.org/10.1177/153476560000600302.

Perry, B. D. (2009). Examining child maltreatment through a neurodevelopmental lens: Clinical application of the Neurosequential model of therapeutics. *Journal of Loss and Trauma, 14*, 240–255. https://doi.org/10.1080/15325020903004350.

Perry, B., & Szalavitz, M. (2017). *The boy who was raised as a dog: And other stories from a child psychiatrist's notebook – What traumatized children can teach us about loss, love, and healing.* New York: Basic Books.

Pfeiffer, E., & Goldbeck, L. (2017). Evaluation of a trauma-focused group intervention for unaccompanied young refugees: A pilot study. *Journal of Traumatic Stress, 30*, 531–536. https://doi.org/10.1002/jts.22218.

Pietrzak, R. H., Goldstein, R. B., Southwick, S. M., & Grant, B. F. (2011). Prevalence and Axis I comorbidity of full and partial posttraumatic stress disorder in the United States: Results from wave 2 of the National Epidemiologic Survey on alcohol and related conditions. *Journal of Anxiety Disorders, 25*(3), 456–465. https://doi.org/10.1016/j.janxdis.2010.11.010.

Powers, M. B., Halpern, J. M., Ferenschak, M. P., Gillihan, S. J., & Foa, E. B. (2010). A meta-analytic review of prolonged exposure for posttraumatic stress disorder. *Clinical Psychology Review, 30*(6), 635–641. https://doi.org/10.1016/j.cpr.2010.04.007.

Price, M., Lancaster, C. L., Gros, D. F., Legrand, A. C., van Stolk-Cooke, K., & Acierno, R. (2018). An examination of social support and PTSD treatment response during *prolonged exposure. Psychiatry, 81*(3), 258–270. https://doi.org/10.1080/00332747.2017.1402569.

Prins, A., Bovin, M. J., Smolenski, D. J., Marx, B. P., Kimerling, R., Jenkins-Guarnieri, M. A., Kaloupek, D. G., Schnurr, P. P., Kaiser, A. P., Leyva, Y. E., & Tiet, Q. Q. (2016). The primary care PTSD screen for DSM-5 (PC-PTSD-5): Development and evaluation within a veteran primary care sample. *Journal of General Internal Medicine, 31*(10), 1206–1211. https://doi.org/10.1007/s11606-016-3703-5.

Raio, C. M., Orederu, T. A., Palazzolo, L., Shurick, A. A., & Phelps, E. A. (2013). Cognitive emotion regulation fails the stress test. *Proceedings of the National Academies of Science, 110*(37), 15139–15144.

Rauch, S., & Foa, E. (2006). Emotional processing theory (EPT) and exposure therapy for PTSD. *Journal of Contemporary Psychotherapy, 36*(2), 61–65. https://doi.org/10.1007/s10879-006-9008-y.

Rauch, S. A., Eftekhari, A., & Ruzek, J. I. (2012). Review of exposure therapy: A gold standard for PTSD treatment. *Journal of Rehabilitation Research and Development, 49*(5), 679–687.

Remch, M., Laskaris, Z., Flory, J., Mora-McLaughlin, C., & Morabia, A. (2018). Post-traumatic stress disorder and cardiovascular diseases: A cohort study of men and women involved in cleaning the debris of the world trade center complex. *Circulation. Cardiovascular Quality and Outcomes, 11*(7), e004572. https://doi.org/10.1161/CIRCOUTCOMES.117.004572.

Resnick, P. A., Monson, C. M., & Chard, K. M. (2014). *Cognitive processing therapy: Veteran/military version: Therapist and patient materials manual.* Department of Veterans Affairs: Washington, DC.

Resnick, P. A., Monson, C. M., & Chard, K. M. (2016). *Cognitive processing therapy for PTSD: A comprehensive manual.* New York: Guilford Press.

Rose, S. C., Bisson, J., Churchill, R., & Wessely, S. (2002). Psychological debriefing for preventing post traumatic stress disorder (PTSD). *Cochrane Database of Systematic Reviews, 2*(2), Art. No.: CD000560. https://doi.org/10.1002/14651858.CD000560.

Rothbaum, B. O., Astin, M. C., & Marsteller, F. (2005). Prolonged exposure versus eye movement desensitization and reprocessing (EMDR) for PTSD rape victims. *Journal of Traumatic Stress, 18*(6), 607–616. [PMID:16382428. https://doi.org/10.1002/jts.20069.

Sannibale, C., Teesson, M., Creamer, M., Sitharthan, T., Bryant, R. A., Sutherland, K., et al. (2013). Randomized controlled trial of cognitive behaviour therapy for comorbid post-traumatic stress disorder and alcohol use disorders. *Addiction, 108*(8), 1397–1410.

Santarnecchi, E., Bossini, L., Vatti, G., Fagiolini, A., La Porta, P., Di Lorenzo, G., Siracusano, A., Rossi, S., & Rossi, A. (2019). Psychological and brain connectivity changes following trauma-focused CBT and EMDR treatment in single-episode PTSD patients. *Frontiers in Psychology, 10*, 129. https://doi.org/10.3389/fpsyg.2019.00129.

Sawhill, I. V., & Karpilow, Q. (2014). *How much could we improve children's life chances by intervening early and often?* Washington, DC: Brookings Institution.

Schnurr, P. P. (2015). Understanding pathways from traumatic exposure to physical health. (Chapter 5; pp. 87–103). In U. Schnyder & M. Cloitre (Eds.), *Evidence-based treat trauma-related psychological disorders: A practical guide for clinicians.* New York: Springer.

Shapiro, F. (2017). *Eye movement desensitization and reprocessing: Basic protocols, principles* (3rd ed.). New York: Guilford.

Silverman, W. K., Ortiz, C. D., Viswesvaran, C., Burns, B. J., Kolko, D., Putnam, F. W., & Amaya-Jackson, L. (2008). Evidence-based psychosocial treatments for children and adolescents exposed to traumatic events. *Journal of Clinical Child & Adolescent Psychology, 37*, 156–183. https://doi.org/10.1080/15374410701818293.

Song, H., Fang, F., Tomasson, G., Arnberg, F. K., Mataix-Cols, D., Fernández de la Cruz, L., Almqvist, C., Fall, K., & Valdimarsdóttir, U. A. (2018). Association of stress-related disorders with subsequent autoimmune disease. *JAMA, 319*(23), 2388–2400. https://doi.org/10.1001/jama.2018.7028.

Spitzer, C., Barnow, S., Völzke, H., John, U., Freyberger, H. J., & Grabe, H. J. (2009). Trauma, posttraumatic stress disorder, and physical illness: Findings from the general population. *Psychosomatic Medicine, 71*(9), 1012–1017. https://doi.org/10.1097/PSY.0b013e3181bc76b5.

Stein, B. D., Jaycox, L. H., Kataoka, S. H., Wong, M., Tu, W., Elliot, M. N., & Fink, A. (2003). A mental health intervention for schoolchildren exposed to violence: A randomized controlled trial. *JAMA, 290*, 603–611.

Strine, T. W., Dube, S. R., Edwards, V. J., Prehn, A. W., Rasmussen, S., Wagenfeld, M., Dhingra, S., & Croft, J. B. (2012). Associations between adverse childhood experiences, psychological distress, and adult alcohol problems. *American Journal of Health Behavior, 36*(3), 408–423.

Substance Abuse and Mental Health Services Administration (SAMHSA). (2014a). SAMHSA's concept of trauma and guidance for a trauma-informed approach. HHS Publication No.(SMA) 14-4884. Rockville: Substance Abuse and Mental Health Services Administration.

Substance Abuse and Mental Health Services Administration (SAMHSA). (2014b). Trauma-informed care in behavioral health services. Treatment improvement protocol (TIP) Series 57. HHS Publication No. (SMA) 13-4801. Rockville: Substance Abuse and Mental Health Services Administration.

van der Kolk, B. A. (2015). *The body keeps the score.* New York: Penguin Books.

Warner, E., Koomar, J., Lary, B., & Cook, A. (2013). Can the body change the score: Application of sensory modulation principles in the treatment of traumatized adolescents in residential settings. *Journal of Family Violence.* https://doi.org/10.1007/s10896-013-9535-8.

Warner, E., Spinazzola, J., Westcott, A., Gunn, C., & Hodgdon, H. (2014). The body can change the score: Empirical support for somatic regulation in the treatment of traumatized adolescents. *Journal of Child and Adolescent Trauma, 7*(4), 237–246. https://doi.org/10.1007/s40653-014-0030-z.

Weathers, F.W., Litz, B.T., Herman, D.S., Huska, J.A., Keane, T.M. (1993). The PTSD checklist (PCL): Reliability, validity, and diagnostic utility. Paper presented at the annual meeting of the International Society for Traumatic Stress Studies. San Antonio, TX.

Weathers, F.W., Litz, B.T., Keane, T.M., Palmieri, P.A., Marx, B.P., Schnurr, P.P. (2013). The PTSD checklist for DSM–5 (PCL-5) 2013 Retrieved from www.ptsd.va.gov

Weathers, F.W., Blake, D.D., Schnurr, P.P., Kaloupek, D.G., Marx, B.P., & Keane, T.M. (2013a). The life events checklist for DSM-5 (LEC-5). Instrument available from the National Center for PTSD at www.ptsd.va.gov

Weathers, F. W., Blake, D. D., Schnurr, P. P., Kaloupek, D. G., Marx, B. P., & Keane, T. M. (2013b). CAPS–5 The clinician-administered PTSD scale for DSM–5 (CAPS–5). Interview available from the National Center for PTSD at www.ptsd.va.gov

Weathers, F. W., Bovin, M. J., Lee, D. J., Sloan, D. M., Schnurr, P. P., Kaloupek, D. G., et al. (2018). The clinician-administered PTSD scale for DSM-5 (CAPS-5): Development and initial psychometric evaluation in military veterans. *Psychological Assessment, 30*, 383–395. https://doi.org/10.1037/pas0000486.

Whitfield, C. L., Anda, R. F., Dube, S. R., & Felitti, V. J. (2003). Violent childhood experiences and the risk of intimate partner violence in adults: Assessment in a large health maintenance organization. *Journal of Interpersonal Violence, 18*(2), 166–185.

Williamson, D. F., Thompson, T. J., Anda, R. F., Dietz, W. H., & Felitti, V. J. (2002). Body weight, obesity, and self-reported abuse in childhood. *International Journal of Obesity, 26*, 1075–1082.

Wortmann, J. H., Jordan, A. H., Weathers, F. W., Resick, P. A., Dondanville, K. A., Hall-Clark, B., et al. (2016). Psychometric analysis of the PTSD Checklist-5 (PCL-5) among treatment-seeking military service members. *Psychological Assessment, 28*, 1392–1403. http://dx.doi.org.ezp.slu.edu/10.1037/pas0000260.

Chapter 8
Screening and Assessment for Depression and Anxiety Disorders

8.1 Overview of Screening and Assessment of Depressive and Anxiety Problems

Major depressive disorder (MDD) and anxiety disorders such as generalized anxiety disorder and panic disorder are some of the most common behavioral health conditions in the world, and they can have an important impact on physical and emotional health (APA 2013). Both sets of disorders are commonly comorbid with each other and with other health and behavioral health conditions, making them significant sources of disability burden worldwide (WHO 2017). The presence of depression and anxiety disorders makes the assessment and treatment of other disorders more difficult because they can overlap and exacerbate the symptoms of other conditions. Depressive and anxiety disorders can also result from several social determinants of health such as poverty, discrimination, lack of secure and stable housing, social isolation, and violence.

Given the medical and social comorbidities associated with depressive and anxiety disorders, collaborative care models that integrate behavioral health and primary care are the best approach to ensure that clients receive care that optimizes their potential for health and well-being. This means that primary care settings need to employ social workers or other behavioral healthcare professionals to routinely assess and treat depressive and anxiety symptoms because doing so can reduce the impact of other medical illness, maximize the impact of medical interventions, and ultimately lead to better overall health. Likewise, behavioral health settings must routinely screen and address physical health issues such as cholesterol, weight, and blood pressure in order to help clients achieve better physical health, which can, in turn, lead to reduced depressive and anxiety symptoms given the bidirectional nature of these conditions with other physical health problems and diseases. In the following sections, several tools, practices, and procedures for the screening, assessment, and differential diagnosis of depressive and anxiety disorders will be

© Springer Nature Switzerland AG 2021

M. A. Mancini, *Integrated Behavioral Health Practice*,

https://doi.org/10.1007/978-3-030-59659-0_8

outlined. We will begin with the screening and assessment of depressive disorders and then move to anxiety disorders in the second half of the chapter.

8.2   Major Depressive Disorder Overview

Major depressive disorder (MDD) is one of the most common behavioral health disorders and has one of the highest levels of disability burden of any disorder in the world, second only to cardiovascular disease (APA 2013; WHO 2017). Depression is also comorbid with many physical and other behavioral health disorders including anxiety, diabetes, hyper- and hypothyroidism, PTSD, inflammatory diseases, cerebrovascular and cardiovascular disease, cancer, and substance use disorders (Gürhan et al. 2019; Scott et al. 2016). Depression can have multiple psychological, physical, social, and environmental etiologies including: (1) maladaptive cognitive beliefs about the self, others, and world, leading to feelings of hopelessness, helplessness, and worthlessness (Beck 2020); (2) genetic and hereditary influences (Caspi et al. 2003); (3) interpersonal trauma and adverse childhood events that include intimate partner violence, community violence, childhood abuse, or neglect (Dube et al. 2001; Felitti et al. 1998); (4) ongoing stressful life events such as poverty, discrimination, relationship discord, loneliness, and social isolation (Cacioppo and Patrick 2008; Cutrona et al. 2006); (5) bodily inflammation due to chronic hyperactivation of the stress response system (Felitti et al. 1998; Kiecolt-Glaser et al. 2015); (6) prescription and nonprescription substance use (SAMHSA 2019); and (7) temperament and personality factors such as high negative affectivity and neuroticism (APA 2013). Depression is often the result of a combination of these intersecting factors, making screening and assessment for depression an important behavioral health practice in integrated practice settings.

8.2.1   Screening and Assessment of Major Depressive Disorder

The two core symptoms of major depressive disorder are a consistent pattern (i.e., almost every day/all day) of *low mood* and a *lack of interest in daily activities* (e.g., anhedonia). Other symptoms that comprise depression include chronic fatigue, appetite, and sleep disturbances, difficulty concentrating, irritability, a sense of worthlessness and guilt, and persistent thoughts of death and suicidal ideation. Table 8.1 lists the core symptoms and diagnostic criteria for major depressive disorder (APA 2013). While depression requires at least five symptoms over a two-week period, it is important to assist people who may be just below the clinical symptom threshold for depression (e.g., "subsyndromal depression") since these symptoms can have serious health consequences for at-risk populations such as older adults and can quickly escalate into full syndromal depression.

Table 8.1 Diagnostic criteria for depressive disorders and related disorders (Based on: APA 2013)

Depressive disorders	Signs and symptoms
Major depressive disorder	(1) Depressed mood most of the day, nearly every day; (2)
Five or more clinically significant depressive symptoms most of the day, nearly every day for two or more weeks. Note: (1) or (2) required. Major depression may be diagnosed during a time of bereavement if criteria for MDD are met.	Markedly diminished interest or pleasure in nearly all activities; (3) appetite and/or weight disturbance; (4) sleep disturbance (insomnia and/or hypersomnia); (5) psychomotor agitation or retardation; (6) fatigue or loss of energy; (7) feelings of worthlessness or guilt; (8) difficulty concentrating, making decisions, or thinking clearly; (9) recurrent thoughts of death or suicide.
Persistent depressive disorder	(1) Poor appetite or overeating; (2) insomnia or hypersomnia;
Depressed mood most of the day, more days than not, for at least two years and with two or more of the following symptoms.	(3) low energy or fatigue; (4) low self-esteem; (5) poor concentration or difficulty making decisions; (6) feelings of hopelessness.

Related disorders that are not classified as depressive disorders

Related disorders	Signs and symptoms
Adjustment disorder with depressed mood	Persistent feelings of (1) low mood; (2) tearfulness; feelings of hopelessness that occur within 3 months of the stressor and do
Development of clinically significant emotional or behavioral symptoms in response to an identifiable stressor. Symptoms should not be better accounted for by bereavement or another disorder.	not persist for more than 6 months past the end of the stressor. Examples of stressors can include: (1) single events (e.g., natural disaster, divorce); (2) multiple events (e.g., marital stress and financial strain); (3) chronic issues (e.g., poverty; prolonged illness, or chronic pain or illness); or (4) developmental milestones (e.g., marriage, going back to school, going to work).
Bipolar I disorder	Distinct period of abnormally and persistently elevated,
Criteria met for at least one-lifetime manic episode	expansive, or irritable mood and increased goal-directed activity or energy lasting at least one week, and three or more of the following: (1) inflated self-esteem or grandiosity; (2) decreased need for sleep; (3) more talkative than usual or pressure to keep talking; (4) flight of ideas or racing thoughts; (5) distractibility; (6) increased goal-directed activity or psychomotor agitation; (7) excessive risky activities.
	Symptoms cause severe impairment in functioning or require hospitalization. Psychotic features may be present.
	An episode of major depressive disorder or hypomania may occur before or after the manic episode but is not required.

(continued)

Table 8.1 (continued)

Bipolar II disorder	Hypomanic episode shares similar symptoms with manic episode except that hypomanic symptoms are less severe and in a shorter duration than manic episodes. A distinct period of abnormally and persistently elevated, expansive, or irritable mood and increased energy and activity lasting at least 4 consecutive days, and three or more of the following: (1) inflated self-esteem or grandiosity; (2) decreased need for sleep; (3) more talkative than usual or pressure to keep talking; (4) flight of ideas or racing thoughts; (5) distractibility; (6) increased goal-directed activity or psychomotor agitation; (7) excessive risky activities.
Criteria met for major depressive disorder and hypomanic episode	
	Episode is a marked departure from normal functioning and noticeable to others, but is not severe enough to impair the functioning or require hospitalization. Psychotic features are never present. If psychotic features are present—the episode should be classified as manic.
	Criteria must be met for a major depressive episode either before or after a hypomanic episode.
Schizoaffective disorder	Criteria A for Schizophrenia: At least two of the following symptoms: delusions (fixed, false beliefs), hallucinations (perceptual disturbance), disorganized speech (incoherence), grossly disorganized or catatonic behavior, negative symptoms (e.g., blunted affect). At last, one symptom must be delusions, hallucinations, or disorganized speech.
Period of illness in which Criteria A for Schizophrenia is met and the person experiences symptoms of either major depressive episode (must include low mood) and/or mania for the majority of the illness.	
	Mood symptoms (mania, major depressive episode) must be experienced alongside schizophrenia-spectrum symptoms for the majority of the illness.
	Person must have experienced psychotic symptoms for at least a two-week period *without* any mood symptoms during a lifetime.
Borderline personality disorder	At least five of the following symptoms: (1) frantic efforts to avoid abandonment; (2) a pattern of unstable, intense relationships; (3) unstable self-image; (4) chronic impulsivity; (5) recurrent suicidal behavior and self-harm; (6) affective instability; (7) chronic feeling of emptiness; (8) frequent, uncontrollable anger; (9) occasional stress-induced paranoia or dissociative symptoms.
A pervasive, global pattern of instability and impulsivity beginning in early adulthood and impacting all areas of life, causing significant distress and impairment	

Instruments that are commonly used to screen for depression include the Patient Health Questionnaire-9 (PHQ-9) (Kroenke et al. 2001) and the Revised Center for Epidemiologic Studies Depression Scale (CESD-R) (Radloff 1977). These two scales screen for the major signs and symptoms of depression. Both scales have excellent reliability and validity, are commonly used in a variety of settings, have been translated into multiple languages, and are easy and fast to complete. The Patient Health Questionnaire (PHQ-9) is an effective and widely used screening tool in primary care settings for depression (Kroenke et al. 2001). It is a 9-item scale that assesses the nine core symptoms of depression. It has excellent psychometric properties. Respondents are asked to report how bothered they have been by nine core depressive symptoms over the last two weeks (e.g., 0 = not at all; 1 = several days; 2 = more than half the days; and 3 = nearly every day). A score of 1–4 indicates symptoms of minimal depression, 5–9 indicates mild symptoms, 10–14 indicates moderate symptoms, and 15+ indicates moderately severe to severe symptoms.

There is also a two-item version of the PHQ-9 scale called the PHQ-2 (Kroenke et al. 2003) that assesses the presence of low mood and anhedonia. The first question of the PHQ-2 asks if patients have often been bothered by feeling down, depressed, or hopeless (e.g., depressed mood). The second question asks patients if they have often been bothered by little interest or pleasure in doing things (e.g., anhedonia) (Arroll et al. 2010). These are the two main depression symptoms in the DSM-5, at least one of which is required for a diagnosis (APA 2013). Using the PHQ-2 allows clinicians to provide a quick initial screen for depression. If a person answers positively to either question they would be asked the remaining 7 questions on the PHQ-9. Deployment of the PHQ-2 has been shown to effectively identify persons in need of further assessment and intervention for depression (Arroll et al. 2010).

The Center for Epidemiological Studies Depression Scale (CES-D) (Radloff 1977) is one of the most reliable, valid, and utilized depression scales in the world. It is relatively fast and easy to score and has excellent psychometric properties (Stockings et al. 2015). The scale was revised in 2004 (Eaton et al. 2004). The scale is also readily available in the public domain. Respondents are asked to rate the past week frequency of 20 items such as, "I felt down or unhappy" and "I didn't sleep as I usually sleep" on a 4-point scale (0 = not at all, 1 = a little, 2 = some, 3 = a lot). Scores can range from 0 to 60 with higher scores indicating higher depression levels. The clinical cut-off score is 16. The scale has a children's version and has been revised to reflect the DSM-5 changes.

8.2.2   Differential Diagnosis of Depression

A major depressive episode is marked by the experience of persistent depressed mood that can take the form of sadness, the "blues" or "blahs," hopelessness, irritability, anger, and hostility as well as feeling anxious. Major depressive disorder (MDD) requires the presence of five out of nine depressive symptom areas. Table 8.1 lists the diagnostic criteria for major depressive disorder and related disorders with depressive symptoms. The condition is characterized by a depressed mood state that exists for most of the day, nearly every day, for at least two weeks. As mentioned previously, this state must include either: (1) a self-reported depressed mood (e.g., sadness, tearfulness, hopelessness); and/or (2) a diminished or absent lack of interest or pleasure in most or all daily activities sometimes referred to as anhedonia. This can include giving up many hobbies or activities of interest and not caring to partake in any activities once deemed pleasurable. Either of these symptoms should be a marked departure from the person's normal baseline functioning (APA 2013). Disturbances in seven other symptom areas may also be present. These include: (1)

appetite disturbance typically experienced as a loss of appetite and/or weight loss; (2) disturbances in sleep that can include either sleeping too much (i.e., hypersomnia) or insomnia. This is commonly manifested as a diurnal cycle of sleep where a person experiences insomnia during the night and hypersomnia during the day; (3) psychomotor agitation (i.e., restlessness) or psychomotor retardation (i.e., listlessness) nearly every day; (4) the experience of fatigue or lack of energy (a universal symptom for depression); (5) chronic feelings of worthlessness and guilt; (6) neurocognitive problems in the areas of planning, memory, concentration, and attention; and (7) persistent and recurrent thoughts of death and persistent suicidal ideation (APA 2013). The main or "core" symptoms of depression that occur across severity levels include: feelings of dysphoria (e.g., depressed, irritable, or anxious mood), anhedonia, fatigue, feelings of worthlessness and guilt, hopelessness, and impaired concentration and decision-making (Rakofsky et al. 2013). The symptoms of MDD must also not be solely due to a general medical condition (e.g., over/underactive thyroid condition, Parkinson's Disease), medication, or other substance. The major depressive disorder should be differentiated from other related behavioral health conditions that have depressive features.

Depression and Adjustment Disorders
Adjustment disorder with depressed mood is the experience of marked emotional distress, such as low mood and hopelessness, due to an *identifiable stressor* that causes significant impairment in functioning. Adjustment disorder should not be diagnosed if a person meets the criteria of another mental disorder. If a person meets the criteria for major depressive disorder, whether or not they experience an identifiable stressor, major depressive disorder should be diagnosed.

Depression and Bipolar Spectrum Disorders
Persons with bipolar spectrum disorders can meet diagnostic criteria for major depressive disorder. In Bipolar I Disorder, a person must exhibit at least one manic episode experienced as a "distinct period of abnormally and persistently elevated, expansive, or irritable mood and abnormally and persistently increased goal directed activity or energy." (APA 2013, pp. 124). Symptoms associated with mania include grandiosity, lack of a need for sleep, reckless behaviors, pressured speech, distractibility, and flight of ideas. Psychotic features such as hallucinations and delusions can also be present. While the major depressive disorder is not required for a diagnosis of Bipolar I Disorder, MDD is often experienced as part of the Bipolar syndrome. In short, if the client has ever experienced mania, Bipolar I Disorder should be the diagnosis. In Bipolar II Disorder, meeting the criteria for MDD is required in addition to the experience of at least one hypomanic episode, which has the same symptoms as mania, but experienced with less severity, shorter duration, and without psychotic symptoms. Careful consideration of hypomania should be utilized before making a diagnostic decision regarding MDD. The symptoms of irritability present in both bipolar spectrum disorders and MDD should also be assessed carefully. For persons with MDD, irritability will be present alongside other symptoms of depression such as persistent sadness and anhedonia. In mania and hypomania, irritability is accompanied by a marked increase in energy and euphoria. Assessment

for a history of mania or hypomania must be conducted to rule out these other possibilities (APA 2013).

Depression and Schizophrenia Spectrum Disorders
Another differential diagnostic concern is schizoaffective disorder. Schizoaffective disorder is a schizophrenia spectrum disorder with frequent overlapping mood symptoms. While persons with major depressive disorder can experience psychotic symptoms such as auditory or visual hallucinations (e.g., hearing voices no one else hears, seeing things no one else can see), disorganized thoughts, and delusional beliefs, these symptoms are only experienced as *features* of active depressive episodes. They are not experienced outside of these episodes. Persons with schizoaffective disorder (SAD) meet the main diagnostic criteria for schizophrenia and must experience psychotic symptoms *in the absence of any mood symptoms* for at least a two-week period. However, persons with SAD also experience significant mood symptoms (e.g., manic or depression) and meet the criteria for major depressive disorder or bipolar disorder for the majority of the duration of the illness. In persons who experience depression with psychotic features, full assessment psychotic symptoms should be conducted to ensure they do not meet the criteria for schizoaffective disorder or another schizophrenia-spectrum disorder.

Depression and Grief
In the past, the major depressive disorder could not be diagnosed while experiencing active bereavement for six to eight weeks. This so-called bereavement exclusion was in place to help practitioners avoid misdiagnosing normative grief as depression. Research has found that depression and normative grief are distinct and can co-occur, making assessment and treatment of depression during an episode of bereavement an important practice. DSM-5 has removed this exclusion. In order to differentiate MDD from normative grief and bereavement, it is important to note that the severity, duration, and impairment experienced in MDD far exceeds what is normally experienced as grief or sadness (APA 2013). In grief, self-esteem is preserved, symptoms generally improve over time, suicidality is absent, and happiness and sadness often come in alternating waves. In MDD, sadness, anhedonia, fatigue, hopelessness, and feelings of worthlessness and death are persistent and worsen over time. Grief and MDD can co-occur, particularly in people with a history of psychiatric illness. Figure 8.1 lists the differences between normative grief and depressive symptoms. If clients meet the diagnostic criteria for MDD during a period of bereavement, MDD can, and should, be diagnosed and treated (APA 2013).

Depression and Borderline Personality Disorder
Borderline personality disorder (BPD) is a long-standing pattern of symptoms that causes significant emotional distress and functional impairments. Persons with BPD experience several interrelated symptom clusters that include: (1) significant emotional dysregulation and affective instability (McGlashan et al. 2005); (2) unstable personal relationships (Gunderson et al. 2018; APA 2013); (3) unstable self-image or identity and a chronic sense of emptiness (Gunderson et al. 2018; Lieb et al. 2004); (4) impulsive and reckless behaviors (Lieb et al. 2004; McGlashan et al.

Grief	Depression
Intense sadness; Feelings of emptiness and loss	Persistent sadness and inability to experience pleasure
Withdrawal from activities	Withdrawal from activities
Sadness comes in waves, decreasing dysphoria over time, and intermixed with positive feelings of the deceased	Moods and thoughts persistently negative. Dysphoria is persistent without preoccupations with the deceased
Self-esteem preserved	Sense of worthlessness and self-loathing common
Preoccupied with thoughts and memories of the deceased	Self-critical and pessimistic ruminations
Guilt around the deceased. Thoughts of joining the deceased	Suicidal ideation due to feeling of worthlessness, undeserving of life, or unable to cope with the pain

Fig. 8.1 Differences between grief and depression (Based on: APA 2013)

2005); and (5) frequent suicidal behavior (e.g., suicidal ideation, planning/intent, attempts, and completion) and non-suicidal self-injury (NSSI) (APA 2013; Zanarini et al. 2013).

Persons with BPD often experience comorbid conditions including major depressive disorder, anxiety disorders, eating disorders, substance abuse, and posttraumatic stress disorder (PTSD) (APA 2013; Lenzenweger et al. 2007; Shea et al. 2004; Zanarini et al. 1998; Zimmerman and Mattia 1999). Borderline personality disorder shares many symptoms with major depressive disorder (MDD). If a client meets the criteria for MDD and BPD, both conditions can be diagnosed.

The symptoms of irritability, low self-worth, negative affect, and suicidal behavior can make a differential diagnosis of major depressive disorder and BPD difficult. One difference is that the negative mood symptoms and suicidality experienced by persons with a major depressive disorder are prolonged (at least two weeks), exist nearly all day/every day, and are accompanied by physical symptoms such as fatigue, sleep problems, and psychomotor retardation that may not be experienced in persons with BPD who do not have MDD. In contrast, negative affect, irritability, and suicidality experienced by persons with BPD often fluctuate throughout the day and are often linked to interpersonal stressors or frantic efforts to avoid abandonment (another hallmark symptom of BPD) (APA 2013). Furthermore, persons with major depressive disorder only do no typically exhibit the other symptoms of BPD such as chronic anger and aggressiveness, efforts to avoid abandonment, chronic emptiness, and unstable identity.

Depression in Young People

Depression is not normal for any age group including teenagers and older adults. Perhaps the most important symptoms across age categories for depression are anhedonia or the loss of interest or pleasure in daily activities. Young persons may experience moodiness and irritability that is a normative part of growing up; however, these experiences usually fluctuate over the course of the day and are often linked to stressors encountered in school, home, or personal relationships. Persistent sadness, loss of interest in daily activities, and organic symptoms such as psychomotor retardation, sleep problems, loss of appetite, and fatigue are not normative experiences for young people. Depression in younger children may also present as excessive irritability, clinginess, school avoidance, anxiousness or worry, and loss of appetite or somatic complaints such as headache, stomachache, and fatigue. When anxiety, particularly when manifested as school refusal or avoidance, is seen in children and adolescents, it should be treated. Children and adolescents who experience excessive anxiety do not typically grow out of it. Rather, they are more likely to develop into depressed and anxious young adults and adults. In adolescents, depression may also manifest as irritability or anger, emotional sensitivity, isolation, poor school performance, excessive feelings of guilt or a sense of worthlessness, hypersomnia, suicidal ideation, and behaviors such as self-harm and alcohol and drug use. It is important to note that suicide is the leading cause of death in adolescents and young adults. Screening for depression and suicide should be a routine part of any health or behavioral health practice setting serving children and adolescents.

Late-Life Depression

Late-life depression (LLD) is common, persistent, and life-threatening. Fortunately, there are many effective approaches to treating late-life depression. Primary care settings are an ideal place to screen and assess for depression in older populations because many older adults often visit their primary care physician several times a year to manage ongoing health conditions. However, detection of depression in older populations can be complicated for three reasons: (1) Depressive symptoms can be masked by other illnesses and somatic complaints or concerns; (2) Older adults may be reluctant to disclose depression or are unaware of the signs and symptoms; and (3) Providers may prioritize other physical complaints over LLD or consider depression as normative given the clinical context of the client. Each of these three reasons is common and avoidable with proper screening, assessment, and education of the provider and client. Understanding the vast health implications of late-life depression is a first step in positioning LLD as an important condition to screen and assess for in older clients.

Late-Life Depression and Health   Late-life depression exerts one of the most powerful impacts on health in older populations. Experiencing late-life depression increases the risk of comorbid physical disorders, suicide, medical service utilization, caregiver burden, and disability (Andreescu and Reynolds 2011). Depression is commonly comorbid with other physical and cognitive disorders, making diagnosis difficult as symptoms of LLD may be masked by symptoms from other disorders

(Mitchell et al. 2010). The presence of depression exacerbates the symptoms of other conditions, making them more intense, harder to treat, and more disabling, leading to increased disability, caregiver burden, healthcare utilization, and mortality (Reynolds et al. 2019). For instance, LLD is associated with a higher risk for cardiovascular and cerebrovascular disease (Alexopoulos et al. 1997; Krishnan et al. 1997; Rudisch and Nemeroff 2003; Valkanova and Ebmeier 2013). Depression often precedes or develops after a stroke or other less noticeable vascular events such as transient ischemic attacks (TIAs) (Robinson, 2003). Depression and cerebrovascular disease may have a bidirectional relationship as having one increases the risk for the other (Thomas et al. 2004). Depression has been associated with undetected vascular infarcts, and it has been proposed that vascular disease and events can lead to and sustain late-onset depression through inflammation and/or damage to brain structures and circuitry (Alexopoulos et al. 1997; Alexopoulos and Kelly 2009).

Another important health area relevant to depression is the relationship between depression and dementia. Depression and dementia share similar symptoms and have a bidirectional relationship. Persons with late-life depression can be at a higher risk for developing dementia, particularly vascular dementia and Alzheimer's disease. In fact, depression is often an early symptom of dementia (Diniz et al. 2013). Late-life depression often accompanies cognitive decline and problems in executive processing and impulse control (Alexopolous 2005). For persons with high blood pressure, the presence of depression and/or memory complaints increases the risk for developing cognitive impairments and decline (Borda et al. 2019).

Older adults with LLD are also less likely to report depressive symptoms because they may not view their symptoms in psychiatric terms. Instead, they may conceptualize LLD symptoms such as anhedonia (lack of interest, pleasure, or activity), memory problems, irritability, weight loss, loss of appetite, fatigue, sleep problems, lack of joy or pessimism for the future, pain, and other somatic symptoms as indicative of other physical disorders or just another part of aging rather than as a treatable behavioral health condition. Providers, too, may join older clients in this line of thinking (Reynolds et al. 2019). Older adults represent one of the highest risk groups for suicide in the United States, making it important for providers to routinely screen for depressive symptoms in older adults. Depression is not a normal part of getting older. In fact, subsyndromal depression (depressive symptoms that do not reach the threshold of a diagnosis) can have a profound impact on the quality of life and health in older adults.

Risk Factors and Treatment for LLD Several psychosocial factors can also lead to depression in older adults including: (1) grief and bereavement; (2) pain; (3) sleep disturbances; (4) loneliness and loss of social roles, activities, and functioning; (5) medical issues related to neurocognitive disorders such as Alzheimer's and Parkinson's disease, cardiovascular conditions, metabolic disorders such as diabetes, and cerebrovascular conditions; (6) social determinants of health including poverty, isolation, and negative life events; and (7) high-risk behaviors (e.g., smoking, drinking, lack of physical activity, obesity) (Almeida et al. 2010; Draper Pfaff, Pirkis et al. 2008; Kraaij et al. 2002; Reynolds et al. 2019).

Given this wide range of risk factors, collaborative care for depression has shown improvement in not only depression scores but also improved cholesterol, blood pressure, and blood sugar levels for patients with depression and comorbid disorders (Katon et al. 2010). One type of collaborative care, the depression care management model, has been shown to be one of the most effective approaches to treating late-life depression (Snowden et al. 2008). Depression care management is based on the chronic disease management model and is a team approach to treating depression. The team of primary care and behavioral health specialists is managed by a social worker or nurse practitioner. The team engages in routine screening and assessment of depression of patients and the implementation of evidence-based treatments designed to effectively treat depression.

The implementation of sequential antidepressant therapy and CBT through a collaborative team approach described above can ensure that older adults have adequate access to effective treatments that address the full range of medical, psychological, and social factors that lead to symptoms (Snowden et al. 2008; Andreescu and Reynolds 2011). For instance, the PROSPECT study showed that providing stepped collaborative care in primary care settings, including interpersonal psychotherapy (IPT) and/or antidepressants, led to significantly reduced suicidal ideation and depressive symptoms and increased remission rates in older patients with major depressive symptoms over standard or usual care (Bruce et al. 2004). Likewise, the IMPACT study showed a significant and sustained reduction in depressive symptoms, an increase in satisfaction with care, and improvement in the quality of life and functioning in primary care patients over the age of 60 who had major depressive disorder (Unutzer et al. 2002).

8.2.3 Depression and Suicide

There are four major risk factors for suicide that stand above all others: (1) the presence of a behavioral health disorder; (2) a previous suicide attempt; (3) access to firearms; and (4) alcohol or substance use. Table 8.2 lists the major risk and protective factors for suicide. The most significant of these four is the presence of a behavioral health disorder. Major depressive disorder and bipolar spectrum disorders have the two highest suicide rates of any psychiatric disorder. Universal suicide assessment is an important practice and should be implemented as a routine part of the assessment in primary care, emergency care, behavioral health, and social service settings. It is vitally important to conduct suicide assessments with clients who have a history of suicide attempts or who present with or have a history of depressive disorder. Suicide assessment should be conducted at intake and when a change is observed in a client's behavioral health status (e.g., symptoms getting worse or suddenly better) or lack of improvement in behavioral health symptoms is observed.

Assessment for suicide is also indicated after the client has undergone or anticipates any major loss, life change, or any stressful or traumatic experience; any time the client undergoes a change in treatment status (e.g. Hospital discharge/admission; admission to outpatient treatment; entering or leaving residential treatment); and after the emergence of a serious physical illness or injury, especially one that is life-threatening, painful, chronic, disfiguring, or disabling (APA 2010).

Suicide Screening Few standardized screening instruments have been shown to be effective. The American Psychiatric Association has developed a full set of guidelines for suicide assessment and treatment (APA 2010). During a full psychiatric evaluation, it is important to include a suicide assessment that examines: (1) a family history of mental illness, dysfunction, and suicide in the client; (2) the current psychosocial stressors in the client's life that may place them at a higher risk for suicide (e.g., financial stress, social isolation, loss of relationships/divorce, job loss, legal problems, bullying); (3) specific stressors that may be experienced by persons (particularly youth) in the LGBTQ community and Black, Indigenous, and People of Color (BIPOC) communities including any form of discrimination, insults, bullying or other forms of violence; and (4) any protective factors such as coping skills, social support, or cognitive flexibility that may mitigate or buffer the person from suicide risk (APA 2010). Table 8.3 lists the main areas of suicide screening and assessment with sample questions.

Suicidal Ideation Suicide assessments begin by assessing for suicidal ideation by asking general questions about life, such as "How is your life right now?," "Have you ever thought that life is not worth living or that you would be better off dead?," and "Have you ever thought about harming yourself or ending your own life?" If the

Table 8.2 Risk and protective factors for suicide

Suicide risk factors	Suicide protective factors
*Presence of any behavioral health disorder	Positive social support
Previous suicide attempts	Having family or children
Easy access to unsecured firearms	Pregnancy
Substance use	Positive coping skills
Experiencing discrimination, harassment, and persecution	Cognitive flexibility/good problem-solving skills
Chronic medical condition or injury characterized by loss of functioning or pain	General life satisfaction
Unemployment/financial stress	Religious beliefs that do not condone violence
High stress	Pets
Social isolation	
Past or current trauma (especially physical or sexual abuse)	
Cognitive inflexibility	
Hopelessness	

person confirms suicidal thoughts, it is important to discuss some contextual details such as when, how often, how intense, and under what circumstances these thoughts emerged. Were they able to control the thoughts or were the thoughts intrusive? Once thoughts have been identified, the provider moves on to assess suicidal intent.

Suicidal Intent and Plan Next, it is important to assess suicidal intent and motivation by asking detailed questions about suicidal plans and any actions or behaviors taken to enact those plans. How motivated or serious is the person about dying? Have they enacted any behaviors to develop the plan such as stockpiling medications or purchasing a firearm? Do they have access to lethal means? Questions include: (1) Have you ever developed a plan to kill yourself? (2) If so, what elements does the plan include? (3) How likely do you think it is that you would enact the plan? (4) How likely do you think it is that you will die if you enact the plan? (5) Have you experienced a recent stressor or loss such as losing a job or a house, experiencing a divorce, or going to jail? and (6) How likely do you think you would enact the plan in the future? (APA 2010).

Access to Unsecured Firearms It is important to assess whether the person has access to an unsecured firearm. If they do, it is vital to discuss with the client the need to remove or secure the firearm. This can be done by having the firearm stored by a family member or law enforcement. Sometimes the firearm can be temporarily stored securely at a shooting range.

Past Attempts If a client has attempted suicide in the past, it is important to gather details about the event such as when it happened, what methods they used, how intent they were to die, whether alcohol or other substances were involved, how they survived (e.g., aborted attempt, rescued, called 911 themselves), and if they received any medical and behavioral health treatment afterward? For persons with repeated attempts, it is important to understand how many times they have attempted suicide, the details about the most recent attempt, the most serious attempt, and the factors or circumstances that most often trigger the urge to die. If a person experiences psychotic symptoms as a result of schizophrenia spectrum disorder or a mood disorder with psychotic features, such as Bipolar I or major depressive disorder, be sure to ask about whether they experience hallucinations. If so, have the hallucinations (e.g., voices) ever suggested to them that they hurt themselves or others, and have they ever acted upon these commands? (APA 2010).

Determining Risk Level Next, it is important to assess the risk level. Table 8.4 lists suicide risk criteria and the appropriate provider response to ensure safety. The first step is to identify major risk factors. The most important is the presence of a psychiatric disorder. Access to a firearm, chronic medical condition or injury, unemployment, high stress, social isolation, hopelessness, impulsivity, experiencing trauma (especially physical or sexual abuse), and substance misuse or substance use disorders are additional important risk factors to assess. Protective factors for suicide include pregnancy, having children or a family, social support, high general life

Table 8.3 Suicide assessment areas and questions (Based on: APA 2010)

Suicide ideation	Has the person ever thought about their own death or suicide? If so, how frequent and intense are the thoughts? How recently have they thought about death or suidie?
	"How is your life right now?"
Assess whether or not client has thought about suicide in the past or recently.	"Have you ever thought that life is not worth living or that you would be better off dead?"
	"Have you ever thought about harming yourself or ending your own life?"
	If client endorses suicidal thoughts, identify contextual details: when, how often, how
	intense, and under what circumstances these thoughts emerged
	Were they able to control the thoughts or were the thoughts intrusive?
Suicidal intent and plan	How motivated or serious is the person about dying? Have they enacted any behaviors to develop the plan such as stockpiling medications or purchasing a firearm? Do they have access to lethal means?
If client endorses suicidal ideation, assess the intent level and whether they have developed a plan.	Have you ever developed a plan to kill yourself? If so, what elements does the plan include?
	How likely do you think it is that you would enact the plan?
	How likely do you think it is that you will die if you enact the plan?
	Have you experienced a recent stressor or loss such as losing a job or a house, experiencing a divorce, or going to jail?
	How likely do you think you would enact the plan in the future?
Assess firearm access	Do you have access to a firearm?
For clients with suicidal ideation, it is important to assess whether the person has access to an unsecured firearm in the home.	If they do, it is vital to discuss with the client the need to remove or secure the firearm.
	This can be done by having the firearm stored by a family member or law enforcement. Sometimes the firearm can be temporarily stored securely at a shooting range.
	At the very least, access to the firearm will need to be restricted by family
Assess past attempts	How many times have you attempted suicide? When was the last time you attempted suicide?

(continued)

Table 8.3 (continued)

If a client has attempted suicide in the past, it is important to gather details about the event as possible	What methods did you use?
	How intent were you to die?
	What precipitated the attempt?
	Was alcohol or drugs involved?
	How did you survive? (e.g., aborted attempt, rescued, called 911 themselves)
	Did you receive any medical and behavioral health treatment afterward?
	For those with multiple attempts: How many times have you attempted suicide? Please tell me the details about your most serious attempt? What are the details about your most recent attempt? What are the factors that most often trigger suicidal ideation?
	For those who experience psychotic symptoms: Do you ever experience hallucinations (e.g., voices, images) that suggest that you harm yourself or other people? If so, have you ever acted on these suggestions or found it difficult to resist them? What do you do to help yourself when these issues come up?

satisfaction, religious or other beliefs that do not condone suicide, positive coping skills, cognitive flexibility, and good problem-solving skills (APA 2010).

Response to Suicidality As a general rule, patients who are suicidal should never be left alone for any period of time and should *at least* be taken to an emergency room for a risk assessment and evaluation or be evaluated by a mobile crisis team. Persons who have attempted suicide should generally be admitted to a hospital setting for further monitoring and evaluation. For persons with suicidal ideation who have not attempted suicide, a person at a high risk for suicide requiring admission to a secure setting includes persons who have attempted suicide in the past, have strong suicidal intent with a lethal plan or suicide rehearsal, have significant psychiatric symptoms or medical conditions, have little or no therapeutic relationship with a provider, and have limited or no social support. Persons who generally have many risk factors and few protective factors should also be admitted to the hospital for observation and treatment. For persons who have suicidal ideation with low intent or a plan that is nonspecific with low lethality, good social support, a safe and stable living environment, no prior attempts, and who are currently in treatment, emergency evaluation, and discharge with a follow-up plan may be indicated. Outpatient treatment may be a better option than hospitalization for people with modifiable risk factors, no prior attempts, and who live in a safe, stable living environment and are engaged in ongoing outpatient treatment (APA 2010).

Documentation After assessment for suicide, it is important to thoroughly document the clinical interaction, collaborate, and coordinate a follow-up care plan for the client. It is also important to provide education and information (e.g., hotline numbers, safety plan) to the client and their family, provide an ongoing reassessment of suicide, monitori psychiatric status, and evaluate treatment effectiveness. Minimally, documentation should include details of the evaluation and risk assessment, rationale for all decisions and the decision-making process, whether firearms were present in the home and the instructions that were given to the client and family about securing firearms, and a record of consultations with other professionals, family, and collateral contacts (APA 2010).

Safety Plan Lastly, it is not advisable for providers to solely rely on the use of suicide prevention contracts, sometimes called "no harm" or "behavioral" contracts, with clients. They don't work. They create a false sense of security without actually reducing suicide risk, and they can expose the provider to liability if the client harms or kills themselves afterward. A more useful alternative to a contract is a safety plan. Table 8.5 lists the components of a suicide safety plan. A suicide safety plan is a set of strategies and resources designed to reduce the risk of harm and increase safety. The safety plan should be developed collaboratively with the client. Part of the plan should include increased follow-up and monitoring of the client, the involvement of other relevant health and behavioral health providers, and an increase in the frequency of sessions (APA 2010).

A safety plan can also include: (1) identification of warning signs of when a crisis is developing; (2) ways the client can make their immediate environment safer such as removing firearms and other lethal means and having someone stay with them; (3) a list of tailored coping strategies the client can use to stay well and deploy when they are in distress such as specific distractions, proper rest and nutrition, using medications, relaxation techniques, and exercise; (4) a list of things that they have to live for; (5) identification of personal social supports and people they can talk to and reach out to for help; (6) professional resources and contact information such as clinicians, hotlines, urgent or emergency care centers, and behavioral response teams.

8.3 Anxiety Disorders Overview

Anxiety is the experience of fear or nervousness in anticipation of a possible threat in the near or distant future (APA 2013). Table 8.2 lists the diagnostic signs and symptoms of several anxiety disorders and related disorders that have anxiety symptoms. It is accompanied by physical feelings associated with the anticipation of threat such as nervousness or jitteriness, muscle tightness, tension, and hypervigilance designed to prepare someone for a perceived threat. In short, anxiety is a state in which one is ready to respond to a threat (e.g., fight, flight, or freeze). Anxiety can invoke caution in the form of behavioral or mental avoidance as a natural response when a person is in a state of anxiety. Anxiety itself is not pathological. Anxiety becomes pathological when it: (1) exists in the absence of a threat; (2) is excessive to a perceived threat; (3) persists well beyond the point when the threat has gone

Table 8.4 Suicide risk and response (Based on: APA 2010)

Suicidality level	Risk/protective factors	Response
Suicide attempt	No further risk factors needed.	+Immediate admission to secure treatment setting with suicide precautions for monitoring and evaluation
Suicidal ideation (without attempt)	With *any* of the following risk factors:	+*Admission to secure treatment setting with suicide precautions for monitoring and evaluation
	Previous attempt	
	High intent (i.e., clear, lethal plan and/or rehearsal)	
	Access to lethal means	
	Behavioral health disorder or symptoms	
	Presence of a medical disorder	
	Lack of therapeutic relationship with a behavioral health provider	
	Lack of social support	
	Substance use	
Suicidal ideation (low intent/plan)	Nonspecific plan with low lethality due to modifiable/precipitating stressors or risk factors.	+Emergency evaluation and discharge with a follow-up plan for outpatient treatment and development of a safety plan
	Example statements:	
	"I just wish the ground would swallow me up."	
	"I would just like to go to sleep and not wake up."	
	"I just want this to end"	
	No access to means	
	No prior attempts	
	Good social support	
	Stable living situation	
	Has good treatment relationship with a provider	
Chronic suicidal ideation and nonsuicidal self-injury	Nonspecific plan with low lethality and no access to means.	+Development of a safety plan with follow-up and ongoing outpatient treatment may be appropriate
	Modifiable risk factors, stressors, or situational issues (e.g., poor test grade, and relationship breakup)	
	No prior attempts	
	Good social support	
	Stable living situation	
	Has good treatment relationship with a provider	

*In general, a person with suicidal ideation who has many risk factors and few protective factors should be admitted for evaluation

+Person should not be left alone for any period of time if suicidal. Consultation with team members necessary. If client does not have social support, emergency evaluation is minimally indicated

away; and (4) leads to maladaptive avoidance behaviors that negatively reinforce and perpetuate the anxious feelings (APA 2013) (Table 8.6).

Anxiety disorders are the most common behavioral health disorders in the United States. Like depression, anxiety is comorbid with a variety of other behavioral health disorders (e.g., depression, substance use disorders, and eating disorders) and a range of physical health disorders including diabetes, cancer, cardiovascular and cerebrovascular disease, stomach problems, and chronic obstructive pulmonary disorder (COPD). There are a range of anxiety disorders that include generalized anxiety disorder (GAD) marked by excessive worry, social anxiety disorder (SAD) marked by fear of being embarrassed in social situations, panic disorder (PD) marked by persistent experiencing and anticipation of panic attacks, and agoraphobia marked by fear and avoidance of places with no escape (APA 2013). In DSM-5, obsessive-compulsive disorder (OCD) was removed from the Anxiety Disorders chapter into its own chapter. However, OCD is still considered a disorder marked by significant anxiety. Like depression, people can also experience lower levels of anxiety that have important impacts on health while not meeting diagnostic criteria for any particular disorder. Symptoms such as excessive worry, intermittent panic symptoms or full-blown panic attacks, and avoidance of situations that might lead to anxiety are common symptoms that can lead to serious functional impairments (APA 2013).

8.4   Screening and Assessment for Anxiety Disorders

A common screening instrument for anxiety in addition to the PHQ-4 listed above (see depressive disorder section) is the Generalized Anxiety Disorder 7-item Scale (GAD-7) (Spitzer et al. 2006). This scale screens for several of the most common symptoms of anxiety including being nervous or on edge, excessive worrying, irritability, restlessness, and being unable to relax. The GAD-7 is often combined with the PHQ-9 to be a relatively simple, comprehensive, and reliable depression and anxiety combination screen ideal for busy clinical settings. However, in settings that cannot sustain the implementation of these two screens, the Patient Health Questionnaire 4-item scale for anxiety and depression (PHQ-4) has shown good psychometrics in a variety of settings (Kroenke et al. 2009). This very brief 4-item scale screens for the presence of the two main symptoms in both anxiety and depression for the last two weeks. Respondents are asked how often they have been bothered (e.g., not at all, several days, more than half the days, nearly every day) over the last two weeks by four symptoms that indicate the presence of possible depression and anxiety disorders that include: (1) feeling nervous or anxious; (2) not being able to stop or control worrying; (3) feeling down, depressed, or hopeless; and (4) little interest or pleasure in doing things (e.g., anhedonia).

Table 8.5 Suicide safety plan (Based on: APA 2013)

A suicide safety plan is a set of strategies and resources designed to reduce the risk of harm and increase safety.

Domain	Examples
Identification of triggers and warning signs of when a crisis is developing	**Crisis triggers:** Anniversaries, certain people, holidays, seasons, criticism, rejection, alcohol or drugs, loss, stress, trauma
	Early warning signs: Low mood, fatigue, negative thoughts, thoughts of death or self-harm, self-harming behavior, isolation, sleep problems, anger/tension, urges to use substances
Ways the client can make their immediate environment safer.	**Removing access to firearms:** Store firearms outside the home with a friend or relative. You can also have a firearm dealer, shooting range, or law enforcement store guns for you.
	Use firearm safes and/or trigger locks, and be sure a person cannot access keys or combinations. Store ammunition in a separate secure location
	Reduce/eliminate other lethal means: Do not keep lethal doses of any medications in the home. This includes acetaminophen (Tylenol), which is particularly lethal due to liver damage, and ibuprofen. Keep only small quantities of over-the-counter medication.
	Lock up all prescription medications—Especially benzodiazepines and pain medications. Dispose of outdated medications.
	Remove or lock up any toxic or poisonous materials. Only keep small amounts of toxic household chemicals (e.g., cleaners, pesticides) in the home.
	Keep little or no alcohol in the home.
	Remove sharp knives, razor blades, or scissors when suicidal.
	Stay connected: Stay connected by having someone stay with you or through frequent check-ins.
	When suicidal, do not be left alone—have a person stay with you at all times.
List of tailored coping strategies the client can use to stay well and deploy when they are in distress. Listed on a coping card or on phone or other digital devices.	Specific distractions: Movies, reading, walking, hobbies, calling people, gaming.
	Proper rest and nutrition
	Staying connected with loved ones
	Avoiding drugs or alcohol
	Taking medications
	Relaxation techniques/reducing stress
	Engaging in hobbies or meaningful activities
	Exercise
	Routinely reviewing a list of people and things to live for

(continued)

Table 8.5 (continued)

A suicide safety plan is a set of strategies and resources designed to reduce the risk of harm and increase safety.

Domain	Examples
Identification of personal social supports and people they can talk to and reach out to for help.	Trusted friends and family
	Sponsors/peer support
	Counselors
	Faith representatives
Professional resources and contact information	Clinicians, hotlines, urgent or emergency care centers, behavioral response teams, poison control lines.
Follow-up	Increased follow-up and monitoring of the client
	Involvement of other relevant health and behavioral health providers
	Frequent provider check-ins
	Increase in frequency of sessions

8.4.1   Differential Assessment of Anxiety Disorders

Generalized Anxiety Disorder

Persons with Generalized Anxiety Disorder (GAD) engage in excessive, uncontrollable worrying about a variety of events. Worry is clinically significant and occurs "more days than not" for at least six months (APA 2013, pp.222). This can include uncontrollable worry about work or school performance, finances, routine activities, the well-being of loved ones, or more abstract concerns about safety and security. Symptoms of GAD include restlessness, fatigue, problems concentrating, irritability, muscle tension, and sleep problems (APA 2013). For a diagnosis of GAD, clients should exhibit at least three of these symptoms (one for children) persistently over a six-month period. GAD shares some predisposing genetic factors with major depressive disorder. Personality characteristics that can increase the risk for GAD include a tendency for higher negative affectivity, behavioral inhibition or timidity in novel situations, and high intolerance for ambiguity. Persons with GAD tend to focus extensively on potentially threatening stimuli, scan the environment for potential threats, and use worrying both as a means to solve problems and avoid fear.

About 3% of the US population will meet the criteria for GAD in any given year. The median age for GAD is 30 years of age. GAD is about twice as prevalent in women than men and is commonly comorbid with depression (APA 2013). Risk factors for GAD include poverty, family history of mental illness, chronic medical and mental health problems, recent or early experience of adverse events or trauma, parental loss or separation, and emotional neglect in childhood (APA 2013; Zhang et al. 2015). GAD is associated with a higher risk for cardiovascular disease, hypertension, and increased blood pressure (WHO 2017; Tully et al. 2013; Butnoriene et al. 2015).

Table 8.6 Diagnostic criteria for anxiety disorders and related disorders (Based on: APA 2013)

Anxiety disorders	Signs and symptoms
Social anxiety disorder Clinically significant fear that is centered on being negatively evaluated or scrutinized in social settings by others. Fear is out of proportion to the actual threat or exaggerated.	(1) Concerned that they will act in a way that will embarrass themselves or offend others, leading to being negatively evaluated or rejected in a social setting (e.g., social gatherings, performances, conversations); (2) social situations almost always lead to feelings of fear; and (3) avoidance of social situations that provoke a fear response or social situations are endured with great distress.
Panic disorder The experience of recurrent panic attacks combined with persistent concern for future attacks or maladaptive attempts to avoid panic attacks.	(1) Recurrent panic attacks or an uncontrollable surge of intense fear or discomfort that can include sweating, rapid breathing or heart rate, shaking, nausea, dizziness, fear one is dying or losing control, etc.; (2) persistent concern for future attacks and what they mean; (3) maladaptive attempts to avoid situations or events where a panic attack might occur.
Agoraphobia Fear and avoidance of several types of situations or spaces for fear of being trapped and developing panic-like symptoms.	(1) Intense fear or anxiety of developing "panic-like" symptoms in at least two situations where escape might be difficult including: (a) Public transportation, (b) enclosed spaces, (c) open spaces, (d) being in crowded spaces, or (e) going outside of the home by oneself; (2) fear is persistent; (3) feared situations are almost always avoided or endured with great distress.
Generalized anxiety disorder Excessive, uncontrollable, and persistent worry (more days than not for 6 months) about a range of issues.	(1) Excessive, persistent, uncontrollable worry about work, school, family, relationships, health, finances, etc.; (2) experience of three or more of the following six symptoms: restlessness, fatigue, difficulty concentrating, irritability, muscle tension, sleep disturbance; (3) worry or concern is not exclusively about health (i.e. this may indicate Illness Anxiety Disoder, a separate condition); (4) worry or concern is clinically significant and out of proportion to actual threats.
Related disorders that are not classified specifically as anxiety disorders	
Related disorders	Signs and symptoms
Adjustment disorder with anxious distress Development of clinically significant emotional or behavioral symptoms in response to an identifiable stressor. Symptoms should not be better accounted for by bereavement or another disorder.	Persistent feelings of nervousness, jitteriness, and worry related to an identifiable stressor. Examples of stressors can include: (1) single events (e.g., natural disaster, divorce); (2) multiple events (e.g., marital stress and financial strain); (3) chronic issues (e.g., poverty, prolonged illness, or chronic pain or illness); or (4) developmental milestones (e.g., marriage, going back to school, going to work).

(continued)

Table 8.6 (continued)

Obsessive compulsive disorder Presence of recurrent, intrusive, and unwanted thoughts, urges, or images that cause significant distress and/or repetitive, time-consuming behaviors the person feels compelled to engage in to reduce anxiety related to obsessions or prevent a feared or dreaded event.	(1) Recurrent and persistent thoughts causing distress; (2) attempts to ignore or neutralize the thoughts through acts or other thoughts; (3) repetitive behaviors such a hand washing, checking, or mental compulsions that the person feels compelled to do in response to an obsession; (4) compulsions are performed to reduce the distress and anxiety caused by the obsessions; (5) the person spends an inordinate amount of time (1+ hours a day) engaging in obsessive thinking or compulsions that cause significant impairment.

Panic Disorder

Panic is a physical state marked by a sudden onset or surge of intense anxiety or fear that can include the experience of uncontrollable rapid heartbeat or palpitations, sweating, shaking, feelings of shortness of breath or choking, lightheadedness, chest pain, nausea, tingling, chills, or the sense that one is losing control or dying (APA 2013). These experiences are obviously very frightening and often lead the person to consult a medical professional. Panic symptoms are not attributable to the effects of a medication or controlled substance, nor are they the result of a general medical condition such as cardiovascular disorders or hyperthyroidism. Persons presenting with panic symptoms should have all relevant medical conditions ruled out. The experience of panic attacks is, by itself, not sufficient to diagnose panic disorder. Panic disorder is an anxiety disorder that includes frequent, recurrent panic attacks, but is also accompanied by persistent concern over additional attacks and/ or the presence of maladaptive behavior designed to avoid the recurrence of panic attacks such as avoiding crowded or enclosed places, situations, or activities (e.g., exercise, driving) that may lead to panic symptoms.

Assessment for panic disorder can lead to a reduction in costly and dangerous unnecessary medical procedures, ER visits, and medications. There is evidence of genetic contributions to panic disorders, particularly if a person has a family history of anxiety or depressive disorders. Age of onset for panic disorder is between 20 and 24 years of age. Personality characteristics marked by increased risk for experiencing negative emotions (e.g., negative affectivity) and sensitivity to anxiety symptoms can increase the risk for panic disorder. A lifetime history of toxis stress and trauma including physical, emotional, and/or sexual abuse can increase the risk for panic disorder (APA 2013).

Panic disorder is commonly comorbid with other anxiety disorders, particularly agoraphobia, as well as major depressive disorder and substance use disorders. Assessment for the presence of these other psychiatric disorders is advised. Panic disorder is also comorbid with medical conditions that include asthma (Favreau et al. 2014), cardiovascular disease (Tully et al. 2015), COPD (WHO 2017), stomach problems such as ulcers (Goodwin et al. 2013), and hypertension (Stein et al. 2014). DSM-5 has introduced the option of a "panic attack specifier" that can be added to any disorder if the person experiences comorbid panic attacks (APA 2013).

Social Anxiety Disorder

Persons with Social Anxiety Disorder (SAD) experience significant fear that is centered on being negatively evaluated in social settings. Persons with SAD are concerned that they will embarrass themselves and/or be rejected by others in a social setting (e.g., social gatherings, performances, conversations), leading to feelings of fear and avoidance of social situations that provoke a fear response. The fear that people experience toward social situations is exaggerated, persistent, and causes significant distress. For instance, a person may refuse to attend parties or go on a date because they are afraid, they will be negatively evaluated or do something to embarrass themselves. Persons with SAD are concerned that they may be judged as incompetent, weak, sick, unattractive, boring, aggressive, or nervous. If a person with SAD does attend a social event, they do so while enduring high amounts of distress, anxiety, or fear. This disorder can often lead to social isolation and loneliness (APA 2013). SAD impacts about 7% of the U.S. population in any given year. Age of onset is usually in childhood and adolescence. SAD differs from normative shyness or introversion in that persons with SAD experience significant psychiatric distress and impairment in occupational, school, and social functioning.

Agoraphobia

Agoraphobia is defined as a fear and avoidance of at least two of five situations that include: (1) Public transportation; (2) open spaces; (3) enclosed spaces; (4) crowds or standing in a line; and (5) being outside of home alone. People fear these situations to a significant degree because escape or rescue may be impossible if they experience panic-like symptoms such as falling, fainting, hyperventilating, incontinence, or other embarrassing symptoms. The fear is excessive and out of proportion to the situation. The situations are always either avoided or endured with excessive fear. The person may also require a companion. If the person meets criteria for both panic disorder and agoraphobia, both disorders can be diagnosed.

Obsessive Compulsive Disorder

Obsessive compulsive disorder (OCD) is no longer part of the Anxiety Disorder chapter in DSM-5. OCD is now part of a separate chapter called Obsessive-Compulsive and Related Disorders. People with OCD suffer from dysfunctional beliefs that lead to maladaptive coping responses. These beliefs include overestimating danger or threat in the environment, the need to control one's thoughts, perfectionism, and an intolerance of uncertainty. Persons with OCD utilize mental or physical compulsions in order to neutralize the anxiety caused by obsessive thoughts. Obsessive-compulsive disorder has two parts: (1) the presence of obsessions defined as intrusive and unwanted thoughts, urges, or images that cause significant anxiety and distress requiring actions by the person to neutralize the anxiety produced by the obsessions through actions or other thoughts; and (2) compulsions defined as repetitive behaviors that the person is compelled to perform in response to the obsessive thoughts in order to reduce the anxiety produced by them. Obsessions or compulsions are excessive, time-consuming (1 hour or more per day), and cause significant distress and impairment in functioning (APA 2013). About 1% of the population in the United States meets diagnostic criteria for

OCD. Age of onset is about 20 years of age. OCD is frequently comorbid with tic disorders, other anxiety disorders, and depression. Symptoms tend to be persistent and long-lasting without treatment (APA 2013).

Adjustment Disorder with Anxious Distress

Adjustment disorders are located in the trauma-and stressor-related disorders chapter. Adjustment disorder with anxious distress involves the emergence of anxiety symptoms in response to an identifiable stressor. The distress is out of proportion to the stressor causing significant functional impairment, yet does not meet the criteria of another anxiety or depressive disorder, nor are symptoms due to bereavement or grief. When the stressor is resolved or otherwise ends, symptoms do not persist for more than six months afterward.

8.5   Summary and Conclusions

Depressive and anxiety disorders represent a diverse set of conditions that have a drastic impact on overall physical and behavioral health. They are highly prevalent in the community and impact every population and group. Despite being very responsive to treatment, these conditions often go untreated, indicating the importance of routine screening and assessment of these conditions in health and behavioral health settings. Screening and assessment for these conditions are easy, fast, inexpensive, and can be conducted with modest training of staff. Integration of screening and assessment procedures for these conditions into billing and medical records systems as well as making them a routine part of the clinical encounter can increase uptake of these practices in health and behavioral settings. Implementation of community- and site-based education about these conditions is a key public health approach that can also build awareness of these conditions and reduce stigma. Expansion of screening and assessment procedures for depression and anxiety can increase treatment access and improve overall health, making them an integral part of integrated behavioral health practice.

Case Study 8.1: Julia Chen-Smith

Julia,[1] 29, is a cisgendered, biracial woman. She is currently a librarian at a large metro high school in San Francisco, California. She is passionate about her work and beloved by students and staff. Julia's mother is Korean-American and her father is Black. Julia has experienced a host of depressive- and anxiety-related symptoms throughout her life including frequent depressive episodes, panic attacks, hyperventilation, sweating, and avoidance of feared social situations. However, since she moved to San Francisco from the Midwest for her current job opportunity a year

---

[1]All names and other identifiers of this case have been changed to protect privacy and confidentiality.

ago, her symptoms have worsened to the point where she is seeking help so that, in her words, she can "live a social life that is normal, calm, engaged, and healthy."

Julia's most feared situation is social gatherings including parties, small get-togethers, happy-hour gatherings after work, dinner or movie engagements, and going on dates. Julia is self-conscious about her ability to engage in interesting conversation and measure up to others since moving to a large metro area on the west coast. She says she fears that she is going to say or do something embarrassing and so avoids gatherings despite wanting to develop friendships. Julia has been invited to various social events by co-workers including parties, after-work gatherings, movie/dinner gatherings, concerts, and the like. She consistently makes up excuses as to why she cannot attend. She is getting worried that she is developing an "antisocial" reputation even though she continues to get invitations and says she has great relationships with her co-workers. She claims that she would like to: (1) develop connections with a small group of friends; (2) find a romantic partner; and (3) feel comfortable in the company of others.

Julia is the youngest of four and has often been the focus of jokes at her expense both in school and at home due to her perceived timid nature. She has also experienced racist stereotypes throughout her life.

Julia states: You know. I get the 'hey, where are you *from*?' I say, Peoria. They say, 'No, no, where are you *really* from?' I say, Peoria. It's in Illinois. Do you want to see my Passport? It's blue like yours. I've got a lot of good comebacks. I've dealt with that my whole life. I've also been called other names I won't mention. I'm Korean and Black. I embrace both parts of my life. My mother spoke Korean around the house and taught me all about Korean culture. I can speak Korean. I know Korean history. I can cook authentic Korean food. I've been to Seoul twice. I love that part of me. My father is Black. He taught me all about Black history. Black culture. Black food. Black artists and musicians. I love all of it. It is who I am. But it's like I don't feel like I fit anywhere. I'm not considered "Black enough." I'm not considered "Korean enough." I'm not considered "American" even though I was born in damn, Peoria, Illinois. I don't know where I fit and maybe I'm self-conscious about it. And now? I've always had to be careful, but I don't feel safe outside my house right now. People say the craziest things to me. I was reading by myself in a park with a mask on and some lady came up to me and said, 'why don't you all go back to China and get your own people sick!' These things are not helping my issues. That's the other thing. People think my anxiety is just shyness. That it's because I'm "Asian" and it's part of my "deferential culture or nature." I'M FROM PEORIA. I'm an anxious, sad librarian who is great at her job and who wants a boyfriend and to go out once in a while and not freak out. School counselors would just say that it's who I am. I am quiet and introverted. But I want to have some friends. I'm interesting. I know stuff. I'm funny one on one with people I trust. I have two best friends back home and a couple college friends that are close. But here? I'm not good at starting fresh and I am lonely and scared to meet new people. I want to go out and have fun. Get married someday. Kids. The whole thing. But I just can't bring myself to go to social gatherings. I get flushed. I go blank. My voice shakes. My heart starts beating fast. I sweat. I feel like I am judged and I'm going to make a mistake and look foolish. So when someone invites me, I say 'no' and then I just stay home and can't get out of bed for the whole weekend because I'm so sad because I said 'no.' I like spending time with myself. I'm a librarian. That's not an accident. But I'd like a few friends, too. Explain how I can do a read-aloud and presentations in front of a bunch of high school kids, no problem, but I freak out when I get invited to a party or asked out on a date? How can I do *this* right here with you and tell you my life story – but I can't do this in a restaurant with a few other people? How does that work?

Despite having opportunities to meet others, achieving her professional goals, and being a successful, bilingual, well-traveled, and well-informed person, Julia is not confident that she can meet new people. She is afraid that she will be all alone in a strange city forever. She has entertained thoughts of moving back home, although she says she loves her job, co-workers, her condo, and the city in general. She has historically been shy and introverted but she has always had two or three friends in the past from high school and college, both of which were in the same Midwestern region she grew up in. However, since moving to this new city she has developed a fear of social situations. She is afraid that people will ignore her or that she will find that she has nothing to say and that once they learn of her true self, they will shun her. She states that when she is asked to go to any event, she feels a rush of panic and then develops an elaborate excuse to avoid the event. If she must go to the event, then she often shows up late, keeps to herself, makes frequent trips to the bathroom, and then leaves as soon as she can. In the time leading up to the event, she experiences panic-like symptoms and finds that while at the event she is anxious as evidenced by feeling out of breath, extensive sweating, feeling dizzy, and fearing that she would pass out. When these symptoms begin to occur, she usually finds an excuse to leave the event where she feels a rush of relief. She fears that if she continues to engage in this behavior that people will think she doesn't like them and will stop asking her to social gatherings.

Julia reports that she does not drink alcohol or use drugs and she has not experienced any traumatic, life-threatening events. Julia also reports depressed symptoms related to her anxiety. She often experienced bouts of sadness and fatigue that keep her in bed all day. She forces herself to work, but she does not enjoy her work during these episodes. When she gets home, she feeds her cat and then collapses into bed until the next day. During these periods she often experiences ruminating thoughts about worthlessness and guilt, offenses, or insults she may or may not have committed against others in the distant past, and the fear that she has let her family down. These periods can last for a week or more, but they eventually fade. These episodes often happen on the weekend when she has little to do. They are often triggered by social events that she avoids.

Julia states that she has had occasional suicidal thoughts in the past, but none in the past two years. Her suicidal thoughts are typically vague, (i.e., "I just wish I could go to sleep and not wake up," "I just wish this would all end"). She reports one suicide attempt in her past when she was in college. Julia attended a local college close to home that she commuted to each day. During a particularly bad depressive episode, she reports taking a hand full of aspirin. She immediately called 911 and was brought to the hospital. She did not suffer any medical issues. She states, "I was in a bad place then and I wasn't really thinking straight. I saw the pills and just thought, let's end this and before I knew it I had finished the bottle – but there were only a handful of pills left. I immediately call 911. I was pretty scared. The doctor said if they had been Tylenol I could have done some damage to myself. I really regret that episode and what it did to my parents. I have not felt that way in a while.

I've had some counseling after that and it kind of helped. That suicide attempt is one of the reasons I don't drink. I'm afraid of what might happen to me."

Julia is motivated to identify and solve her problems. She states that common thoughts that run through her head include: "What's wrong with me?," "no one will find me interesting," "I won't know what to say," "I'll freeze and look stupid," "I'm just not as interesting as these people," and "They're going to laugh at me." Julia states that a group of friends from work meet for a happy-hour every Thursday after work and have given her a standing invitation. In addition, with the holidays coming up, Julia states that there are several holiday parties that she hopes (and fears) she will be invited to including an annual holiday party at her Principal's house in a couple of months. It will be outside, socially distanced and masks will be required. She has also been invited to a book club starting next week outside in a park by an acquaintance at work that she would like to join but is afraid to because, as she states, "I work with these people. They will have expectations. What if I show up and look stupid or say something inappropriate. What if they think I'm an idiot? How will I ever face them again? I know this is probably an overreaction – but I'm getting flushed just thinking about it. How would I go into this close, intimate situation with no place to hide and hold it together for two hours? What if I pass out or freak out? The masks make it worse because of the difficulty breathing and having to really speak up, but the social distance thing makes is a bit easier. Ugh! I don't know. It seems impossible."

Case Analysis Questions

What is your case conceptualization of Julia based on the information in the vignette?

What symptoms does she experience?

Do Julia's symptoms meet the criteria for one or more behavioral health disorders and, if so, which one(s)?

What risk factors does Julia possess in regard to suicide?

What is your assessment of Julia's suicide history and how would you respond (e.g., safety plan)?

What are three to five treatment goals and objectives that would make a good treatment plan for Julia?

What symptoms would you target?

Looking ahead to Chap. 9, what interventions would you deploy to help Julia achieve her goals?

What strengths and resources does Julia have that she can rely on to solve her problems?

What kind of situations can be used to help Julia address her fears and depressive symptoms?

References

Alexopolous, G. S. (2005). Depression in the elderly. *Lancet, 365*, 1961–1970.

Alexopoulos, G. S., & Kelly, R. E. (2009). Research advances in geriatric depression. *World Psychiatry, 8*, 140–149.

Alexopoulos, G. S., Meyers, B. S., & Young, R. C. (1997). 'Vascular depression' hypothesis. *Archives of General Psychiatry, 54*, 915–922.

Almeida, O. P., Alfonso, H., Hankey, G. J., & Flicker, L. (2010). Depression, antidepressant use and mortality in later life: The health in men study. *PLoS One, 5*, e11266.

American Psychiatric Association. (2010). *Practice guidelines for the assessment and treatment of patients with suicidal behaviors*. Washington, DC: American Psychiatric Association. Downloaded May, 17th, 2020 at: https://psychiatryonline.org/pb/assets/raw/sitewide/practice_guidelines/guidelines/suicide.pdf

American Psychiatric Association. (2013). *Diagnostic and statistical manual of mental disorders, fifth edition (DSM-5)*. Arlington, VA: American Psychiatric Association.

Andreescu, C., & Reynolds, C. F. (2011). Late-life depression: Evidence-based treatment and promising new directions for research and clinical practice. *Psychiatric Clinics of North America, 34*, 335–355.

Arroll, B., Goodyear-Smith, F., Crengle, S., Gunn, J., Kerse, N., Fishman, T., Falloon, K., & Hatcher, S. (2010). Validation of PHQ-2 and PHQ-9 to screen for major depression in the primary care population. *Annals of Family Medicine, 8*(4), 348–353. https://doi.org/10.1370/afm.1139.

Beck, J. S. (2020). *Cognitive behavior therapy: Basics and beyond* (3rd ed.). New York: Guilford Press.

Borda, M. G., Santacruz, J. M., Aarsland, D., Camargo-Casas, S., Cano-Gutierrez, C. A., Suarez-Monslave, S., Campos-Fajardo, S., & Perez-Zepeda, M. U. (2019). Association of depressive symptoms and subjective memory complaints with the incidence of cognitive impairment I older adults with high blood pressure. *European Geriatric Medicine, 10*(3), 413–420. https://doi.org/10.1007/s41999-019-00185-1.

Bruce, M. L., Ten Have, T. R., Reynolds, C. F., Katz, I. I., Schulberg, H. C., Mulsant, B. H., Brown, G. K., McAvay, G. J., Pearson, J. L., & Alexopoulos, G. S. (2004). Reducing suicidal ideation and depressive symptoms in depressed older primary care patients: A randomized controlled trial. *JAMA, 291*, 1081–1091.

Butnoriene, J., Bunevicius, A., Saudargiene, A., Nemeroff, C. B., Norkus, A., Ciceniene, V., & Bunevicius, R. (2015). Metabolic syndrome, major depression, generalized anxiety disorder, and ten-year all-cause and cardiovascular mortality in middle aged and elderly patients. *International Journal of Cardiology, 190*, 360–366. https://doi.org/10.1016/j.ijcard.2015.04.122.

Cacioppo, J. T., & Patrick, W. (2008). *Loneliness: Human nature and the need for social connection*. New York: W.W. Norton and Co.

Caspi, A., Sugden, K., Mofftt, T. E., Taylor, A., Craig, I. W., Harrington, H., et al. (2003). Influence of life stress on depression: Moderation by a polymorphism in the 5-HTT gene. *Science, 301*(5631), 386–389.

Cutrona, C. E., Wallace, G., & Wesner, K. A. (2006). Neighborhood characteristics and depression—An examination of stress processes. *Current Directions in Psychological Science, 15*(4), 188–192.

Diniz, B. S., Butters, M. A., Albert, S. M., Dew, M. A., & Reynolds, C. F. (2013). Late-life depression and risk of vascular dementia and Alzheimer's disease: Systematic review and meta-analysis of community-based cohort studies. *British Journal of Psychiatry, 202*, 329–335.

Draper, B., Pfaff, J. J., Pirkis, J., Snowdon, J., Lautenschlager, N. T., Wilson, I., Almeida, O. P., & Depression and Early Prevention of Suicide in General Practice Study Group. (2008). Long-term effects of childhood abuse on the quality of life and health of older people: Results from the

Depression and Early Prevention of Suicide in General Practice Project. *Journal of the American Geriatrics Society, 56*(2), 262–271. https://doi.org/10.1111/j.1532-5415.2007.01537.x.

Dube, S. R., Anda, R. F., Felitti, V. J., Chapman, D. P., Williamson, D. F., & Giles, W. H. (2001). Childhood abuse, household dysfunction, and the risk of attempted suicide throughout the life span: Findings from the adverse childhood experiences study. *JAMA, 286*(24), 3089–3096. https://doi.org/10.1001/jama.286.24.3089.

Eaton, W. W., Muntaner, C., Smith, C., Tien, A., & Ybarra, M. (2004). Center for Epidemiologic Studies Depression scale: Review and revision (CESD and CESD-R). In M. E. Maruish (Ed.), *The use of psychological testing for treatment planning and outcomes assessment* (3rd ed., pp. 363–377). Mahwah, NJ: Lawrence Erlbaum.

Favreau, H., Bacon, S. L., Labrecque, M., & Lavoie, K. L. (2014). Prospective impact of panic disorder and panic-anxiety on asthma control, health service use, and quality of life in adult patients with asthma over a 4-year follow-up. *Psychosomatic Medicine, 76*(2), 147–155. https://doi.org/10.1097/PSY.0000000000000032.

Felitti, V. J., Anda, R. F., Nordenberg, D., Williamson, D. F., Spitz, A. M., Edwards, V., Koss, M. P., & Marks, J. S. (1998). Relationship of childhood abuse and household dysfunction to many of the leading causes of death in adults: The Adverse Childhood Experiences (ACE) study. *American Journal of Preventive Medicine, 14*, 4.

Goodwin, R. D., Talley, N. J., Hotopf, M., Cowles, R. A., Galea, S., & Jacobi, F. (2013). A link between physician-diagnosed ulcer and anxiety disorders among adults. *Annals of Epidemiology, 23*(4), 189–192. https://doi.org/10.1016/j.annepidem.2013.01.003.

Gunderson, J. G., Herpertz, S. C., Skodol, A. E., Torgersen, S., & Zanarini, M. C. (2018). Borderline personality disorder. *Nature Reviews. Disease Primers, 4*, 18029. https://doi.org/10.1038/nrdp.2018.29.

Gürhan, N., Beşer, N. G., Polat, Ü., et al. (2019). Suicide risk and depression in individuals with chronic illness. *Community Mental Health Journal, 55*, 840–848. https://doi.org/10.1007/s10597-019-00388-7.

Katon, W. J., Lin, E. H., Von Korff, M., Ciechanowski, P., Ludman, E. J., Young, B., Peterson, D., Rutter, C. M., McGregor, M., & McCulloch, D. (2010). Collaborative care for patients with depression and chronic illnesses. *The New England Journal of Medicine, 363*(27), 2611–2620. https://doi.org/10.1056/NEJMoa1003955.

Kiecolt-Glaser, J. K., Derry, H. M., & Fagundes, C. P. (2015). Inflammation: Depression fans the flames and feasts on the heat. *The American Journal of Psychiatry, 172*(11), 1075–1091. https://doi.org/10.1176/appi.ajp.2015.15020152.

Kraaij, V., Arensman, E., & Spinhoven, P. (2002). Negative life events and depression in elderly persons: A meta-analysis. *The Journals of Gerontology. Series B, Psychological Sciences and Social Sciences, 57*(1), P87–P94. https://doi.org/10.1093/geronb/57.1.p87.

Krishnan, K. R. R., Hays, J. C., & Blazer, D. G. (1997). MRI-defined vascular depression. *American Journal of Psychiatry, 154*, 497–500.

Kroenke, K., Spitzer, R. L., & Williams, J. B. W. (2001). The PHQ-9: Validity of a brief depression severity measure. *Journal of General Internal Medicine, 16*(9), 606–613. https://doi.org/10.1046/j.1525-1497.2001.016009606.x.

Kroenke, K., Spitzer, R. L., & Williams, J. B. (2003). The patient health questionnaire-2: Validity of a two-item depression screener. *Medical Care, 41*, 1284–1292.

Kroenke, K., Spitzer, R. L., Williams, J. B., & Löwe, B. (2009). An ultra-brief screening scale for anxiety and depression: The PHQ-4. *Psychosomatics, 50*(6), 613–621.

Lenzenweger, M. F., Lane, M. C., Loranger, A. W., & Kessler, R. C. (2007). DSM-IV personality disorders in the National Comorbidity Survey Replication. *Biological Psychiatry, 62*, 553–564.

Lieb, K., Zanarini, M. C., Schmahl, C., Linehan, M. M., & Bohus, M. (2004). Borderline personality disorder. *Lancet, 364*, 453–461.

McGlashan, T. H., Grilo, C. M., Sanislow, C. A., Ralevski, E., Morey, L. C., Gunderson, J. G., et al. (2005). Two-year prevalence and stability of individual DSM-IV criteria for schizotypal, borderline, avoidant, and obsessive-compulsive personality disorders: Toward a hybrid model of axis II disorders. *American Journal of Psychiatry, 162*, 883–889. https://doi.org/10.1176/appi.ajp.162.5.883.

Mitchell, A. J., Rao, S., & Vaze, A. (2010). Do primary care physicians have particular difficulty identifying late life depression? A meta-analysis stratified by age. *Psychotherapy and Psychosomatics, 79*(5), 285–294.

Radloff, L. S. (1977). The CES-D scale: A self-report depression scale for research in the general population. *Applied Psychological Measurement, 1*, 385–401.

Rakofsky, J. J., Schettler, P. J., Kinkead, B. L., Frank, E., Judd, L. L., Kupfer, D. J., Rush, A. J., Thase, M. E., Yonkers, K. A., & Rapaport, M. H. (2013). The prevalence and severity of depressive symptoms along the spectrum of unipolar depressive disorders: A post hoc analysis. *The Journal of Clinical Psychiatry, 74*(11), 1084–1091. https://doi.org/10.4088/JCP.12m08194.

Reynolds, C. F., Lenze, E., & Mulsant, B. H. (2019). Assessment and treatment of major depression in older adults. In S. T. DeKosky & S. Asthana (Eds.), *Handbook of clinical neurology (3rd series) Geriatric neurology* (pp. 429–435). Amsterdam: Elsevier. https://doi.org/10.1016/B978-0-12-804766-8.00023-6.

Rudisch, B., & Nemeroff, C. B. (2003). Epidemiology of comorbid coronary artery disease and depression. *Biological Psychiatry, 54*, 227–240.

Robinson, R. G. (2003). Poststroke depression: prevalence, diagnosis, treatment, and disease progression. *Biological psychiatry, 54*(3), 376–387. https://doi.org/10.1016/s0006-3223(03)00423-2

Scott, K. M., Lim, C., Al-Hamzawi, A., Alonso, J., Bruffaerts, R., Caldas-de-Almeida, J. M., Florescu, S., et al. (2016). Association of mental disorders with subsequent chronic physical conditions: World mental health surveys from 17 countries. *JAMA Psychiatry, 73*(2), 150–158. https://doi.org/10.1001/jamapsychiatry.2015.2688.

Shea, M. T., Yen, S., Pagano, M. E., Morey, L. C., McGlashan, T. H., Grilo, C. M., et al. (2004). Associations in the course of personality disorders and Axis I disorders over time. *Journal of Abnormal Psychology, 113*(4), 499–508. https://doi.org/10.1037/0021-843X.113.4.499.

Snowden, M., Steinman, L., & Frederick, J. (2008). Treating depression in older adults: Challenges to implementing the recommendations of an expert panel. *Prevention of Chronic Disease, 5*, A26.

Spitzer, R. L., Kroenke, K., Williams, J. B. W., & Lowe, B. (2006). A brief measure for assessing generalized anxiety disorder. *Archives of Internal Medicine, 166*, 1092–1097.

Stein, D. J., Aguilar-Gaxiola, S., Alonso, J., Bruffaerts, R., de Jonge, P., Liu, Z., Miguel Caldas-de-Almeida, J., O'Neill, S., Viana, M. C., Al-Hamzawi, A. O., Angermeyer, M. C., Benjet, C., de Graaf, R., Ferry, F., Kovess-Masfety, V., Levinson, D., de Girolamo, G., Florescu, S., Hu, C., Kawakami, N., et al. (2014). Associations between mental disorders and subsequent onset of hypertension. *General Hospital Psychiatry, 36*(2), 142–149. https://doi.org/10.1016/j.genhosppsych.2013.11.002.

Stockings, E., Degenhardt, L., Lee, Y. Y., Mihalopoulos, C., Liu, A., Hobbs, M., & Patton, G. (2015). Symptom screening scales for detecting major depressive disorder in children and adolescents: A systematic review and meta-analysis of reliability, validity and diagnostic utility. *Journal of Affective Disorders, 174*, 447–463. https://doi.org/10.1016/j.jad.2014.11.061.

Substance Abuse and Mental Health Services Administration. (2019). *Key substance use and mental health indicators in the United States: Results from the 2018 National Survey on Drug Use and Health (HHS Publication No. PEP19-5068, NSDUH Series H-54)*. Rockville, MD: Center for Behavioral Health Statistics and Quality, Substance Abuse and Mental Health Services Administration. Retrieved from https://www.samhsa.gov/data/

Thomas, A. J., Kalaria, R. N., & O'Brien, J. T. (2004). Depression and vascular disease: What is the relationship? *Journal of Affective Disorders, 79*, 81–95.

Tully, P. J., Cosh, S. M., & Baune, B. T. (2013). A review of the affects of worry and generalized anxiety disorder upon cardiovascular health and coronary heart disease. *Psychology, Health & Medicine, 18*(6), 627–644. https://doi.org/10.1080/13548506.2012.749355.

Tully, P. J., Turnbull, D. A., Beltrame, J., Horowitz, J., Cosh, S., Baumeister, H., & Wittert, G. A. (2015). Panic disorder and incident coronary heart disease: A systematic review and meta-regression in 1131612 persons and 58111 cardiac events. *Psychological Medicine, 45*(14), 2909–2920. https://doi.org/10.1017/S0033291715000963.

Unutzer, J., Katon, W., & Callahan, C. M. (2002). Collaborative care management of late-life depression in the primary care setting: A randomized controlled trial. *JAMA, 288*, 2836–2845.

Valkanova, V., & Ebmeier, K. P. (2013). Vascular risk factors and depression in later life: A systematic review and meta-analysis. *Biological Psychiatry, 73*, 406–413.

World Health Organization (WHO). (2017). *Depression and other common mental disorders: Global health estimates*. Geneva: License: CC BY-NC-SA 3.0 IGO. Accessed 20 June 2019 at https://apps.who.int/iris/bitstream/handle/10665/254610/WHO-MSD-MER-2017.2-eng.pdf

Zanarini, M. C., Frankenburg, F. R., Dubo, E. D., Sickel, A. E., Trikha, A., Levin, A., & Reynolds, V. (1998). Axis I comorbidity of borderline personality disorder. *American Journal of Psychiatry, 155*, 1733–1739.

Zanarini, M. C., Laudate, C. S., Frankenburg, F. R., Wedig, M. M., & Fitzmaurice, G. (2013). Reasons for self-mutilation reported by borderline patients over 16 years of prospective follow-up. *Journal of Personality Disorders, 27*(6), 783–794. https://doi.org/10.1521/pedi_2013_27_115.

Zhang, X., Norton, J., Carrière, I., Ritchie, K., Chaudieu, I., & Ancelin, M. L. (2015). Risk factors for late-onset generalized anxiety disorder: Results from a 12-year prospective cohort (the ESPRIT study). *Translational Psychiatry, 5*(3), e536. https://doi.org/10.1038/tp.2015.31.

Zimmerman, M., & Mattia, J. I. (1999). Axis I diagnostic comorbidity and borderline personality disorder. *Comprehensive Psychiatry, 40*, 245–252.

Chapter 9
Brief Approaches to Treating Depression and Anxiety

9.1 Overview of Anxiety and Depression Treatment

The World Health Organization has identified depression and anxiety disorders as one of the most significant sources of disability burden worldwide (2017). Depression is the largest contributor to disability burden and is frequently comorbid with a range of health and mental health conditions (Moussavi et al. 2007). Anxiety disorder, the sixth source of worldwide disability and one of the most prevalent psychiatric disorders in children and adults, can lead to a range of health and mental health conditions. These conditions also differentially impact persons in poverty, particularly women (2017). Persons with depression and anxiety are also at greater risk of experiencing comorbid substance use disorders and often struggle to access treatment (Han et al. 2017).

Brief cognitive behavioral therapy has been identified as an effective psychotherapeutic treatment for depression and anxiety (Beck 2020; Dobson and Dobson 2018; Greenberger and Padesky 2015; Wright et al. 2017). This form of psychotherapy has been found to be just as effective or even more effective than medication and far more effective than usual care. Cognitive behavioral therapy (CBT) is a collaborative evidence-based model of psychotherapy where the therapist and client work together to identify and reframe maladaptive thinking patterns and beliefs (Dobson and Dobson 2018). CBT should be considered a primary, frontline treatment for depression and anxiety in adult and child populations. CBT has been shown to be effective in reducing symptoms of depression and anxiety (Hunot et al. 2007). CBT works best with motivated clients suffering mild-to-moderate depression. For clients suffering from moderate-to-severe depression, a combination of

---

[1] All names and other identifiers of this case have been changed to protect privacy and confidentiality.

[2] All names and other identifiers of this case have been changed to protect privacy and confidentiality.

© Springer Nature Switzerland AG 2021
M. A. Mancini, *Integrated Behavioral Health Practice*,
https://doi.org/10.1007/978-3-030-59659-0_9

CBT and antidepressant medication should be considered. The use of lay health counselors in low- and middle-income countries as well as in high-need areas in the United States to provide common elements to treatment in primary care settings such as behavioral activation (BA), exposure-based therapy, and problem-solving therapy has shown significant reductions in the symptoms of common mental disorders (Patel et al. 2010).

The core theory behind cognitive behavioral therapy is that feelings of depression and fear are due to the activation of persistent, automatic negative thinking patterns and cognitive distortions that emerge from maladaptive beliefs clients have about themselves, other people, and the outside world. These cognitive distortions are activated by outside events and situations and lead to intense depressed or anxious feelings, which then result in maladaptive behaviors (e.g., lashing out, social withdrawal, giving up, avoidance). In short, thoughts lead to feelings and then behaviors (Beck 2020; Greenberger and Padesky 2015). Therapy is designed to target maladaptive thinking patterns. If you can change how people think through new information, you can change how they feel and behave (Greenberger and Padesky 2015). Therapy, then, is designed to reduce depressed and anxious feelings by identifying maladaptive thinking patterns and reframing or replacing them with more realistic and evidence-based thoughts about the self, others, and world. For depression, this may mean identifying negative thinking patterns or cognitive distortions and then changing them through the identification and evaluation of contrary evidence (Beck 2020; Greenberger and Padesky 2015; Wright et al. 2017).

For persons with anxiety disorders, anxious feelings triggered by feared stimuli result in erroneous and maladaptive thoughts that the anxious feelings will overwhelm or lead to harm (e.g., I am going to die…go crazy…get hurt). These "false alarms" often result in escape or avoidance behaviors that are subsequently negatively reinforced through a false sense of relief. Treatment often involves learning relaxation skills and undergoing gradual imaginal and/or in vivo exposure to the feared stimulus under safe conditions in order to incorporate new information and develop mastery (e.g., I am not going to die…go crazy…get hurt. I can manage these feelings). CBT also involves learning coping skills to better solve problems, manage anger, and plan for emergencies (e.g., decatastrophize).

Collaborative care is an effective way to treat anxiety and depression in clients (Archer et al. 2012). Collaborative care (see Chap. 1) is a form of integrated interprofessional care that involves multiple professionals including a medical doctor, care managers with behavioral health expertise such as a social worker or nurse, and psychiatrist who work together to meet the multidimensional needs of clients. In a review of 79 randomized control trials, collaborative care led to improvements in mental health, treatment adherence, and patient satisfaction (Archer et al. 2012). There is support for transdiagnostic approaches in the treatment of depression and anxiety disorders in healthcare settings such as the Unified Protocol of Transdiagnostic Treatment of Emotional Disorders (UP) (Barlow et al. 2011a, 2011b; Farchione et al. 2012) and the Coordinated Anxiety Learning and Management (CALM) approach to treatment (Bomyea et al. 2015; Roy-Byrne et al. 2010; Craske et al. 2009; Craske et al. 2011; Williams et al. 2018).

The UP is a CBT-based protocol designed to address the symptoms of anxiety and depressive disorders. The UP has shown to significantly reduce symptoms in patients with anxiety and depressive disorders) (Farchione et al. 2012). The UP has shown to be comparable in reducing symptoms across depression and anxiety disorders to single-disorder protocols indicating that a single, unified protocol can be used to address a range of disorders (Barlow et al. 2017).

CALM is also a CBT approach to behavioral health treatment in primary care settings that can address various forms of anxiety disorders including social anxiety disorder, panic disorder, and generalized anxiety disorder. This computerized model combines a stepped approach to anxiety treatment within a collaborative care model in which clients have access to medication, CBT, or both. Clients can choose the format for their treatment and the approach that makes the most sense for them. CALM learning tools are implemented by staff that are a part of the collaborative case team. These interventions are designed to require only minimal levels of training and can be easily implemented in a variety of settings by a range of staff members across disciplines. These CBT approaches include psychoeducation about anxiety disorders, developing a fear hierarchy, imaginal and in vivo exposure therapy, breathing re-training, relaxation, and cognitive restructuring delivered in 8 to 10 one-hour modules. Providers help clients learn and utilize tools, practice skills and monitor progress. Clinical trials of CALM have shown significant reductions in anxiety and depressive symptoms (Bomyea et al. 2015; Roy-Byrne et al. 2010; Craske et al. 2009; Craske et al. 2011; Williams et al. 2018). CALM has also been shown to be cost-effective (Joesch et al. 2012) and was effective in persons with medication-resistant anxiety disorders (Campbell-Sills et al. 2016). An adaptation of CALM (CALM ARC) for persons with comorbid anxiety and substance use disorders has also shown decreases in anxiety symptoms and alcohol use (Wolitzky-Taylor et al. 2018).

In the sections that follow, I provide a comprehensive review of brief psychotherapeutic approaches and treatments for depressive and anxiety disorders. Case examples are used to illustrate important practice concepts and approaches.

9.2 Cognitive Behavioral Therapy

The basic cognitive behavioral model posits that behavioral health issues are the result of negative thinking patterns that are automatic and rooted in maladaptive core beliefs about the self, others and world (Beck 2020; Dobson and Dobson 2018; Greenberger and Padesky 2015; Wright et al. 2017). A person's pattern of negative thinking leads to emotional responses such as fear, sadness, or anger that then lead to problematic behaviors such as withdrawal, avoidance, substance use, or aggression. Figure 9.1 displays the basic cognitive model. In this model, a situation leads to a negative automatic thought, which then leads to a feeling or emotion. This feeling or emotion can then lead to a behavior, which then leads to another thought, and the cycle continues. The target of therapy is changing how a person thinks about a particular situation. Changing how a person thinks about a situation can then impact

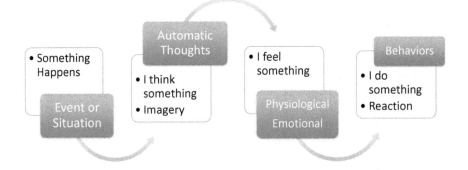

Fig. 9.1 The cognitive model (Based on: Beck 2020; Greenberger and Padesky 2015; Wright et al. 2017)

how they feel and behave. For instance, for a mother who gets into an argument with her adult children, she may automatically think that, "They don't love me." This thought leads to feelings of anger, resentment, and sadness. These feelings then result in behaviors such as lashing out and then withdrawing by staying in bed for 3 days. Persons with depression can also ruminate on negative thoughts, triggering the same thought process over and over. If the mother had a more rational or realistic thought about the argument such as, "This is a simple disagreement. It is not a referendum on my parenting or my children's love for me. We'll figure it out and move on," she may have had a much different emotional and behavioral response. Changing maladaptive thoughts to more adaptive, realistic thoughts are the main tenet of cognitive behavioral therapy (Beck 2020; Greenberger and Padesky 2015). In the next sections, we will review this model in more depth and identify specific cognitive and behavioral strategies designed to address negative automatic thinking patterns and enhance more effective coping responses.

9.2.1 The Cognitive Model of Depression

The cognitive theory of depression positions depressed feelings and behaviors such as low mood, low self-worth, lack of interest or pleasure in daily activities, social withdrawal, and suicidality as resulting from cognitive distortions related to three common core beliefs about the self relating to: (1) worthlessness, (2) unlovability, and (3) helplessness (Beck 2020; Wright et al. 2017). Figure 9.2 illustrates the relationship between core beliefs and automatic thoughts. Beliefs of worthlessness include thoughts such as, "I am no good, bad, evil, or broken"; "others are better than me"; "the world doesn't care about me and would be better off without me in it"; and "I don't deserve to live." These beliefs can lead to withdrawal, low mood and energy, and suicidality. Beliefs of unlovability can include thoughts such as "I am unlikeable, unwanted, disgusting, or abandoned," "others do not care about me or love me," "I

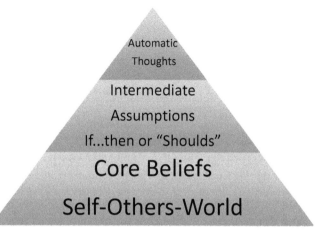

Fig. 9.2 Core beliefs and automatic thoughts (Based on: Beck 2020; Wright et al. 2017)

will always be alone," "the world is cold and heartless," and "I am defective or not good enough to be loved." These thoughts can lead to anger, despair, suicidality, and persistent low mood. Helpless core beliefs include thoughts such as: "I am powerless and out of control," "I am a loser or weak," "Nothing I do matters," "I am vulnerable and need protection," and "My fate is decided by others or is out of my control."

In addition to these core beliefs, people with depression may operate under certain firmly held rules or assumptions about themselves, others, and the world that can also lead to depression and anger. These assumptions are usually in the form of "if…then" statements that can include themes of power, perfection, status, and self-esteem. Examples can include: "if you are going to do something you must be the best or you're a failure," "If I back down or give in or compromise (even a little), then others will think I'm weak and vulnerable and try to take advantage of me," "Bad things happen to bad people so I must be bad," "I am nothing without a significant other," "It is all my fault," "If I fail at something, then it means I'm a loser and broken," and "I must have 100% control in all situations." Operating under these and other maladaptive, unrealistic, and unsupported beliefs and assumptions can lead to a range of problematic feelings and behaviors associated with depression and anxiety. Therapeutic work with clients includes psychoeducation about how thoughts impact feelings and behaviors, helping them identify, challenge, and replace maladaptive thoughts with more realistic alternatives and teaching coping skills related to problem-solving, self-soothing, and relaxation (Wright et al. 2017).

9.2.2   Cognitive Model of Anxiety

The cognitive model of anxiety also posits that maladaptive thoughts lead to anxious feelings and avoidant behavior. Maladaptive thoughts often involve overestimation of risk and danger in situations, and emotional reasoning or misperceiving anxious feelings as indications of possible danger. *Emotional processing theory* is a theory of anxiety and PTSD that positions anxiety disorders as the result of the development of a fear structure that consists of associations between anxious feelings, sensations, and maladaptive thoughts related to a feared stimuli or situation (Foa and Kozak 1986; Rauch and Foa 2006). Figure 9.3 outlines the emotional processing theory of anxiety. When an individual comes into contact with a feared stimuli or environmental cue, the fear structure is activated and triggers: (1) a physiological stress response (e.g., rapid breathing, shaking, increased heart rate, sweating); (2) intrusive, maladaptive thoughts or images (e.g., "I am going to die!," "I can't handle this!," "Something really bad is going to happen!," "This is really dangerous!"); and (3) avoidance behaviors (e.g., running away or leaving a situation, social withdrawal, saying "no" to an invitation to dinner, washing hands, maladaptive avoidance of feared situations, places, or things). The avoidance behaviors then remove the tension and lead to a temporary sense of relief, which acts to negatively reinforce the avoidant behavior in the future and further establish the fear structure. Furthermore, the person typically enacts avoidance behaviors preemptively, or so quickly after experiencing anxiety, that they never have a chance to learn new information about their fears. In other words, people do not stay in the anxiety-producing situations long enough to learn new information such as that they are, in fact, not in danger, or that their symptoms are not life-threatening, or that they actually can manage their symptoms and are in control.

From this perspective, treatment involves imaginal and in vivo exposure of the person to feared stimuli in a safe environment without engaging in typical avoidant behavior. Doing so dismantles the fear structure and reduces anxiety through a process of *habituation* as the body and mind get used to the feared situation and learn that feared consequences are not realized. When people stay with their anxiety for an extended period of time, their anxiety naturally decreases through this habituation process. The activation of the fear structure through repeated exposure to the fear stimuli in a safe situation without experiencing feared consequences creates opportunities for learning new information that can deactivate the fear structure by breaking the conditioned responses leading to a reduction in anxious feelings when

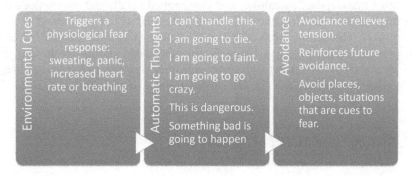

Fig. 9.3 Emotional processing theory of anxiety (Based on: Foa and Kozak 1986; Rauch and Foa 2006)

the stimuli are present. This can lead to opportunities to develop alternative thoughts and perceptions about the feared stimuli (Foa et al. 2006).

9.2.3 Common Cognitive Distortions

People who are depressed or anxious have problems processing information that interfere with learning and problem-solving. The basic principles of cognitive behavioral therapy are that problems are rooted in how we think (e.g., cognitive distortions). How we think about and conceptualize our experiences impact how we feel and behave. Our behavior, then, strongly influences and reinforces our thinking patterns and subsequent emotions. Therefore, the key to changing how we feel is to change how we think and behave. The intervention target is identifying and modifying distorted and maladaptive thinking patterns. Persons with depression and anxiety are likely to engage in distorted thinking patterns that can reinforce their symptoms. For instance, persons who are actively depressed are more likely to take excessive blame for negative events and attribute positive events to luck or chance. An anxious person is more likely to view negative events as inevitable and are less likely to see themselves as having any agency to stop or avoid those events from happening or underestimate their ability to cope with negative events. Persons who are depressed see negative events as having far-reaching global consequences, while persons who tend to be anxious overestimate the likelihood of risk and exaggerate the potential harm that could come to them. Persons who are depressed or anxious are overly pessimistic and are likely to see negative events as fixed and unchangeable and see themselves as unable to avoid, influence, alter, or recover from perceived negative events.

Several cognitive distortions have been identified that can lead to overly negative evaluations of the self, others, and world (Beck 2020; Greenberger and Padesky 2015; Wright et al. 2017). Table 9.1 lists the most common cognitive distortions along with their definition and an example. Often, people engage in several cognitive distortions. These can often reinforce each other and lead people to make unsupported conclusions that run contrary to the evidence. Providers of CBT services seek to identify cognitive distortions or maladaptive thinking patterns in their clients and then seek to reframe those thinking patterns into more adaptive and accurate ways of thinking about an event or situation (Beck 2020; Wright et al. 2017).

9.2.3.1 Selective Abstraction (Negative Filtering)

A person engages in selective abstraction when they pay attention to only part of the evidence available such as negative information about themselves, others, the world, or the future that confirms their negative core belief about themselves. They tend to ignore other information or evidence that offers an alternative view. An example can include a person who has been highly successful in their job as evidenced by the

Table 9.1 Cognitive distortions, definitions, and examples

Cognitive distortion	Definition	Example
Negative Filter, Selective Abstraction, Ignoring the Evidence	Pays attention only to information that confirms negative beliefs. Ignores disconfirming or positive information about the self.	Rochelle (from this chapter) believes she will get a negative teaching evaluation based on one student's complaint.
		Julia (from Chap. 8) ignores qualities and talents about herself that she is interesting and focuses only on her perceived negative attributes or faults.
Emotional Reasoning (False Alarms)	Misinterpret physiological or emotional experiences as evidence of danger or doom. Leads to avoidance behaviors.	Man experiences shortness of breath and believes he is going to have a panic attack that leads him to stay home from work.
		Person experiences nervousness in a crowded store and immediately leaves believing that danger is imminent.
		Julia experiences anxiety when getting ready to go to a party and believes this is evidence that she will embarrass herself and makes an excuse to cancel.
		Rochelle experiences anxiety related to her evaluation and sees this as evidence she will be fired. Craves a drink to cope.
Arbitrary inference	Persons come to a conclusion with no evidence and/or in the face of contradicting evidence	Rochelle believes she will get a poor evaluation despite no evidence that this is the case and ignores evidence indicating her good to exemplary performance.
		Julia believes she is boring and people will make fun of her despite no objective evidence and in spite of evidence that she is interesting and likable (i.e., people ask her to parties and on dates, students favor her).
Overgeneralization	Taking a small piece of isolated evidence and then using it to make conclusions about a broad range of life domains.	Doctoral student gets critical feedback from a mentor and says, "I am never going to finish this program. I am a failure. I will never find a job or a partner or amount to anything in my life."
Magnification or minimization	Exaggerating failures or defects or minimizing accomplishments/attributes	A client with a Ph.D. and several teaching awards focuses on minor mistakes and attributes them as proof he is a "loser" and a "failure."

(continued)

Table 9.1 (continued)

Cognitive distortion	Definition	Example
Personalization	Taking too much responsibility for events or circumstances beyond one's control or unrelated to the person.	A client who was forced to fire a staff member blames themselves when they learn that the staff member defaulted on their mortgage and lost their home several years later.
All-or-Nothing Thinking	Perfectionistic thinking. Viewing the self, other, and world through an absolutistic lens (i.e., all good or all bad).	Rochelle focuses on mildly negative evaluations from one or two students as evidence of poor teaching.
Mind Reading or Fortune Telling (Catastrophizing)	Assuming one knows what is going to happen or what another person is thinking without evidence.	A person's boss ignores them at the office holiday party and they think that they are out of favor or going to get fired.

Based on: Beck (2020), Greenberger and Padesky (2015), Wright et al. (2017)

existence of rewards and strong evaluations but ignores this evidence and solely focuses on one or two negative evaluations to conclude that they are going to lose their job or that they are not good enough leading to anxious and depressive symptoms.

9.2.3.2 Emotional Reasoning (False Alarms)

This distortion is when a person feels physical symptoms of anxiety, guilt, fatigue, inadequacy, or low mood and automatically assumes that there is actual danger present or that something about them is true without any evidence. The concept of "false alarms" is useful here. People who are anxious have physical alarm bells that can go off and trigger the belief that the person is unsafe without any evidence resulting in increased anxiety and conditioned responses (e.g., avoidance behaviors). For instance, a person may feel nervous and then think, "There must be danger here, I need to get out." For persons who are depressed may *feel* guilty and assume, "I must have done something wrong" or they may feel fatigue and assume, "I am lazy, weak, and worthless."

9.2.3.3 Arbitrary Inference

A similar distortion is when a person comes to a conclusion in spite of evidence to the contrary. An example would be when a person is convinced that they will die in an elevator, plane, or train crash despite overwhelming evidence that this is a safe mode of transport. This may be due to unresolved fears or from learning of an isolated incident.

9.2.3.4   Overgeneralization

This occurs when a person makes broad claims about an area of functioning based on a small piece of evidence from an isolated incident. For example, a person states, "I will never find anyone to love me" after they do not receive a return text from a person they recently went out on a date with the week before.

9.2.3.5   Magnification/Minimization

Clients who are depressed or anxious may magnify or minimize the significance of a particular event, experience, or attribute. For example, a person with generalized anxiety disorder may experience high anxiety when they call a loved one to check on them and they do not answer the phone despite there not being any obvious reason to worry.

9.2.3.6   Personification

A person engages in personification when they take on too much responsibility or blames for negative events. Depressed persons tend to take on too much responsibility for poor outcomes. A common example of this occurs when after a break up a person gets depressed because they think it was all their fault. Another example is that a person may blame themselves for when their child does not perform well on a test because they did not prepare them enough and they view themselves as a bad parent. This could also be combined with other distortions such as magnification (exaggerating the meaning and consequences of their child performing poorly) and selective abstraction (ignoring alternative evidence that they are a good parent or that their child chose to goof off several nights before the test instead of studying.)

9.2.3.7   Absolutistic (All-or-Nothing) Thinking

This is often related to perfectionistic thinking. Persons use this distortion when they engage in black-and-white thinking or view oneself and others as either a total failure or a total success. For example, a client may see themselves as a total failure because they failed at something once and view another person as complete success because they perceived them as succeeding at the same task. Another common thought is that you are either the best at something or you are a total loser.

9.2.3.8   Mind Reading/Fortune Telling/Catastrophizing

This set of distortions involves the belief that one knows what another or others may be thinking about them or what the future holds. These beliefs are always exaggerated negative outcomes with little supportive evidence. A client passes by their boss in the hallway who does not look up from their report and say good morning, leading the person to think their boss does not like them or thinks they are incompetent. Mind reading and fortune telling can also lead a person to engage in catastrophizing when they imagine the worst-case scenario and believe that scenario is going to happen without any consideration of other more likely alternatives that are positive or less catastrophic (e.g., a person is late to work and they are convinced they are going to be fired).

9.2.4   Basic Skills of Cognitive Behavioral Therapy

Cognitive behavioral therapy has several techniques and approaches that have been found to be effective in reducing depressive and anxious symptoms. CBT has several common practices and intervention approaches that will be reviewed next. Common practices that cut across CBT practices include the following elements:

9.2.4.1   Use of the Case Conceptualization

CBT is a present- and problem-focused intervention approach that addresses thinking patterns in the "here and now" to deal with current issues and counter hopelessness, helplessness, avoidance, and procrastination. The case conceptualization draws together information about the client into a coherent hypothesis for the client's problems that then leads to the development of a treatment plan that identifies intervention techniques to solve specified problems and acheive goals (Wright et al. 2017). Elements of the case conceptualization include (1) diagnosis and symptom information; (2) formative experiences related to the development of negative thought patterns; (3) interpersonal issues; (4) medical, genetic, and family history; (5) strengths and attributes; and (6) problematic or maladaptive thinking patterns and beliefs about the self, others, and world.

9.2.4.2   Psychoeducation

Providers take on a teacher or coaching role and seek to educate clients about the relationship between depressed and anxious moods and related thoughts and behaviors. The therapeutic relationship is predicated on a shared sense of acceptance, nonjudgmental understanding, collaboration, and warmth. Psychoeducation involves providing clients with information about the cognitive model of depression and/or anxiety. Psychoeducation is something that is very important in the first one to three sessions as it accompanies screening and assessment. During psychoeducation, clients are informed about the cognitive model, how automatic thoughts impact feelings and moods, which then impact behaviors. Practitioners can also provide clients with handouts, brochures, and bibliographic information about CBT to take home and review. Practitioners should also inform clients about the various strategies of CBT and the format of each CBT session. CBT is a type of intervention that is collaborative, practical, and requires active participation from the client to address depressive thinking patterns and behaviors (Beck 2020).

9.2.4.3   Behavioral Experiments

CBT values clients practicing skills and conducting behavioral experiments between sessions. These are often referred to as "homework." Clients are asked in between sessions to practice skills taught in session such as using a thought record to identify and correct maladaptive thinking patterns, engaging in behavioral activation and activity scheduling, practicing relaxation techniques or other coping skills learned in treatment, and engaging in exposure activities. These between-session activities are vitally important to reinforce skills learned within sessions (Beck 2020; Wright et al. 2017).

9.2.4.4   Agenda Setting and Mood Checks

CBT is a very structured approach. At the start of each session, the provider reviews the previous week's assignments and session topics and then sets the stage for the rest of the current session identifying problem areas and coping skills to develop and explore. Agenda-setting helps keep sessions on track and focused. Providers also conduct "mood checks" and utilize subjective units of distress scales (SUDS ratings) throughout the session to establish baseline moods, to measure how moods shift as the session progresses and how the client is responding to in-session techniques. When taking a SUDS rating, clients are asked to measure their distress using a 10- or 100-point scale with higher numbers indicating more distress. Clients will typically measure and rate distress before, during, and after an activity, intervention, or session to examine reactions and evaluate practice (Beck 2020).

9.2.4.5   Socratic Questioning

Didactic statements and reassurance do not lead to changes in thinking or acting. The provider and client explore and critically challenge negative assumptions, beliefs, and thinking patterns. Rather than reassuring or giving advice or tell the clients what to think, Socratic questioning is a style of questioning that asks clients to explore and interrogate their thoughts and behaviors from a stance of curiosity. Providers ask clients to consider the evidence that supports and does not support a particular thought and to explore more rational ways of thinking about problems. Table 9.2 lists several examples of Socratic questions (Beck 2020; Dobson and Dobson 2018; Greenberger and Padesky 2015; Wright et al. 2017).

Table 9.2 Socratic questions and examples

Type of Socratic question	Examples
Examining the evidence	What evidence do you have to support this idea?
	What is the evidence for that thought and how would you rate its quality?
	What evidence have you considered that does not support that thought or supports a different thought?
	What do we do with this new information?
	How does this new information change how you think?
Exploring alternatives	What would you say to a friend who was experiencing the same way? If a close friend thought this way, what would you tell him or her? What advice would you give your best friend in this situation?
	What would be another way to look at this situation?
	What cognitive distortions do you suppose might be operating here? Are any distortions present in the thought you identified?
	How might thinking differently about this change how you feel and act?
	If you told a close friend about this thought, what would he or she say?
	When you have felt differently in the past, what would you have said about this thought?
Exploring impact	What do you suppose has been the effect on you for thinking this way?
	How does this thought affect how you feel and act?
	How has thinking this way impacted your relationships?
Evaluating strength of belief	Can you describe experiences when this thought was not completely true?
	How strongly do you believe this now?
	On a scale from 0%–100%, where does your belief fall?

Based on: Beck (2020), Dobson and Dobson (2018), Greenberger and Padesky (2015), Wright et al. (2017)

9.2.4.6 Addressing Maladaptive Thoughts

Providers collaborate with clients to identify and modify maladaptive thinking patterns through thought change methods. These are typically accomplished through thought change records. Thought change records consist of five columns: (1) Event, (2) Automatic Negative Thought(s), (3) Feelings and Distress Level, (4) The Cognitive Distortion Underlying the Negative Automatic Thought and An Alternative Thought or Response, and (5) The Result (e.g., change in distress level or behavior) (Beck 2020; Dobson and Dobson 2018; Greenberger and Padesky 2015; Wright et al. 2017).

9.2.4.7 Behavioral Activities

Providers help clients boost self-efficacy and reduce feelings of helplessness, anxiety, and avoidance behaviors through behavioral methods such as behavioral activation, relaxation, breathing retraining, and imaginal and in vivo exposure techniques (Wright et al. 2017).

9.2.4.8   Skill Building

Providers teach clients skills related to anger management, problem-solving, assertiveness, and adaptive coping to reduce relapse and improve functioning.

9.3   Behavioral Approaches

Several behavioral approaches have been identified that help reduce depressive and
anxiety symptoms. These approaches are often used as part of cognitive behavioral
therapy. Behavioral approaches are often used first in depression as they can assist
in reducing symptoms of fatigue and melancholy and prepare people for approaches
that address cognitive symptoms. For persons with anxiety, providers first explore
maladaptive thinking patterns and teach coping skills before engaging in exposure
techniques that can be distressing. Behavioral approaches for depression include
behavioral activation, activity scheduling, graded task assignments, and relaxation.
Behavioral approaches for anxiety also include relaxation, breathing retraining,
response prevention, imaginal exposure, and in vivo exposure.

9.3.1   Behavioral Activation

Behavioral activation (BA) is used to break cycles of avoidance, inactivity, and
helplessness and help persons who are depressed to build a bit of self-efficacy and
break self-defeating thinking and behavior. BA is a low-threshold approach specially designed to get people moving and break depressive cycles of low mood,
withdrawal, and isolation. BA and physical movement and exercise have been found
to be an effective approach to reducing depressive and anxiety symptoms. (Boswell
et al. 2017; Kvam et al. 2016). BA involves engaging in simple, time-limited, valued
tasks in order to gain sense of momentum, accomplishment, mastery, and positive
emotion. Behavioral activation is one of the simplest and effective therapeutic strategies for the treatment of depression (Chan et al. 2017). In addition to sadness,
people who are depressed experience physical fatigue; difficulty concentrating,
making decisions, and organizing activities; and a constant drumbeat of negative
thoughts. This experience can lead to withdrawal and inactivity. The depressed person then become overwhelmed by the build-up of neglected responsibilities, and
they can experience loneliness due to their social withdrawal. The experience of
perceived loneliness can have serious negative consequences for health leading to
increase morbidity and even early morality (Cacioppo and Patrick 2008; Holt-
Lunstad et al. 2015). And because clients often engage in cognitive distortions, they
can engage in self-blame and can become angry with themselves, others, and the
world. They then retreat further into themselves, avoiding the stress of having to
complete a growing pile of tasks and face their family and friends. In short, people

who are depressed can become paralyzed or stuck, leading to prolonged symptoms and delayed remission.

For the behavioral health specialist, it may be tempting to begin addressing the person's negative thinking patterns. But the inertia and pessimism of depression can interfere with the ability and motivation of people to look at their negative thinking patterns. Instead, it can be more helpful to get people moving by helping people to re-engage (slowly) with activities they once thought interesting and pleasurable and to also complete some relatively easy tasks in order to help establish a sense of momentum. Engaging in pleasurable tasks can lead to positive emotions and a sense of accomplishment and competence.

BA involves several components that can be considered behavioral interventions in their own right. BA also has a structure and intentionality. It is appropriate for persons who are having trouble becoming active and who are discouraged, pessimistic, overwhelmed, and paralyzed. The key to behavioral activation is to start small and proceed slowly. Design activities that the client views as achievable and not too overwhelming and then move on to more complex activities as the person gains momentum. Figure 9.4 lists the different components of behavioral activation. The focus of BA should include problematic activities in daily living (e.g., chores such as light housework, washing dishes, laundry, paying bills, sorting mail), work or school tasks, pleasurable activities, and socializing (e.g., coffees, phone calls/texts, walks, picnics, lunch, dinners, or parties/social gatherings). For anxious clients, BA can be used to counter anxious avoidance behavior through the (re)-engagement with valued activities and routines (Boswell et al. 2017). It is best to start with pleasurable activities that can be reasonably accomplished by the client that are not overwhelming. These activities are strategically selected and tailored to the needs, choices, and situation of the client. Providers can also use this to identify activities such as hobbies, activities, or other interests that a client finds enjoyable or gives them a sense of accomplishment (Wright et al. 2017). These activities will inform the BA approach.

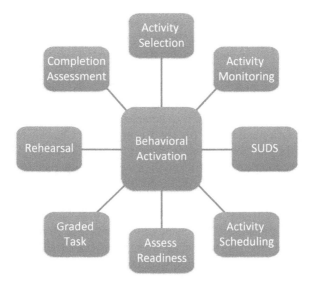

Fig. 9.4 Components of behavioral activation (Based on Wright et al. 2017)

Activity Monitoring One of the key elements of BA is activity monitoring. This involves having clients log their activities each hour of the day over the course of a 1- to 2-week period. Clients will also take a SUDS rating for each activity to identify their experience such as their sense of pleasure, accomplishment, or self-efficacy regarding the activity. These logs can also be used to identify when a client may be engaged in procrastination or avoidance, engaged in activities too often (e.g., sitting on the couch watching television, sleeping), times of inactivity, or times of the day or week where the client feels either particularly depressed or when they feel energetic. This log can then be used to strategically identify and deploy activities that may assist the client in feeling better (Beck 2020; Wright et al. 2017).

Activity Scheduling Activity scheduling is used to gently encourage a client to perform simple, enjoyable activities to boost mood and time-limited and achievable tasks that can give a client a sense of control and mastery over their lives. These activities are planned by using information from the activity monitoring log. For instance, if a client finds that they have low energy during the early afternoon and this results in them sitting on the couch watching television for the rest of the day and into the evening, the client and therapist may schedule an activity that interrupts this cycle of inactivity. Clients may also complain of tasks that are piling up (e.g., paying bills, dishes in the sink or household chores, neglect of friendships, lack of eating properly). This information can also be used to prioritize a list of activities and then schedule those activities at specific times of the day. Clients will also record SUDS ratings before and after they complete each task in order to monitor their level of pleasure or accomplishment. Figure 9.4 lists a range of BA tasks and activities than can be helpful for clients suffering from depression. There are several ways to enhance the success of BA. These include:

1. *Give a Rationale.* BA should be introduced to the client as a way to feel better. Give a clear rationale that explains that engaging in pleasurable activities and completing certain routine tasks can increase mood and energy, and improve sleep.
2. *Pick low hanging fruit.* Success through completion is the key. When selecting activities to include in the scheduling list be sure to have a good understanding of the current level of functioning of the client. Clients who are depressed often want to select activities that are too difficult because the client thinks they *should* be able to complete them. It is very important that activities are selected early in therapy to have a greater chance of completion (e.g., low hanging fruit). They should be a little challenging, but not overwhelming. Clients who are unable to complete tasks may blame themselves and view this as another "failure," further deepening their negative view of self. It is therefore important to start where the client actually is and not where they think they should be. For example, having a client that has been immobilized and sitting on the couch for 2 months to "go to the gym" will likely lead to failure. Going to the gym can be too overwhelming (for anyone). Instead, have the client go for a walk for 10 minutes or do some light stretching. Likewise, instead of having the client "clean the house," suggest that they do one load of laundry or just make some soup.

3. *Be concrete, specific, and time-limited...and write it all down.* It is important to be very specific and concrete when selecting tasks and activities. Be sure to plan ahead for potential obstacles by asking clients "what do you think could get in your way?" in order to devise a plan to address such obstacles. Activities should be planned out in advance with a client, identifying action steps to complete the activity or task. Clients who are depressed have trouble with memory. It is important to review activities and plans at the end of the session and have the client leave the session with a detailed, written plan for achieving these activities including a plan for what to do when they feel overwhelmed or are encountering obstacles (e.g., call for help, review notes, take a step back and reduce the activity time or effort level, don't blame yourself).

4. *Break down tasks using graded task assignments.* Graded task assignments break one task into several smaller steps. Clients who are depressed and anxious can have difficulty organizing tasks and can also become easily overwhelmed. Practitioners work with clients to break a task that initially seems overwhelming down into a series of smaller steps. It is important that each step, when completed, will lead to the completion of the entire task (e.g., don't leave out a step). Use graded task assignments in conjunction with activity scheduling to increase mastery experiences and enhance self-efficacy. Practitioners need to listen for and address negative automatic thoughts that may interfere with task completion (e.g., black-and-white thinking, catastrophizing). Be sure to praise progress and assess readiness for the next task (e.g., how confident are you on a scale from 1 to 100 that you can complete this task?).

5. *Set a date and time for completion and follow up if you can.* Write down the task or activity, steps, and a date and time for completion. Review what happened at the next session or ask permission to call and follow up with the client after the task was to be completed. This can help clients build motivation, remind clients of the tasks, and problem-solve in the moment to assist clients in overcoming obstacles. Encouraging the client to call for help or guidance in between sessions may also be helpful.

6. *Measure distress and give credit.* When clients successfully complete activities and tasks it is important to assess how they felt before and after completion of each task through SUDS ratings. Be sure that clients give themselves credit for accomplishing these tasks. Clients often report that they felt better after completion. This can be used to build momentum and reinforce the rationale of the intervention.

7. *Problem-solve non-completion before and after tasks.* As activities are identified and broken down into achievable chunks it is important for providers to work with clients to identify potential roadblocks to completion. Asking, "What might prevent you from completing this activity?" can help open up a conversation to help plan for overcoming obstacles. Despite this planning, many times clients are unable to complete the assigned tasks. This is a good opportunity to assess what obstacles prevented the client from completing the task and provides an opportunity for further problem solving and strategizing. A question to ask clients is: "What got in your way?" and "How can we plan around this obstacle in

the future." When clients report that they did not complete tasks it is important to not frame this as a failure or lack of compliance, but as a normal part of the recovery process and that this is an opportunity to learn what happened and plan for a better outcome. Work together to identify obstacles and to problem-solve ways around the task. Were the tasks too long or complicated? Did they miss an important step? Did the client forget or become distracted? Did they feel over-whelmed? Did they experience negative automatic thoughts and if so what were they telling them? How did this make them feel? Use this information to plan for the next round of BA. It may be that clients need more encouragement between sessions or that they require rehearsal or accompaniment in order to complete the task. Work with clients collaboratively to help them complete each task in order to build momentum and mastery (Beck 2020; Dobson and Dobson 2018; Greenberger and Padesky 2015; Wright et al. 2017).

9.3.1.1 The Act "As if..." Exercise

The Act "As if" exercise is a form of behavioral activation that asks clients to act as if they are confident or happy or some other positive attribute. In this exercise you ask the client to identify what they are like when they are happy or confident. What do they do? How do they look? How do they act? Clients are then asked to act these characteristics out regardless of how they feel inside. This may include things like smiling at the first 10 people they see that day (which often leads to people smiling back at them, which has then been found to lead to improved mood), to walk with a straight back, making good eye contact, saying positive things about themselves or their experiences to others, and using a pleasant or upbeat tone of voice. These simple behaviors can lead to mood changes in the same way that thinking more positive thoughts can also change mood. Mood can be impacted by making changes to thoughts and/or behaviors.

9.3.2   Relaxation and Mindfulness Skills

Teaching mindfulness and relaxation skills are core strategies to help people who are anxious and depressed manage distress, develop body awareness, reduce stress, and prevent relapse. Teaching relaxation skills can reduce symptoms of depression (Jorm et al. 2008). Relaxation training has been found to be effective in reducing the symptoms of anxiety (Manzoni et al. 2008). Relaxation and yoga both have been found to reduce stress and anxiety, increase physical and mental health, and improve sleep. These interventions can have a positive impact in a short amount of time, they are easily incorporated into daily routines, and when practiced regularly they can lead to sustained positive outcomes (Smith et al. 2007). Figure 9.5 lists several types of relaxation training. Each of these are explored in more detail next.

9.3.2.1 Relaxation Skills and Breathing Retraining

Relaxation skills often include Jacobson's progressive muscle relaxation (PMR) techniques (1938). The theory behind this technique is that the mind and body are connected and a state of physical relaxation resulting from the tensing and relaxation of the body will naturally lead to a state of mental calmness (1938). PMR can lead to reduced anxiety and improved sleep. PMR involves the slow, sustained, and repetitive tensing and releasing of separate muscle groups starting at one end of the body and moving to the next group until all muscle groups have been addressed. Muscle groups often start at the lower extremities such as the feet and toes, moving up to the legs and buttocks, abdomen, fingers, arms, chest, shoulders, head, neck, and face. Muscle groups are tightened from 5 to 10 seconds and then released. Clients are instructed to inhale while tightening and exhale while relaxing. Each muscle group can be tensed and released in sets of 1–3 repetitions. Sessions can last 10–20 min. The approach can be combined with relaxing music and slow, deep breathing. However, the approach can also be done in multiple positions (e.g., sitting, standing, or lying on the floor) and situations (e.g., home, work, school), making it easy to incorporate into everyday routines. The tightening and relaxation of the muscles helps in focusing attention on the body and bodily cues and distracting from anxious thoughts. The deployment of basic yoga stretches and positions can

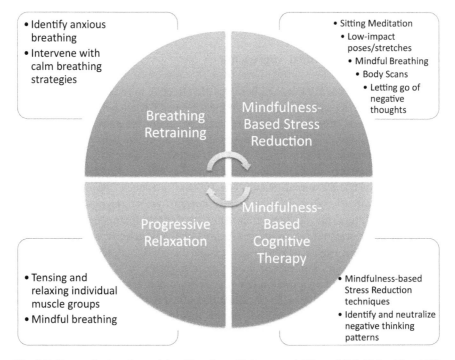

Fig. 9.5 Types of relaxation training (Based on: Hofmann and Gómez 2017; Kabat-Zinn 1990; Segal et al. 2013; Smith et al. 2007; Wright et al. 2017)

also be utilized by clients and have been found to have comparable impact on sleep and psychiatric symptoms as PMR (Smith et al. 2007).

Deep breathing exercises or "breathing retraining" can be used to assist people in inducing a state of calm and in managing breathing difficulties related to hyperventilation or overventilation often experienced during states of anxiety and panic. Breathing retraining can help people recognize and prevent panic attacks or reduce their intensity as well lead to a more overall sense of calm. Anxious breathing involves short, rapid, and shallow breaths that can deepen anxiety and cause fatigue and irritability. Breathing retraining involves helping clients practice establishing deep, slow, and sustained breathing patterns to combat the short, shallow, and rapid breathing that accompanies anxiety. Teaching clients deep breathing techniques can include having them lie on the floor or sit in a chair with their hand on their stomach to feel how taking deep breaths can expand and contract their abdomen. When they breathe deeply, clients should be doing so through their abdomen (not their chest) and be able to see their hand move up and down; they can practice this at times when they feel anxious. During breathing retraining, providers teach clients how to breathe in deeply and more slowly. Clients practice breathing in for 3–4 seconds, holding for 1 seconds or 2, and then releasing for 4–6 seconds. Practice with clients in session and encourage them to do this 2–3 times per day to improve breathing practice. Combining this with mindful practice, where the client focuses only on the breath, can also help improve calmness. Providers can also combine this as part of a behavioral activation exercise.

9.3.2.2 Mindfulness-Based Approaches

Mindfulness and meditation-based therapies are effective in reducing stress and the symptoms of anxiety and depression (Chen et al. 2012; Khoury et al. 2013). Mindfulness-based approaches combine meditative philosophies and practices such as sitting meditation, tai chi, or yoga practices, with cognitive behavioral treatment elements (Hofmann and Gómez 2017). Mindfulness is a state of present-focused attention, awareness, openness, and acceptance of bodily sensations, thoughts/ beliefs, emotions, and external stimuli. Mindfulness is a state of openness and non-judgmental awareness (Bishop 2004). When mindful, one's thoughts do not wander to the past or future, nor do they jump from one thing to the next. Being mindful means that one does not react or judge thoughts, feelings, actions, or beliefs of oneself or of others one way or another—but accepts them without judgment. This state and practice is in stark contrast to the constant negative ruminations, harsh self-judgments, and fearful anticipation that characterize depressed and anxious thinking. Mindful-based practice is the combination of the practice of mindful awareness with the skills of cognitive behavioral therapy that helps clients notice and reframe their negative thinking patterns and try out new ways of thinking (Bishop 2004; Creswell 2017; Hofmann and Gómez 2017; Kabat-Zinn 2003).

The two most common forms of mindfulness-based practice for the treatment of anxiety and depression are Mindfulness-Based Stress Reduction (MBSR) developed by Jon Kabat-Zinn (1990) and Mindfulness-Based Cognitive Therapy (MBCT) developed by Teasdale and colleagues (Segal et al. 2013; Teasdale et al. 2000). Mindfulness-based therapies such as MBSR and MBCT are effective in reducing distress and enhancing well-being in healthcare professionals (Burton et al. 2017; Spinelli et al. 2019).

Mindfulness-Based Stress Reduction was initially developed to treat chronic pain, but has been found to be effective in reducing depressive and anxious symptoms. MBSR is an 8-week group program for 2- to 2.5-hour sessions that teach clients mindfulness practices such as sitting meditation, body scans, and low-impact yoga exercises and stretches. Audio listening programs for home practice and retreats are also used. Clients learn how to monitor bodily sensations; accept thoughts, feelings and sensations in a non-judgmental manner; stay aware and focused on the present moment; and regulate emotions by noticing and letting go of stressful thoughts and feelings. The core focus is how to reduce stress and negative thinking and how to incorporate practice into daily life. MBSR has been found to be superior to many forms of treatment in systematic reviews and randomized controlled trials in reducing anxiety and stress in a range of populations in medical and other settings (Bohlmeijer et al. 2010; Fjorback et al. 2011; Hoge et al. 2013).

Mindfulness-Based Cognitive Therapy (MBCT) is an approach heavily influenced and informed by MBSR (Segal et al. 2013). MBCT follows the approach of MBSR and adds additional cognitive therapy components designed to address depressed thinking (Beck et al. 1979). These include helping clients identify and neutralize negative thinking patterns that lead to low mood. Clients learn how to notice how mood is impacted by negative thinking patterns. They then learn to observe those patterns without judging or reacting to them and then to let them go. MBCT has been found to be effective in reducing symptoms of anxiety and stress (Evans et al. 2008). MBCT has also been found to reduce anxiety and depressive symptomology in primary care settings (Finucane and Mercer 2006; Creswell 2017). MBSR may reduce emotional reactivity and improve the ability to regulate emotions (Goldin and Gross 2010; Kober et al. 2019). MBCT has been most effective in reducing depressive symptoms and relapse in persons with recurrent depression (Creswell 2017; Williams et al. 2014).

9.4   Exposure-Based Therapies

Exposure is a core CBT technique for anxiety, depression, and post-traumatic stress disorder based on emotional processing theory. In anxiety disorders, exposure is designed to activate fear structures that fuel anxious distress and avoidance behaviors and then challenge and weaken them through the introduction of incompatible information (e.g., safety, mastery) and the process of *habituation* or the tendency to become less anxious in the repeated and prolonged presence of anxiety-producing stimuli (Foa and Kozak 1986; Rauch and Foa 2006). In depression, exposure techniques are designed to challenge procrastination and self-doubt through energizing activities. Exposure-based therapeutic techniques, then, require clients to confront their fears in a safe situation without engaging their usual avoidant behavior. Repeatedly doing so over time results in a reduction in anxious reactivity and physiological arousal (e.g., habituation) to feared stimuli, and increased sense of coping self-efficacy and control and subsequently less avoidant behavior. In order for exposure therapy to be effective, the fear structure must be activated, producing anxiety symptoms that can be measured through SUDS scores from the client. The client must then learn new corrective information that is incompatible with the fear structure. This can be done through imaginal exposure where the person re-imagines a feared situation, object, or experience, or through in vivo exposure, which involves real-life exposure to fear situations within a safe environment. The client must also learn new information that counters information in the fear structure. This involves information regarding the ability of the person to manage anxious symptoms, that anxious symptoms are not harmful, and that feared consequences do not come to pass. As this new information is added to the fear structure, the fear structure begins to break apart and over time clients should experience within-session and between-session habituation or a reduction in anxious distress (Foa et al. 2007; Gillihan et al. 2012; Rauch et al. 2012).

9.4.1   In-Vivo Exposure and Fear Hierarchies

In in vivo exposure therapies clients face fear situations and objects in real-life circumstances. In vivo exposure is best used for specific phobias such as fear objects (e.g., snakes, spiders, dogs) or situations (e.g., flying in planes, elevators, social gatherings, or reminders of trauma). When utilizing in vivo exposure the provider and client first develop a *graded fear hierarchy* that is developed using SUDS scores. The hierarchy is a graded list of feared elements (e.g., situations, objects, actions) that are rated on a scale of 1–100. The list rates the feared situations in order from least to most fear-producing. For instance, a person who is afraid of using elevators may develop a fear hierarchy that looks something like this:

Look at a picture of an elevator	SUDS = 10
Watch movie with scenes of people in elevators	SUDS = 30
Imagine taking an elevator ride	SUDS = 40
Go to an elevator and touch the button or the door	SUDS = 60
Walk into elevator and then walk out	SUDS = 75
Take a short elevator ride with a with a friend	SUDS = 90
Take a ride alone	SUDS = 100

The provider and the client work through the hierarchy, slowly increasing the exposure of the client to the various elements (Foa et al. 2007; Rauch et al. 2012). Clients continue this work on their own between sessions. When clients are able to tolerate each element and demonstrate a reduction in distress (as measured through

SUDS scores), they can then move on to the next element. For clients who engage in avoidance of places, situations, or objects due to trauma, the provider and client work together to increase exposure of the client to those elements as long as they are safe. For instance, if a client was robbed in a park and now fears going to any park alone the client would work toward going to a relatively safe park by themselves through a hierarchy that might include driving through the park, walking in the park with a friend for an increasing amount of time, and then eventually going to a park alone for an increasing amount of time until habituation is achieved. These activities could be done with the therapist at first, with the client transitioning to accomplish these tasks in-between sessions while the client and therapist utilize imaginal exposure within sessions to work on the trauma symptoms associated with the robbery itself. Two important elements in in vivo exposure are utilizing real-life spaces and duration of exposure. Ideally clients would engage in in vivo exposure in between sessions in actual, real-life environments at home or in public spaces rather than in the provider's office or a clinic. Second, it is important for clients to endure in vivo exposure exercises for a period of time that is long enough for them to experience a reduction in distress (i.e. habituation). This is very important because the client will learn that staying in anxiety-producing situations will eventually lead to a reduction in distress. They will, therefore, be less likely to engage in avoidance behaviors (Foa et al. 2007; Gillihan et al. 2012; Rauch et al. 2012).

9.4.1.1   Imaginal Exposure

In imaginal exposure, the client repeatedly imagines themselves in a fear-provoking situation while narrating the event or writing about the event. Imaginal exposure is commonly used with PTSD, OCD, generalized anxiety disorder, and social anxiety disorder. For PTSD treatment, imaginal exposure is often used to help clients reduce anxious distress. Clients re-imagine the details of the traumatic event and narrate the event out loud to the therapist or in writing. Repeated imaginal exposure can then lead to a reduction in anxious distress related to the cues of the event that may trigger PTSD symptoms. Clients with OCD will imagine situations that trigger their obsessional thinking patterns and anxiety and then imagine what would happen if they did not engage in the ritualistic compulsions they typically use to neutralize their anxious distress. In social anxiety disorder treatment, clients are asked to imagine social situations that cause a significant amount of distress as a means to prepare them for in vivo exposure exercises. During imaginal exposure exercises the client describes the details of the event, the physical sensations they experience, and the feelings and thoughts that come to them as they engage in the exercise (Foa et al. 2007; Gillihan et al. 2012; Rauch et al. 2012; Wright et al. 2017).

Panic Disorder and Agoraphobia   Persons with panic disorder or agoraphobia fear physical sensations and are often afraid they will have a panic attack or panic-like symptoms in certain situations and engage in avoidance behaviors (APA 2013). In vivo exposure for panic disorder and/or agoraphobia may include having the client be exposed to feared situations (e.g., enclosed spaces, open space, public spaces, crowds) for increasing amounts of time using enclosed spaces or an elevator in the provider's office before moving to more public venues such as malls, stores, crowded spaces, or public transportation. This will depend on the client's fear hierarchy. For between-session homework it may be necessary for the client to engage in these behaviors with trusted others before doing so on their own.

Persons with panic disorder are often afraid of certain bodily sensations because they fear they may lead to a panic attack or signal imminent danger or even death. These include increased heartbeat, lightheadedness, rapid breathing, or dizziness. Providers often use an exposure technique called interoceptive exposure to re-enact these physical experiences in session in order to help clients understand that simply experiencing these physical sensations is not harmful. When using interoception clients are asked to run in place or go up a flight of stairs to induce a more rapid heartbeat, breathe through a straw to mimic shortness of breath, spin in a chair or shake the head from side to side to induce dizziness, or breathe rapidly to mimic the feeling of hyperventilation. The activities activate the fear structure in the client. The provider and client then stay with the anxiety until habituation or a reduction in distress is achieved despite the presence of these physical symptoms. Repeated exposure to the fear stimuli then leads to a reduction of fear associated with the sensation (Gillihan et al. 2012; Wright et al. 2017).

Social Anxiety Disorder   Persons with social anxiety disorder (social phobia) may be frightened of going to a large social gathering, engaging in small talk, going on a date, or giving a speech (APA 2013). The provider and client would develop a fear hierarchy-related to social interaction and then begin imaginal and in vivo exposure to those elements in the hierarchy that cause a moderate level of distress. Imaginal exposure may be used first to help the client better tolerate the anxiety related to situations that will later be the target of in vivo exposure exercises. One important consideration is understanding the safety behaviors that clients utilize to manage distress in social situations such as standing still so as to be "unseen," moving around to avoid interaction or small talk, asking rapid-fire questions, hiding, staying with only one or two trusted friends and avoiding strangers, pretending to talk on the phone to avoid conversations, or using an excuse to either avoid the event (e.g., canceling) or leaving soon after arrival. Clients would be asked to avoid these safety behaviors and instead to practice new, more useful behaviors in session. This might include role-playing, initiating a conversation and engaging in small-talk conversation in session, rehearsing a speech or presentation, and video analysis of body language and behavior (Gillihan et al. 2012; Wright et al. 2017).

For example, if a person is terrified of attending a work holiday party, but wants to go because it is the norm that all employees attend, the provider may help the client in the following ways: (1) rehearsing small-talk strategies; (2) role-playing different scenarios that are particularly anxiety-provoking such as entering the party, leaving the party and saying goodbye, initiating conversations with strangers, how to extricate oneself if they are being "cornered" in a conversation; (3)

identifying specific things to talk about (e.g., talking points) in a conversation that are in the news or relevant to the people at the party; (4) outlining an emergency escape plan if the anxiety becomes too overwhelming or the person is "stuck" in a conversation and doesn't know what to say next; and (5) outlining a plan for the party that may include how long to stay (e.g., 1 hour) that is manageable for the client, how many conversations to initiate, or staying away from alcohol and controversial subjects. These in-session strategies then prepare the client for the exposure event. The provider and client then discuss what went well, what did the person think and feel, and what could have gone better after the exposure to process the experience, and correct any cognitive distortions that might be in play such as negative filtering, ignoring the evidence, or minimizing success or magnifying failure (Gillihan et al. 2012; Wright et al. 2017).

Obsessive Compulsive Disorder In clients with OCD, imaginal exposure is first used to help the clients visualize and consider what it would be like to not engage in compulsive rituals when faced with obsessive thoughts. For instance, for a client with obsessive fear of germs who spends large amounts of time engaging in hand washing, the client might be asked to imagine using a public restroom and washing their hands for 20 seconds and then leaving without engaging in any other washing behavior. These imaginal exposure exercises prepare the client for the eventual in vivo exposure exercises they will engage in later in therapy. For persons with OCD, in vivo exposure involves *response or ritual prevention* or EX/RP. Response prevention is the prevention of ritualistic, compulsive behavior used to neutralize the anxiety triggered by obsessional thoughts. In EX/RP the client is asked to expose themselves to situations that activate obsessional thoughts and anxiety and to *not* engage in their typical rituals (e.g., hand washing, checking behavior, mental compulsions). Using the above example, the client would eventually be asked to use a public restroom (a high-anxiety situation) and wash their hands once for 20 seconds only (far less than they normally would) and to endure the anxiety they experience without engaging in a later ritualizing such as going home that evening and washing their hands repeatedly or engaging in mental compulsions. They will be asked simply to sit with their anxiety without ritualizing. This demonstrates to clients with OCD that thoughts themselves do not lead to feared outcomes and that anxiety decreases over time (Gillihan et al. 2012; Wright et al. 2017).

9.5 Cognitive Approaches

9.5.1 Identifying and Changing Maladaptive Thinking Patterns

Negative automatic thoughts, the typical targets for cognitive treatment, emerge from maladaptive core beliefs that develop through formative experiences in childhood and adolescence (Beck 2020; Greenberger and Padesky 2015). Core beliefs or "schemas" are the rules, principles, and templates we use when processing large amounts of information, and while generally out of our consciousness, they exert extraordinary influence in how we perceive the world and ourselves. Core beliefs can be adaptive or maladaptive. They are how we define ourselves in certain situations. More specifically, they consist of any number of adjectives that follow the statement, "I am..." For instance, "I am worthy...powerful...or loveable." Maladaptive core beliefs are formed from negative formative experiences. These experiences may include toxic stress; traumatic events; complex trauma due to physical, sexual, and/or emotional abuse and neglect; as well as stress from hypercritical caregivers. Common maladaptive core beliefs can include, "I am helpless... worthless...broken...or unlovable."

We form core beliefs about other people and the world from the same influential formative experiences that form and inform the core beliefs we develop about ourselves. Adaptive core beliefs about other people can include "other people are... good...kind, or...decent." Adaptive core beliefs about the world can include "The world is...just...beautiful...or interesting." Maladaptive core beliefs about other people can include things such as "other people are...out to get me...selfish...or untrustworthy." Maladaptive core beliefs about the world might be that the "world is...cold...unfair or dangerous." These core beliefs direct how we perceive ourselves, others, the world, and the future and can have a profound impact on our thoughts, feelings, and behaviors.

While *core beliefs* are often out of our consciousness, the *automatic thoughts* generated by those core beliefs are believed to exist at the "preconscious" level. That is, if we pay attention, we can identify thoughts that arise in any given situation. Automatic thoughts are part of a stream of private, unspoken cognitive processing that we engage in as we evaluate the significance of an event in our lives. They can be recognized and understood if we pay attention to them. People with depression and anxiety experience a flood of automatic thoughts that are distorted or maladaptive. These thoughts generate painful feelings and can lead to destructive behaviors. Automatic thoughts might be present if there is the presence of strong emotions. For depression, automatic thoughts focus on hopelessness, low self-esteem, and failure. People with anxiety often overestimate the danger in a situation or perceive danger where there is none. They also overly focus on uncontrollable danger and their inability to manage perceived threats (Beck 2020; Dobson and Dobson 2018; Greenberger and Padesky 2015; Wright et al. 2017).

For example, if I hold the core belief that there is something wrong with me or that I am worthless, I might react to getting an poor grade on an exam with an automatic thought of: "I'm never going to graduate," or "I am just not good at this," or "I am stupid." If I have a more positive core belief about myself that says I am competent, I might think to myself after receiving the same grade: "I am going to have to study harder for the next exam," or "I guess I need some extra tutoring," or "I should not have stayed out so late the night before the exam. I am going to have to try harder next time." It is easy to see how each of these two sets of thinking patterns about the event can lead to different feelings and subsequent behaviors. The first person might drop out of school, give up, get depressed, or withdraw. The second person is likely to take more proactive steps that will lead to a different outcome on the next exam.

9.5.1.1 Using Thought Change Records to Identify and Reframe Maladaptive Thoughts

Thought change records are a tool to help clients identify negative thinking patterns and cognitive distortions that lead to depressed or anxious mood and avoidance behaviors. Thought records consist of several columns that coincide with the cognitive model of depression and anxiety (Beck 2020; Greenberger and Padesky 2015; Wright et al. 2017). Table 9.3 provides an example of a thought change record for Rochelle (the case in this chapter) and Julia (the case from Chap. 8). The first column identifies a specific situation, image, or memory identified by the client that preceded a negative emotional experience (i.e., receiving a party invitation that resulted in anxiety; seeing a Facebook post from a friend who got a promotion that resulted in a mixture of depression and anxiety). The second column asks the client to identify the thought(s) that were going through their mind at the time (e.g., I will make a fool of myself; Why would they ask me to the party; I am such a loser; I should be doing better; there is something wrong with me). Clients are also asked to rate the level of belief in the thought or how true the thought is from their perspective 0% (not at all true) to 100% (completely true). A common scale can include:

0—10—20—30—40—50—60—70—80—90—100
None   Slight Moderate   Very   Extreme

It is important to identify thoughts or situations that lead to particularly extreme emotional intensity or belief as well as times when emotional intensity (positive or negative) is not as strong or the person doesn't believe the negative thought as much. What's different in those situations? Variability in belief ratings of negative beliefs shows the client that the belief is not absolute, that there is some doubt in the negative belief, and to always look for ways to challenge the thought with evidence. For instance, why was the belief that you're defective so strong in that situation than in the other situation? What's different about the thoughts you're having in those situations?

The third column asks clients to identify the emotion they experienced as well as the level of intensity (0% not intense/distressing at all) to 100% (extremely intense/overwhelming). Clients can also identify the behavioral response that they had to the emotion such as avoidance, crying, going to bed, drinking, drug use, screaming, self-harm. In the fourth column, clients are asked to identify the cognitive distortion that might be in operation and give a rational alternative thought that is more accurate to describe or explain the situation. Once an automatic thought has been identified using the thought change record, the practitioner and client can explore the presence of cognitive distortions such as overgeneralizing or catastrophizing, minimizing, selective abstraction (paying attention only to bad news or negative

Table 9.3 Thought change record (Rochelle and Julia examples)

Situation or event	Thoughts	Emotions/ Feelings	Rational response	Outcome
A situation or event that is associated with strong emotion.	Thoughts a person has in the moment and a belief rating (1-100).	Emotions experienced with a SUDS level (1-100) and the behavioral response.	Identify potential cognitive distortions and a rational response	The result of this new thought, such as a different behavioral response or a reduction in distress level.
	Indicate the thought that led to the strongest emotion.			
[Rochelle] My annual evaluation meeting with my boss	I am going to get a poor evaluation (100).	Anxious (95)	Selective Abstraction Fortune-telling	I feel relieved. I am still nervous, but that is normal.
	She is going to be disappointed in me. (90).	Sadness (90)	Arbitrary Inference	I think that I will probably get at least a good (if not great) evaluation this year.
	I am never going to get promoted (85).		Rational response: My performance numbers are some of the best I have had, and are better than most in my department. I had only one or two negative reviews and dozens of positive ones.	
	I should have had better numbers this year (90).			
	I had some negative reviews this year (80).			
[Julia] My coworkers asked me to be part of a book club.	I am going to be nervous and not know what to say (100).	Anxious (95); Sadness (because I want to go) (85).	Selective Abstraction	I feel less nervous and a little excited at going out and socializing.
	They are going to think I am weird (90).		Arbitrary Inference	
	They will never ask me to another event (85),		Mind reading	
	I will have to quit my job (75).		Fortune-telling	
			Rational response: My coworkers are good people, and I have a lot of interesting things to say on a lot of topics. I can go for an hour and handle some light conversation.	
			Rational response: I am a librarian. This is in my zone.	

All names and other identifiers of these cases have been changed to protect privacy and confidentiality outcomes and ignoring positive evidence), self-blame or taking on too much responsibility, and mind reading, among others (Beck 2020; Wright et al. 2017).

After identifying possible cognitive distortions that may be operating in relation to the negative thought, it may be useful to explore and list advantages and disadvantages of continuing the thought. What does the client benefit from continuing the thought? What disadvantages are there for continuing to think this way? This sets up the ability to then reframe the negative thought to something more relevant and grounded in the evidence—a more rational alternative to thinking about the situation. This could be added in another column and you would again ask the client to rate their level of belief in this new thought from a scale of 0–100. Once these distortions have been identified, the practitioner and the client can work together to determine a more rational response (Wright et al. 2017).

Lastly, in the fifth column clients are asked to give the result of this new thought such as a different behavioral response or a reduction in distress level. Clients should also rate their belief in this new thought on a scale from 1 to 100 and re-evaluate their belief level in the maladaptive thought they identified in the second column (Wright et al. 2017).

9.5.1.2 Eliciting Automatic Thoughts from Clients

Identifying negative thoughts can be challenging for clients. In order to help clients accurately identify negative thoughts the practitioner can employ several methods. One method is to help clients identify the "hot" thought; that is, the thought that leads to the most intense negative emotion or elicits a swift and intense physical reaction such as sadness, hurt, and anger. Sometimes focusing on these events can yield significant information. Another way to elicit automatic thoughts is to identify the specific situation associated with an intense emotion and then guess what the thought might be by offering suggestions or examples of possible thoughts. A third way to elicit thoughts is to try the "complete the thought" method by having the client complete the sentence such as the following:

> "I felt angry when my partner disagreed with me because I thought…"
> "I felt sad when my friend didn't call on my birthday because I thought…"
> "I felt nervous when my boss ignored me in the hallway because I thought…"

Automatic thought records can be used to challenge and reframe negative automatic thoughts. Practitioners can use thought records to identify activating events, thoughts, and their emotional and behavioral consequences. Thought change records can be used as homework assignment to address any negative thinking patterns identified in the case conceptualization. They can also be used in conjunction with other approaches that help clients challenge and reframe negative thinking patterns and thoughts (Beck 2020; Dobson and Dobson 2018; Greenberger and Padesky 2015; Wright et al. 2017).

9.5.1.3   Evaluating the Evidence for the Thought (e.g., the Defense Attorney)

Once negative thoughts have been identified, practitioners can then ask clients to check negative thoughts against all the facts. This process is called evaluating the evidence or the "defense attorney" method (Wright et al. 2017). The client must identify a negative automatic thought and then list all of the objective evidence in support of that thought and then all the objective evidence against the thought. List all the evidence you can find that either supports the thought or disproves the automatic thought. The quality of the evidence on each side should also be considered. Socratic questions that can be used to explore the evidence for and against the automatic thought can include:

- What objective evidence is there that firmly supports this thought?
- What evidence can you find that does not support this thought?
- If you imagined yourself as your own defense attorney, how would you mount a defense in support of yourself that goes against this charge (negative thought)?
- What do you think is the quality of the evidence that supports this negative thought that you are incompetent, unlovable, defective?
- What do you think other people would say about this evidence? What would your best friend say about this?
- If your best friend presented this information about themselves, what would you tell them?

When taking a "defense attorney" approach, ask your client to take the role of their own defense attorney opposite their negative thoughts (prosecuting attorney). Ask your client to mount a vigorous defense against the negative automatic thought claims. For instance, ask "If you were to act as your own defense attorney, what would you say in your own defense?" As the practitioner, take on the role of the prosecutor and be sure to tell the client they do not have to believe in their own "innocence," just that they take the job as attorney seriously.

It is very important to ask clients to practice these exercises or "experiments" in real-world settings at home or work, between sessions as "homework." Be sure to write everything down in a therapy log or journal and give handouts so that the client can remember what exactly to do between sessions. Clients can also be asked to complete "positive data logs". These logs are used by clients to record evidence in their environments that support more positive conceptualizations and beliefs about themselves, others, and the world. It is often helpful to ask clients to identify how they would like to view themselves and then have them specifically seek out and record objective evidence in support of that belief between sessions (Beck 2020).

9.5.1.4   Reattribution

Depressed persons tend to internalize blame and take more than their fair share for negative outcomes leading to unnecessary or exaggerated feelings of guilt and shame. Reattribution exercises help people examine a situation, brainstorm likely contributors to the problem, and re-assign a more appropriate level of responsibility to themselves. Ask clients to give a percentage (out of 100) of their responsibility for a paricular event. Using the pie chart method, you can have the client imagine a pie with different pieces in it. Then have them consider all of the different causes of a particular event being represented by each piece of the pie. How big a piece (ask for a percentage) of the pie is represented by each of these causes? Then ask the client to determine how much of the pie are they responsible for and compare that percentage they originally identified. Reattribution is often used to help clients take a more appropriate level of responsibility for negative events. But it can also help clients who tend to minimize their positive contributions to take a more appropriate level of credit for positive events that they help generate (Wright et al. 2017).

9.5.1.5 Decatastrophizing

Persons who are depressed or anxious often make catastrophic predictions about events that are frequently influenced by cognitive distortions. Decatastrophizing can help clients build confidence to face feared outcomes or situations more competently. Decatastrophizing asks people to imagine the *worst-case* scenario of a particular situation and examine how different elements of their life would be different or changed. Clients are then asked to list the *best*-case scenario and then the *most likely* case scenario. This exercise can be combined with the *examining the evidence exercise* in order to help clients identify more rational or likely scenarios or outcomes to events. An added element to this exercise is helping clients recognize that if the "catastrophic" event did in fact happen, it often will not have as big a negative impact on their lives as they originally thought. After reviewing all of the evidence, ask the client to re-estimate the likelihood of the worst-case scenario of the event occurring. This exercise helps the client to develop a more realistic (and probably less frightening) picture of the situation. The next step in the process is to help the client assess their perceived level of control over the occurrence of the event and create an action plan by brainstorming strategies to reduce the likelihood of the event occurring. In other words, what can they do to help avoid the event from happening? Finally, help the client develop an action plan for coping if the event should occur and then reassess the client's level of fear regarding the event. Usually, having a more realistic idea of possible scenarios and their impact, combined with an action plan to prevent and/or cope with negative events, leads to developing a better sense of mastery and control and reduced distress (Wright et al. 2017).

9.5.1.6 Coping Cards

Use coping cards in conjunction with decatasrophizing and have the client create a coping card that lists all of the action steps the client can take to both avoid the event from happening and how to cope with the event should it happen. This can be done on an index card or on a person's phone or other digital device so they have easy access. Coping cards can also be used to identify all the skills the client can use to cope with depressive or anxious thinking. Clients can utilize cards to write down instructions to give to themselves in order to help them cope with significant issues or situations in the moment. Box 9.1 provides an example of a coping card for Rochelle. To help a client create coping cards, choose a situation important to the client and develop and practice developing coping cards in-session. At first, assess readiness to implement strategies and focus on achievable goals that aren't too over-whelming. Be specific in defining the situation and the steps taken to manage the problem and boil instructions down to small, highly memorable segments. Advocate use of coping cards in real-life situations and assign their use and deployment as homework (Beck 2020; Dobson and Dobson 2018; Greenberger and Padesky 2015; Wright et al. 2017).

Box 9.1: Coping Card Example: Rochelle[1]
Situation: My annual review is coming up to go over my performance over the last year.

Coping Strategies:
- Remind myself that I have achieved most of what I set out to do this year.
- Spot my negative thinking patterns such as perfectionism, mind reading, and catastrophizing.
- Remember to look at all the evidence. I have done well in some areas and not as well as I would have liked in others—but I have not "failed" in any one area.
- My performance is better than most in my department.
- There is no evidence that my boss has it in for me or that I will lose my job.
- This is an evaluation so I need to expect some criticism. I need to stand back and remember that this is normal and will help me perform better.

9.6   Coping Skill Development

9.6.1   Problem-Solving Skills

A key skill area that is rooted in cognitive behavioral practice is problem-solving and is even its own therapy approach (D'Zurilla and Nezu 2007). Persons with depression and anxiety often have trouble concentrating and thinking flexibly. They are often paralyzed with indecision, which hampers their ability to identify prob-lems, recognize the relevant solutions, and make the best decision on a path forward (Wright et al. 2017). Problem-solving strategies involve several common elements that include: (1) problem identification, definition, and prioritization; (2) generating a list of alternative solutions; (3) evaluating the pros and cons of each solution;

(4) selecting the best perceived solution; (5) deploying or executing the solution; and (6) evaluating whether or not it worked.

Problem solving begins by accurately and succinctly identifying the problem. Problems should be clearly defined and measurable so the provider and client know if progress is being made. Complex problems with multiple components need to be broken down into their separate parts so they can be manageable and not overwhelming. Providers should help clients prioritize problems that are achievable and have the most impact. For clients with severe depression it may be advisable to go after low hanging fruit first to build momentum. In general, try to help the client focus on the central issue. Next, the provider helps the client brainstorm a list of potential solutions. The data that is generated in session from notes, thought change records, assessments, case conceptualizations, and the daily journal could be used to inform solutions and generate the list. The client may also need to do some research on the best possible solutions. Providers should use Socratic questions to help clients think about potential solutions. Questions include: What would you advise a friend to do about this? What would your friend say to do? What have you done in the past to solve similar problems? A solution may also be to do nothing or delay the decision.

After a list of solutions has been generated, the provider and client work together to identify the pros and cons of each potential solution. It may be useful to first eliminate any solutions that are unreasonable, unachievable, costly, ineffective, more trouble than they're worth, or clearly not the best choice. The goal is to narrow down the selections to just two to four options and then focus on the potential pros and cons of each choice. The final choice should be a solution that is effective, attractive, and most likely to succeed. The next phase is to plan out the implementation of the solution and troubleshoot potential barriers. Questions in this phase include: What tasks have to be done and in what order? Who has to do what? What is the timeline for completion of tasks? What barriers exist that need to be negotiated? How will barriers be overcome? And most importantly, how will we know if we succeeded? Lastly, clients and providers evaluate the impact of the solution. Providers should examine the automatic thoughts that were experienced during implementation and if they helped or hindered the client. What made success possible? If the client was not completely successful, what got in their way? What can be done to increase the likelihood of success next time? Be sure to celebrate successes and be supportive if clients fall short. Be sure to frame failure as a learning opportunity for growth and development.

9.6.2 Assertiveness Skills

Learning how to communicate assertively can help persons who suffer from depression and anxiety ask for what they need more effectively. These skills can also help them more clearly communicate their needs to others and clarify other comments that may otherwise be misinterpreted. Teaching assertive communication involves five elements. First, providers help clients clearly identify what they want to say to another person, Second, they help the client generate a clear statement of purpose— the central theme of what the person wants the other person to know. Third, the provider teaches the "good news, bad news, good news" approach to communication. This approach has the client start with a positive statement (e.g., Thanks for meeting with me about my evaluation). This is then followed by the assertive demand (e.g., I disagree with what you said about my performance. I feel it was inaccurate because…). This statement is then followed by a positive closing (e.g., thanks for listening to me). Fourth, the provider and the client role-play the whole scenario/interaction. During the role-play phase, the provider and client discuss the targets, communication style, and role play best, worst, and most-likely case scenarios and give feedback and fine-tune the approach. It sometimes helps for the provider and client to switch roles and play both sides to give the client multple perspectives and to hear the statement comeing from another person. Video recording role plays and playing them back can also be effective teaching tools. The last phase is eliciting predictions from the client for the event and brainstorming ways to maximize effectiveness in terms of timing, location, and tone (Monti et al., 2002)

9.6.3   Anger Management Skills

Anger is a common symptom of many behavioral health conditions including depression, anxiety, stress, and PTSD. Anger can also be a powerful cue or trigger for alcohol and substance misuse (Monti et al., 2002). Anger is often fueled by negative thoughts and misinterpretation of the communication of others. Providers first help clients identify situations that commonly lead to anger and the automatic thoughts that accompany those situations. For instance, during disagreements with partners a client may often misread a person's body language or words that lead to automatic thoughts focused on abandonment (e.g., they are going to leave me, they don't love me anymore, they think I'm stupid). Identifying these cognitive distortions during a review of thought change records can help clients identify situations and negative automatic thoughts. Second, once clients are aware of thoughts that cause anger, they can use this information to identify more rational alternative thoughts by examining the evidence for more rational alternatives. Clients can then review negative consequences of their anger and identify alternative thoughts (e.g., my partner is just arguing their point) that are more appropriate to the situation. Lastly, clients can learn more healthy responses such as taking a break, taking a deep breath or engaging in relaxation exercises, calling someone or engaging in a distraction activity. Clients can also learn more responsive communication strategies to employ with their partners reviewed in Chap. 3.

9.7 Psychoeducation Approaches: Illness Management and Family Psychoeducation

Illness management and family psychoeducation are two approaches to treatment that have been found to improve outcomes in persons with behavioral health disorders including serious mental illnesses such as schizophrenia, bipolar disorder, and major depressive disorder. Illness management approaches teach clients skills and personal strategies to maintain wellness, understand symptoms, identify and respond to early warning signs for relapse, and plan for crises. Family psychoeducation approaches provide education and support to caregivers and close family members of persons with behavioral health disorders so that they can be better informed about what their loved one is experiencing and be better able to support their loved one's recovery. Both approaches can help persons with behavioral health disorders achieve and maintain wellness and recovery.

9.7.1 Illness Management Strategies

9.7.1.1 Illness Self-Management and Recovery

Illness Management and Recovery (IMR) is an intervention designed to help persons with behavioral health disorders learn strategies to achieve and maintain wellness (Mueser and Gingerich 2013). IMR is a type of modular program that can be effectively implemented in community mental health settings and has been found to increase people's ability to understand and cope with their behavioral health symptoms and how to identify and respond to worsening symptoms. IMR uses psychoeducation modules designed to educate people about their disorders and help them design action plans to identify and achieve their recovery-oriented goals. Providers of IMR rely on motivational and cognitive-behavioral approaches to help clients design and achieve recovery-oriented goals. They use psychoeducation to teach clients about their mental illness and recovery strategies. They use motivational strategies to help clients weigh the benefits and costs of making behavior changes (Mueser and Gingerich 2013). They also use CBT methods such as rehearsal, role modeling, and behavioral tailoring to help clients develop and practice social skills, relaxation skills, assertiveness, and problem-solving strategies. Psychoeducation has also been found to reduce relapse and readmission rates and improve medication adherence in persons with schizophrenia (Xia et al. 2011).

IMR is often delivered in a group format over several weekly or biweekly sessions. IMR is often provided by peer specialists or teams of peers and non-peer professionals. Utilization of peer providers help clients recognize that recovery is possible and provide real-world evidence (e.g., credibility) to the strategies discussed. Specific topics covered in IMR include: (1) understanding recovery concepts and recovery goal-setting; (2) psychoeducation about the signs, symptoms, and treatments for serious mental illness and the stress vulnerability model of mental illness (Chap. 3); (3) recognizing and addressing external and internal stigma; (4) the importance of social support and how to develop social support networks; (5) treatment strategies and the effective use of medications and managing their side effects; (6) the impact of drugs and alcohol use on recovery; (7) identifying when symptoms get worse and developing relapse prevention strategies and plans; (8) developing problem-solving strategies and other skills for coping with persistent symptoms (e.g., relaxation, distraction, using social support) and other life stresses; and (9) advocating for yourself and understanding how to use the mental health system.

9.7.1.2   Wellness Recovery Action Plan (WRAP)

Another popular illness self-management strategy is the Wellness Recovery Action Plan or WRAP. WRAP was developed by Mary Ellen Copeland, a person who has experienced mental illness, and is designed to help people develop detailed plans for managing mental illness symptoms and designing strategies to achieve recovery and well-being. WRAP plans are broken down into several parts and require clients to design specific plans for each part that they keep in a binder or folder they can reference as needed. Ideally, WRAP plans are developed in collaboration with peer providers and shared with the client's social support network and other treatment providers. The use of WRAP has been found to lead to a reduction in overall service utilization and need (Cook et al. 2013).

The first part of the WRAP plan involves clients developing their recovery tool box that lists all of the activities and strategies they can draw on to stay well. This list can include hobbies and pastimes, social activities and important people, things to avoid such as alcohol or negative people, exercise routines, and strategies to cope with troubling voices or negative thinking. The second aspect of WRAP plans has clients identify the daily activities they need to do in order to stay well. These activities are expected to be accomplished daily and can include things such as waking up at a specific time, eating breakfast, taking a bath, exercising, using medication, calling a friend, going to work, listening to music, or other activities that maintain well-being. The third aspect of the plan is a list of factors that can exacerbate symptoms. These are basically things to avoid in order to maintain wellness. They can include specific daily stressors; negative people, thinking, or activities; drinking or using substances; isolation; or overwork (or under work) that can lead to an exacerbation of mental health symptoms. Fourth, clients list the early warning signs that the symptoms of the mental illness are getting worse. These are the specific signs that indicate a worsening of symptoms. Increased intensity of internal stimuli such as voices or a change in tone of voices; increased fatigue, agitation, or lack of a need for sleep; problems concentrating; thoughts of self-harm; increased use of alcohol or drugs; and other signs that may indicate an impending problem. Once these signs have been identified the person also develops responses or activities that can be engaged in to counter these signs such as making an appointment with their doctor, talking to a professional or peer, calling someone important, exercising or enjoying nature, taking a day off, or getting enough sleep. It is also a good idea for the client to share these signs with others so that other people can notify the person if they see any troubling signs. Fifth, clients describe what they are like when symptoms have gotten so bad that they are a danger to themselves or others and there needs to be intervention or "when things have broken down." This is a late stage of symptoms exacerbation that may indicate the need for outpatient treatment, hospitalization, or medication adjustment. This can include increased psychosis, self-harm, aggressiveness, drug or alcohol use, or disorganized, risky, or dangerous behavior. This step is followed by the last step: the crisis plan. The crisis plan is similar to a psychiatric advanced directive and is something that should be shared with providers and family. This helps the client have a voice when they may have lost the ability to make choices for themselves. The crisis plan directs specific caregivers and providers as to what the client preferences are when they have suffered a mental break down. This includes who and who should not be involved in care, the type of care that is preferred, preferred medications, and a list of items that help and do not help the person's recovery, such as how to be spoken to, what helps and does not help the person feel better, and, in general, how the person wishes to be treated. This plan is an important way to help people achieve and maintain their wellness as well as empower clients who may, from time to time, lose the ability to care for themselves and make decisions on their own behalf. Crisis intervention can be effective in reducing re-admission rates, reduces family burden, and improves the mental state of clients (Murphy et al. 2015).

9.7.2 Family Psychoeducation

Families are often the central caretaker for persons with serious mental illness and endure high amounts of emotional and financial stress, confusion, and isolation. Family dysfunction and high expressed emotion can also lead to poor outcomes for persons with serious mental illnesses. Family psychoeducation has been identified as a core evidence-based practice for the treatment of schizophrenia (Dixon et al. 2009). Family interventions can reduce relapse rates and hospitalizations and lead to a range of positive functional outcomes (Jewell et al. 2009; Pharoah et al. 2010) (See McFarlane 2016 for a review).

The purpose of family psychoeducation is based on the assumption that family caregivers of persons with mental illness need information, coping and communication skills, and support to help their loved ones. Family psychoeducation programs can take many forms. Two of the most researched and effective models are the multi-family group psychoeducation model (McFarlane 2002), and the family support model provided by the National Alliance for Mental Illness (NAMI), which uses support groups led by peer providers and family members who have a loved one with serious mental illness (SMI) (Dixon et al. 2011). While family psychoeducation can include single-family or multifamily groups, the range of content covered in these models typically includes: (1) information on mental illness, medication and treatment, and services; (2) strategies to work with treatment providers to provide the best care for loved ones; (3) skills training on effective communication, problem-solving, and decision-making; (4) emotional support for families and developing coping strategies and techniques; (5) information on available services and treatments in the community; (6) crisis planning; and (7) strategies for enhancing social support and respite. Collaborating with families and providing ongoing education, skills training, and support can enhance functional outcomes in clients and increase quality of life in families. These interventions can be integrated into case management models as part of their usual care, provided as ongoing group sessions at hospital or residential settings, or provided in the community at a local NAMI Chapter or by individual behavioral health providers. Family models should be considered especially in the earliest phases of illness, when lack of information, confusion, and stress can be highest, in order to assist families in providing effective care as soon as possible (Lucksted et al. 2012).

9.8 Summary and Conclusion

Depressive and anxiety disorders are highly prevalent behavioral health disorders that are often comorbid with each other and other behavioral and physical health disorders. As such, they are responsible for a tremendous amount of disability burden worldwide. The good news is that these disorders are highly treatable with a range of effective approaches. The bad news is that these conditions often go untreated. Two ways to improve this trend are to: (1) integrate routine and universal screening procedures for anxiety and depression into behavioral health, primary care, education, criminal justice, and social service settings and (2) integrate brief psychotherapeutic approaches into these settings. While these approaches are often provided by highly trained psychotherapists, research indicates that they can also be effectively provided by a range of staff and peer providers with modest training.

Cognitive approaches to depression and anxiety include helping clients identify and challenge cognitive distortions and negative thinking patterns in order to improve mood and reduce fear, avoidance, and social withdrawal. Behavioral approaches to these conditions such as behavioral activation and teaching relaxation, mindfulness, and coping skills help get clients moving and teach them how to (re)engage with the work and themselves. Exposure-based therapies help clients with anxiety challenge maladaptive or pathological fears leading to a reduction in physiological and emotional symptoms and avoidance behaviors. Illness management and family psychoeducation approaches help teach clients and families how to better understand their conditions and deploy strategies designed to achieve and maintain wellness and recovery. Each of these approaches can be implemented in a variety of settings and by a range of transdisciplinary staff, making them highly portable and effective in improving the physical and behavioral health of clients.

Case Study 9.1 Rochelle Richmond

You are a social worker at a behavioral health outpatient clinic that provides community-based mental health counseling services. Rochelle,[2] a cisgender woman, was referred to you by her nurse practitioner for counseling in order to address behavioral health issues impacting her health. Rochelle came to therapy with the goal of feeling better about herself and is seeking help to continue maintaining her sobriety. She came because she would like to (in her own words) "be healthier, happier, less depressed and anxious, calmer, to have a more realistic and kinder view of myself, and to quiet down the voices in my head telling me I'm not good enough and to accept myself for who I am today." The following are excerpts from the initial encounter with Rochelle that you can use to develop your case conceptualization and treatment plan.

Rochelle Richmond is a successful, 46-year-old associate advertising sales manager for a local television station. She is assertive, organized, and effective. She has strong leadership capabilities and is also kind and committed to justice. She, her brother, and her mother emigrated from Nigeria to the United States when she was 9 years old after the death of her father and due to the threat of violence and political and economic turmoil. Her mother was a history professor at the University of Nigeria in Lagos. Her birth father was a journalist. When Rochelle was 7, she, her mother, brother, and father were driving to a family gathering. On a deserted stretch of the trip, they were forced off the road. Their father was dragged from the vehicle and beaten by the roadside by a group of assailants. He died at a hospital a few hours later due to his injuries. Rochelle and her family witnessed the entire event. The police determined the event was a robbery, but most people believe that Rochelle's father was assassinated due to his reporting of government corruption. Soon thereafter they applied for visas to the United States because her mother had contacts at a local university. Her mother was later re-married to a white engineer at a large aerospace firm. Rochelle reports that she loved her biological father very much and that he was kind, but was very strict. She says her stepfather and mother were also all very strict and religious. She describes her stepfather as a "problem drinker." He would come home from drinking after work and would often be verbally abusive to Rochelle and her mother, less so to her brother John. He would sometimes threaten that if her mother did not obey him that he would have her and her two children "sent back to Africa." Despite these racist and violent episodes, and being otherwise strict, Rochelle wanted to please her stepfather and earn his respect. She often stated that she felt that he looked down on her and favored her brother, John, both because he was a boy and because he had a lighter skin color. Rochelle's mother struggled to find work when she came to the United States.

> Rochelle states: "My mother was a respected history professor when we lived in Nigeria. People would come over to the house and talk about critical issues, philosophy, history, everything. It was wonderful. The conversations were so rich. She was brilliant. She would hold court. It was so impressive. I was so proud even though I had no idea what she was talking about. Then she came here and people wouldn't even look at her. No one would hire her at first – it was like everything she did in Nigeria didn't count. She had a Ph.D., but wouldn't even get an interview for positions she was overqualified for. She became very

bitter and resentful. She would come home discouraged because people thought that her education was somehow inferior. They sometimes talked to her like she was a child. She did eventually get an adjunct teaching position in an African studies department, but she never regained her status even though she was just the most brilliant woman I ever met in my life. She died too young from a stroke when I was 25. I think it had to do with the stress she felt, not just from my stepdad's constant berating and all that happened to our life in Nigeria, but also from the perpetual disrespect she experienced here wherever she went. It broke her heart. It broke her down. My coming out as a lesbian probably didn't help in that regard. I carry a strange sense of guilt even though I know that it is unfair for me to think this way. But it's there nonetheless."

Rochelle's stepdad passed away 2 years before her mom from lung and liver cancer. Today, Rochelle is a citizen of the United States and she speaks three languages. She graduated near the top of her class. She and her partner Maxine, a high school English teacher, have been together for over 20 years. Five years ago they got married in an Episcopal Church. They have two adopted children, Ade (now 22) and Yvonne (now 20). Ade graduated with honors from the University of Chicago. He is getting his masters to become a high school math teacher. Yvonne plans to get her Juris Doctorate from Northwestern, where she is currently top of her class. She plans to work for a large legal firm serving non-profit organizations in Chicago. Rochelle has been an athlete her whole life. She was a softball and basketball stand-out in high school and played both sports at the collegiate level as a member of the second string. She has run several marathons prior to age 40 and is currently an avid golfer and tennis player. Rochelle loves her wife and children deeply. She speaks freely of her devotion to Maxine who she says, "saved my life more times than I can count. She stood by me through all the tough times in my life. She never left my side, even when she had every right to. She's the reason I am sober today." Rochelle credits Maxine with her success in life. She is eager to discuss her children, proudly ticking off their accomplishments, skills, and talents.

Rochelle has experienced periods of depressed and anxious moods for several years. Her depressed periods are marked by extreme fatigue, lack of pleasure in activities, withdrawal, irritation, and sadness. Her anxiety is marked by periods of intense worry and occasional panic attacks. She also reports occasionally that she has intrusive memories of the day her father was killed and wakes up in the middle of the night sweating and heart racing from nightmares. She also reports intrusive memories from her stepfather's abuse—but she states that this is often manifested by an "over-alertness" to threats in the environment.

Rochelle states: "I am afraid sometimes for no reason. I feel like when you're watching a horror film and the person is trying to start the car and the car won't start and the dude with the chainsaw is coming in the rearview mirror. Like that, for no reason. This happens a couple times a week. It is just something that I live with now. I think that it is because of what happened to my father. That day. I can remember all of it. My brother was too young, I think. But me and my mother saw everything. I think they wanted us to. We never talked about it in detail – but it sometimes haunts me and I think the nightmares are a part of it. I remember the blood. The smell. The way he looked when his eyes rolled up in the back of his head. How they beat him. Kicked him. I remember the sounds of their boots on him. My eyes were closed for most of it. And then I remember the silence when they stopped. I remember how I felt like it was now our turn and I remember the relief I felt when they took off and left. How I felt when their car started. How relieved I felt even though my father lay half dead in the road. And I hold that guilt of the relief I felt to this day. Sometime even when I feel relief for whatever reason – it can take me back there. I cry sometimes when I feel it because it reminds me of that day and how I felt when I realized they were not going to do to me what they did to him. The guilt can be crippling. I think that is one of the legacies of that day that haunts me the most. Sometimes I think that they will come back for me. But the guilt of just sitting there while they beat him to death and I did nothing except feel relief when I knew it wasn't going to be me next. This is the most I have talked about it with anyone ever. I don't talk about it – but the memories come anyway."

Rochelle is also in recovery from problem drinking that she experienced for several years. She attends an Alcoholics Anonymous (AA) group for LGBTQ persons sporadically and has a sponsor. She has not had a drink in 5 years. Rochelle experiences urges to drink occasionally but manages to control them through, "willpower, Maxine, and Gerry (her sponsor)." She states, "I don't ever want to go back to that life. I would drink almost every day after work for "happy hour" just like my stepdad. Then I would come home and yell at Maxine or pick fights…just like my stepdad. I didn't think I had a problem because I would only have two or three, but that was enough to make me mean, verbally abusive, and argumentative. But a near breakup made me realize that I had a huge problem with alcohol. And anger. I was basically buzzed every night and I was detached from my wife, my kids and my life. Just cut off. And I couldn't deal with anything. We worked so hard to get married. We fought for this right, literally in the streets. The day we got married we wept because we felt recognized as a couple by our adopted family, friends, society. We mattered. We wept for all the years we lost and weren't recognized. The hiding. The self-loathing. The terror. And I nearly threw it all away. One moment during a fight I saw myself, like from above, from outside myself and I said 'you're just like he was. My stepdad. You're just like him.' We were standing in the kitchen discussing our plans for the weekend. I tell Maxine that I made plans to work on my report on Saturday. She makes this face like she is irritated and I just go bonkers. I'm like, 'well if you don't care about my job then I don't care either!' and I slam my fist on the table. Maxine's like, 'You're crazy! What's wrong with you?' And that was my turning point. I must have said something he used to say and it triggered something. It wasn't our worst fight – but it was the day I realized I needed to do something before it was too late."

Rochelle has done better since her recovery. Her health has improved; however, she continues to experience hypertension (BP is 140/90) and high cholesterol. She struggles to manage these conditions with medicine that she sometimes does not take regularly. Her doctors warn her that she must get these two things under control or she is at risk for a later stroke or heart attack.

Her relationship with her family and her work production has improved since sobriety. However, Rochelle continues to experience periods of depression and anxiety and is prone to angry outbursts. Rochelle describes her depressed mood as feeling like she is "a failure and a loser." During these times Rochelle has trouble sleeping, eating, and concentrating; consumed by her constant ruminations about her worthlessness and how a drink would help her feel better and more confident.

She also experiences stomach upset during these times. She reports feeling "nervous and jittery." She states that she is terrified that she will be denied promotion to vice president or be fired from her job due to low production and performance despite a long history of good evaluations that exceeded expectations. Her customer evaluations are routinely excellent and she receives regular awards and accolades. She has a good sales record that is at or above those of her colleagues. Rochelle states, "If I don't get promoted to VP, then it means that I am a failure. It means I've let myself and my family down. If I let my family down that it means I'm not a good wife, mother, or professional. It is my greatest fear and I stay awake at night dreading it. I sometimes dread going to work because I know I'm going to get fired or get a poor evaluation. If not today, then tomorrow. One time my director stood in my office and read one of my reports. She nodded her head, and then says 'thanks' and walked out of my office. Pretty mundane right? Well, I thought I was going be fired. I had no doubt. I was practically packing up my office. I was nervous and sad for days and I was just a mean person to Maxine and my assistant for a week. I had to apologize to my assistant in an e-mail it was so bad. And then I got my evaluation and had the highest productivity in the department that year. I mean – what a waste of energy."

Rochelle grew up with an older brother, John, whom she claims his parents favored. She would later state, "John made my parents so proud. He made all of us proud. He was a golden child. Me? I was pretty good. I was a good girl – well above average, exceptional even. Didn't get into trouble. But I was a girl. A dark-skinned girl. And then, a lesbian. That did not fit in with the religious perspective of my family. I'm not sure which was worse for them. My being a girl, having dark skin, or being a lesbian. My coming out did not go well as you can imagine. They threw me out of the house. My mom cried. I thought my stepdad was going to hit me. But he didn't. He just never talked to me again. Which was probably worse. I think both my fathers were perpetually disappointed in me. My mother was detached. She was focused on John. But my stepfather rode me. He taught me and John, "if you're going to do something, be the best. You're either first, or your last." There was no in between. He said, 'You're either perfect or you're a failure.' In my stepfather's eyes, even though I was an athlete and a good student, near the top of my class, it didn't count because I was not number 1. I would come in second, or be second string and that was like being last. None of it counted. I know intellectually that is nonsense. But that is not what I feel inside. I feel like a loser. And when I came out it was finally the last straw. Or maybe it was a relief for him. He could finally let it all go. Let me go. It was OK to give up on me, because I was nothing in his eyes at that point. That's the message I got when he looked at me. I did not speak to him again. Not even when he was sick. He died slow and he never wanted to see me. John says he never even mentioned me when he would go and visit him. It was like I died to him. It was like a light switch that night when I told them. I was now officially 'off.' John doesn't talk to me much either. We don't talk about my being a married lesbian mother. We talk about *his* wife and *his* children. But not mine. I guess my family isn't real for him. Or maybe I'm making that up. I just don't know. But he's got his own issues. He was not left unscathed. My mom is dead, too, and she never forgave me either. Am I over it? Sometimes I think so – but that stays with you forever. I'm not sure which day was worse for me. The day my father was beaten in front of my own eyes or the day I came out to my parents. I have nightmares about both. My mother looked me in the eyes and said to me: 'Thank god your father is dead so that he cannot feel the shame that I feel right now. Get out of my sight.' I will never forget it. I'm angry. The older I get, the angrier I get about how easily they let me go. How easy it was for them to discard me. Can you be traumatized by silence? By lack of action? By a void? An absence? That's what I have nightmares about – just their silence. But regardless of how angry I feel, I continue to carry the lesson my whole life that you have to be the best at everything or you're nothing."

Case Analysis Questions

What is your case conceptualization of Rochelle based on the information in the vignette?

What symptoms does she experience?

Do Rochelle's symptoms meet criteria for one or more behavioral health disorders and, if so, which one(s)?

What are 3–5 treatment goals and objectives that would make a good treatment plan for Rochelle?

What symptoms would you target?

What interventions would you deploy to help Rochelle achieve her goals?

What strengths and resources does Rochelle have that she can rely on to solve her problems?

What kind of situations can be used to help Rochelle address her fears and depressive symptoms?

How will you ensure your treatment approach is affirming and supportive given her multiple identities?

References

American Psychiatric Association. (2013). *Diagnostic and statistical manual of mental disorders* (DSM-5) (5th ed.). Arlington: American Psychiatric Association.

Archer, J., Bower, P., Gilbody, S., Lovell, K., Richards, D., Gask, L., Dickens, C., & Coventry, P. (2012). Collaborative care for depression and anxiety problems. *Cochrane Database of Systematic Reviews, 10.*, Art. No.: CD006525. https://doi.org/10.1002/14651858. CD006525.pub2.

Barlow, D. H., Farchione, T. J., Bullis, J. R., Gallagher, M. W., Murray-Latin, H., Sauer-Zavala, S., Bentley, K. H., Thompson-Hollands, J., Conklin, L. R., Boswell, J. F., Ametaj, A., Carl, J. R., Boettcher, H. T., & Cassiello-Robbins, C. (2017). The unified protocol for transdiagnostic treatment of emotional disorders compared with diagnosis-specific protocols for anxiety disorders: A randomized clinical trial. *JAMA Psychiatry, 74*(9), 875–884. https://doi.org/10.1001/jamapsychiatry.2017.2164.

Barlow, D. H., Ellard, K. K., Fairholme, C. P., Farchione, T. J., Boisseau, C. L., Allen, L. B., & Ehrenreich May, J. (2011a). *The unified protocol for transdiagnostic treatment of emotional disorders: Client workbook.* New York: Oxford University Press.

Barlow, D. H., Farchione, T. J., Fairholme, C. P., Ellard, K. K., Boisseau, C. L., Allen, L. B., & Ehrenreich, M. J. (2011b). *The unified protocol for transdiagnostic treatment of emotional disorders: Therapist guide*. New York: Oxford University Press.

Beck, J. S. (2020). *Cognitive behavior therapy: Basics and beyond* (3rd ed.). New York: Guilford Press.

Beck, A. T., Rush, A. J., Shaw, B. F., & Emery, G. (1979). *Cognitive therapy of depression*. New York: Guilford.

Bishop, S. R. (2004). Mindfulness: A proposed operational definition. *Clinical Psychology: Science and Practice, 11*(3), 230–241. https://doi.org/10.1093/clipsy/bph077.

Bohlmeijer, E., Prenger, R., Taal, E., & Cuijpers, P. (2010). The effects of mindfulness-based stress reduction therapy on mental health of adults with a chronic medical disease: A meta-analysis. *Journal of Psychosomatic Research, 68*(6), 539–544. https://doi.org/10.1016/j.jpsychores.2009.10.005.

Bomyea, J., Lang, A., Craske, M. G., Chavira, D. A., Sherbourne, C. D., Rose, R. D., Golinelli, D., Campbell-Sills, L., Welch, S. S., Sullivan, G., Bystritsky, A., Roy-Byrne, P., & Stein, M. B. (2015). Course of symptom change during anxiety treatment: Reductions in anxiety and depression in patients completing the coordinated anxiety learning and management program. *Psychiatry Research, 229*(1–2), 133–142. https://doi.org/10.1016/j.psychres.2015.07.056.

Boswell, J. F., Iles, B. R., Gallagher, M. W., & Farchione, T. J. (2017). Behavioral activation strategies in cognitive-behavioral therapy for anxiety disorders. *Psychotherapy, 54*(3), 231–236.

Burton, A., Burgess, C., Dean, S., Koutsopoulou, G. Z., & Hugh-Jones, S. (2017). How effective are mindfulness-based interventions for reducing stress among healthcare professionals? A systematic review and meta-analysis. *Stress and Health, 33*(1), 3–13. https://doi.org/10.1002/smi.2673.

Cacioppo, J. T., & Patrick, W. (2008). *Loneliness: Human nature and the need for social connection*. New York: W. W. Norton.

Campbell-Sills, L., Roy-Byrne, P. P., Craske, M. G., Bystritsky, A., Sullivan, G., & Stein, M. B. (2016). Improving outcomes for patients with medication resistant anxiety: Effects of collaborative care with cognitive behavioral therapy. *Depression and Anxiety, 33*, 1099–1106. https://doi.org/10.1002/da.22574.

Chan, A. T. Y., Sun, G. Y. Y., Tam, W. W. S., Tsoi, K. K. F., & Wong, S. Y. S. (2017). The effectiveness of group-based behavioral activation in the treatment of depression: An updated meta-analysis of randomized controlled trial. *Journal of Affective Disorders, 208*(1), 345–354. https://doi.org/10.1016/j.jad.2016.08.026.

Chen, K. W., Berger, C. C., Manheimer, E., Forde, D., Magidson, J., Dachman, L., & Lejuez, C. W. (2012). Meditative therapies for reducing anxiety: A systematic review and meta-analysis of randomized controlled trials. *Depression and Anxiety, 29*(7), 545–562. https://doi.org/10.1002/da.21964.

Cook, J. A., Jonikas, J. A., Hamilton, M. M., Goldrick, V., Steigman, P. J., Grey, D. D., et al. (2013). Impact of wellness recovery action planning on service utilization and need in a randomized controlled trial. *Psychiatric Rehabilitation Journal, 36*(4), 250–257.

Craske, M.G., Stein, M.B., Sullivan, G., Sherbourne, C., Bystritky, A., Rose, R.D., Lang, A.J.,… Roy-Byrne, (2011). Disorder-specific impact of coordinated anxiety learning and management treatment for anxiety disorders in primary care. Archives of General Psychiatry, 68(4), 378–388. doi: https://doi.org/10.1001/archgenpsychiatry.2011.25.

Craske, M. G., Rose, R. D., Lang, A., Welch, S. S., Campbell-Sills, L., Sullivan, G., Sherbourne, C., et al. (2009). Computer-assisted delivery of cognitive behavioral therapy for anxiety disorders in primary-care settings. *Depression and Anxiety, 26*, 235–242. https://doi.org/10.1002/da.20542.

Creswell, J. D. (2017). Mindfulness interventions. *Annual Review of Psychology, 68*, 491–516. https://doi.org/10.1146/annurev-psych-042716-051139.

Dixon, L. B., Lucksted, A., Medoff, D. R., Burland, J., Stewart, B., Lehman, A. F., et al. (2011). Outcomes of a randomized study of a peer-taught family-to-family education program for mental illness. *Psychiatric Services, 62*(6), 591–597.

Dixon, L. B., Dickerson, F., Bellack, A. S., Bennett, M., Dickinson, D., Goldberg, R. W., et al. (2009). The 2009 schizophrenia PORT psychosocial treatment recommendations and summary statements. *Schizophrenia Bulletin, 36*(1), 48–70.

Dobson, D., & Dobson, K. S. (2018). *Evidence-based practice of cognitive behavioral therapy* (2nd ed.). New York: Guilford Press.

D'Zurilla, T. J., & Nezu, A. M. (2007). *Problem-solving therapy: A positive approach to clinical intervention* (3rd ed.). New York: Springer.

Evans, S., Ferrando, S., Findler, M., Stowell, C., Smart, C., & Haglin, D. (2008). Mindfulness-based cognitive therapy for generalized anxiety disorder. *Journal of anxiety disorders, 22*(4), 716–721. https://doi.org/10.1016/j.janxdis.2007.07.005

Farchione, T. J., Fairholme, C. P., Ellard, K. K., Boisseau, C. L., Thompson-Hollands, J., Carl, J. R., Gallagher, M. W., & Barlow, D. H. (2012). Unified protocol for transdiagnostic treatment of emotional disorders: A randomized controlled trial. *Behavior Therapy, 43*(3), 666–678. https://doi.org/10.1016/j.beth.2012.01.001.

Finucane, A., & Mercer, S. W. (2006). An exploratory mixed methods study of the acceptability and effectiveness of mindfulness-based cognitive therapy for patients with active depression and anxiety in primary care. *BMC Psychiatry, 6,* 14. https://doi.org/10.1186/1471-244X-6-14.

Fjorback, L. O., Arendt, M., Ornbol, E., Fink, P., & Walach, H. (2011). Mindfulness-based stress reduction and mindfulness-based cognitive therapy: A systematic review of randomized controlled trials. *Acta Psychiatrica Scandinavica, 124*(2), 102–119. https://doi.org/10.1111/j.1600-0447.2011.01704.x.

Foa, E. B., Hembree, E., & Rothbaum, B. O. (2007). *Prolonged exposure therapy for PTSD: Emotional processing of traumatic experiences: A therapist guide.* New York: Oxford University Press.

Foa, E. B., & Kozak, M. J. (1986). Emotional processing of fear: Exposure to corrective information. *Psychological Bulletin, 99*(1), 20–35. https://doi.org/10.1037/0033-2909.99.1.20.

Foa, E. B., Huppert, J. D., & Cahill, S. P. (2006). Emotional Processing Theory: An Update. In B. O. Rothbaum (Ed.), Pathological anxiety: Emotional processing in etiology and treatment (p. 3–24). The Guilford Press.

Gillihan, S. J., Hembree, E. A., & Foa, E. B. (2012). Behavior therapy: Exposure therapy for anxiety disorders. In M. J. Dewan, B. N. Steenberger, & R. P. Greenberg (Eds.), *The art and science of brief psychotherapies: An illustrated guide.* Arlington: American Psychitric Publishing.

Goldin, P. R., & Gross, J. J. (2010). Effects of mindfulness-based stress reduction (MBSR) on emotion regulation in social anxiety disorder. *Emotion, 10*(1), 83–91. https://doi.org/10.1037/a0018441.

Greenberger, D., & Padesky, C. A. (2015). *Mind over mood: Change how you feel by changing the way you think* (2nd ed.). New York: Guilford Press.

Han, B., Compton, W. M., Blanco, C., & Colpe, L. J. (2017). Prevalence, treatment and unmet treatment needs of US adults with mental health and substance use disorders. *Health Affairs (Millwood), 36*(10), 1739–1747. https://doi.org/10.1377/hlthaff.2017.0584.

Hofmann, S. G., & Gómez, A. F. (2017). Mindfulness-based interventions for anxiety and depression. *The Psychiatric Clinics of North America, 40*(4), 739–749. https://doi.org/10.1016/j.psc.2017.08.008.

Hoge, E. A., Bui, E., Marques, L., Metcalf, C. A., Morris, L. K., Robinaugh, D. J., et al. (2013). Randomized controlled trial of mindfulness meditation for generalized anxiety disorder: Effects on anxiety and stress reactivity. *Journal of Clinical Psychiatry, 74*(8), 786–792. https://doi.org/10.4088/JCP.12m08083.

Holt-Lunstad, J., Smith, T. B., Baker, M., Harris, T., & Stephenson, D. (2015). Loneliness and social isolation as risk factors for mortality: A meta-analytic review. *Perspectives on Psychological Science, 10*(2), 227–237.

Hunot, V., Churchill, R., Teixeira, V., & Silva de Lima, M. (2007). Psychological therapies for gen-eralised anxiety disorder. *Cochrane Database of Systematic Reviews, 1*, Art. No.: CD001848. https://doi.org/10.1002/14651858.CD001848.pub4.

Jacobson, E. (1938). *Progressive relaxation*. Chicago: University of Chicago.

Jewell, T. C., Downing, D., & McFarlane, W. R. (2009). Partnering with families: Multiple fam-ily group psychoeducation for schizophrenia. *Journal of Clinical Psychology, 65*, 868–878. https://doi.org/10.1002/jclp.20610.

Joesch, J. M., Sherbourne, C. D., Sullivan, G., Stein, M. B., Craske, M. G., & Roy-Byrne, P. (2012). Incremental benefits and cost of coordinated anxiety learning and management for anxiety treatment in primary care. *Psychological Medicine, 42*, 1937–1948. https://doi.org/10.1017/S0033291711002893.

Jorm, A. F., Morgan, A. J., & Hetrick, S. E. (2008). Relaxation for depression. *Cochrane Database Systematic Reviews, 4*, CD007142. Published 2008 Oct 8. https://doi.org/10.1002/14651858.CD007142.pub2.

Kabat-Zinn, J. (1990). *Full catastrophe living: Using the wisdom of your body and mind to face stress, pain, and illness*. New York: Delacorte Press.

Kabat-Zinn, J. (2003). Mindfulness-based interventions in context: Past, present, and future. *Clinical Psychology: Science and Practice, 10*(2), 144–156. https://doi.org/10.1093/clipsy/bpg016.

Khoury, B., Lecomte, T., Fortin, G., Masse, M., Therien, P., Bouchard, V., et al. (2013). Mindfulness-based therapy: A comprehensive meta-analysis. *Clinical Psychology Review, 33*(6), 763–771. https://doi.org/10.1016/j.cpr.2013.05.005.

Kober, H., Buhle, J., Weber, J., Ochsner, K. N., & Wager, T. D. (2019). Let it be: Mindful accep-tance down-regulates pain and negative emotion. *Social Cognitive and Affective Neuroscience, 14*(11), 1147–1158. https://doi.org/10.1093/scan/nsz104.

Kvam, S., Kleppe, C. L., Nordhus, I. H., & Hovland, A. (2016). Exercise as a treatment for depres-sion: A meta-analysis. *Journal of Affective Disorders, 202*, 67–86. https://doi.org/10.1016/j.jad.2016.03.063.

Lucksted, A., McFarlane, W., Downing, D., & Dixon, L. (2012). Recent developments in family psychoeducation as an evidence-based practice. *Journal of Marital and Family Therapy, 38*(1), 101–121.

Manzoni, G. M., Pagnini, F., Castelnuovo, G., & Molinari, E. (2008). Relaxation training for anx-iety: A ten-years systematic review with meta-analysis. *BMC Psychiatry, 8*, 41. https://doi.org/10.1186/1471-244X-8-41.

McFarlane, W. R. (2002). *Multifamily groups in the treatment of severe psychiatric disorders*. New York: Guilford Press.

McFarlane, W. R. (2016). Family interventions for schizophrenia and the psychoses: A review. *Family Process, 55*, 460–482. https://doi.org/10.1111/famp.12235.

Monti, P., Kadden, R., Rohsenow, D., Cooney, N., Abrams, D. (2002). Treating alcohol depen-dence: A coping skills training guide. (2nd Ed). New York: Guildford Press.

Moussavi, S., Chatterji, S., & Verdes, E. (2007). Depression, chronic diseases, and decrements in health: Results from the World Health Surveys. *Lancet, 370*, 851–858.

Mueser, K. Y., & Gingerich, S. (2013). Illness management and recovery. In V. Vandiver (Ed.), *Best practices in community mental health*. Chicago: Lyceum Books.

Murphy, S. M., Irving, C. B., Adams, C. E., & Waqar, M. (2015). Crisis intervention for peo-ple with severe mental illnesses. *Cochrane Database of Systematic Reviews, 12.*, Art. No.: CD001087. https://doi.org/10.1002/14651858.CD001087.pub5.

Patel, V., Weiss, H. A., Chowdhary, N., Naik, S., Pednekar, S., Chatterjee, S., De Silva, M. J., et al. (2010). Effectiveness of an intervention led by lay health counselors for depressive and anxiety disorders in primary care in Goa India (MANAS): a cluster randomised controlled trial. *Lancet, 376*(December (9758)), 2086–2095.

Pharoah, F., Mari, J. J., Rathbone, J., & Wong, W. (2010). Family intervention for schizo-phrenia. *Cochrane Database of Systematic Reviews, 12.*, Art. No.: CD000088. https://doi.org/10.1002/14651858.CD000088.pub3.

Segal, Z. V., Williams, J. M. G., & Teasdale, J. D. (2013). *Mindfulness-based cognitive therapy for depression: A new approach to preventing relapse* (2nd ed.). New York: Guilford.

Smith, C., Hancock, H., Blake-Mortimer, J., & Eckert, K. (2007). A randomized comparative trial of yoga and relaxation to reduce stress and anxiety. *Complementary Therapies in Medicine, 15*(2), 77–83.

Spinelli, C., Wisener, M., & Khoury, B. (2019). Mindfulness training for healthcare profession-als and trainees: A meta-analysis of randomized controlled trials. *Journal of Psychosomatic Research, 120,* 29–38. https://doi.org/10.1016/j.jpsychores.2019.03.003.

Teasdale, J. D., Segal, Z. V., Williams, J. M. G., Ridgeway, V. A., Soulsby, J. M., & Lau, M. A. (2000). Prevention of relapse/recurrence in major depression by mindfulness-based cog-nitive therapy. *Journal of Consulting and Clinical Psychology, 68*(4), 615–623. https://doi.org/10.1037/0022-006X.68.4.615.

Rauch, S. A., Eftekhari, A., & Ruzek, J. I. (2012). Review of exposure therapy: A gold standard for PTSD treatment. *Journal of Rehabilitation Research and Development, 49*(5), 679–687.

Rauch, S., & Foa, E. (2006). Emotional Processing Theory (EPT) and exposure therapy for PTSD. *Journal of Contemporary Psychotherapy, 36*(2), 61–65. https://doi.org/10.1007/s10879-006-9008-y.

Roy-Byrne, P., Craske, M. G., Sullivan, G., Rose, R. D., Edlund, M. J., Lang, A. J., Bystritsky, A., Welch, S. S., Chavira, D. A., Golinelli, D., Campbell-Sills, L., Sherbourne, C. D., & Stein, M. B. (2010). Delivery of evidence-based treatment for multiple anxiety disorders in primary care: A randomized controlled trial. *JAMA, 303*(19), 1921–1928. https://doi.org/10.1001/jama.2010.608.

Williams, J. M. G., Crane, C., Barnhofer, T., Brennan, K., Duggan, D. S., Fennell, M. J. V., Hackmann, A., et al. (2014). Mindfulness-based cognitive therapy for preventing relapse in recurrent depression: A randomized dismantling trial. *Journal of Consulting and Clinical Psychology, 82*(2), 275–286. https://doi.org/10.1037/a0035036.

Williams, M. D., Sawchuk, C. N., Shippee, N. D., Somers, K. J., Berg, S. L., Mitchell, J. D., Mattson, A. B., & Katzelnick, D. J. (2018). A quality improvement project aimed at adapting primary care to ensure the delivery of evidence-based psychotherapy for adult anxiety. *BMJ Quality Improvement Report, 7,* e000066. https://doi.org/10.1136/bmjoq-2017-000066.

Wolitzky-Taylor, K., Krull, J., Rawson, R., Roy-Byrne, P., Ries, R., & Craske, M. (2018). Randomized clinical trial evaluating the preliminary effectiveness of an integrated anxiety dis-order treatment in substance use disorder specialty clinics. *Journal of Consulting or Clinical Psychology, 86*(1), 81–88. https://doi.org/10.1037/ccp0000276.

World Health Organization (WHO). (2017). *Depression and other common mental disorders: global health estimates.* Geneva: License: CC BY-NC-SA 3.0 IGO. Accessed 20 June 2019 at https://apps.who.int/iris/bitstream/handle/10665/254610/WHO-MSD-MER-2017.2-eng.pdf

Wright, J. H., Brown, G. K., Thase, M. E., Ramirez Basco, M., & Gabbard, G. O. (2017). *Learning cognitive behavioral therapy: An illustrated guide* (Core competencies in psychotherapy) (2nd ed.). Arlington: American Psychiatric Publishing.

Xia, J., Merinder, L. B., & Belgamwar, M. R. (2011). Psychoeducation for schizophrenia. *Cochrane Database of Systematic Reviews, 6.*, Art. No.: CD002831. https://doi.org/10.1002/14651858.CD002831.pub2.

Chapter 10
Screening, Assessment, and Brief Interventions for Substance Use

10.1 Overview of Alcohol and Substance Use

The misuse of alcohol and other substances commonly occurs in the general population and is linked to a range of negative health consequences. In 2018, according to the National Survey on Drug Use, approximately 60% of the US population over the age of 12 (165 million people) reported using substances, including alcohol, in the past month. Of that number, 67 million reported binge drinking (41%), 43.5 million reported marijuana use (26%), over 10 million people reported opioid misuse (6%), and 5.5 million reported cocaine use (3%) (SAMHSA 2019). In 2018, 23 million people had a substance use disorder (SUD), two-thirds of which were alcohol-related (SAMHSA 2019). Overall, 10% of the US population will experience a substance use disorder in their lifetime and 4% will experience an SUD within the next 12 months (Grant et al. 2016). Approximately 8% or 1 in 13 people in the United States over the age of 12 will need treatment for an alcohol or substance use disorder (SAMHSA 2019). Despite these figures, treatment rates remain low. Only a quarter of people with an SUD will receive any treatment (Grant et al. 2016) and only 10% will receive specialized substance abuse treatment services (SAMHSA 2019).

Problematic alcohol and substance use rates among older populations are expected to rise in the coming years due to the aging of the baby boomer population who have reported higher rates of substance use than previous generations (Blazer and Wu 2009; Han and Moore 2018; Kuerbis et al. 2014; Moore et al. 2009; Youdin 2019). In 2013–2014, nearly two-thirds of the older adult population reported alcohol use and a fifth reported binge drinking. Furthermore, approximately 5% of older men and 2.5% of older women reported alcohol use disorders. This represents nearly a 20% increase in binge drinking and a 25% increase in alcohol use disorder for this population in less than 10 years (Han et al. 2017a). While the use of marijuana has also increased in older adult populations (Han et al. 2017b), the most concerning increase has been the rise in prescription opioid and benzodiazepine use

© Springer Nature Switzerland AG 2021
M. A. Mancini, *Integrated Behavioral Health Practice*,
https://doi.org/10.1007/978-3-030-59659-0_10

in this population. These drugs pose significant risks for older adult populations in the form of falls, accidental overdoses, and delirium. The increased use of these drugs combined with increased poly-pharmacy and alcohol misuse creates a context for increased service utilization, morbidity, and mortality (Achildi et al. 2013; Han and Moore 2018; Larney et al. 2015; Sullivan and Howe 2013; Youdin 2019). This increase in prevalence has important health implications and will require the implementation of universal and robust screening and assessment procedures in routine medical and behavioral health settings (Han and Moore 2018).

These statistics, again, point to a need for the integration of behavioral health care and primary care and an expansion of substance use screening, assessment, and treatment in routine clinical settings. In the sections that follow, specific approaches to providing these services will be reviewed and discussed. These approaches include the deployment of universal screening for alcohol and substance misuse, the assessment and diagnosis of substance use disorders, and the use of brief interventions for harmful alcohol and substance use. Each of the approaches that are considered can be utilized by a range of multidisciplinary providers in a variety of settings including primary care settings, inpatient and outpatient behavioral health settings, and community mental health organizations.

10.2   Screening and Assessment for Substance Misuse and Substance Use Disorders

Alcohol and substance use have tremendous impact on health and are commonly comorbid with depression, anxiety, PTSD, personality disorders such as borderline and antisocial personality disorders. Alcohol and substance use is also associated with accidents, and a full range of health conditions impacting the functioning of the liver, brain, gastrointestinal tract, kidneys, and heart. It is important for service providers to ask all clients if they drink alcohol or use substances, and if so, how much and how often they typically do so. Substance misuse is defined as harmful, problematic, or risky use of substances that include recreational drugs (i.e. cannabis, cocaine, heroin, amphetamines, hallucinogens), prescribed and unprescribed medications (i.e. opioids, painkillers, benzodiazapines) and alcohol. Substance misuse carries significant health consequences. For some substances like opioids and cocaine there are no safe limits. For alcohol and cannabis, misuse (sometimes referred to as problem or harmful drinking/use) is when clients routinely exceed recommended limits or drink/use in a hazardous manner (e.g., while driving). A person has a substance use disorder when they exhibit a pattern of use that causes significant impairment in various life domains and that indicates a lack of control over use and/or continued use despite significant negative health, psychological, and social consequences.

Federal guidelines indicate that men who consume, on average, more than two drinks per day or 14 drinks per week, and women or persons 65 years of age and older who consume on average more than one drink per day or 7 drinks per week, may experience negative health consequences from their drinking. Currently, there are no guidelines specifically designed for transgender and gender nonconforming (TGNC) persons. Also, drinking four to five or more drinks in a single episode or outing is considered harmful or hazardous drinking or a binge drinking event. Clients should be notified that questions about use are standard and asked of all persons receiving treatment. Questions should be posed in a matter-of-fact, non-judgmental manner (USDHHS 2015; NIAAA 2020a, b). Figure 10.1 lists the daily and weekly alcohol use limits.

In regard to cannabis use, several guidelines have been developed that signify lower-risk use. Like alcohol, abstinence is the most effective way to avoid health risks related to cannabis use. Other recommendations to avoid health risks for cannabis use include: (1) not using cannabis products high in Tetrahydrocannabinol (THC); (2) avoiding daily cannabis use; (3) using only occasionally (at most once per week or weekend use); (4) avoiding combusted cannabis use and deep inhalation or holding practices; (5) avoiding use while driving; and (6) avoiding all synthetic cannabis products. Early initiation of cannabis use (before the age of 16) is associated with increased risk of negative health and social outcomes. Further, cannabis use should be avoided by people with a family history or are currently diagnosed with substance use or psychotic disorders as well as by pregnant or nursing women (Fischer et al. 2017).

The integration of routine, brief universal screening for harmful drinking and drug use in primary care and community-based settings such as hospitals, outpatient

What Counts as ONE Standard Drink?		
Beer	**Wine**	**Spirits**
12oz of 5% = 1 standard drink (SD)	5oz. of 12% = 1 (SD)	1.5oz 40% = 1 (SD)
Note: 16oz (Pint) of 5% = 1.3 drinks 12oz of 7%+ = 1.5 drinks 16oz (Pint) of 7%+ = 2 drinks	Note: Regular size bottle (750ml) = 5 drinks	e.g., gin, rum, tequila, whiskey, vodka

Alcohol Use	Max Daily Limit	Max Weekly Limit	Binge Drinking Limit (# drinks within one occasion)
Women and Anyone Over 65 Years of Age	3 Drinks	7 Drinks	4 Drinks
Men Under 65 Years of Age	4 Drinks	14 Drinks	5 Drinks

Fig. 10.1 Alcohol use limits

behavioral health centers, primary care settings, emergency departments, community health clinics, and urgent care centers is used to identify persons who may be at risk of health problems or other negative consequences due to their drinking and substance use behavior. Screening goes beyond identifying people with active alcohol and drug problems and is expanded to include risky forms of use that may not reach the limit of serious addiction problems (Babor et al. 2007). Several screening instruments can be used in primary care settings. I will review several of the most common screening forms next.

Michigan Alcoholism Screening Test (MAST) The MAST is a reliable and valid screen – but it is long (28 items) (Selzer 1971). One of the problems with the MAST is that it targets persons who engage in various serious alcohol problems rather than at-risk drinkers. There is a shorter 13-item version, the S-MAST (Pokorny et al. 1972; Selzer et al. 1975). The S-MAST asks 13 "yes" or "no" questions about alcohol use over the previous 12 months. Sample questions include: "Does your wife, husband, parent or other near relative ever worry or complain about your drinking?", "Are you able to stop drinking when you want to?," "Have you ever gotten in trouble at work because of your drinking?," "Have you ever gone to anyone for help about your drinking?," "Have you ever attended an AA meeting?," "Have you ever been in a hospital because of drinking?," and "Have you ever been arrested for drunken driving or driving under the influence of alcoholic beverages?" A score of 3 or more "yes" answers indicates the need for further investigation or assessment (Selzer et al. 1975).

Drug Abuse Screening Test (DAST) The DAST is a 28-item self-report screening instrument that assesses for problematic and hazardous drug use (Yudko et al. 2007; Skinner 1982). There is also a brief, 10-item version, the DAST-10, that has good sensitivity and specificity (Yudko et al. 2007; Gavin et al. 1989). The DAST-10 asks directly about prescription and nonprescription substance use with 10 "yes" and "no" questions. Sample questions include: "Are you able to stop abusing drugs when you want to?", "Do you ever feel guilty about using drugs?,", "Have you neglected your family because of your drug use?," "Have you ever experienced withdrawal symptoms when you stop taking drugs?," "Have you used drugs other than those required for medical reasons?," "Have you had medical problems as a result of your drug use?," and "Does your spouse (or parents) ever complain about your involvement with drugs?" One or two "yes" responses indicate mild drug problems. Three to five "yes" responses indicate moderate drug problems. Five or more "yes" responses indicate substantial or severe problems with drugs (Skinner 1982). Combining the S-MAST and DAST can provide a very useful combination screen for alcohol and drugs.

Cut Down, Annoyed, Guilty, Eye-Opener, Adapted to Include Drugs (CAGE-AID) The CAGE-AID is a very brief four-item screen used to assess problem drinking and drug use (Brown and Rounds 1995). Persons who answered "yes" to two or more questions should be referred for further assessment. The CAGE asks if a client has ever tried to *C*ut back on their use, had others *A*nnoyed with them regarding their use, have ever felt *G*uilty over their use, or have ever had to have a drink or use a substance upon waking as an "*E*ye-opener" in the morning in order to relieve withdrawal symptoms. A positive response to one or more questions indicates a positive screen for problematic alcohol or drug use. The CAGE-AID may fail to identify at-risk drinkers since its questions focus on criteria that would indicate higher-level alcohol use problems rather than at-risk drinking patterns. However, it is a very common screen used in a variety of settings due to its brevity and relatively good psychometrics.

Alcohol Use Disorder Identification Test (AUDIT) The AUDIT is a brief, comprehensive 10-item screen that focuses on: (1) problem drinking (PD) such as exceeding daily drinking guidelines; (2) binge drinking or drinking when it is hazardous to do so such as when driving; (3) the presence of a possible alcohol use disorder (AUD) indicating an inability to stop or control drinking despite harmful consequences; and (4) alcohol dependence (AD) when drinking patterns indicate a physical and psychological dependence on alcohol as evidenced by the presence of withdrawal and tolerance symptoms (Babor et al. 2001; Saunders, Aasland et al. 1993). The first three questions measure hazardous alcohol use by asking questions about consumption (e.g., frequency, quantity, and frequency of heaving drinking). Questions 4–6 measure alcohol use disorders or dependency symptoms such as the inability to exert control over drinking behavior, problems meeting obligations and roles due to drinking, and the need to have a drink in the morning to mitigate withdrawal symptoms. The last four questions measure harmful alcohol use through assessing guilt after drinking; the presence of blackouts, injuries, or others; and the experience of having family, friends, partners, and healthcare workers voicing concern about drinking behavior. Each question has five choices with scores ranging from 0 to 4 points for each item. In general, a score below 8 indicates low-risk drinking. A score of 8–15 indicates that drinking that exceeds recommended guidelines. Clients in this range should be given advice that they should consider cutting down or stop drinking completely. Scores from 16 to 19 indicate high-risk drinking that is likely to lead to significant health issues. Clients should be informed that they should cut down or stop drinking and be offered assistance or information on how to do so. Scores of 20 and above indicate the likely presence of an alcohol use disorder requiring referral to an addiction specialist (Babor et al. 2001).

The AUDIT-C is a brief, three-question version of the full AUDIT that has shown to be very effective in identifying PD and moderately effective in identifying AUD and AD. The AUDIT-C asks clients three questions with five choices with scores that range from 0 to 4. The following questions and responses are asked (points for each item in parentheses): (1) How often do you have a drink containing alcohol? [Never = (0), Monthly = (1), 2–4 times a month = (2), 2–3 times a month = (3), 4 or more times a month = (4)]; (2) How many standard drinks containing alcohol do you have on a typical day? [1–2 = (0), 3–4 = (1), 5–6 = (2), 7–9 = (3), 10 + =(4)]; and (3) How often do you have six or more drinks on one occasion? [Never = (0),

Less than Monthly = (1), Monthly = (2), Weekly = (3), Daily or Almost Daily = (4)]. A score of 4 or more in men and 3 or more in women or adults over the age of 65 indicates the likely presence of a drinking problem requiring further assessment (Bush et al. 1998; Bradley et al. 2003).

Cars, Relax, Alone, Forget, Friends/Family, Trouble (CRAFFT)   The CRAFFT is a brief drug and alcohol screen designed to detect the possible presence of problematic alcohol or drug use in adolescents requiring further assessment (Knight et al. 1999; Knight et al. 2002). The CRAFFT has two parts. Part A asks the client if they have ever (1) used alcohol; (2) smoked marijuana or hashish; and (3) used anything else to get high. Part B consists of six "yes" and "no" questions: (1) Have you ever ridden in a *C*ar driven by someone (including yourself) who was "high" or had been using alcohol or drugs?; (2) Do you ever use alcohol or drugs to *R*elax, feel better about yourself, or fit in?; (3) Do you ever use alcohol or drugs while you are by yourself, or *A*lone?; (4) Do you ever *F*orget things you did while using alcohol or drugs?; (5) Do your *F*amily or *F*riends ever tell you that you should cut down on your drinking or drug use?; and (6) Have you ever gotten into *T*rouble while you were using alcohol or drugs? A "No" response to all of the questions in Part A would require the provider to only ask the first question about whether the person has ever ridden in a *C*ar driven by someone who was "high" or has been using alcohol or drugs. A "yes" to any question in Part A would require the provider to ask all six of the CRAFFT questions. Each "yes" response to the CRAFFT questions is worth one point. A score of two or more points would indicate the need for further assessment. A person who scores a two has been shown to have a 50% probability for having a substance use disorder. A score of four has been shown to have an 80% probability for a substance use disorder (Knight et al. 1999; Knight et al. 2002).

Alcohol, Smoking, and Substance Involvement Screening Test (ASSIST)   The ASSIST is a brief screening measure developed by the World Health Organization (WHO) and is designed to be deployed in healthcare settings to identify persons in need of intervention for unhealthy drinking, smoking, and drug use behaviors. The ASSIST is designed to help clients recognize health problems due to tobacco, alcohol, and drug use (Humeniuk et al. 2010a; WHO 2002). The ASSIST effectively screens for problematic use behaviors related to alcohol, tobacco, cannabis, cocaine, amphetamine, sedatives, hallucinogens, inhalant, and opioids. It also tests for current and past use, problems associated with use, risks for harm, dependence, and injecting drug use. The ASSIST is a good screening tool that can be linked with the FRAMES brief intervention approach (Bien et a. 1993; Miller and Sanchez 1994) and other motivational interviewing interventions or methods (Humeniuk et al. 2010b; Miller and Rollnick 2002, 2013; Miller 1995).

Substance Use Disorder Diagnostic Criteria
Table 10.1 lists the specific DSM-5 criteria for a substance use disorder. An alcohol or substance use disorder diagnosis is warranted if a person demonstrates a sustained pattern of drug or alcohol use that leads to "clinically significant impairment

or distress" (APA 2013, pp.490) and identifies two or more symptoms from a list of 11 symptom criteria. The 11 symptoms include: (1) taking larger amounts of the substance than intended; (2) failed attempts to cut down or stop use; (3) a great deal of time spent obtaining and using substances and recovering from its effect; (4) craving of substance when not available; (5) failure to adequately fulfill responsibilities and roles due to substance use; (6) continuing to use substance despite continually experiencing negative consequences in the areas of interpersonal relationships, occupational functioning, and other social areas; (7) giving up or neglecting important activities due to use; (8) using when it is physically hazardous to do so; (9) continuing substance use despite persistent negative physical, social, and psychological physical problems; (10) experiencing tolerance or the need for more of the substance to achieve intoxication; and (11) experiencing withdrawal or the negative physical and psychological effects of not using a substance. (APA 2013). A person who experiences two or three of the above criteria would qualify for mild substance use disorder and experiencing four to five symptoms would qualify for moderate substance use disorders. More than five symptoms would indicate a severe disorder. DSM-5 also lists specific symptoms for substance intoxication and substance withdrawal. Figure 10.2 lists the most common intoxication and withdrawal symptoms for each substance.

Table 10.1 Substance use disorder criteria (Based on: APA 2013)

A sustained pattern of drug or alcohol use that leads to "clinically significant impairment or distress" and identifies 2 or more symptoms from a list of 11 criteria occurring within a 12-month period:
(1) Taking larger amounts of the substance than intended
(2) Failed attempts to cut down or stop use
(3) A great deal of time spent obtaining and using substances and recovering from its effect
(4) Craving of substance when not available
(5) Failure to adequately fulfill responsibilities and roles due to substance use
(6) Continuing to use substance despite continually experiencing negative consequences in the areas of interpersonal relationships, occupational functioning, and other social areas
(7) Giving up or neglecting important activities due to use
(8) Using when it is physically hazardous to do so
(9) Continuing substance use despite experiencing persistent negative physical, social, and psychological physical problems
(10) Experiencing tolerance or the need for more of the substance to achieve intoxication
(11) Experiencing withdrawal or the negative physical and psychological effects of not using a substance
Severity levels: 2–3 Symptoms = Mild 4–5 Symptoms = Moderate 6+ Symptoms = Severe

10.3   Screening, Brief Intervention, and Referral to Treatment (S-BIRT)

The use of tobacco, drugs, and alcohol account for a significant proportion of morbidity and mortality and can lead to a range of interpersonal, social, financial, and legal problems for clients. Integrating effective screening and brief interventions in primary care settings represents an important opportunity to identify persons at risk for harm due to substance use and to provide brief, easily accessible interventions and treatment (World Health Organization (WHO) 1996). One such model that has shown good efficacy is screening, brief intervention, and referral to treatment (S-BIRT). S-BIRT has been shown to be an effective, efficient, and cost-effective public health approach to reduce harmful drinking and substance use for nearly 40 years (Babor et al. 2007; Bernstein et al. 2007; Kaner et al. 2018; Pringle et al. 2018). The program started in the early 1980s and was found to be an effective approach for helping large groups of people reduce smoking and risky drinking in a short period of time with limited professional contact (Kristenson et al. 1983; Russell et al. 1988). A key aspect of S-BIRT is that it formally integrates alcohol and substance use services within primary care settings to change risky behavior and increase service engagement for clients with alcohol and substance use issues (Babor et al. 2007). Multisite evaluations of S-BIRT have found the approach effective in screening patients in high-volume settings and was associated with substantial reductions in substance and alcohol use (Aldridge et al. 2017a; Babor et al. 2017). The focus of the S-BIRT program is to provide universal screening and brief

Substance	Intoxication Symptoms	Withdrawal Symptoms
Alcohol	Slurred speech, incoordination, unsteady gait, blurred vision, impaired attention or memory, stupor, coma	Autonomic hyperactivity, hand tremor, insomnia, nausea/vomiting, transient hallucinations, psychomotor agitation, anxiety, seizures
Cannabis	Blood shot eye, increased appetite, dry mouth, tachycardia	Irritability, anger, aggression, anxiety, sleep difficulty, decreased appetite/weight loss, restlessness, depressed mood, at least one of the following (abdominal pain, tremors, sweating, fever, chills, headache)
Stimulant	Tachycardia or bradycardia, pupil dilation, elevated/lowered blood pressure, perspiration, chills, nausea, vomiting, weight loss, psychomotor agitation/retardation, muscle weakness, respiratory depression, chest pain, arrhythmia, confusion, seizures, dystonia, coma	Fatigue; vivid, unpleasant nightmares; insomnia; increased appetite; psychomotor retardation
Opioid	Drowsiness, coma, slurred speech, impairment of attention or memory	Dysphoric mood, nausea, vomiting, muscle aches, lacrimation or rhinorrhea, sweating, pupil dilation, diarrhea, yawning, fever, insomnia

Fig. 10.2 Symptoms of intoxication and withdrawal from substances (Based on: APA 2013)

motivational interventions in routine primary care settings to address problematic or harmful drinking and alcohol and substance use disorder.

There are several key clinical practices that define S-BIRT. These include: (1) universal annual screening of all adults for problematic or harmful alcohol and substance use and alcohol or substance use disorders; (2) the provision of brief interventions for clients who screen positive. Brief interventions typically involve sharing screening results with clients, reviewing recommended limits on drinking and drug use, identifying the risks associated with use, and giving advice to clients about cutting down or eliminating use; (3) referral to specialty treatment services, peer support/self-help, medications, and individual or group counseling for those clients identified as having an alcohol or substance use disorder; and (4) routine follow-up and monitoring with those clients. Organizational elements that are critical for the effective implementation of S-BIRT services include clinical and administrative support at all levels of care, routine evaluation of the program through continuous quality improvement (CQI), providing ongoing professional development opportunities for staff, and integration of S-BIRT protocols into medical records and billing systems (Bradley et al. 2018; Mancini and Miner 2013).

S-BIRT is very appropriate for interprofessional and collaborative care team settings. Effective implementation of S-BIRT approaches requires several practices. First, it is important to identify early adopters and champions for S-BIRT within the organization. Second, ongoing training that outlines each step of the S-BIRT protocol helps keep providers fully trained and competent in all S-BIRT operations. Third, it is important to fully integrate S-BIRT into the routine practices of the site such as having more time in clinical interactions to deliver S-BIRT and having prompts in the electronic medical record guiding providers in screening and assessment practices. Lastly, it is important for sites to have formal relationships with outside agencies that can provide substance use disorder counseling services in order to enhance the referral process (Hargraves et al. 2017; Mancini and Miner 2013).

Brief motivational interventions that are often used in S-BIRT have been shown to be cost-effective ways to reduce drinking in persons who drink heavily in primary care populations compared to no intervention. Brief interventions of only 15–30 min integrated as a part of standard clinical care encounters have been shown to be just as effective as longer interventions (Aldridge et al. 2017a,b; Babor et al. 2017; Barbosa et al. 2017; Kaner et al. 2018; Paltzer et al. 2017; Pringle et al. 2018).

For persons whose screening suggests a severe drinking or substance use disorder, referral to treatment by an outside specialty program or intra-agency/team program offers the client an opportunity for more in-depth assessment and diagnostic services, detoxification services, and longer-term inpatient or outpatient treatment for moderate to severe alcohol and substance use disorders. The referral process is facilitated by formal agreements with specialized treatment agencies or professionals within the organization who provide services or via formal relationships with trusted outside service providers. This facilitates a seamless, effective, and collaborative referral to other services. Research indicates that screening, the deployment of brief interventions, and referral to treatment can increase engagement and retention in specialized treatment for persons with alcohol and substance use problems

(Bernstein et al. 1997; D'Onofrio et al. 1998; Dunn and Ries 1997; Elvy et al. 1988; Hillman et al. 2001; Rochat et al. 2004).

10.4   Brief Motivational Interventions

Brief motivational interventions (BI) can be deployed in primary care settings such as emergency departments and health clinics as well as community-based behavioral health and social service settings. Brief interventions have consistently been found to help reduce problem drinking and to be as effective as longer-term treatment, particularly, in persons with mild or moderate drinking or substance use problems (Bien et al. 1993; Kahan et al. 1995; Wilk et al. 1997; Ballesteros et al. 2004; Moyer et al. 2002; Alvarez-Bueno et al. 2015; Barata et al. 2017; D'Onofrio et al. 2012). D'Onofrio and colleagues found that the use of the brief negotiation interview (BNI), combined with universal screening in the ED, reduced harmful drinking and hazardous drinking episodes at 6- and 12-month follow-up (D'Onofrio et al. 2005, 2012). Table 10.2 lists the core components and sample script for the BNI. A systematic review of brief interventions in primary care settings found that they were moderately effective in reducing alcohol consumption in people who engage in hazardous or harmful drinking compared to no intervention (Kaner et al. 2018).

Brief motivational interventions have also been found to be effective for reducing cocaine and opioid use and opioid overdoses when deployed in clinical community health settings such as urgent care centers, women's health clinics and clinics for persons who are homeless, emergency departments, and primary care sites (Bernstein, Bernstein et al. 2005; Bohnert et al. 2016; Madras et al. 2009). Brief interventions can also reduce tobacco use rates. When brief interventions were combined with access to nicotine replacement therapy and referral to a nicotine quit line in an emergency department, tobacco use decreased and abstinence rates increased at three and 12 months (Lemhoefer et al. 2017). Further, since most overdoses are accidental and without intent to self-harm, hospitals and EDs represent important places to implement brief interventions for hazardous drug and alcohol use, particularly for hazardous opioid use (Bohnert et al. 2018).

Brief interventions (BI) rely on motivational approaches to inform clients of the consequences of their drinking or drug use and to inquire and encourage reduced use or abstinence (Babor et al. 2007). The approach involves providing feedback to clients about unhealthy drinking and drug use behaviors and helping motivate them to set goals, develop strategies to reduce their drinking patterns, and take action to modify their drinking and drug use behaviors (Fleming and Baier-Manwell 1999). These interventions consist of short conversations that last 10–20 min and can be integrated into routine clinical encounters. In these meetings, providers give feedback on screening scores, attempt to increase motivation to take action (e.g., reduce or eliminate use), and offer advice and teach skills about reducing or eliminating use. These brief interventions are most often provided to persons who score in the low-to-moderate use range and do not require intensive forms of treatment (Babor

Table 10.2 Brief negotiation interview and script (Based on: D'Onofrio et al. 2005, 2012)

Raise the subject	Explain your role Ask permission to discuss screening forms Ask for use patterns Listen and reflect understanding	Would you like to review your screening results? What does a typical day look like for you? When you use X, what does that look like? When do you use and how often? How much would you drink/use on a typical occasion?
Give feedback	Share results, review low-risk drinking limits, and explore reaction Explore the connection to health and social consequences	Current guidelines for drinking indicate that [5 or more drinks (M)/(4 or more drinks (F/65+)] or more than [14 drinks (M)/7 drinks (F & 65+)] drinks in a week or use of X substance can lead to significant health and social problems, and can place you at a higher risk of illness and injury (give handout on impacts). It looks like your drinking/use could have significant negative consequences for you. What are your thoughts about that?
Enhance motivation	Ask about pros and cons of using and not using (e.g., decisional balance) Explore readiness to change and reasons for change using a "readiness ruler"	What are the good things about using? What are the not-so-good things? Sounds like on the one hand (add pros), and on the other hand (add cons). On a scale from 1 to 10, with 1 being not at all ready and 10 being totally 100% ready, how ready are you to change your use? Great! You're X% ready. Why did you choose that number and not a lower number?

Negotiate action plan	If motivated:
	  Summarize (repeat reasons for change mentioned by client)
	  Ask: What do you think you will do? Or what steps can you take to cut back?
	If not ready: (1) stop intervention, thank patient, and hand out information; (2) encourage patient to cut back; (3) negotiate follow-up visit; (4) offer options for change
	If motivated for referral: (1) explore understanding of different options for treatment and (2) warm handoff—make call for an appointment or walk to colleague for further assessment.
		If motivated:
		It sounds like you have some good reasons to change such as (list the ones the client identified). What are some action steps you could take today to help you stay healthy and safe (or to cut back on your use)? I think you have identified some great ideas. Let me write them down for you so you have a reminder. Could you summarize those for me again? Here are some additional resources that can help. Would you like to learn about them? [self-help, counseling, support groups, medication assistance, social services, peer support, advocacy groups]. Would you like to call now or walk to meet one of the counselors who can set you up with an appointment?
		If not ready:
		Thanks for listening. Take this information with you in case you change your mind. I advise you to consider cutting back on your use to within the guidelines we reviewed to keep you healthy and safe. Let's set up another appointment.

et al. 2007). Brief interventions can be a part of an S-BIRT style intervention in a primary care setting, or they can be used independently and combined with screening and assessment procedures. BI is designed for persons who engage in problem drinking, but are not yet experiencing consistent problems. BIs are ideal for persons who have not yet identified their drinking as a problem and are not currently seeking help for their drinking.

FRAMES

FRAMES is a 10- to 15-min intervention targeted to low-to-moderate risk drinkers or substance users. The FRAMES approach stands for Feedback, Responsibility, Advice, Menu of Options, Empathic, and Self-Efficacy (Humeniuk et al. 2010b). Table 10.3 lists the main components and script for the FRAMES interview. The FRAMES approach gives providers guidelines for their treatment interactions with clients who engage in problematic or harmful drinking or substance use. The approach begins by giving nonjudgmental *feedback* to clients based on the results of their screening forms (e.g., AUDIT, MAST, DAST, Patient Health Questionnaire (PHQ) 2 or Patient Health Questionnaire (PHQ) 9 or Generalized Anxiety Disorder (GAD) 7). Feedback involves providing scores on screening instruments, notifying the client that their score exceeded recommended drinking guidelines, and then informing clients that they are at a higher risk of health problems due to their use. Providers also give client's handouts and brochures that outline these health risks (e.g., falls, accidents, hypertension, liver damage, depression, stomach problems, cancer, and interpersonal problems). Lastly, providers ask the client open-ended questions about their thoughts and reactions to this information (Bien et al. 1993; Miller and Sanchez 1994; Miller and Rollick 2002; Humeniuk et al. 2010b).

It is important for providers to communicate to the clients that they are *responsible* for the decisions they make about their health and the consequences of those decisions. This involves asking clients if they want to see their scores, and whether they are concerned about their scores. This can give clients a sense of control and reduce resistance (Bien et al. 1993; Miller and Sanchez 1994; Miller and Rollick 2002; Humeniuk et al. 2010b).

Providers should also give clients *advice* about what to do about the behavior. This often entails telling the person to stop using or cutting back to recommended levels. This advice should be clear, unequivocal, and delivered in a nonjudgmental manner. Providing advice is designed to bring awareness to the client about their behavior and the risks associated with it. Advice should be followed up with open-ended questions asking the clients what they think about changing their behavior, how important it is for them to change their behavior, and how confident they are that they can make the change. This could then be followed up with a menu of options for the client. It is generally unhelpful to tell people "you should stop drinking" or "I'm concerned about your drinking," because this can be taken as judgmental and lead to defensiveness and resistance (Bien et al. 1993; Miller and Sanchez 1994; Miller and Rollick 2002; Humeniuk et al. 2010b).

Table 10.3 FRAMES approach and script (Based on: Humeniuk et al. 2010b)

Practice	Definition	Example script
Feedback	Give clients nonjudgmental feedback on their screening scores and the health risk posed by their behavior. Provide clients with handouts identifying guidelines and health effects	Do you want to know how you scored on the questionnaire? Your scores indicate that your drinking (or drug use) exceeds recommended daily limits and that you are at risk of several health and behavioral health problems such as (list specific health effects such as lung cancer, HIV, HCV, liver damage, diabetes, accidents, social problems, depression). How concerned are you about this information?
Responsibility	Tell clients that they have responsibility and control over their health behaviors	
Advice	Give clients advice about changing their behaviors	The best way you can reduce your health risks of (depression, anxiety, cancer, health problems) is to cut back or stop using altogether. Based on what I just told you, how important is it for you to change your behavior? How confident are you that you can make a change? What would help you make a change? Sounds like you are not interested in changing today even though you are aware that there are significant consequences to your health. How concerned are you about these consequences? Sounds like you are unsure about whether you want to make a change today. Can we talk about some of the good things and not-so-good things you experience from your drinking/drug use/ gambling? What are some of the good things? What are some of the not-so-good things? What are some good things that could happen if you make a change?
Menu of options	Give clients a range of choices, resources, and alternatives to guide their decision to change their behaviors.	We have a number of different options for you if you decide you want to make a change. Provide several options and give handouts, then ask: Which option do you think makes the most sense for you? Options can include: onsite support groups or educational groups, referral to treatment, information about peer support tor self-help, medications, or meeting with a counselor to address interpersonal, social, or other mental health issues. Referrals should be structured and "warm."
Empathic style	Summarize using a quiet, respectful, and nonjudgmental counseling style	Sounds like you are concerned about your health. There are things you can do now that can make a positive difference in your health. I can help. Which ones are you interested in choosing and pursuing today?
Self-efficacy	Communicate to clients that they can make changes and there is hope.	

Clients are then presented with a *menu of options* from which they can choose various treatment alternatives. Providing a range of alternatives helps clients decide which approach fits their perspective and preferences, which can increase the likelihood of change, decrease resistance, and enhance motivation to change. Providing a menu of options also helps clients take responsibility for their actions through informed decision-making. Asking clients about what they have tried in the past and how things worked out is a good way to open up the conversation. Each option on the menu should be clear, relevant, and fully described. Options can include (1) attending an informational group at the clinic; (2) taking a referral to treatment; (3) making a commitment to reduce or eliminate use and strategizing about how best to cut down or quit; (4) using medications to control cravings; (5) attending self-help groups; or (6) meeting with a counselor or attending coping skills groups for problem-solving, anger management, family therapy, or depression/anxiety management. These groups can be provided by the agency, co-located on site, or provided by outside community agencies. If they are referrals to outside agencies, a formal relationship with the organization should be in place to facilitate a "warm handoff" of the client to the agency. Cold referrals are discouraged due to their decreased likelihood for follow-through.

10.5   Summary and Conclusion

The US Preventive Services Task Force (2018) has recommended that screening and brief interventions be implemented in health settings for persons over the age of 18 years, including pregnant women, due to moderate evidence that suggests doing so can reduce hazardous and harmful drinking. This recommendation is supported by other research suggesting that while moderately effective, additional research on BIs using more rigorous designs is needed (Kaner et al. 2018).

Research is also needed to better understand the processes, mechanisms, and barriers related to the implementation of screening and brief interventions for substance use in various health settings. Research in this area has already begun (Rahm et al. 2015). For instance, Singh et al. 2017 found that the presence of organizational champions, managing staffing challenges such as turnover, training, and communication to ensure providers can competently deliver the intervention, and securing funding, is vital to sustaining brief intervention practices within an organization (Singh et al. 2017). Further, research has identified that consistent organizational leadership support and integration of screening and BI practices into existing processes and procedures within the agency are important, as time constraints, conflicting priorities, and lack of communication have been identified as barriers to implementation (Mancini and Miner 2013). While universal screening has been found to be supported generally by clients, concerns about privacy and cultural competence of practitioners have been identified. This indicates that training of staff regarding proper and sensitive deployment of screening that is culturally tailored to meet the needs of all clients and communication and targeted messaging about the purpose of these interventions will be needed (Rahm et al. 2015). Creating policies that allow for billing of SBIRT services is vital to the implementation and sustainment of these practice in primary care and other health settings (Hinde et al. 2017; Singh et al. 2017). For instance, whether states activate S-BIRT reimbursement codes is often a political matter. States that are more politically progressive, spend on substance abuse treatment, and value parity are more likely to activate S-BIRT Medicaid reimbursement codes. Reliance on federal block grant funding reduces the likelihood of activation of codes, and grant dollars have been shown to have little to no impact on whether states enact the codes (Hinde et al. 2017). Despite these challenges, the research is clear that providing screening and brief interventions as a routine part of clinical practice is an efficient and cost-effective way to significantly reduce harmful drinking patterns in clients and increase access to treatment services for alcohol and other substance use disorders.

Case Study 10.1: Mike Daly

Mike Daly[1] is a white, 32-year-old cisgender male. He was brought to the ER by an ambulance after driving his car into a ditch at low speed. He suffered a cut on his forehead which required four stitches. Mike's alcohol level was over the legal limit and he will be charged with driving under the influence of alcohol (DUI) (his second such offense in the last five years). Mike had the equivalent of four or five drinks in his system. He reports being at a barbecue with friends and drinking beer steadily from about 6 pm to 10 pm. Mike scored positive on two CAGE questions (Have people ever gotten annoyed by your drinking and Have you ever felt guilty about your drinking). He also scored a 15 on the AUDIT indicating clinically positive for harmful drinking. He reports drinking three to four times a week and approximately three to four drinks per occasion. He also reports having five or more drinks on at least six occasions within the last six months.

Scenario 1: Dr. Eric Larson

Dr. Eric Larson, an ER resident, is currently stitching up Mike. They have this exchange.

> Dr. Larson: So looks like you got drunk and really messed up. But this could have been much worse. What happened?
>
> Mike: "Look Doc. I've been locked up in the house for four months with this COVID thing. I just wanted to see some friends in person. I didn't mean to overdo it. I wasn't fall down drunk or anything—just a little buzzed—I forgot about the drainage ditch and I was checking a message and just went in. I wasn't going fast. Only about 5 miles an hour. It's Friday. It's not a big deal. Nobody got hurt. It was just an accident.
>
> Dr. Larson: Just an accident? Looks like somebody got hurt. Who am I stitching up? You were drunk and you were driving. You could have killed yourself or someone else. What were you thinking?

---

[1]All names and other identifiers of this case have been changed to protect privacy and confidentiality.

Mike: Like I said—I was at a barbecue. There was beer. I drank some. It was an accident. I wasn't drunk—just a little buzzed.

Dr. Larson: Five beers, which probably means 6 or 7, is way over the limit for safe drinking. It's almost double the recommended limit. Your screening results indicate that you actually have a drinking problem. You need help. The standard limit is two drinks a day.

Mike: Maybe for someone like you, Doc. For me—4 or 5 drinks is pretty standard.

Dr. Larson: You think this is a joke? You're at risk for some serious health problems. And you already have plenty of legal problems. You need to get this problem under control. You're stitches are all set. This should heal with minor scarring. But as for your drinking—But you better get some help.

Mike: Thanks Doc. Sure thing.

Analysis

Mike's scores indicate that his drinking could lead to some negative health and social effects. He has already experienced negative consequences given his accident and pending DUI charge. Mike could benefit from cutting back or eliminating his drinking. He may even benefit from some outside assistance (e.g., counseling, self-help). However, Dr. Larson's confrontational approach is obviously not helpful. His approach actually pushes Mike to resist and defend his drinking.

Scenario 2: Dr. Jonathan Garrison

Dr. Jonathan Garrison, an ER resident, is currently stitching up Mike. They have this exchange.

Dr. Garrison: So it looks like you have a pretty nasty cut here—but I don't think it will scar too bad and you'll heal quickly. What happened?

Mike: I went to see some friends at a barbecue I haven't seen in a while. I've been cooped up at home with this COVID thing for months. I just wanted to see some friends. I guess I got a little buzzed. I forgot about the drainage ditch and I was checking a message and just went in. I wasn't going fast. It was just an accident.

Dr. Garrison: I can certainly understand wanting to see some friends. Luckily no one else got hurt and you'll be OK. So, it sounds like you had this accident because of you're drinking. Do you mind if we talk about your drinking for a couple of minutes?

Mike: I guess so. What do you want to talk about?

Dr. Garrison: Can you tell me what are some of the good things you get from drinking?

Mike: Good things? I mean—its something I do with my friends. I don't really think about it. We talk about stuff, you know, sports, work whatever. We pay softball. We bowl. Normal stuff. Sometimes we have some beers. Sometimes we don't. I mean, I enjoy having a few beers with friends or after work to relax. That's all.

Dr. Garrison: So you enjoy drinking as a way to relax and it's something you do to socialize with your friends. That sounds reasonable. What are some not so good things that you've experienced because of your drinking?

Mike: Well, this would be one thing—the accident. I had another accident a few years ago—not serious—but still damaged my car and got a ticket and had to pay a lot of money. Looks like I'm going to have to go through it all over again. I mean, my girlfriend sometimes gets on my case about it. She is going to be pretty upset. Sometimes I can be a bit of a jerk and say things I don't mean if I've had too much. Hangovers, I guess. Those aren't fun.

Dr. Garrison: So on the one hand drinking is a way for you to relax and socialize with your friends, and on the other hand drinking has caused some problems in your relationship, and other negative consequences like crashing your car, getting into trouble, paying lots of money and dealing with hangovers. Those are some pretty significant consequences. Your scores on your screening forms indicate that you are at a higher risk for some health consequences based on your drinking. It looks like you're experiencing some of those now. So what do you think about this?

Mike: I don't know. I probably shouldn't have gotten behind the wheel of the car tonight. Maybe I could cut back a bit or be safer about my drinking.

Dr. Garrison: Sounds like good idea. I recommend reducing your drinking to standard limits, which are four or less drinks on any occasion and no more than 14 drinks per week. Any more than that and you can experience some increased problems. Obviously, I'd also recommend to avoid driving while drinking. Have you ever tried to cut back before? How confident are you that you can cut down.

Mike: I am pretty confident I can do it on my own.

Dr. Garrison: OK. If you find that you're still drinking more than the guidelines after a month, I recommend you get some outside help. I have some brochures here that can point you in the right direction. We also have some support groups and counseling programs here at the hospital. I can give you the number of someone you can talk to or if you want a referral I can walk you over to the counselor right now and we can get you an appointment.

Mike: Thanks Doc. But I can do it on my own. But I will let you know if I have any trouble. Thanks for the information. And thanks for your help.

Analysis

How does Dr. Garrison's approach differ from Dr. Larson's?

How did Mike's reaction differ?

What elements of motivational interviewing did you notice?

What screening and brief intervention strategies (e.g., FRAMES and BNI) were deployed?

How were the outcomes different?

What if Mike's drinking indicated he had an alcohol use disorder? How might the interaction have been different?

References

Achildi, O., Leong, S. H., Maust, D. T., Streim, J. E., & Oslin, D. W. (2013). Patterns of newly-prescribed benzodiazepines in late life. *American Journal of Geriatric Psychiatry, 21*(Suppl. 1(3)), S90–S91. https://doi.org/10.1016/j.jagp.2012.12.117.

Aldridge, A., Linford, R., & Bray, J. (2017a). Substance use outcomes of patients served by a large US implementation of Screening, Brief Intervention, Brief Treatment and Referral to Treatment project (SBIRT). *Addiction, 112*(Suppl. 2), 43–53.

Aldridge, A., Dowd, W., & Bray, J. (2017b). The relative impact of brief treatment versus brief intervention in primary health-care screening programs for substance use disorders. *Addiction, 112*(Suppl. 2), 54–64.

Álvarez-Bueno, C., Rodríguez-Martín, B., García-Ortiz, L., Gómez-Marcos, M. Á., & Martínez-Vizcaíno, V. (2015). Effectiveness of brief interventions in primary health care settings to decrease alcohol consumption by adult non-dependent drinkers: A systematic review of systematic reviews. *Preventative Medicine, 76*, S33.

American Psychiatric Association (APA). (2013). *Diagnostic and statistical manual of mental disorders, fifth edition (DSM-5)*. Arlington: American Psychiatric Association.

Babor, T. F., Higgins-Biddle, J. C., Saunders, J. B., & Monteiro, M. G. (2001). *The alcohol use disorders identification test: Guidelines for use in primary care* (2nd ed.) World Health Organization. Retrieved 3/27/20 at: https://www.who.int/publications-detail/audit-the-alcohol-use-disorders-identification-test-guidelines-for-use-in-primary-health-care

Babor, T., McRee, B., Kassebaum, P., Grimaldi, P., Ahmed, K., & Bray, J. (2007). Screening, brief intervention, and referral to treatment (SBIRT). *Substance Abuse, 28*, 7–30.

Babor, T. F., Del Boca, F., & Bray, J. W. (2017). Screening, brief intervention and referral to treatment: Implications of SAMHSA's SBIRT initiative for substance abuse policy and practice. *Addiction, 112*(Suppl 2), 110–117.

Ballesteros, J., Duffy, J. C., Querejeta, I., Ariño, J., & González-Pinto, A. (2004). Efficacy of brief interventions for hazardous drinkers in primary care: Systematic review and meta-analyses. *Alcoholism, Clinical and Experimental Research, 28*(4), 608–618. https://doi.org/10.1097/01.alc.0000122106.84718.67.

Barata, I. A., Shandro, J. R., Montgomery, M., Polansky, R., Sachs, C. J., Duber, H. C., Weaver, L. M., Heins, A., Owen, H. S., Josephson, E. B., & Macias-Konstantopoulos, W. (2017). Effectiveness of SBIRT for alcohol use disorders in the emergency department: A systematic review. *The Western Journal of Emergency Medicine, 18*(6), 1143–1152. https://doi.org/10.5811/westjem.2017.7.34373.

Barbosa, C., Cowell, A., Dowd, W., Landwehr, J., Aldridge, A., & Bray, J. (2017). The cost-effectiveness of brief intervention versus brief treatment of screening, brief intervention, and referral to treatment (SBIRT) in the United States. *Addiction, 112*(Suppl. 2), 78–81.

Bernstein, E., Bernstein, J., & Levenson, S. (1997). Project ASSERT: An ED-based intervention to increase access to primary care, preventive services, and the substance abuse treatment system. *Annals of Emergency Medicine, 30*, 181–189.

Bernstein, J., Bernstein, E., Tassiopoulos, K., Heeren, T., Levenson, S., & Hingson, R. (2005). Brief motivational intervention at a clinic visit reduces cocaine and heroin use. *Drug and Alcohol Dependence, 77*(1), 49–59. https://doi.org/10.1016/j.drugalcdep.2004.07.006.

Bernstein, E., Bernstein, J., Feldman, J., Fernandez, W., Hagan, M., Mitchell, P., et al. (2007). An evidence based alcohol screening, brief intervention and referral to treatment (SBIRT) curriculum for emergency department (ED) providers improves skills and utilization. *Substance Abuse, 28*(4), 79–92.

Bien, T. H., Miller, W. R., & Tonigan, S. (1993). Brief intervention for alcohol problems: A review. *Addiction, 88*, 315–336.

Blazer, D. G., & Wu, L. (2009). The epidemiology of substance use and disorders among middle aged and elderly community adults: National survey on drug use and health. *American Journal of Geriatric Psychiatry, 17*, 237–245.

Bohnert, A. S., Bonar, E. E., Cunningham, R., Greenwald, M. K., Thomas, L., Chermack, S., Blow, F. C., & Walton, M. (2016). A pilot randomized clinical trial of an intervention to reduce overdose risk behaviors among emergency department patients at risk for prescription opioid overdose. *Drug and Alcohol Dependence, 163*, 40–47. https://doi.org/10.1016/j. drugalcdep.2016.03.018.

Bohnert, A., Walton, M. A., Cunningham, R. M., Ilgen, M. A., Barry, K., Chermack, S. T., & Blow, F. C. (2018). Overdose and adverse drug event experiences among adult patients in the emergency department. *Addictive Behaviors, 86*, 66–72. https://doi.org/10.1016/j. addbeh.2017.11.030.

Bradley, K. A., Bush, K. R., Epler, A. J., Dobie, D. J., Davis, T. M., Sporleder, J. L., et al. (2003). Two brief alcohol-screening tests from the Alcohol Use Disorders Screening Test (AUDIT): Validation in a female veterans affairs patient population. *Archives of Internal Medicine, 163*, 821–829.

Bradley, K., Chung, H., Brown, R. L., Farley, T., Fischer, L., Goplerud, E., et al. (2018). *Implementing care for alcohol and other drug use in medical settings: An extension of SBIRT.* National Council for Behavioral Health. Substance Abuse and Mental Health Services Administration.

Brown, R. L., & Rounds, L. A. (1995). Conjoint screening questionnaires for alcohol and other drug abuse: Criterion validity in a primary care practice. *Wisconsin Medical Journal, 94*(3), 135–140.

Bush, K., Kivlahan, D. R., McDonell, M. B., Fihn, S. D., & Bradley, K. A. (1998). The AUDIT Alcohol Consumption Questions(AUDIT-C): An effective brief screening test for problem drinking. *Archives of Internal Medicine, 58*(16), 1789–1795.

D'Onofrio, G., Bernstein, E., Bernstein, J., Woolard, R. H., Brewer, P. A., Craig, S. A., & Zink, B. J. (1998). Patients with alcohol problems in the emergency department, part 2: Intervention and referral. SAEM substance abuse task force. *Society for Academic Emergency Medicine. Academic emergency medicine: official journal of the Society for Academic Emergency Medicine, 5*(12), 1210–1217. https://doi.org/10.1111/j.1553-2712.1998.tb02697.x.

D'Onofrio, G., Pantalon, M. V., Degutis, L. C., Fiellin, D. A., & O'connor, P. G. (2005). Development and implementation of an emergency practitioner-performed brief intervention for hazardous and harmful drinkers in the emergency department. *Academic Emergency Medicine: Official Journal of the Society for Academic Emergency Medicine, 12*(3), 249–256. https://doi.org/10.1197/j.aem.2004.10.021.

D'Onofrio, G., Fiellin, D. A., Pantalon, M. V., Chawarski, M. C., Owens, P. H., Degutis, L. C., Busch, S. H., Bernstein, S. L., & O'Connor, P. G. (2012). A brief intervention reduces hazardous and harmful drinking in emergency department patients. *Annals of Emergency Medicine, 60*(2), 181–192. https://doi.org/10.1016/j.annemergmed.2012.02.006.

Dunn, C. W., & Ries, R. (1997). Linking substance abuse services with general medical care: Integrated, brief interventions with hospitalized patients. *The American Journal of Drug and Alcohol Abuse, 23*(1), 1–13. https://doi.org/10.3109/00952999709001684.

Elvy, G. A., Wells, J. E., & Baird, K. A. (1988). Attempted referral as intervention for problem drinking in the general hospital. *British Journal of Addiction, 83*(1), 83–89. https://doi. org/10.1111/j.1360-0443.1988.tb00455.x.

Fischer, B., Russell, C., Sabioni, P., van den Brink, W., Le Foll, B., Hall, W., Rehm, J., & Room, R. (2017). Lower-risk cannabis use guidelines: A comprehensive update of evidence and recommendations. *American Journal of Public Health, 107*, e1_e12. https://doi.org/10.2105/AJPH.2017.303818.

Fleming, M. F., & Baier-Manwell, L. B. (1999). Brief intervention in primary care settings: A primary treatment method for at-risk, problem, and dependent drinkers. *Alcohol Research and Health, 23*(2), 128–137.

Gavin, D. R., Ross, H. E., & Skinner, H. A. (1989). Diagnostic validity of the DAST in the assessment of DSM-III drug disorders. *British Journal of Addiction, 84*, 301–307.

Grant, B. F., Saha, T. D., Ruan, W. J., Goldstein, R. B., Chou, S. P., Jung, J., Zhang, H., Smith, S. M., Pickering, R. P., Huang, B., & Hasin, D. S. (2016). Epidemiology of DSM-5 drug use disorder: Results from the National Epidemiologic Survey on alcohol and related conditions-III. *JAMA Psychiatry, 73*(1), 39–47. https://doi.org/10.1001/jamapsychiatry.2015.2132.

Han, B. H., & Moore, A. A. (2018). Prevention and screening of unhealthy substance use by older adults. *Clinical Geriatric Medicine, 34*(1), 117–129. https://doi.org/10.1016/j.cger.2017.08.005.

Han, B. H., Moore, A. A., Sherman, S., Keyes, K. M., & Palamar, J. J. (2017a). Demographic trends of binge alcohol use and alcohol use disorders among older adults in the United States, 2005-2014. *Drug and Alcohol Dependence, 170*, 198–207. https://doi.org/10.1016/j.drugalcdep.2016.11.003.

Han, B. H., Sherman, S., Mauro, P. M., Martins, S. S., Rotenberg, J., & Palamar, J. J. (2017b). Demographic trends among older cannabis users in the United States, 2006-13. *Addiction, 112*(3), 516–525. https://doi.org/10.1111/add.13670.

Hargraves, D., White, C., Frederick, R., Cinibulk, M., Peters, M., Young, A., & Elder, N. (2017). Implementing SBIRT (screening, brief intervention and referral to treatment) in primary care: Lessons learned from a multipractice evaluation portfolio. *Public Health Reviews, 38*, 31. https://doi.org/10.1186/s40985-017-0077-0.

Hillman, A., McCann, B., & Walker, N. P. (2001). Specialist alcohol liaison services in general hospitals improve engagement in alcohol rehabilitation and treatment outcome. *Health Bulletin, 59*, 420–423.

Hinde, J., Bray, J., Kaiser, D., & Mallonee, E. (2017). The influence of state-level policy environments on the activation of the Medicaid SBIRT reimbursement codes. *Addiction, 112*(Suppl 2), 82–91. https://doi.org/10.1111/add.13655.

Humeniuk, R. E., Henry-Edwards, S., Ali, R. L., Poznyak, V., & Monteiro, M. (2010a). *The Alcohol, Smoking and Substance Involvement Screening Test (ASSIST): Manual for use in primary care*. Geneva: World Health Organization.

Humeniuk, R. E., Henry-Edwards, S., Ali, R. L., Poznyak, V., & Monteiro, M. (2010b). *The ASSIST-linked brief intervention for hazardous and harmful substance use: Manual for use in primary care*. Geneva: World Health Organization.

Kahan, M., Wilson, L., & Becker, L. (1995). Effectiveness of physician-based interventions with problem drinkers: A review. *CMAJ: Canadian Medical Association Journal, 152*(6), 851–859.

Knight, J. R., Shrier, L. A., Bravender, T. D., Farrell, M., Vander Bilt, J., & Shaffer, H. J. (1999). A new brief screen for adolescent substance abuse. *Archives of Pediatrics & Adolescent Medicine, 153*(6), 591–596. https://doi.org/10.1001/archpedi.153.6.591.

Kaner, E. F., Beyer, F. R., Muirhead, C., Campbell, F., Pienaar, E. D., Bertholet, N., Daeppen, J. B., Saunders, J. B., & Burnand, B. (2018). Effectiveness of brief alcohol interventions in primary care populations. *The Cochrane database of systematic reviews, 2*(2), CD004148. https://doi.org/10.1002/14651858.CD004148.pub4

Knight, J. R., Sherritt, L., Shrier, L. A., Harris, S. K., & Chang, G. (2002). Validity of the CRAFFT substance abuse screening test among adolescent clinic patients. *Archives of Pediatrics & Adolescent Medicine, 156*(6), 607–614. https://doi.org/10.1001/archpedi.156.6.607.

Kristenson, H., Ohlin, H., Hultén-Nosslin, M. B., Trell, E., & Hood, B. (1983). Identification and intervention of heavy drinking in middle-aged men: Results and follow-up of 24-60 months of long-term study with randomized controls. *Alcoholism, Clinical and Experimental Research, 7*(2), 203–209. https://doi.org/10.1111/j.1530-0277.1983.tb05441.x.

Kuerbis, A., Sacco, P., Blazer, D. G., & Moore, A. A. (2014). Substance abuse among older adults. *Clinics in Geriatric Medicine, 30*(3), 629–654. https://doi.org/10.1016/j.cger.2014.04.008.

Larney, S., Bohnert, A. S., Ganoczy, D., Ilgen, M. A., Hickman, M., Blow, F. C., & Degenhardt, L. (2015). Mortality among older adults with opioid use disorders in the Veteran's health administration, 2000-2011. *Drug and Alcohol Dependence, 147*, 32–37. https://doi.org/10.1016/j.drugalcdep.2014.12.019.

Lemhoefer, C., Rabe, G. L., Wellmann, J., Bernstein, S. L., Cheung, K. W., McCarthy, W. J., Lauridsen, S. V., Spies, C., & Neuner, B. (2017). Emergency department-initiated tobacco control: Update of a systematic review and meta-analysis of randomized controlled trials. *Preventing Chronic Disease, 14*, E89. https://doi.org/10.5888/pcd14.160434.

Mancini, M.A. & Miner, C.S. (2013). Learning and change in a community mental health setting. *Journal of Evidence Based Social Work, 10*(5), 494–504

Madras, B. K., Compton, W. M., Avula, D., Stegbauer, T., Stein, J. B., & Clark, H. W. (2009). Screening, brief interventions, referral to treatment (SBIRT) for illicit drug and alcohol use at multiple healthcare sites: Comparison at intake and 6 0s later. *Drug and Alcohol Dependence, 99*(1–3), 280–295. https://doi.org/10.1016/j.drugalcdep.2008.08.003.

Miller, W. R. (1995). *Motivational enhancement therapy manual: A clinical research guide for therapists treating individuals with alcohol abuse and dependence.* Rockville, Maryland: DIANE Publishing.

Miller, W. R., & Rollnick, S. (2002). *Motivational interviewing: Helping people change* (2nd ed.). New York: Guilford Press.

Miller, W. R., & Rollnick, S. (2013). *Motivational interviewing: Helping people change* (3rd ed.). New York: Guilford Press.

Miller, W., & Sanchez, V. (1994). Motivating young adults for treatment and lifestyle change. In G. Howard (Ed.), *Issues in alcohol use and misuse by young adults*. Notre Dame IN: University of Notre Dame Press.

Moore, A. A., Karno, M. P., Grella, C. E., Lin, J. C., Warda, U., Liao, D. H., & Hu, P. (2009). Alcohol, tobacco, and nonmedical drug use in older U.S. adults: Data from the 2001/02 national epidemiologic survey of alcohol and related conditions. *Journal of the American Geriatrics Society, 57*(12), 2275–2281. https://doi.org/10.1111/j.1532-5415.2009.02554.x.

Moyer, A., Finney, J. W., Swearingen, C. E., & Vergun, P. (2002). Brief interventions for alcohol problems: A meta-analytic review of controlled investigations in treatment-seeking and non-treatment-seeking populations. *Addiction, 97*(3), 279–292. https://doi.org/10.1046/j.1360-0443.2002.00018.x.

National Institute on Alcohol Abuse and Alcoholism. (2020a). *What is a standard drink?* Accessed on June 28, 2020 at: https://www.niaaa.nih.gov/what-standard-drink

National Institute on Alcohol Abuse and Alcoholism. (2020b). *Drinking levels defined.* Accessed on June 28, 2020 at: https://www.niaaa.nih.gov/alcohol-health/overview-alcohol-consumption/moderate-binge-drinking

Paltzer J., Brown R.L., Burns M., Moberg D.P., Mullahy J., Sethi A., & D., W. (2017). Substance use screening, brief Intervention, and referral to treatment among Medicaid patients in Wisconsin: impacts on healthcare utilization and costs. Journal of Behavioral Health Services and Research, 44, 102–112.

Pokorny, A. D., Miller, B. A., & Kaplan, H. B. (1972). The brief MAST: A shortened version of the Michigan alcoholism screening test. *The American Journal of Psychiatry, 129*(3), 342–345.

Pringle, J. L., Kelley, D. K., Kearney, S. M., Aldridge, A., Dowd, W., Johnjulio, W., Venkat, A., Madden, M., & Lovelace, J. (2018). Screening, brief intervention, and referral to treatment in the emergency department: An examination of health care utilization and costs. *Medical Care, 56*(2), 146–152. https://doi.org/10.1097/MLR.0000000000000859.

Rahm, A. K., Boggs, J. M., Martin, C., Price, D. W., Beck, A., Backer, T. E., & Dearing, J. W. (2015). Facilitators and barriers to implementing Screening, Brief Intervention, and Referral to Treatment (SBIRT) in primary Care in Integrated Health Care Settings. *Substance Abuse, 36*(3), 281–288. https://doi.org/10.1080/08897077.2014.951140.

Rochat, S., Wietlisbach, V., Burnand, B., Landry, U., & Yersin, B. (2004). Success of referral for alcohol dependent patients from a general hospital: Predictive value of patient and process characteristics. *Substance Abuse, 25*(1), 9–15. https://doi.org/10.1300/J465v25n01_03.

Russell, M. A., Stapleton, J. A., Hajek, P., Jackson, P. H., & Belcher, M. (1988). District programme to reduce smoking: Can sustained intervention by general practitioners affect prevalence? *Journal of Epidemiology and Community Health, 42*(2), 111–115. https://doi.org/10.1136/jech.42.2.111.

Saunders, J. B., Aasland, O. G., Babor, T. F., de la Fuente, J. R., & Grant, M. (1993). Development of the Alcohol Use Disorders Identification Test (AUDIT): WHO collaborative project on early detection of persons with harmful alcohol consumption--II. *Addiction, 88*(6), 791–804. https://doi.org/10.1111/j.1360-0443.1993.tb02093.x.

Selzer, M. L. (1971). The Michigan Alcoholism Screening Test (MAST): The quest for a new diagnostic instrument. *American Journal of Psychiatry, 3*, 176–181.

Selzer, M. L., Vinokur, A., & van Rooijen, L. (1975). Self-Administered Short Version of the Michigan Alcoholism Screening Test (SMAST). *Journal of Studies on Alcohol, 36*, 117–126.

Singh, M., Gmyrek, A., Hernandez, A., Damon, D., & Hayashi, S. (2017). Sustaining screening, brief intervention and referral to treatment (SBIRT) services in health-care settings. *Addiction, 112*(Suppl 2), 92–100. https://doi.org/10.1111/add.13654.

Skinner, H. A. (1982). The drug abuse screening test. *Addictive Behavior, 7*(4), 363–371.

Substance Abuse and Mental Health Services Administration (SAMHSA). (2019). Key substance use and mental health indicators in the United States: Results from the 2018 National Survey on drug use and health (HHS publication no. PEP19–5068, NSDUH series H-54). Rockville: Center for Behavioral Health Statistics and Quality, Substance Abuse and Mental Health Services Administration. Retrieved from https://www.samhsa.gov/data/.

Sullivan, M. D., & Howe, C. Q. (2013). Opioid therapy for chronic pain in the US: Promises and perils. *Pain, 154*(01), S94–S100.

U.S. Department of Health and Human Services and U.S. Department of Agriculture. (2015–2020). *Dietary Guidelines for Americans.* 8th ed. Available at https://health.gov/our-work/food-and-nutrition/2015-2020-dietary-guidelines/

U.S. Preventive Services Task Force, Curry, S. J., Krist, A. H., Owens, D. K., Barry, M. J., Caughey, A. B., Davidson, K. W., Doubeni, C. A., Epling, J. W., Jr., Kemper, A. R., Kubik, M., Landefeld, C. S., Mangione, C. M., Silverstein, M., Simon, M. A., Tseng, C. W., & Wong, J. B. (2018). Screening and behavioral counseling interventions to reduce unhealthy alcohol use in adolescents and adults: US Preventive Services Task Force Recommendation Statement. *JAMA, 320*(18), 1899–1909. https://doi.org/10.1001/jama.2018.16789.

U.S. Department of Health and Human Services (USDHHS) and U.S. Department of Agriculture. (2015). 2015–2020 Dietary Guidelines for Americans. 8th Edition. December 2015. Available at http://health.gov/dietaryguidelines/2015/guidelines/.

Wilk, A. I., Jensen, N. M., & Havighurst, T. C. (1997). Meta-analysis of randomized control trials addressing brief interventions in heavy alcohol drinkers. *Journal of General Internal Medicine, 12*(5), 274–283.

World Health Organization (WHO) Brief Intervention Study Group. (1996). A cross national trial of brief intervention with heavy drinkers. *American Journal of Public Health, 86*, 948–955. https://doi.org/10.2105/ajph.86.7.948.

World Health Organization (WHO). (2002). WHO ASSIST Working Group. The Alcohol, Smoking and Substance Involvement Screening Test (ASSIST): Development, reliability and feasibility. *Addiction, 97*, 1183–1194.

Youdin, R. (2019). *Old and high: A guide to understanding the neuroscience and psychotherapeutic treatment of baby-boom adults' substance use, abuse and misuse.* New York: Oxford University Press.

Yudko, E., Lozhkina, O., & Fouts, A. (2007). A comprehensive review of the psychometric properties of the drug abuse screening test. *Journal of Substance Abuse Treatment, 32*(2), 189–198. https://doi.org/10.1016/j.jsat.2006.08.002.

Chapter 11
Stage-Based Treatment Approaches for Substance Use Disorders

11.1 Overview of Stage-Based Approaches to Treatment

Addiction to alcohol and other drugs has taken a vast toll on individuals, families, and communities across the United States for decades. Currently, the United States is experiencing a crisis in opioid addiction and overdose deaths. For instance, overdose deaths from opioid drugs, including prescription pain medications, heroin, and synthetic opioids such as fentanyl, have increased sixfold in the last 20 years and claimed almost 47,000 lives in 2018. A third of those deaths were the result of prescription opioids (CDC 2020; Wilson et al. 2020). In addition to opioids, negative consequences from the misuse of alcohol, stimulants, and cannabis continue to devastate the lives of our clients and their families.

Persons with substance use disorders (SUDs) engage in a continuous pattern of excessive alcohol and/or other drug use despite experiencing significant negative consequences in the domains of health, personal relationships, occupation, or other functional domains. Persons with SUDs continue to use substances despite these negative effects due to: (1) a loss of control over use due to physical dependency and/or strong psychological cravings and/or (2) a lack of motivation or desire to change behavior. There are several treatment approaches that are effective in treating substance use disorders (APA 2013). Unfortunately, many people with substance use disorders do not get the treatment they need (SAMHSA 2019). The decriminalizing of addiction and the dismantling of the war on drugs policy combined with an expansion of behavioral health services in the community and the integration of behavioral health practice in health, school, criminal justice, and social service settings represent an effective means to increase access to treatment. For instance, utilization of the collaborative care model that integrates behavioral health in primary care settings increases the likelihood that persons with alcohol and opioid use disorders will utilize evidence-based treatments such as brief psychotherapy and medication-assisted treatment (MAT) and will achieve abstinence within 6 months over usual care (Watkins et al. 2017).

© Springer Nature Switzerland AG 2021

M. A. Mancini, *Integrated Behavioral Health Practice*,
https://doi.org/10.1007/978-3-030-59659-0_11

In order for treatment to be effective, approaches should be matched to a client's stage of change for a particular substance. According to the Transtheoretical Model of Change (TTM) (Prochaska et al. 1992), the decision to change behavior is often contingent upon a person's motivation and readiness to change. Readiness and intention to change often move through a series of stages depending on internal and external factors such as the amount and quality of information available to the client, perceived self-efficacy of the client, external pressure to change, the perceived relative benefits and risks associated with change, and the resources available to the person that may assist change efforts, among others.

There are five general stages of change ranging from the least amount of readiness to the most amount of readiness: (1) precontemplation, (2) contemplation, (3) preparation, (4) action, and (5) maintenance (Prochaska et al. 1992). Clients in precontemplation do not believe they have a problem and have no intention to change their behavior. Clients in contemplation may recognize they have a problem, but are ambivalent about whether or not they can or should change. The preparation stage of change generally describes clients who have less ambivalence about change and are preparing to change their behavior or have taken some initial steps in changing behavior such as reducing the amount and/or frequency of their use. The action stage of change refers to clients who are committed to changing their behavior and are actively engaged in treatment strategies to reduce or eliminate their use. Clients in the maintenance stage have achieved their substance use treatment goals (e.g., abstinence or reduced use) and no longer experience negative consequences related to their use for a sustained period (Prochaska et al. 1992).

Stage-based approaches to treatment coordinate and sequence treatment to match a client's stage of change (Prochaska et al. 1992). For instance, harm reduction (HR) and brief motivational approaches to treatment are often used for persons in the precontemplation and early contemplation stages of change (e.g., clients with no or little intention to change behavior). Motivational interviewing (MI) is often most appropriate for persons in contemplation and early preparation stages of change (e.g., persons who have increasing ambivalence about change or who are moving toward making changes in their behavior). Blending motivational interviewing and cognitive behavioral approaches are often best for persons in the preparation and action stages of change (e.g., persons with less ambivalence and who are committed to making a behavioral change in the near future or those who have already begun making changes). Cognitive behavioral approaches may be best for persons in the action and maintenance stages of change (e.g., persons who are making changes to their behavior and who require relapse prevention strategies and support).

In order for treatment to be effective, providers must continually assess and recognize a person's stage of change and align treatment interventions to match that stage. In this chapter, I will focus on the theoretical orientations, philosophies, principles, and practices of three sets of interventions: (1) harm reduction approaches for persons in the precontemplation stage; (1) motivational interviewing for clients in contemplation and preparation stages; and (3) brief cognitive behavioral treatments for clients in the action and maintenance stages of change. The principles, philosophies, theoretical orientations, and practices for each approach will be reviewed in detail and illustrated using case vignettes.

11.2 Harm Reduction Approaches

11.2.1 Overview and Definition

Harm reduction (HR) is a public health approach to high-risk behaviors. It is a form of tertiary prevention that consists of a constellation of practices and interventions designed to reduce the negative consequences that stem from harmful or high-risk health behaviors involving drug and alcohol use without directly focusing on the alcohol or drug use itself (Denis-Lalonde et al. 2019; Des Jarlais 1995; Hawk et al., 2017; Mancini et al. 2008a, b; Mancini and Linhorst 2010; Mancini and Wyrick-Waugh, 2013). Harm Reduction International (HRI) defines harm reduction as the, "policies, programmes and practices that aim to minimize negative health, social and legal impacts associated with drug use, drug policies and drug laws. Harm reduction is grounded in justice and human rights-it focuses on positive change and on working with people without judgment, coercion, discrimination, or requiring that they stop using drugs as a precondition of support." (HRI 2020).

Harm reduction approaches are most often utilized for persons in the precontemplation and early contemplation stages of change and who currently have little or no intention or motivation to stop substance use. Harm reduction approaches can be blended with motivational approaches so that providers can prevent or reduce harm, while also helping to motivate people toward change. In contrast to medical and moralistic models of substance use, providers using harm reduction approaches take a decidedly public health approach that focuses on reducing the harmful consequences of drug use (Des Jarlais 1995). HR providers accept the person's drug-using behaviors in a nonjudgmental manner and focus on helping them set and achieve goals (Marlatt 1996). While abstinence from substances is a goal in HR approaches, it is a goal that is placed at the far end of a spectrum of other intermediate goals designed to reduce harms associated with substance use such as overdoses, disease transmission, victimization, incarceration, poverty, homelessness, and public intoxication. HR focuses mainly on substance use, but can be used to address a variety of health issues such as obesity, smoking, sex work, and domestic violence and is a very appropriate approach for healthcare settings (Hawk et al. 2017).

11.2.2 Harm Reduction History

Resistance to harm reduction has a long history in the United States for a number of reasons. The field of substance use treatment and policy has long been dominated by moralistic views about substance use condemning intoxication and use of substances as morally reprehensible and addiction as a moral failing. Prevention and treatment programs serving persons who use substances that promote anything other than strict abstinence are often viewed as enabling or encouraging of substance use. This view has also been influenced and magnified by the stigmatization of persons of color in the United States, and the long history of criminalization of drug use initiated and maintained by the failed "war on drug" policy in the United States which began in the 1970's.

Harm reduction approaches came into wide prominence across the world in response to the HIV/AIDS pandemic in the early part of the 1980s. However, the resistance toward harm reduction approaches in the United States prevented the widespread use of practices such as needle and syringe exchange programs during this time, resulting in a high number of avoidable HIV transmissions. For instance, needle and syringe exchange programs were implemented in the United States and supported by funding from states and localities and the North American Syringe Exchange Network in the late 1980s almost a full decade *after* the start of the AIDS pandemic as a way to reduce HIV transmission among people who inject drugs (PWID). Furthermore, needle and syringe exchange programs were not permitted by federal guidelines until 2016 (Des Jarlais 2017).

Harm reduction approaches, including drug decriminalization, needle and syringe exchange programs (NSP), safe injection sites (SIS), opioid substitution therapy (OST), housing-first programs, condom distribution, and naloxone (i.e. Narcan) availability, have been shown to be cost-effective ways to save lives by reducing overdoses, increasing safety and access to health care and treatment, and reducing the spread of infectious diseases such as HIV and hepatitis C virus (HCV) (Csete et al. 2016). Given the rise in opioid deaths in the United States, these programs have never been more essential (Des Jarlais 2017).

11.2.3 Harm Reduction Principles

Harm reduction consists of a range of values that include public health, social justice, and human rights. Harm reduction requires providers to practice in a way that is nonjudgmental, evidence-based, egalitarian, pragmatic, and adaptable, and preserves clients' self-determination and individuality. Harm reduction has been found to be wholly compatible with practice that is person-centered, trauma-informed, and recovery-oriented (Denis-Lalonde et al. 2019; Hawk et al. 2017; Mancini et al. 2008a). The harm reduction principles of *humanism, individualism, autonomy, accountability, and justice* make the approach inherently recovery-oriented and trauma-informed when practicing harm reduction providers prioritize humanistic care that is respectful, nonjudgmental, compassionate, and collaborative (Hawk et al. 2017). Due to the stigma that surrounds substance use and addiction, it is important for providers to avoid stereotypic language (e.g., users, offenders, addicts, junkies) and use humanizing, people-first, and recovery-oriented language when describing and working with persons who use substances. This includes referring to people as "persons with substance use disorders or addictions" or "persons who misuse substances" (Broyles et al. 2014; Sharma et al. 2017). Furthermore, providers should avoid legalistic or moralistic language to describe use such as "clean," "dirty," "drug-free," or "illicit or illegal drugs." Preferable terms include "substances," or saying someone is "negative" or "positive" for substance use (Broyles et al. 2014; Olsen and Sharfstein 2014). Likewise, using recovery-oriented language such as avoiding "adherent," "resistant," or "noncompliant," and referring to people as "in recovery" or "currently receiving or not receiving treatment" is important. When in doubt, providers should ask people how they wish to be considered (Broyles et al. 2014).

Harm reduction providers also hold people *accountable*. This means that clients take responsibility for their choices and the natural consequences for their actions. Providers practicing harm reduction do not endorse or enable drug use behavior. Providers understand that clients have a right to make unhealthy choices and may suffer consequences. Providers help clients understand how their behaviors have led to negative consequences and continue to support clients despite relapses or a lack of treatment progress. Clients are not discharged or punished if they relapse or choose to not complete goals (Hawk et al. 2017; Mancini, et al., 2008; Mancini and Wyrick-Waugh 2013).

The harm reduction principles of *individualism and autonomy* require accepting people where they are in their recovery journey and not where providers think they should be. This also makes harm reduction approaches inherently person-centered and trauma-informed since providers seek to understand the clients' perspective, preferences, and needs and the social determinants that may be driving their substance use. Harm reduction providers offer a range of options and support clients' self-determination through a shared decision-making orientation. Harm reduction is also a recovery-oriented approach to practice because it requires providers to respect client autonomy and choice as clients make their own informed decisions based on knowledge of the available options and their benefits and drawbacks (Denis-Lalonde et al. 2019; Hawk et al. 2017; Mancini et al. 2008a). Providers of harm reduction services hold the view that people who use substances should be free from cruelty and coercion and have adequate access to effective social and health services. All of these principles align with care that is recovery-oriented, trauma-informed, and person-centered.

The principles of *pragmatism, incrementalism,* and *evidence* require providers to collaborate with clients to set realistic goals designed to reduce the harm that clients do to themselves and society without focusing on abstinence. Client goals often involve addressing the social determinants of health around housing and resource access. Practicing from this perspective may require providers to address the internal tensions caused by their socialization around drug use and persons who use substances (Denis-Lalonde et al. 2019; Hawk et al. 2017; Mancini and Wyrick-Waugh 2013; Mancini et al. 2008a, b; Mancini and Linhorst 2010). Providers also celebrate any incremental step forward toward positive change. Recognition that change takes a long time and relapse is part of the process requires providers to plan for relapse and use it as an opportunity to learn new strategies. Harm reduction practices are also evidence-based and have been shown to be efficacious, practical, and cost-effective, making them appropriate for person-centered care. These approaches are public health-oriented and focused on preventing social, legal, and health-related harms to individuals, families, and communities (Des Jarlais 2017; Wilson et al. 2015).

11.2.4   Harm Reduction Programs

Resistance to harm reduction persists despite the clear effectiveness of the approach (Wilson et al. 2015). Several harm reduction practices have been found to be effective in reducing overdoses and disease transmission as well as improving clinical outcomes. Next, I will review several of the most widely utilized and studied practices of harm reduction.

Needle and Syringe Exchange Programs (NSP)   These programs provide people who inject drugs (PWID) with clean and sterile needles and exchange used equipment with new, clean equipment to reduce needle and syringe sharing. Needle and syringe exchange programs are effective at reducing HIV, HCV, and other infections (Aspinall et al. 2014; MacArthur et al. 2014; Wodak and Cooney 2004; Wodak and Maher 2010). These program have also been found to improve access to medical and social care, condoms, behavioral health treatment, overdose education, HIV and HCV education, counseling and testing, drug checking and education, and access to naloxone to prevent overdoses without increasing drug use or drug traffic in communities where exchange programs operate (Des Jarlais 2017; Strathdee et al. 2006).

Opioid Substitution Therapy (OST)   Opioid substitution therapy uses noninjecting, long-lasting opioids such as methadone and buprenorphine as a substitute for heroin or fentanyl. Methadone and buprenorphine, while still opioids with addiction potential, are safer alternatives to heroin due to their longer half-life, more gradual onset of effect, and availability in noninjectable forms such as pills, sublingual dissolvable tablets, and transdermal patches. Pill forms of some substitution therapies can be misused by being crushed, dissolved and injected. To discourage this practice, a combination of buprenorphine and naloxone is now available (e.g., Suboxone). Naloxone is an opioid antagonist used in overdose reversal and taking it can lead to immediate withdrawal symptoms. OST can also be used by pregnant women, increasing their health and reducing harm to the fetus. OST can reduce infection-related infections and overdoses while helping people work and stay housed because the medications can help control cravings and are longer lasting, while not leading to rapid highs and withdrawal associated with heroin. In short, OST leads to more stability and has been extraordinarily effective in helping people reduce infections and live healthier lives in the community (MacArthur et al. 2012; Tsui et al. 2014; Turner et al. 2011).

Safe/Supervised Injection Sites (SIS)   Supervised injection sites (SIS) are legally sanctioned, indoor spaces where people can inject drugs under medical supervision in order to discourage needle sharing, reduce overdoses, and provide a safe injection location for vulnerable people. These sites also provide people with a variety of resources and services including clean injecting equipment, medical and behavioral health care, condoms, the overdose reversal drug Naloxone, drug-checking services, education on how to reduce infections, and referrals to OST programs.

SIS have been effective in increasing access to drug treatment and primary care (Kerr et al. 2010), reducing HIV infections and needle sharing (Milloy and Wood 2009; Pinkerton 2011), and decreasing overdoses, public injecting, and dropped needles, while not being associated with increased drug trafficking, drug injecting, or crime (Potier et al. 2014; Kerr et al. 2010). A cohort study of over 800 PWID in Vancouver, Canada, found that all-cause mortality rates were significantly lower for frequent users of SIS than nonfrequent users (Kennedy et al. 2019).

Drug Checking Drug checking involves using testing strips to test the quality and purity of drugs to ensure drugs do not contain harmful chemicals, agents, or fentanyl, a highly potent and lethal synthetic opioid associated with increased overdose potential and deaths. These services are often available at SIS and at parties or raves where ecstasy and other drugs with high overdose or contamination potential are consumed. The recent rise of fentanyl in the United States and across the globe has led to a surge in overdose deaths, making these programs incredibly important. In a study at one supervised injection site, about 80% of drugs checked were contaminated with fentanyl. Implementation of drug checking at SIS may, therefore, also reduce the potential for overdoses in PWID (Karamouzian et al. 2018). The use of drug testing strips to identify illicit manufactured fentanyl in drugs has also shown good uptake in PWID (Krieger et al. 2018).

Providing Noncontingent Employment and Housing Services Programs such as *Housing First* that provide housing to people with addictions without mandating abstinence have been effective in increasing treatment engagement (Larimer et al. 2009; Tsemberis et al. 2004) and improving health for persons who are homeless with HIV/AIDS (Hawk and Davis 2012). These programs are particularly effective in persons with co-occurring serious mental illness and substance use disorders who are un-housed. This population often struggles to conform to the demands of high-threshold treatment programs that mandate abstinence as a prerequisite to services. As a result, this group tends to have high treatment dropout rates and very high rates of morbidity and early mortality (Mancini and Wyrick-Waugh, 2013). Housing First programs address social determinants of health by providing safe, secure housing and access to medical care and behavioral health treatment though case management. Housing First has been found to lead to less homelessness, greater access to treatment, and higher rates of client satisfaction (Tsemberis et al. 2004). Housing First programs are effective in helping people live longer lives that are healthier, safer, and more dignified.

11.2.5 Intensive Case Management

Harm reduction programs serve people's needs without directly addressing substance use. Providing practical support and access to resources is a fundamental harm reduction approach. Intensive case management services are specifically designed to serve populations with complex needs such as persons with co-morbid serious mental illness and substance use disorders who struggle to stay housed, employed, and healthy. Intensive case management can be provided by a single case manager or by a team of service providers. Intensive case managers provide time-unlimited, intensive, individualized wrap-around services designed to increase stability, improve health, and enhance community tenure and recovery. Intensive case management typically has a low client-to-professional ratio of around 10 to 1. Intensive case management services are comprehensive and include assessment and care planning, benefits management, housing, occupational and social rehabilitation, addiction services, psychiatric symptom management, and physical health/disease management (Salyers et al. 2013). All or most services are provided directly by members of the case management team. Intensive case management services are continuous and time-unlimited. Intensive case management has been found to reduce hospitalization, increase retention in care, and improve functioning as compared to standard care (Dieterich et al. 2017).

Harm Reduction in Primary Care Settings While most harm reduction programs are provided in community settings, use of harm reduction approaches have also been promoted in hospital settings as a way to engage persons who use drugs (PWUD) in treatment (Sharma et al. 2017). Several strategies have been identified that can help to increase patient access to substance use disorder treatment. One approach is using *peer providers* who have lived experience with addictions and mental health issues to engage PWUD in treatment and to include peer providers in developing humanistic and nonstigmatizing organizational policies and procedures for PWUD (Sharma et al. 2017).

Another approach is for hospitals to develop formal organizational relationships with outside addiction providers and organizations to coordinate treatment referrals and engage in consultation and cross-training of staff. For instance, hospitals could provide addiction centers with training in health screening, while addiction specialists could assist healthcare providers in a number of areas related to treating persons with opioid and other addictions. This includes training in administration and disbursement of naloxone (i.e., Narcan) for overdose reversal. Early evidence has demonstrated that providing education about overdose risk prevention and distributing naloxone to at-risk patients and their family and friends are effective in reducing opioid overdoses in the community (Adams 2018).

Providing education referral and initiating opioid substitution therapy (OST) and other medication-assisted treatments (MAT) to assist patients with withdrawal or craving management is another effective approach. Initiating buprenorphine/naloxone treatment in primary care settings such as hospital emergency departments (ED) and clinics can increase the likelihood of using medication-assisted services, reduce the likelihood of nonprescribed opioid use after discharge (Hawk and D'Onofrio 2018; D'Onofrio et al. 2015; Liebschutz et al. 2014), and can lead to increased treatment engagement (Hawk and D'Onofrio 2018; D'Onofrio et al. 2015). Providing buprenorphine in the ED has also shown significant cost-effectiveness by reducing overall healthcare utilization costs (Busch et al. 2017).

In another example, hospital staff often deny opioids to patients with opioid addiction resulting in withdrawal, unnecessary pain, and leaving the hospital against medical advice. Addiction consultants could provide guidance on how to properly prescribe opioids or nonopioid alternatives to assist with pain management while patients are in the hospital (Sharma et al. 2017). Addiction consultants can also assist hospital providers in deploying brief interventions with patients and their families. This includes how to have motivating, nonstigmatizing, educational conversations with persons with substance use disorders and their families. These conversations can include providing patients with advice about how to notice and manage cravings and withdrawal symptoms and information on safe drug use practices. These brief interventions could also include referrals to needle and syringe exchange programs, drug-checking services, self-help, behavioral health treatment programs, and services that address housing, employment, and benefits (Sharma et al. 2017).

Case Study 11.1 Mia

Mia[1] is a 21-year-old, cisgendered woman. She was brought to the emergency room by the fire department after suffering an acute opioid overdose. She was injecting heroin laced with fentanyl (unknown to her) with friends when she and another friend passed out and would not wake up. The others who had not yet injected called 911.

Mia has a history of depression and PTSD. She was sexually abused as a child by her ex-stepfather. She was kicked out of her house at age 17, when she told her mother and her second stepfather that she was bisexual. She subsequently stayed at friend's houses and shelters. She eventually dropped out of school and started working as a server in several restaurants. She made good money and was able to rent a small apartment. She started using prescription opioids when she was in high school. After she was kicked out of the house, she was exposed to other means to use opioids and quickly moved to injecting heroin. She states, "The oxy was everywhere in high school so I never thought I would inject because we would crush them and snort them. I was probably addicted then. But I got kicked out and started hanging around some people from work and they taught me how to smoke it, and then how to doing skin poppers just under the skin and then the next thing I knew I was injecting. They changed the formula of oxy so you couldn't make it into a solution to cook or shoot so we switched to heroin. It didn't take long. The feeling was like a warm hug that I never got from anyone. It was like nothing I ever experienced. And then I couldn't stop myself. Every day. The withdrawals were terrible."

Mia received a nasal injection of an opioid antagonist Narcan (naloxone) from a first responder that reversed her overdose and saved her life. While she was recovering in the hospital, the police officer who responded to the scene called a peer support worker, Jade, employed by the hospital to try to engage Mia in treatment. The peer worker, a person with lived experience of addiction and recovery, met Mia at

---

[1]All names and other identifiers of this case have been changed to protect privacy and confidentiality.

her bedside. She told Mia, "You're young, you have got your whole life ahead of you. I was in the same boat as you – I was raped, blamed for it, kicked out of my damn house by the person who raped me, got addicted, loved it at first, then I overdosed, overdosed again, tried to kill myself, and then a peer came to my bedside in this very hospital and told me I had my whole life ahead of me and asked me if I want to try to turn it around? You know what I said to her? I told her to 'fuck off.' So she left. And then I sat with it for a night and I called her and she came and she helped me save myself." Jade informed Mia of some program options available and asked if she would like to enroll, get some treatment, earn her GED, and get a job or go to college.

Mia refused and said that she was OK. That she just got a bad batch. She'd be more careful. So the peer worker gave Mia her own Narcan nasal dispenser, fentanyl test kit, and taught her how to use both. She also gave her some clean syringes, her card with her phone number and told Mia to call her anytime day or night. Mia refused the Narcan and clean needles at first. The peer worker became firm: "No. You don't know it yet – but you are going to call me and I need you to live to do that. You take these. You need to stay healthy and maybe you'll need these to help someone else." Mia took the items. Two weeks later her best friend overdosed and Mia was able to use the Narcan to save her. After this incident Mia called Jade and met her for coffee. Jade told Mia more about the program and how she could enroll. Jade would stand by her throughout the process.

Mia enrolled in the program. She received an opioid substitution medication (buprenorphine) that helped control her cravings and go back to work as a cashier. Mia would briefly relapse twice more that year before achieving her first 6 months of sobriety. After each relapse she and Jade would see what went wrong and develop skills to cope. They determined that boredom, seeing people she used to use with, having money, and depressed symptoms were her main triggers. They worked together to develop coping skills (e.g., craving management, refusal skills, and planning for emergencies), budgeting skills, and activity scheduling to fill her time. Mia also completed a 10-session sequence of eye movement desensitization and reprocessing (EMDR) therapy to help target her intrusive thoughts and negative self-evaluation related to her trauma. At night she studied for her GED. Mia eventually titrated off of the buprenorphine and moved to naltrexone to control her cravings. While in treatment Mia learned how to control her cravings using relaxation and distraction techniques. She received some antidepressant medication and CBT to control her depressed moods and change her negative thinking patterns. She would eventually earn her GED and is now attending college courses to earn her social work degree. She has a new girlfriend and they are considering moving in together. She is also considering being a peer support worker to help others. Jade has moved into a management position and is a supervisor for several peer workers across the city. She and Mia are still close.

Case Analysis Questions
- What is your case conceptualization and hypothesis of Mia?

Describe how Mia moved through the various stages of change and how the treatment approaches she experienced shifted across these different stages.
Describe how Jade was able to help Mia. What strategies did she use?
Why was Jade successful in engaging Mia?
What harm reduction principles and practices are evident in this case?
What role did harm reduction play in Mia's eventual sobriety?

11.3 Motivational Interviewing

11.3.1 Motivational Interviewing: Philosophy, Basic Skills, and Techniques

Motivational interviewing (MI) was developed by William R. Miller and Stephen Rollnick in the 1980s. MI is a person-centered, collaborative style of practice that helps people explore their ambivalence about changing health behaviors related to alcohol and substance use, diet and exercise, using medication, and safe sexual practices (Miller and Rollnick 2013). Motivational interviewing is a "client centered, directive method, for enhancing intrinsic motivation to change by exploring and resolving ambivalence." (Miller and Rollnick 2002; pg. 25). The basic skills of motivational interviewing can be useful in each stage of change. However, the approach is most useful in the contemplation and early preparation stages of change where ambivalence toward change is high and insight and knowledge can tip the motivational scales in the direction of change. MI approaches focus on being nonjudgmental, accepting, and empathic, which can also assist in building relationships and engaging clients in the precontemplation stage of change where intention to change is low or nonexistent. Clients in precontemplation may be uninterested in change or are unconcerned about any negative effects of their behavior. Being accepting and offering some information about the potential risks of use and strategies to reduce harm in a gentle, empathic, and nonjudgmental way through reflections and open-ended questions can help people think about their use differently and diffuse conflict and defensiveness. Receptivity to this kind of approach is more likely to be higher than using confrontation which can lead the person to shut down or "dig in" to their view (Humeniuk et al. 2010b; Miller and Rollnick 2013; Prochaska et al. 1992).

The goal of MI is to invite people to consider change through a supportive relationship (Miller and Rollnick 2002). Three concepts animate the spirit of motivational interviewing approaches (Miller and Rollnick 2013). The first is *collaboration*. Providers work closely with clients using a warm, nonjudgmental, accepting, and empathic approach. Providers avoid confrontation, which can lead to resistance. Instead, providers create an open and warm context and seek to be in attunement with clients' dreams, goals, and aspirations. This helps them identify discrepancies between clients' stated goals and current behavior. Providers seek to help clients identify and resolve ambivalence about change and help direct them toward behaviors that are best aligned with their readiness and confidence (Miller and Rollnick 2002, 2013). The second is *evocation*. Rather than impart unwanted advice, MI providers use reflective listening to elicit or draw out information from the client in order to help them develop an understanding of the discrepancies between their current behavior and their desires and goals for the future. MI providers strive to elicit a person's intrinsic motivation for change and then reflect that back to the person so that they can decide whether or not to seek change. MI providers avoid preaching, ordering, persuading, praising, sympathizing, or interpreting. MI is a quiet, eliciting approach to counseling (Miller and Rollnick 2013). The third is *autonomy*. For MI providers, change is viewed as a natural process that is the responsibility of the client. MI providers avoid coercion or telling clients what they must or should do. Practitioners communicate to the client that the direction and amount of change is their responsibility (Miller and Rollnick 2013). These principles make motivational interviewing inherently aligned with care that is person-centered, recovery-oriented, and supportive of shared-decision-making approaches.

Motivational interviewing also has four general principles that act as a foundation to the approach. The first general principle is *empathy*. MI providers recognize the people are doing the best they can, given their experiences and circumstances. Therefore, the MI approach is predicated on respect, acceptance, and sensitivity. MI providers understand that change is difficult for everyone and recognize that ambivalence toward change is natural and expected. MI providers avoid judgments, labels (e.g., addict, user, alcoholic), blame, and confrontation, and instead accept clients exactly as they are, and where they are, in the change process. Providers foster this accepting environment through the use of open-ended questions and reflective listening as a means to understand and evoke client ambivalence about change and to seek out client goals, dreams, and aspirations. To put it more bluntly, no one likes to be judged or pushed around. Showing empathy and acceptance allows the client to feel comfortable and understood. This is more likely to facilitate change by giving clients a chance to see the discrepancy between their actions and their goals. The approach gives clients the space they need to consider change without feeling like they are "giving in," reducing resistance and frustration for both the client and the provider (Miller and Rollnick 2002; Humeniuk et al. 2010b).

The second general principle is *developing discrepancy*. MI is a directive approach in that providers seek to help clients develop motivation toward change. This is accomplished through the development of discrepancy. Discrepancy is the gap between a person's current behavior and their personal goals and values (Miller and Rollnick 2013). The goal of an MI provider is to help create, identify, or amplify discrepancy between the client's present situation and where and who they want to be in the future. As discrepancy increases, the importance for change also rises. When a person sees how their current behavior interferes with their personal goals related to relationships, identity, roles, health, and success within an open and accepting environment, they will be the ones advocating for change. In order to develop discrepancy between client goals and current behavior, MI providers use a range of practices that include open-ended questions, reflections, and strategies such as decisional balance exercises to help clients identify the pros and cons of changing and not changing behavior.

The third general principle is *rolling with resistance*. People naturally resist change and are ambivalent about making changes in their life. This is normal, and the MI provider accepts this as part of the change process. The goal is to invite the person to take in new information and knowledge about their substance use or other unhealthy behavior. MI providers do not argue for change. Rather, they help the *client* argue for change. When resistance does come, rather than fighting it, MI providers roll with resistance by reflecting the resistance back at clients by asking more open-ended questions (Miller and Rollnick, 2013; Humeniuk et al. 2010b). Signs of resistance include: (1) discounting the importance of change; (2) arguing and challenging your expertise; (3) interrupting you, talking over you, and cutting you off; (4) minimizing the problem, denying there is a problem, and blaming others; and (5) "checking out" or not paying attention. Resistance is to be expected and signals to the provider to slow down and explore (Miller and Rollnick 2002, 2013). The fourth general principle is *supporting self-efficacy*. Self-efficacy involves how much the person believes they have the ability and competence to be successful in a particular task or solve a problem. In order for change to proceed, providers must communicate to clients that they can change and that change is up to them. One way to communicate this is to inform the person that change can take many forms. Offering the person a menu of treatment options can help the person identify and select the best pathway for change (Miller and Rollnick 2002, 2013).

11.3.2   Motivational Interviewing Practices

By establishing and nurturing a caring and nonjudgmental relationship the provider can increase the intrinsic motivation for change by gently pointing out how the person is at odds with something they value (e.g., stability, health, employment, positive relationships). When this discrepancy has been acknowledged a person's intrinsic motivation for change rises. In the MI tradition, change is a natural process that is most likely to occur when: (1) there is a *discrepancy* between the client's current situation and how they want their life to be; (2) the *importance* of change is high; (3) a person understands what they have to do to change and has *confidence* that they can make the change; and (4) the client is *ready* to make the change and that change is more important than maintaining the status quo. Healthcare providers can enhance a person's motivation for change by providing information and pointing out the discrepancy between their stated goals and their current behavior, communicating the importance of change, and providing a clear pathway for change through information and a menu of treatment options (Miller and Rollnick 2013).

11.3.2.1 Avoiding Traps

Confrontation and the use of shame, humiliation, or other punishments can act to create defensiveness in the person and can often lead to immobilization and a sense of hopelessness. It can also create anger that may cause the person to resist change. For instance, Miller and Rollnick (2002, 2013) have identified several "traps" that get in the way of increasing client's intrinsic motivation to change. I will explore several of these traps below.

The Q & A Trap This trap is when the provider asks a series of closed-ended questions that invites the client to give easy, short answers that require no introspection, exploration, or analysis. This trap is common for new or rushed professionals. This situation reinforces the providers as the authority (i.e., the interrogator) and the client as passive. It also creates a nonempathic environment that is predictable and shallow. Avoid this trap by gathering checklist type information in the intake form and reserve enough time in the clinical interaction to share and explore change in a relaxed atmosphere. During the clinical interaction, only rely on open-ended questions, reflections, and affirmations. The client should be doing most of the talking and the clinician should rely on multiple reflections for each open-ended question asked.

Taking Sides This is when providers tell the client they have a problem and argue for the changes the client *should* be making. This naturally leads to defensiveness or passivity and puts the client in the position of arguing *against* change (i.e., resistance). This is the opposite of MI. It is the client, not the provider, who should be arguing for change. It is important for the provider to not defend one side of the argument but to help the client explore the pros and cons of *both* sides: change and not changing.

Expert Trap This is when the provider sends the message that they have all the answers. This leads to passive resistance. This trap is endemic in treatment planning processes that are not person-centered and is obvious when the provider both identifies the problem and generates the solutions while the client sits passively, waiting to go home and ignore the plan the provider has so expertly developed for them. It is important to open up space for the client to explore their ambivalence about the problem. Ambivalence is best summarized in the "Yes, but…" statements clients may give in response to change. Ambivalence is both wanting to change and not wanting to change at the same time. Use reflections to identify this ambivalence and then ask, "What do you make of this? How can you resolve this and move forward?"

Labeling Trap The labeling trap is when providers feel it is important for the client to admit they have a problem or a particular diagnosis (e.g., depressive, alcoholic, addict), and if they don't they pronounce them as "in denial." This approach is mostly ineffective and can drive people who are ambivalent about change away from help. It engenders resistance in the highest form because you are forcing people to accept a label they do not necessarily agree with or are interested in accepting. This also leads directly into a struggle for power and authority in the interview. Avoid this trap by de-emphasizing labels and focus instead on behavior and how it may be in conflict with a person's values and goals.

Premature Focus Trap The premature focus trap can happen due to a busy environment and an eagerness to help. The provider attempts to focus in on the problem behavior too soon in the interview and creates resistance. In this trap, the provider seeks to force the conversation to focus on what they think the problem is. This can lead to defensiveness with the client and an ensuing struggle. In MI, you want to go where the client takes you, gently selecting and amplifying any comments focused on change and ambivalence. Clients often want to talk about things that are related to the problem. This can be an opportunity to learn about how the problem behavior is affecting the client's life and provide an opportunity to develop discrepancy. For instance, the client may score highly on harmful drinking behavior, but wants instead to focus on his anger and how it is destroying his relationship with his partner more so than the drinking. This is an opportunity to explore how his drinking and anger are linked. Focusing on addressing his anger and relationship issues first may represent in indirect way to address drinking by developing discrepancy by asking later in the interview something like, "It sounds like your anger is something that you want to work on changing. I'm also curious to know if you think there may be a relationship between your drinking and your anger. What are your thoughts about that?" (Miller and Rollnick 2002, 2013).

11.3.2.2   Common Practice Skills for Motivational Interviewing: OARS

There are four common practice skills that serve as the foundation to motivational interviewing that make the acronym OARS: (1) *O*pen-ended Questions, (2) *A*ffirmations, (3) *R*eflections, and (4) *S*ummaries. OARS can be used to create and amplify ambivalence around change and highlight discrepancies between: (1) what clients would like their life to be; (2) what is happening now; and (3) how their substance use is interfering in their pursuit of their goals and impacting their health. The use of OARS can help evoke these discrepancies and help the client identify their own reasons for change from their point of view (Humeniuk et al. 2010b; Miller and Rollnick 2002, 2013).

Open-Ended Questions Open-ended questions invite the client to explore a particular topic and to do most of the talking. Open-ended questions usually begin with stems such as: "Tell me about...," "I'm curious to know....," or "Help me understand." Open-ended questions create a context that is marked by acceptance, respect, and exploration. Open-ended questions invite people to explore their lives or topics. As a general guideline, you should follow up on an open-ended question with a series of reflections and affirmations and then a summarization of the topic before moving on to another area (Humeniuk et al. 2010b; Miller and Rollnick 2002, 2013; SAMHSA 1999).

Examples of Open-Ended Questions
- What brought you here today?
- How did the problem start?
- What concerns do you have about your use?
- What concerns do others have about your use?
- I curious, what do you think about your use?
- How has your drinking been a problem for you? For other people?
- What are some of the benefits you get from using? What are the "not-so-good things" about drinking or drugs?
- In what ways does your score on the drinking scale concern you?
- What makes you sure that you can make a change if you decided to do it?

Affirmations Providers can occasionally use *affirmations* that highlight client strengths and qualities and acknowledge a positive development or action. Affirmations should be used sparingly and acknowledge client attempts, their strength in surviving any adversity they may share, and the courage to be talking to you at all. For instance, a question one might ask to affirm and to elicit change could be, "You being here shows me that at least in some ways you think it is time to do something different. What reasons do you have for changing? What makes you think you need to make a change?" The emphasis should be on genuineness and authenticity (e.g., don't fake it) and focused on courage, competence, strengths, and endurance (Miller and Rollnick 2013; SAMHSA 1999).

Reflective Listening Reflective listening is the most important skill in MI. Reflective listening requires practitioners to listen intently to a person's words, body language, and tone of voice in order to infer the explicit *and* implicit meaning of their statement and to reflect that information back to them in the form of a statement. This involves not only listening to what the person is saying, but then also reflecting back the underlying *meaning* of what they said. Table 11.1 lists examples of several types of reflective statements. In *simple reflections* providers reflect the words a client has said back to them to elicit more talk. More *complex reflections* use words that get at the deeper meaning beyond a client's statement. Slightly *underestimating* the intensity of a comment by using words such as "a bit" or "a little" may lead a person to continue to explore their feelings and thoughts, while over-estimating or *amplifying* will cause a person to stop or go in the other direction. A *double-sided reflection* (e.g., On the one hand…and on the other hand…) is a good tool to reflect a client's ambivalence about change. When the client uses a "Yes, but" statement to refer to a problem, this is often a signal that it is a good time for a double-sided reflection. See the following example.

> *Client:* My family is probably right. I sometimes overdo it on the weekends and I know I should probably cut down.
> *Provider uses simple reflection*: So it sounds like you agree that you need to cut down on your drinking?"
> Client: Yes, but I enjoy it. I like going out with my friends and having a good time. I deserve it. I work hard.

Provider uses double-sided reflection: So it sounds like on the one hand, you recognize that your drinking is causing you some problems with your health and family and you should cut down, *and on the other hand* you feel that you deserve to have some fun with your friends. It sounds like there are some benefits to drinking that you're not sure you want to give up.

In this example, the client's "yes, but" statement revealed some important information that could lead to a discussion of how the client could continue to socialize and enjoy the benefits of his friends, while also cutting down on his drinking and preserving his health. Note the use of "and" instead of "but" in the double-sided reflection. You do not want to use "but" because it negates the statement that came before it. Instead, use "and" or "yet" in double-sided reflections to recognize the importance and validity of *both* statements. In MI, providers must decide which of the statements from the client they will reflect. These usually involve statements focused on ambiguity and change talk. It is wise to follow open-ended questions with two to three reflections (Miller and Rollnick 2013). Using simple, amplifying, and double-sided reflections are important ways to help people develop discrepancy using their own words. It also keeps the conversation moving (Humeniuk et al. 2010b; Miller and Rollnick, 2013).

Summarizing Summarizing, or "picking the flowers," can be used to collect and consolidate information, reinforce what has been said, check accuracy of information, and transition to another topic. At their best, summaries communicate to the client that you have listened to them, and reinforce important information in one place so the client can reflect and move forward to the next step. Summaries can be used periodically to collect information that has been said on a topic and to link one set of information with another set. Lastly, summaries can transition to another topic area. As with double-sided reflections, when summarizing a client's statements, avoid using "but" as this can be confusing. Instead use "and," "on the one hand *and* then on the other hand," or "at the same time." These statements more accurately capture the ambivalence around change. Both things can be true: wanting to change and wanting to continue the status quo (Miller and Rollnick 2013).

11.3.2.3 Eliciting Change Talk

Eliciting change talk is a directive way to resolve ambivalence toward change. It is important to first be able to recognize change talk when you hear it. There are several types. Table 11.2 lists the main strategies for eliciting change talk. The first type of change talk is *acknowledging disadvantages* of the status quo or of things staying as they are. These are statements of recognition and insight. The client has indicated that they recognize that their current trajectory is untenable and that there are clear consequences and disadvantages to the status quo (Miller and Rollnick 2013).

A second form of change talk is *recognizing the advantages of making a change*. Clients may acknowledge that change would be good for them and recognize that making a change would have some positive consequences (Miller and Rollnick 2013). A third type of change talk is when clients *express optimism for change*. This

Table 11.1 Examples of reflections in motivational interviewing (Based on Miller and Rollnick 2013)

Client comment	Provider response	Reflection type and purpose
I don't need help. I can quit on my own.	You have the ability to do this by yourself.	Simple reflections: Using reflection to recognize what the person is saying and feeling in the moment. This can repeat using the same words or, even better, to capture the feeling and perspective of the person.
I'm not interested in quitting smoking.	You don't think quitting smoking would work for you right now.	
My partner is exaggerating. My drinking isn't that bad.	So there are no problems in your relationship because of your drinking.	Amplified reflection: Amplifies or exaggerates what the person says. Used to get people to tone down a statement or argue the other side. Be careful to not go too far. Use judiciously or you will get resistance.
	Your drinking isn't causing any problems in your life.	
	Your partner has no reason to be worried about your drinking.	
My grandfather smoked his whole life and he lived until he was 85.	So smoking doesn't really lead to any health problems.	
	You don't expect any health problems no matter how long you smoke.	
	Your grandfather didn't experience any health problems due to his smoking, and so you won't either.	
I know I may drink too much sometimes, but I work hard and like to spend time unwinding with my friends.	On the one hand you realize your drinking is causing problems in your marriage, yet on the other hand it is important for you to spend time with your friends and unwind after work.	Double-sided reflection: Attempts to capture the full range of ambivalence about a problem. In this approach you identify ambivalence for and against a health behavior. The key is to use "and," "yet," or "on the one hand…yet/and on the other hand." by avoiding the "but," you do not cancel what came before. Instead you capture both sides of the issue. You may have to use information the client has given you in the past regarding the behavior.

type of change talk goes beyond recognizing the disadvantages of things staying as they are and the advantages of making a change, to demonstrating the recognition that the person could make the change. This type of change talk includes notes of *confidence and intention* (Miller and Rollnick 2013). The last form of change talk includes *expressing clear intentions to change.* This type of change talk indicates the importance of change and *signals to the therapist that the person is entering the preparatio/action stage of change* (Miller and Rollnick 2013). Table 11.3 lists some examples of change talk that you may hear from clients and different types of responses that can elicit more change talk.

11.3.2.4 Using Rulers to Assess Readiness, Importance, and Confidence

Readiness implies a level of confidence and importance. In order to understand a client's level of readiness to change it is useful to know how *important* a person thinks it is to change, how *confident* they are that they can make a change, and how *ready* they are to make a change. Using "rulers" can help you know whether you need to help the person see the importance of making a change, or whether you need to help build up the person's self-efficacy for making a change. The use of rulers to measure these aspects can shed light on a client's level of ambivalence and readiness to change as well as open up some conversations about making changes. It may also guide the provider on where to go next. Some clients have high confidence, but do not see the need or importance of making a change. For others, they know they should make a change and the importance is high, but they have low confidence due to failed past attempts or they do not see a way forward (i.e., they don't know how). For others, they have low importance and low confidence indicating they are not ready to make a change. For those with high confidence and high importance, they are ready to take action and providers should begin planning for next steps.

Implementing change rulers is a relatively straightforward process. Providers ask clients three questions (they may also show the client the ruler so they can see a visual): (1) How important is making this change for you on a scale of one to ten with one being not at all important and ten being extremely important. Where would you say you fall on this scale?; (2) How confident are you that you could make the change? On a scale from one to ten with one being not at all confident and ten being extremely confident, where would you say you fall on this scale?; and (3) How ready are you that you could make the change? On a scale from one to ten with one being not at all ready and ten being extremely ready, where would you say you fall on this scale? It is not necessary to ask clients each question in a row, but providers can use the rulers at different times during the session or across multiple sessions. Providers can also start with the importance and confidence rulers first to indicate where to focus efforts (e.g., on building importance or building confidence).

After using each ruler, it is important to ask the client why they chose the number they did and not a *lower* number. This can open up opportunities for change talk and helps emphasize to people that they are ready to change. Asking them why they are not at a higher number suggests that they *should* be at a higher number (i.e., Taking-Sides Trap) and can lead to defensiveness and resistance. After you discuss why they weren't at a lower number, ask them what it would take for them to go from their current number to a higher number. This opens up an opportunity to identify areas to focus treatment, build skills, or increasing knowledge about how their behavior is impacting their lives.

Table 11.2 Strategies for eliciting change (based on Miller and Rollnick 2013)

Strategy	Definition
Elaborating	Reinforce motivation to change by having the client elaborate on why they want to change. Ask questions like: Why now? What have you done in the past? What are some things that you would do differently now to change? Linger here for a while and resist the urge to move on to other areas. This helps the client consolidate motivation and offer additional change talk. Ask, "What else?" to elicit more change talk about a particular topic.
Asking about extremes	Ask clients about the long-term and short-term consequences of making or not making a change. Ask people, "What do you think will happen in the next 5 or 10 years if you do not reduce or stop drinking or drug use?" On the other side, ask clients what they think will happen if they changed right now and were successful? What would be the best outcome?
Looking back	Create discrepancy between the past and present by asking about a time when the problem was not present or not as severe.
	Ask, "Tell me about a time when you didn't have this problem (e.g., alcohol, drugs, gambling) or when it was better? What was your life like then?"
Looking forward	Similar to elaborating, build hope and motivation by helping clients look ahead into the future and ask them to imagine their lives after making a change. Ask: What would your life be like if you didn't use drugs or drink or gamble? What would be different? What if you don't make the change? What will your life be like in the future? If you did not make any changes in your life, what do you think things will be like 10 years from now?
Explore what is important to people	This is really about spirituality and developing discrepancy between current behavior and goals or values. Ask clients what is most important in their lives. What gives them joy? Ask: What do you care about the most? What dreams or aspirations do you have for the future? Who is most important to you? And then ask: How do you think your drinking or drug use or gambling is impacting these areas of your life now?

11.3.2.5   Decisional Balance Exercises

In the decisional balance exercise providers explore four domains (in this order): (1) the advantages of the status quo (e.g., drinking, using drugs), (2) the disadvantages of status quo, (3) the disadvantages of changing, and (4) the advantages of changing (Mueser et al. 2003; Miller and Rollnick 2013). Figure 11.1 provides an example of the decisional balance exercise. These domains can be positioned as four quadrants on a sheet of paper and the client can list their answers within each quadrant. Providers should go clockwise starting from the top left quadrant (e.g., advantages of status quo) and end with the "advantages of change" quadrant in the bottom left. Decisional balance is a way to develop discrepancy and explore the importance of change. The decisional balance sheet can provide an opportunity for the client to explore the advantages and disadvantages of the status quo and change in a non-judgmental environment so that they can consider the importance of change and their level of readiness. It can also reveal a client's motivations for their use and the ways to help clients mitigate their concerns about change (Miller and Rollnick 2013).

Table 11.3 Examples of change talk and eliciting questions (based on Miller and Rollnick 2013)

Type of change talk	Examples	Eliciting questions
Acknowledging disadvantages	"This is having an impact on my family."	"Tell me the ways in which this information worries you?"
	"I can't go on like this much longer."	"What are some of the negative consequences you've experienced by your use?"
	"Things are getting pretty bad now."	"What do you think will happen if things don't change?"
	"Maybe I need to do something different."	"What are some of the disadvantages of not making a change?"
Recognizing the advantages of making a change	"My family would sure appreciate it."	"What would be some good things about making a change?"
	"People would get off my back."	"How would your life be different if you made a change?"
	"I'd have more money."	"What are some of the advantages of making a change?"
	"I probably would feel better."	
	"I'd be able to enjoy my children more."	
	"I'd be a better role model for my kids."	
Expressing optimism for change	"If I put my mind to it, I can do it."	"How confident are you that you could make a change?"
	"I did it before and so I can probably do it again."	"What or who do you need to be successful in making a change?"
	"I'm pretty sure I can do it with some help."	"What qualities or strengths do you already possess that will help you make a change?"
		"When were other times that you have made a change?"
		"What do you think could help?"
		"Who do you think would help?"
Expressing clear intentions to change	"I'm tired, it's time to make a change."	"How important is making a change for you right now?"
	"I've had enough, it is time I did something."	"What things would you be willing to try to make a change?"
	"I can't keep going on like this, I need to change."	"What do you think about your drinking right now?"
		"What are you going to do about this?"

Case Study 11.2 James

James[2] is a 27-year-old white, cisgendered male who works in an IT department at a large pharmaceutical company. He is speaking to a social worker at an individual

---

[2]All names and other identifiers of this case have been changed to protect privacy and confidentiality.

intake interview as part of a 10-week program of couples counseling initiated by his partner to improve communication. James has reluctantly agreed to participate in the program. His partner has told him that she is considering leaving the relationship unless they receive help in communicating better and to address his problem drinking. James has experienced a long history of problem drinking. He drinks about 3–4 times per week and during those episodes he drinks 4 or 5 beers at a time. He has been fighting with his girlfriend of 3 years (whose father was a severe alcoholic) about his drinking. She says if he doesn't cut down she's leaving. As a child, he grew up in a large extended family that engaged in regular drinking during celebrations and crises. James's father would regularly consume 3–5 beers per day after work and more on the weekends. "I work hard. I deserve it. Give me a break," he would say. His parents would often fight due to his father's drinking because of extended time spent in bars (all Saturday afternoon) and that James's father would come home in an argumentative mood. James, himself, spent his youthful years drinking with friends in the woods when they were underage and in bars 3–4 times per week when they were older. He has had a history of minor bar fights, broken relationships, and one driving under the influence (DUI) citation (i.e. drunk driving) approximately 1 year ago.

> Provider: James, thank you for coming. What brought you here today?
> James: I guess my girlfriend has had enough and wants to see if we can figure this out or she's moving on.
> Provider: I'm curious to know what your perspective is on this? Why do you think you're here?
> James: My drinking, I guess. Her father was a drunk and she is sensitive about my drinking. She thinks I drink too much and when I do drink I can be argumentative. Verbally. Not

Advantages Not Changing/Status Quo	Disadvantages of Not Changing/Status Quo
• People have seemingly good reasons for use • Short circuits resistance • Identifies barriers to change	• Where ambivalence/change talk begins
Advantages of Changing	**Disadvantages of Changing**
• Most of change talk happens here • Elicits client's own arguments for change • Short circuits resistance • New areas may come up	• Short circuits resistance • Elicits fears around changing behavior

Fig. 11.1 Decisional balance (based on: Miller and Rollnick 2013; Mueser et al. 2003)

physically. I guess she's tired of it.

Provider: Sounds like she's concerned about your use of alcohol. Based on your screening results you are at a higher risk of health problems, relationships problems, and accidents. I'm curious to know what you think about your drinking?

James: I'm not a drunk. You probably hear that a lot, but I work, I don't drink every day. I don't even drink a lot. I drink less than all my friends. But when we go out to a party or have a party at our house or I go out with my friends everything goes well for a while, but then I start drinking and one becomes two, and two becomes four, and the next thing I know me and my girlfriend are fighting about something and then I apologize the next day for something stupid I said. I don't have more than four drinks when she is around (she won't let me). But when I start, I find it is hard to stop. I always go to four. Always. And I'd probably go five or six. Since she has been on me I've noticed this 'tug' when I drink. I just want another one. Maybe that's what she sees since her father was a lousy drunk. I don't like that feeling. I also find that when I drink more than three beers I magically turn into my father. Which is to say, I become an argumentative asshole, if you will. I like my girlfriend and I want to stay in the relationship. I hope we'll get married some day and have children. I don't want to be my father (when he drinks). He's fine when he is not drinking, but three beers in and he starts to turn. You can see it. And I guess I do the same thing.

Provider: So it sounds like you value your relationship and that you recognize that your drinking has caused some problems in that area of your life. I'm also hearing that you are concerned about some not very positive similarities you're seeing between your drinking behavior and your father's. What are some positive things you get from drinking?

James: I've been drinking with the same guys my whole life—since high school, which is now 10 years. We've all done the same thing each weekend. Our girlfriends all know each other. We're all good friends. I love my friends. We've always got each other's backs. I want to drink less but when I start I can't seem to stop without some help like my girlfriend's dirty looks, but I don't want my relationship with my friends to get screwed up either. They wouldn't be kind to me if suddenly I stopped drinking or got weird or something. What am I supposed to do? I don't need AA or any of that stuff and I don't want to change my friends or routines. I want this relationship to work. I probably need to cut down, but I don't want to lose my friends either.

Provider: So it sounds like on the one hand you recognize that your drinking is a problem and you want to do something about it, and on the other hand you're not sure what to do and you're afraid if you change you will lose some friends. Is that right?

James: Yeah, I guess that is right.

Provider: What are some concerns you have for the future if you do not change your drinking?

James: I'm afraid that my girlfriend will leave me and I will be all alone. I have this image that I'm going to be that older guy at the bar all alone and that all my friends will have successful jobs, and marriages and kids and I'll be the loser that still does the same shit 20 years later. It's already starting. People are making their moves with careers and getting more serious. Two of my friends are now engaged and talking house and kids. I start thinking about how I'll be left out because who wants to hang out with "that guy." I imagine I'll be in the same apartment, same job, same life and everyone else will move on and I admit, I get really panicky about it. Hyperventilate and all that. I sometimes wake up in a cold sweat at night thinking about it. My girlfriend threatening to leave me doesn't help. I get real upset when I think about that and I worry about it all the time. You'd think this would motivate me – but I just feel paralyzed sometimes. I don't know what to do. I guess things are more messed up than I thought before I came in here.

Questions

- How would you characterize James's drinking?

What is your working hypothesis for James's drinking, depression, and anxiety problems?

What stage of change is James in right now in regard to his drinking? What is your evidence?

Can you identify the different OARS skills used by the provider?

What are some examples of additional open-ended questions, reflections, and affirmations that could be used with James in this interview?

What would a summary of this interview look like?

What other elements of motivational interviewing could be used in this interview such as strategies to elicit change talk, decisional balance exercise, and readiness and confidence rulers?

What are some traps to avoid in this interview?

What are some motivational and/or cognitive behavioral intervention options that would be appropriate to include in your menu of options for James?

11.4   Brief Cognitive Behavioral Treatment Approaches

Cognitive behavioral therapy (CBT) for substance use disorders is an effective approach to substance abuse treatment. Providers use CBT to teach people skills to manage addictive thoughts, feelings, and behaviors in order to establish and maintain sobriety and prevent relapse (Carroll and Kiluk 2017; Darker et al. 2015; Gates et al. 2016; Magill and Ray 2009; Magill et al. 2019; McHugh et al. 2010; Naar and Safren 2017). CBT has also been found to be effectively combined with psychopharmacology, contingency management, and motivational approaches to help people with substance use disorders achieve and maintain treatment gains (Carroll and Kiluk 2017; Naar and Safren 2017). Combining CBT with motivational approaches that prepare people for change represents a powerful and effective combination of interventions designed to address substance misuse and substance use disorders (Carroll and Kiluk 2017; Chan Osilla et al. 2016; Gates et al. 2016; McHugh et al. 2010; Naar and Safren 2017). CBT approaches, including functional analysis, psychoeducation, skills training, and substance abuse counseling, are most often deployed in persons who are in the *action* and *maintenance* stages of change. Persons in the action stage are fully committed to change, have achieved some success, and are fully engaged in behaviors designed to lead to recovery. People in the maintenance stage of change seek to prevent relapses and develop long-term changes to promote a healthier lifestyle.

Four CBT techniques help people recover in a number of ways. These include: (1) functional analysis to analyze and understand the factors that trigger substance use and the consequences of use; (2) psychoeducation to learn the role substance use has played in their life and how addictive behavior develops over time through expectancies and reinforcement; (3) skills training to help manage addictive behavior and maintain sobriety such as understanding and responding to triggers for use, craving management techniques, communication, and problem-solving skills to recognize and manage situations that may lead to relapse, planning for emergencies, and anger management; and (4) teaching people how to incorporate new activities and develop sober social networks (Chan Osilla et al. 2016; Kadden et al. 2003; McHugh et al. 2010; Monti et al. 2002). In the next sections, we will explore the cognitive behavioral model for change and review the four specific cognitive behavioral practices that have been found to be effective in treating substance use disorders described above.

11.4.1   Cognitive Behavioral Model of Substance Use Disorder

The cognitive behavioral model of substance use disorders has two main considerations. First, problematic substance use is a learned behavior that is the result of powerful physical and psychological conditioning and reinforcement patterns. When the physiological and psychological effects of a substance are repeatedly associated with contextual cues in the person's environment or subjective experience (e.g., emotions, thoughts, physiological reactions), the person can be conditioned to experience craving responses in the presence of the substance or cues associated with the substance (e.g., classical conditioning) (McHugh et al. 2010; SAMHSA 2012). For persons with substance use disorders, being in the presence of alcohol, drugs, or any cues associated with use (e.g., certain people, places, or things such as money, equipment, advertisements, emotions such as anxiety, joy, depression) can act as cues that trigger a physiological withdrawal response (i.e., craving) and thought patterns (e.g., one drink won't hurt anyone) that can lead to relapse or problematic use patterns. Furthermore, substance use is negatively and positively reinforced through operant learning principles. Substance use can be positively reinforced by invoking positive feelings of euphoria, social bonding, and warmth that the person may be susceptible to due to past trauma and neglect, or genetic or other biological risk factors (Mate 2010). The immediate and temporary alleviation of psychological and physical pain associated with distress, dysphoria, craving, or withdrawal that substance use brings to the person also negatively reinforces substance use behavior. This rewarding of substance using behavior can lead to problematic use patterns over time (Koob 2017; SAMHSA 2012). Second, the decision to use substances is heavily influenced by maladaptive thinking patterns. These thinking patterns include: (1) negative beliefs about the self as helpless, unlovable, worthless; (2) irrational global expectancies about substances as a good way to solve problems; (3) low distress tolerance; and (4) thinking patterns that are generally rigid/inflexible, dichotomous (e.g., black or white/all or nothing), and automatic.

These two factors when combined with the effects of physical dependence can lead to problematic patterns of substance use marked by a loss of control, intense cravings when substances are not present or when cues to substances emerge, and use despite experiencing negative health and social consequences. In order to break these patterns of abuse and dependence, providers using CBT rely on the following approaches: (1) psychoeducation, functional analysis, and cognitive reframing to help clients identify and change maladaptive thinking patterns that can lead to problematic use; (2) contingency management strategies to reward abstinence and reduce use in order to break the pattern of positive and negative reinforcement that leads to substance abuse; and (3) teaching and practicing coping skills designed to help manage cravings and recognize and negotiate situations that can lead to use and relapse (McHugh et al. 2010). These approaches can address the main neurocognitive issues associated with addiction such as executive functioning deficits that impair problem-solving and impulse control, chronic dysphoria, negative emotions, and incentive salience or strong associations between substances and reward. These approaches can improve skills associated with problem-solving, planning, threat recognition, decision-making, and overall executive functioning. Coping skills designed to manage cravings and recognize and change negative thoughts can improve negative emotions by improving cognitive flexibility, increasing positive affect, and improving the ability to tolerate distress. Learning refusal skills and preparing for seemingly irrelevant decisions and emergencies can improve assertiveness, the ability to deal with stress, and reduce cravings (Carrol and Kiluk, 2017; Kwako et al. 2016). There are four main elements of cognitive behavioral therapy for substance use disorders: (1) functional analysis; (2) craving management; (3) coping skills development; and (4) relapse prevention. These strategies will be discussed briefly in the sections that follow.

11.4.2 Functional Analysis

Therapy usually begins by conducting a functional analysis (FA) of substance use behavior. The FA is designed to help the provider and the client understand the antecedents (e.g., internal and external triggers or cues) that can lead to substance use and the consequences of substance use in the person's life such as negative health impacts, interpersonal problems, and problems in occupational and other functioning areas (Chan Osilla et al. 2016; Kadden et al. 2003; McHugh et al. 2010; Monti et al. 2002; Mueser et al. 2003). A functional analysis can begin with a conversation about stress. What kinds of situations, people, or events cause stress in the client's life? What are some typical things that the client does to handle or relieve stress? What stressful situations, feelings, or thoughts commonly lead to drinking or substance use? How does using substances relieve stress? These questions can lead to a conversation about cues or triggers for substance use.

Providers inform clients that triggers or cues are the external people, places, things, and internal emotions and thoughts that can lead to substance use. Triggers can lead the person to crave a substance physically or psychologically and then initiate automatic thoughts (e.g., rationales for use) that justify substance use. Providers work with clients to identify high-risk drinking or substance use situations that often or always lead to problematic substance use. They explore the thoughts, feelings, and behaviors that occur before, during, and after these situations to better understand the external and internal contexts that led to substance use and the consequences of that use. Figure 11.2 lists some common internal and external cues or triggers for substance use.

It may be helpful to identify specific thoughts that the client has when they experience internal and external triggers. Providers conducting an FA can use the three-column thought record (see Chap. 9) for this purpose that identifies: (1) a situation or event; (2) the automatic thoughts triggered by the situation; and (3) the feelings (e.g., anger, sadness, panic) and behaviors (e.g., use) that result from the thoughts. This can be done as an imaginal exercise where the client recounts an experience of a trigger and tries to reimagine the thoughts they had before they engaged in substance use, or as an in vivo exercise they can do in between sessions. Once internal and external triggers that lead to substance use are identified, it is helpful to collaborate with the client to identify ways to avoid external triggers and positive and healthy ways to deal with internal triggers that can replace substance use.

11.4.3 Craving Management

An important way to help people with substance use disorders reduce or eliminate their use and prevent relapse is through helping them manage their cravings (SAMHSA 2012; Marlatt and Gordon 1985; Kadden et al. 2003; Monti et al. 2002; McHugh et al. 2010). A craving is a strong desire and compulsion to use a substance. Cravings are most often triggered by cues associated with using substances. Like waves, cravings generally tend to build in intensity, peak, and then dissipate over the course of 10–15 min. During a craving a person may think of nothing else and believe that the strong urge for substances will only grow rather than dissipate. This fundamental misperception of craving can lead to substance use. People with substance use disorders have difficulty tolerating distress, making decisions, planning, and controlling impulses. These deficits compound the challenges in helping people manage cravings (Kwako et al. 2016). However, cravings are common, and clients who experience them can learn how to manage them in different ways. Cravings also tend to lessen in frequency and severity over time with continued abstinence or reduced use.

Providers can teach clients a number of skills designed to help them manage cravings. First, the functional analysis is used to identify high-risk situations and harmful activities that can trigger cravings and lead to drinking or drug use such as gatherings where alcohol or drugs will be consumed and/or situations where there will be pressure to drink or use substances. The provider and the client work together to identify ways the client can anticipate and avoid those situations and use healthy alternative activities and strategies instead. These activities can be used as a substitute for engaging in activities and situations deemed to be risky, or they can also be relied upon to help the client cope with cravings when they happen. The client and the provider also identify any potential barriers to doing healthier alternatives and brainstorm ways to overcome those barriers. Barriers can include low motivation,

Internal Cues (e.g., Thoughts, Feelings)	External Cues (People, Places, Things, Events)
Stress	Being in the presence of alcohol, drugs, or injection equipment
Depression	Celebrations or holidays
Loneliness	Being with friends or intimate partners that use
Boredom	Before or after sex
Anger	A certain time (e.g., "happy hour," the weekend, or payday)
Anxiety	Having money
Guilt/Shame	Arguments with family
Joy	Remembering the "good old days" of drinking with friends
Excitement	Being by oneself

Fig. 11.2 Common triggers for substance use (based on: Chan Osilla et al. 2016; Kadden et al. 2003; Monti et al. 2002)

problematic thoughts, low confidence, or cost (Chan Osilla et al. 2016; McHugh et al. 2010; Carroll and Kiluk 2017; Marlatt and Gordon 1985).

Activities to manage cravings are numerous. One model is called "urge surfing" or "white knuckling it." This is a *mindfulness-based strategy* in which the person focuses on the urge as it increases in intensity and then dissipates (i.e., like a wave) over time. In this strategy the client notices, without judgment, how the craving feels, thoughts that come to their mind, and how the craving passes in a nonjudgmental way. This strategy can be practiced in session through rehearsal and imaginal exposure approaches. The use of *distraction* is the most common way to manage cravings. When a client identifies that they are experiencing a craving they engage in predetermined activities to distract them from the craving until it passes. There are hundreds of simple activities that can be used to distract from a craving. The provider and the client work together to generate a list of healthy activities the client has done in the past, uses currently, or wants to try out. They can be as simple as taking a walk, calling a friend or sponsor, exercising, listening to music, praying, completing a household chore, or running an errand, to more complex and ongoing activities such as attending a self-help meeting, solving a personal problem, or learning a new language or musical instrument. The key is for clients to: (1) know what cravings are; (2) realize they are common, normal, and temporary; (3) know how to avoid situations that can lead to cravings; (4) recognize when cravings happen; and (5) be prepared to engage in specific healthy alternatives to using when cravings occur.

11.4.4 Coping Skills Training

Psychoeducation Coping skills training begins with psychoeducation about the cognitive behavioral therapy model and how substance use is conceptualized from a CBT perspective. This can be done through handouts that describe the model and then through questioning the client about the thinking patterns that can lead to substance use. As mentioned, the cognitive behavioral model positions substance use as learned behavior that is reinforced over time. Persons who use substances are often triggered by external cues in the environment (e.g., people, places, and things) as well as internal cues such as strong emotions (e.g., anxiety, anger, joy, distress, depression) and irrational thinking patterns (e.g., one drink can't hurt, drinking will take away this pain, I will never be able to do this, I am worthless). A person, when faced with one or more of these triggers, will then be more likely to use substances because this behavior is reinforced over time. The goal of cognitive behavioral therapy is to understand and interrupt these patterns of negative thinking and reinforcement, help the client notice when triggers are present, and give them the coping skills and tools to respond to those triggers in healthy ways (SAMHSA 2012).

Refusal Skills and Assertive Communication Strategies Certain people can represent a significant trigger for substance use. It is important to help clients learn effective communication strategies including assertiveness and drug and alcohol refusal skills when confronted with people who may trigger their use. First, providers work with clients to identify how people can trigger their use through cravings and who those persons may be. This can include friends who the person may have used with in the past (e.g., an old drinking buddy) and who may ask or pressure them to use again, or it may also include family or friends who are overly critical or otherwise cause the person distress that can then lead to cravings and relapse. Second, the provider and the client then work together to identify how the client can utilize assertive communication strategies to avoid use situations, get their needs met, and prevent relapse (Chan Osilla et al. 2016; Carroll and Kiluk 2017; Kadden et al. 2003; Monti et al. 2002; SAMHSA 2012).

Assertive communication involves reviewing three types of communication: Passive, Aggressive, and Assertive. Passive communication strategies involve deferring or withholding one's own emotional needs, opinions, and desires in order to please or not upset another person. In this type of communication strategy, the client assumes they are powerless to change the situation and either withdraws or "goes along" with the other person *sacrificing their own needs and goals, in exchange for respecting the needs of someone else.* Anger, helplessness, shame, and self-loathing are often associated with this type of communication style. Aggressive communication uses strategies such as shouting, expressing anger, hurling insults, arguing, or using threats or violence to express one's thoughts and emotions. *The person using aggressive communication gets what they want through disrespecting the needs of others.* Anger and guilt are often associated with this communication style. Both strategies are rooted in fear, insecurity, and a lack of skills. Both are wholly ineffective and can lead to relapse since helplessness, self-loathing, guilt, and anger are all common internal cues that can lead to drinking or substance use as a coping strategy.

Assertive communication, on the other hand, respects the needs of both parties. In this type of communication style, clients learn how to express their needs in a way that is effective, clear, and respectful to the other person. The style is devoid of negative emotion, is direct, and provides a clear message. Assertive communication uses "I" statements to communicate needs, emotions, thoughts, and desires in a clear, nonjudgmental, and direct way. The use of assertive communication relies on the following steps: (1) identify who the person is who you want to communicate to; (2) use "I" statements to describe and express thoughts and feelings such as, "I feel…" or "I think…"; (3) give a clear request; and (4) provide a statement at the beginning or end that acknowledges the other person's situation and communicates appreciation such as, "I know you're busy" or simply "Thank you."

It is helpful for providers to help clients anticipate situations where they may be approached to drink or use drugs (e.g., being asked to go out to a bar, someone buying them a drink, being offered drugs) and to rehearse and practice refusal skills. Assertive refusal skills include the following: (1) refuse alcohol or substances with a clear and unequivocal "No"; (2) change the subject or suggest an alternative activity; and (3) request a behavior change if the person persists (e.g., please stop asking me, the answer is "no," let's do something else). If the person persists it is advised that the client inform the person that it was good to see them, but that they are going to have to leave and say goodbye. It is not advised for the client to offer excuses or give false information such as, "I don't feel like it," "I have to work in the morning," "I'm not feeling good," or "maybe some other time." This is passive and indirect communication that invites the other person to try to convince or persuade the client to see their side. A clear, firm, and polite "No" combined with a request to change the subject or a behavior change is the best course (Chan Osilla et al. 2016; Carroll and Kiluk 2017; Kadden et al. 2003; Monti et al. 2002; SAMHSA 2012).

Managing Negative Thoughts People with substance use disorders often engage in negative thinking patterns that can lead to anxiety or depression and trigger substance use. Negative self-talk can often include focusing only on negative events or traits (e.g., mistakes, failures, shortcomings, "the bad" in a given situation) and ignoring positive evidence (e.g., refusal to take credit for successes, positive attributes, accomplishments, or see "the good" in a situation). Clients may also "catastrophize" or exaggerate negative attributes and failures and minimize success and positive developments and engage in "all-or-nothing" or "black-and-white" thinking (e.g., things will never improve, I can't do anything right, I'm never going to be able to stop drinking). Negative thinking patterns can trigger substance use directly (e.g., "just one drink won't hurt," "I deserve this drink," or "No one cares about me so I might as well drink") or indirectly by triggering depressed or anxious mood states. It is important to help clients catch and challenge negative self-talk and replace it with more realistic statements combined with a behavior change (Chan Osilla et al. 2016; Carroll and Kiluk 2017; Kadden et al. 2003; Monti et al. 2002;

SAMHSA 2012). Persons with substance use disorders tend to have attributional styles that are internal (it's all my fault), global (I'm completely worthless or a bad person), and stable (I will always be a drunk/addict). They also tend to hold negative expectancies about themselves, others, the world, and the future, and positive expectancies about alcohol or drugs ("I've had a bad day and I need a drink" or "Drinking will solve this problem"). It is important help clients identify and challenge these thinking patterns (SAMHSA 2012).

Thought change records can be used to help clients identify and interrogate negative automatic thoughts and cognitive distortions that lead to distressful emotions and replace them with more realistic thoughts. When using thought change records, clients clearly identify a situation that preceded a drinking or drug-use episode. The client identifies the different thoughts that emerged in their head as the episode unfolded. The provider explores the emotions that each thought produced (e.g., anger, sadness, anxiety) and the subsequent behavior. A "hot thought" is identified that led to the most intense negative emotion and was most likely the thought that resulted in substance use. The client and the provider explore any cognitive distortions and problematic expectancies that may have been operating and then examine the evidence supporting and challenging the thought (see Chap. 9 for more information on this technique). Based on the data that is collected, the provider and the client work together to identify a more realistic way of thinking about what happened that is more balanced, healthy, and positive. This constitutes the replacement thought. The client then identifies a more healthy behavior that could replace drinking or drug use. This exercise could be role-played in-session and could also be used in hypothetical scenarios to plan for the future. The approach can be combined with coping cards that identify negative thought patterns that lead to substance use and that remind the client of more positive ways to think about a situation along with some distraction activities to help avoid relapse.

Seemingly Irrelevant Decisions and Planning for Emergencies It is often the case that relapse occurs as a result of seemingly minor and irrelevant decisions. It is important to help people plan for when cravings may strike and how to evaluate situations with high-risk potential, so they can be avoided if possible. If avoiding the situation is not possible, then it is important for people to anticipate emergencies and plan ahead (Chan Osilla et al. 2016; Kadden et al. 2003; Monti et al. 2002; SAMHSA 2012). This involves two components. First, providers work with clients to play the "what if game" for every seemingly irrelevant decision. For instance, if a client wants to attend a wedding, funeral, reunion, or celebration, the provider may ask a series of "what if" questions—what if you are offered a drink? What if you see X, your old drinking buddy, and he asks if you want to have a drink? What if X is there and starts to criticize you? What if you're in the bathroom and an old friend asks if you want to get high? What if you are handed a glass of champagne during the toast? What if they go to the family reunion and have a fight with a sibling? What if they are asked to go to the afterparty at a bar? What if they are at the grocery store and they bump into a former partner who asks them out for a drink? It is not unreasonable to want to attend a friend's wedding or a family gathering; however, it is precisely these decisions that can leave people unprepared for situations in which they find themselves triggered by external cues. People need to evaluate every decision, assess the risk, and make one of two decisions: (1) to avoid the situation entirely or (2) to not avoid the situation but anticipate and mitigate risk by having a plan. Help clients identify all possible scenarios that may lead to relapse and then help them plan for emergencies. It is a good idea to have clients rehearse what they will say and practice assertive communication and refusal skills through role-plays and reverse the role-plays where they play the other side, so they can see assertive communication in action. Help clients plan for other ways they can cope if they are triggered. Several strategies include: (1) limiting their time at the event; (2) choosing to be seated away from alcohol and away from former drinking partners; (3) making a preemptive announcement that they are not drinking and are the designated driver; (4) going with a supportive friend; (5) rewarding themselves afterward for not drinking with a healthy activity, meal, or buying something nice; or (6) having a friend or sponsor be ready to take your call if you need some support.

It is also useful for people to anticipate unavoidable situation that may trigger a relapse. These might include events that cause stress such as evaluations, planned events, court dates, project deadlines, reunions, anniversaries, deaths, or times of the year (e.g., seasonal, holidays) that may be times of increased emotionality or stress (positive or negative) that could increase cravings. It may be helpful for the person to engage in mitigating actions such as increasing pleasant activities, going to self-help meetings, increasing therapy appointments, and engaging in activities designed to manage emotions such as meditation, eating healthy, mindfulness, exercise, and socializing with healthy and supportive people during these times.

11.4.5 Relapse Prevention

The fourth important component in CBT for substance use disorders is relapse prevention. Relapse prevention includes four elements: (1) building self-efficacy; (2) changing expectancies about substances; (3) managing slips; and (4) developing healthy lifestyles. Relapse prevention strategies rely on the functional analysis by identifying high-risk situations for relapse (Chan Osilla et al. 2016; Carroll and Kiluk 2017; Kadden et al. 2003; Monti et al. 2002; SAMHSA 2012).

Build Self-Efficacy Providers use the FA to help clients understand their cues for cravings and to identify high-risk relapse situations. The provider then helps the client avoid those situations or plan for how to manage those situations and the cravings that result when they occur. Providers can help clients build self-efficacy by encouraging them to slowly expose themselves to situations that may trigger cravings and use the strategies developed in-session to manage high-risk situations. For instance, the provider may encourage the client to attend the wedding of their friend knowing that alcohol will be readily available and former drinking companions will be present. Using strategies and plans developed and rehearsed in-session, clients can then go out and try those strategies in real-world situations. Successful implementation can lead to a more developed sense of self-efficacy. Clients should only engage in these exposure experiences when they feel they are adequately prepared and able to handle the situation competently. They should not engage in activities or situations that are too overwhelming.

Changing Expectancies   Another strategy is to challenge clients' strongly held positive expectancies about alcohol and substance use. Clients holding strong positive expectancies about alcohol and drugs are more prone to relapse than clients who recognize the negative impact alcohol and drugs can have on their physical, emotional, and social health. It is important for providers to explore positive expectancies around drugs and alcohol and to help clients develop more balanced expectancies. This involves gathering evidence that challenges positive expectancies of substance use and that highlights the negative consequences that alcohol and drugs have had on the person's physical and social well-being. Decisional balance exercises as part of motivational interviewing strategies reviewed previously can be useful in exploring expectancies (Miller and Rollnick 2013).

Managing Slips   A third area of relapse prevention is managing slips. Drug and alcohol relapse is the expectation rather than the exception. Clients should be informed that relapse presents an opportunity to learn new strategies and to develop better relapse prevention plans. One problem that clients often experience is when slips (e.g., having a drink, smoking a joint or cigarette) become full-blown relapses due to negative thinking patterns. For instance, a client may have a fight with a spouse or partner that triggers an urge to use. The client may then have one drink. The client then starts to feel powerless over their alcohol use and ashamed that they "failed." These feelings of being out of control may lead to stronger urges to drink and so the person gives up (i.e., Oh, the hell with it!) and drinks to intoxication, having decided that they are incapable of controlling their use. This process is called the *abstinence validation effect* and is a powerful driver of relapse that is rooted in a lack of self-efficacy and negative thinking patterns that include the person thinking that they are a total failure and that their drinking problem is permanent and out of their control.

Providers can help clients manage these situations by helping them to realize that: (1) a "slip" is a normal part of recovery and can be avoided or mitigated; (2) there is wisdom to be learned in analyzing what caused this slip; (3) a slip is not evidence of failure, permanency of the problem, or requires the person to have to "start all over again"; and (4) after a slip it is important to talk about what happened and plan for the future. Providers can help clients avoid slips by planning for emergencies and ensuring that clients have tools at their disposal in case they do have a slip. These tools include: (1) knowing the warning signs of craving and being triggered; (2) having contact information of helpful people whom they can call for support or intervention such as a sponsor, family member or friend, or counselor; and (3) a concrete list of activities to engage in to manage any cravings or slips in order to prevent further relapse (Kadden et al. 2003; Monti et al. 2002; SAMHSA 2012; Marlatt and Gordon 1985).

Developing Healthy Lifestyles The last important area of relapse prevention is ensuring that the person has developed healthier lifestyle habits and activities. The development of these activities leads to a reduction in triggers such as boredom or loneliness and can lead to an increase in positive feeling and self-efficacy. The establishment of solid, healthy daily routines is important. These may include exercise, eating healthy meals, praying or meditation, and managing stress through a balanced lifestyle that has adequate time for work, leisure, and social relationships. The establishment of a network of sober social support is also important. This involves cultivating healthy relationships with friends and family that boost sobriety, letting go of relationships that are risks for relapse, and managing the grief that may accompany letting those people go. Lastly, people can integrate routine professional support to help them become more psychologically healthy such as individual, family, or group therapy as well as self-help and peer support to continue to establish and maintain healthy lifestyles (Marlatt and Gordon 1985).

Case Study 11.3 Ms. Carla Delgado

Carla[3] is a 32-year-old, cisgendered white woman. She has been referred to your outpatient behavioral health treatment team by the courts for assessment and treatment for major depressive disorder and substance abuse. Carla is a bright and engaging individual with a dry sense of humor. Carla likes to be in the outdoors, walking in the park or otherwise being in nature. She has been taking martial arts lessons off and on for 10 years as a release, although she has not trained in the last 2 years. In the past, she has also found yoga to be helpful in clearing her mind and relaxing. She is a voracious reader and enjoys journaling and writing poetry and short stories. She also likes to "dabble" in art, particularly in the use of oil paints and multimedia sculpture when she can afford it. She was an English major at a small liberal arts college. She dropped out in her junior year. She refers to this as, "my biggest mistake. I loved it there. But I can never seem to finish anything." She has dreamed of teaching creative writing or art to high school students, or at a community college someday. At this point she says, "I would like to get a job, move into a safe, affordable apartment, find a partner, and lead a calm, stable life without any drama." In the past year, Carla has lost three jobs due to her substance use. Twice she was fired for not showing up to work due to her substance use, and another time she was fired for being verbally aggressive with other co-workers who criticized her work performance. She currently lives in a studio apartment and is unemployed. Earlier this year she was homeless and staying with various friends. She is currently living on savings and unemployment benefits.

Carla has a history of severe stimulant use disorder, moderate alcohol use disorder, major depressive disorder (recurrent), and she suffers from symptoms of partial

---

[3]All names and other identifiers of this case have been changed to protect privacy and confidentiality.

PTSD (nightmares, intrusive thoughts, negative alteration in cognitions and mood, and hypervigilance). She does not currently meet full diagnostic criteria for PTSD, but these symptoms are present and distressing. Carla is also 20 pounds overweight, has a history of asthma, and is prediabetic. During the initial intake assessment Carla reveals that she recently relapsed after 2 years of sobriety from cocaine. Her relapse was initiated after she lost her last job as a clerk in an art supply store after verbally insulting her supervisor following a poor review. Carla states that after she was fired she went to a local bar and drank to the point of intoxication. After the bar closed she left with a group of friends and used cocaine for the remainder of the night and into the morning. She states that she then went on a cocaine, marijuana, and alcohol binge for the next several days.

> Carla: I have real friends that are close and that support me and love me. And then I have these other friends that I get high with like at the bar. I had cut these friends off while I was sober – but then I went to the bar, had a few and texted them. Big mistake. I only went to the bar to blow off some steam and have a couple of beers. But then I made the mistake of texting one of them because I was afraid to go back home. I was afraid I was going to go home and sulk and mope and get depressed and I just didn't want to do that. I wanted to have some fun. So I texted them they came up and that's when all hell broke lose. I didn't text them to get high…I don't think. I texted them because they are a fun crowd to be with and they won't let you mope around feeling sorry for yourself. I wanted to have a couple more beers and commiserate and laugh and forget. I guess I should have texted my other friends. But I texted, they came, we laughed and then the drugs came out and that's when I should have left – but I wanted to keep going and so first we smoked weed, and then the cocaine comes out and away we went. I guess that's the pattern.

During that binge, she was arrested for getting into a fight in a bar with another patron a few days later. She was arrested and was referred to behavioral health and drug treatment at your agency.

Carla has a history of major depressive disorder and symptoms and PTSD. Carla reports she was sexually abused by her mother's live-in boyfriend when she was 12 for 2 years. She was also physically assaulted when she was 21 in a robbery. That precipitated her taking martial arts lessons. When she is depressed, she often sleeps all day, refuses to see anyone, does not eat, and becomes suicidal. Carla has attempted suicide on two previous occasions. She often drinks and uses cocaine more when she is in a depressed state.

> "When I go through one of those periods my life is blown to pieces, yeah. And then my friends and family have to come and clean it up just like now. And then once it's cleaned up and I think I'm doin' OK, the darkness comes again and I go under. It's like I'm trying to keep my head above water in the darkest, scariest place on earth and there is no one there to save you. It swallows you up." She states, "I just shut myself off from the world. I don't eat. I turn the phone off. I stop showering and I just sit and cry all day when I'm not sleeping. I just can't do anything. Then at night I stay up and think about what a piece of garbage I am. All that goes through my head is: 'Everyone hates me.' 'I can't do anything right.' 'I'd be better off dead.' 'I'm the biggest fuck-up in the whole world.' Like a recording in my head. I get these bouts of nerves too. I feel like I can't breathe and I pace around the house freaking out, smoking, and shaking and worrying about everything. It's not a pretty picture."

Carla states that she began using cocaine when she was 16. By the time she was 19 she was using it every day and needing more and more of it to get high. Once she starts using, it is hard for her to stop. She says, "it takes over my life. I can't think about anything else but getting high. Cocaine helps me feel alive. When I'm depressed, I just want to crawl up and die. All I think about is the abuse and what a piece of crap I am and cocaine always helps lift me out of that. The problem is, once I start, I can't stop."

Carla says that she has always used alcohol since she was 14.

"Alcohol helps me sleep and helps loosen me up. It's cheap and it helps me feel better. It's true that I get a little crazy when I've had too much, but I like the way it makes me feel. I'm not a drunk. I don't drink everyday. Sometimes I don't drink for a couple of weeks. I don't think about it or crave it. I can have one or two and stop. I am not a drunk no matter what my file says. A cocaine addict? Yes. But I'm working on that. I can have a few beers or cocktails and stop whenever I want. It's when I start to use cocaine, or sometimes weed, that things start to spiral. I should be careful, but I don't need to quit drinking. Cocaine is my problem. I need help staying clean from cocaine. I crave it (cocaine) when I feel bad. I crave it when I feel good. When I'm balanced and occupied – I'm OK. When I use it, my life gets really bad. I can't stop myself. I crave it. I'm really tired of this. I need to learn how to avoid it, how to keep it out of my life so I can just get on with it. I have not used it in like almost two months. I'm ready to never use it again. I know how to *get* clean. I need to learn how to *stay* clean. So I can do what I want to do with my life. Can you help me do that?"

Case Analysis Guiding Questions

What is your case conceptualization of Carla based on the information in the vignette?

What symptoms does she experience?

Do Carla's symptoms meet criteria for one or more behavioral health disorders and, if so, which one(s)?

What are 3–5 treatment goals and objectives that would make a good treatment plan for Carla?

What symptoms would you target?

How would you describe the inter-relationship between Carla's depression, cocaine, marijuana, and alcohol use?

What stage of change is Carla in with regard to her cocaine use? Alcohol use? Depressive symptoms?

Discuss the treatment strategies that would be appropriate for Carla's substance use and depressive symptoms—particularly in regard to helping her maintain sobriety from cocaine use. What interventions would be helpful?

How might these interventions be sequenced?

What strengths and resources does Carla have that she can rely on to solve her problems?

What kind of situations can be used to help Carla address her fears and depressive symptoms?

What is your assessment of Carla's risks for suicide and how will you respond to this risk assessment?

11.5 Summary and Conclusions

Substance use disorders exert a tremendous toll on physical and behavioral health. Three important approaches to treating substance use in integrated behavioral health settings are harm reduction, motivational interviewing, and cognitive behavioral therapy. These approaches are brief and highly adaptable to a range of health and behavioral health settings. They also span the stages of change. Knowing when to deploy these interventions is vital to effective treatment. The global COVID-19 pandemic has changed how health care is practiced. To mitigate the risk of spreading the virus, health and behavioral health settings are increasingly turning toward virtual telehealth and computer/web/app-mediated approaches. Fortunately, substance abuse treatment has been exploring these approaches for several years. For instance, virtual interventions for screening, brief intervention, and relapse prevention, including internet or web-based approaches (Boumparis et al. 2017), computerized brief interventions (Gryczynski et al. 2015), and smartphone applications (Gustafson et al. 2014), are showing promise. Computerized versions of CBT (e.g., CBT4CBT), a virtual CBT treatment with minimal clinical interaction or monitoring for substance abuse treatment, have shown the approach to be comparable to face-to-face, professionally delivered CBT. The approach was efficacious, durable, and had high satisfaction and low dropout rates compared to standard treatment (Kiluk et al. 2016, 2018). These approaches as well as other innovations, such as delivery of opioid substitute medication and clean injecting equipment and virtual self-help meetings, are expected to grow in use in future years, perhaps transforming how we deliver behavioral health care. Regardless, effective substance abuse treatment will continue to be predicated on relationships that are warm, nonjudgmental, and accepting. These relationships enhance treatment engagement and retention, which is associated with better outcomes and more durable recoveries.

References

Adams, J. M. (2018). Increasing naloxone awareness and use: The role of health care practitioners. *JAMA, 319*(20), 2073–2074. https://doi.org/10.1001/jama.2018.4867.

American Psychiatric Association. (2013). *Diagnostic and Statistical Manual of Mental Disorders* (DSM-5) (5th ed.). Arlington: American Psychiatric Association.

Aspinall, E. J., Nambiar, D., Goldberg, D. J., Hickman, M., Weir, A., Van Velzen, E., Palmateer, N., Doyle, J. S., Hellard, M. E., & Hutchinson, S. J. (2014). Are needle and syringe programmes associated with a reduction in HIV transmission among people who inject drugs: A systematic review and meta-analysis. *International Journal of Epidemiology, 43*(1), 235–248. https://doi.org/10.1093/ije/dyt243.

Boumparis, N., Karyotaki, E., Schaub, M. P., Cuijpers, P., & Riper, H. (2017). Internet interventions for adult illicit substance users: A meta-analysis. *Addiction, 112*(9), 1521–1532. https://doi.org/10.1111/add.13819.

Broyles, L. M., Binswanger, I. A., Jenkins, J. A., Finnell, D. S., Faseru, B., Cavaiola, A., Pugatch, M., & Gordon, A. J. (2014). Confronting inadvertent stigma and pejorative language in addiction scholarship: A recognition and response. *Substance Abuse, 35*(3), 217–221. https://doi. org/10.1080/08897077.2014.930372.

Busch, S. H., Fiellin, D. A., Chawarski, M. C., Owens, P. H., Pantalon, M. V., Hawk, K., Bernstein, S. L., O'Connor, P. G., & D'Onofrio, G. (2017). Cost-effectiveness of emergency department-initiated treatment for opioid dependence. *Addiction, 112*(11), 2002–2010. https://doi. org/10.1111/add.13900.

Carroll, K. M., & Kiluk, B. D. (2017). Cognitive behavioral interventions for alcohol and drug use disorders: Through the stage model and back again. *Psychology of Addictive Behaviors: Journal of the Society of Psychologists in Addictive Behaviors, 31*(8), 847–861. https://doi. org/10.1037/adb0000311.

Centers for Disease Control and Prevention (CDC). (2020). *Wide-ranging online data for epidemiologic research (WONDER)*. Atlanta: CDC, National Center for Health Statistics; 2020. Available at http://wonder.cdc.gov

Chan Osilla, K., D'Amico, E. J., Lind, M., Ober, A. J., Watkins, K. E. (2016). *Brief treatment for substance use disorders: A guide for behavioral health providers*. Santa Monica, CA: RAND Corporation. Retrieved on April 28, 2020 at: https://www.rand.org/pubs/tools/TL147.html

Csete, J., Kamarulzaman, A., Kazatchkine, M., Altice, F., Balicki, M., Buxton, J., Cepeda, J., Comfort, M., Goosby, E., Goulão, J., Hart, C., Kerr, T., Lajous, A. M., Lewis, S., Martin, N., Mejía, D., Camacho, A., Mathieson, D., Obot, I., Ogunrombi, A., et al. (2016). Public health and international drug policy. *Lancet, 387*(10026), 1427–1480. https://doi.org/10.1016/ S0140-6736(16)00619-X.

Darker, C. D., Sweeney, B. P., Barry, J. M., Farrell, M. F., & Donnelly-Swift, E. (2015). Psychosocial interventions for benzodiazepine harmful use, abuse or dependence. *Cochrane Database of Systematic Reviews, 5*, CD009652.

Denis-Lalonde, D., Lind, C., & Estefan, A. (2019). Beyond the buzzword: A concept analysis of harm reduction. *Research and Theory for Nursing Practice, 33*(4), 310–323. https://doi. org/10.1891/1541-6577.33.4.310.

Des Jarlais, D. C. (1995). Harm reduction—A framework for incorporating science into drug policy. *American Journal of Public Health, 85*, 10–12.

Des Jarlais, D. C. (2017). Harm reduction in the USA: The research perspective and an archive to David purchase. *Harm Reduction Journal, 14*(1), 51. https://doi.org/10.1186/ s12954-017-0178-6.

Dieterich, M., Irving, C. B., Bergman, H., Khokhar, M. A., Park, B., & Marshall, M. (2017). Intensive case management for severe mental illness. *The Cochrane Database of Systematic Reviews*. https://doi.org/10.1002/14651858.CD007906.pub3.

D'Onofrio, G., O'Connor, P. G., Pantalon, M. V., Chawarski, M. C., Busch, S. H., Owens, P. H., Bernstein, S. L., & Fiellin, D. A. (2015). Emergency department-initiated buprenorphine/naloxone treatment for opioid dependence: A randomized clinical trial. *JAMA, 313*(16), 1636–1644. https://doi.org/10.1001/jama.2015.3474.

Gates, P. J., Sabioni, P., Copeland, J., Le Foll, B., & Gowing, L. (2016). Psychosocial interventions for cannabis use disorder. *Cochrane Database of Systematic Reviews, 5*, CD005336. https:// doi.org/10.1002/14651858.CD005336.pub4.

Gryczynski, J., Mitchell, S. G., Gonzales, A., Moseley, A., Peterson, T. R., Ondersma, S. J., O'Grady, K. E., & Schwartz, R. P. (2015). A randomized trial of computerized vs. in-person brief intervention for illicit drug use in primary care: Outcomes through 12 months. *Journal of Substance Abuse Treatment, 50*, 3–10. https://doi.org/10.1016/j.jsat.2014.09.002.

Gustafson, D. H., McTavish, F. M., Chih, M. Y., Atwood, A. K., Johnson, R. A., Boyle, M. G., Levy, M. S., Driscoll, H., Chisholm, S. M., Dillenburg, L., Isham, A., & Shah, D. (2014). A smartphone application to support recovery from alcoholism: A randomized clinical trial. *JAMA Psychiatry, 71*(5), 566–572. https://doi.org/10.1001/jamapsychiatry.2013.4642.

Hawk, M., Coulter, R., Egan, J. E., Fisk, S., Reuel Friedman, M., Tula, M., & Kinsky, S. (2017). Harm reduction principles for healthcare settings. Harm reduction journal, 14(1), 70. https:// doi.org/10.1186/s12954-017-0196-4

Harm Reduction International. (2020). *What is harm reduction?* Retrieved from https://www.hri.global/what-is-harm-reduction on April 1, 2020.

Hawk, K., & D'Onofrio, G. (2018). Emergency department screening and intervention for substance use disorders. *Addiction Science and Clinical Practice, 13*, 18. https://doi.org/10.1186/s13722-018-0117-1.

Hawk, M., & Davis, D. (2012). The effects of a harm reduction housing program on the viral loads of homeless individuals living with HIV/AIDS. *AIDS Care, 24*(5), 577–582. https://doi.org/10.1080/09540121.2011.630352.

Humeniuk, R. E., Henry-Edwards, S., Ali, R. L., Poznyak, V., & Monteiro, M. (2010b). *The ASSIST-linked brief intervention for hazardous and harmful substance use: Manual for use in primary care.* Geneva: World Health Organization.

Kadden, R., Carroll, K., Donovan, D., Cooney, N., Monti, P., Abrams, D., Litt, M., & Hester, R. (2003). *Cognitive behavioral coping skills therapy manual. A clinical research guide for therapists treating individuals with alcohol abuse and dependence.* National Institute on alcohol and alcoholism: Project MATCH monograph series volume 3. NIH Publications No. 94-3724.

Karamouzian, M., Dohoo, C., Forsting, S., McNeil, R., Kerr, T., & Lysyshyn, M. (2018). Evaluation of a fentanyl drug checking service for clients of a supervised injection facility, Vancouver, Canada. *Harm Reduction Journal, 15*(1), 46. https://doi.org/10.1186/s12954-018-0252-8.

Kennedy, M. C., Hayashi, K., Milloy, M. J., Wood, E., & Kerr, T. (2019). Supervised injection facility use and all-cause mortality among people who inject drugs in Vancouver, Canada: A cohort study. *PLoS Medicine, 16*(11), e1002964. https://doi.org/10.1371/journal.pmed.1002964.

Kerr, T., Small, W., Buchner, C., Zhang, R., Li, K., Montaner, J., & Wood, E. (2010). Syringe sharing and HIV incidence among injection drug users and increased access to sterile syringes. *American Journal of Public Health, 100*(8), 1449–1453. https://doi.org/10.2105/AJPH.2009.178467.

Kiluk, B. D., Devore, K. A., Buck, M. B., Nich, C., Frankforter, T. L., LaPaglia, D. M., Yates, B. T., Gordon, M. A., & Carroll, K. M. (2016). Randomized trial of computerized cognitive behavioral therapy for alcohol use disorders: Efficacy as a virtual stand-alone and treatment add-on compared with standard outpatient treatment. *Alcoholism, Clinical and Experimental Research, 40*(9), 1991–2000. https://doi.org/10.1111/acer.13162.

Kiluk, B. D., Nich, C., Buck, M. B., Devore, K. A., Frankforter, T. L., LaPaglia, D. M., Muvvala, S. B., & Carroll, K. M. (2018). Randomized clinical trial of computerized and clinician-delivered CBT in comparison with standard outpatient treatment for substance use disorders: Primary within-treatment and follow-up outcomes. *The American Journal of Psychiatry, 175*(9), 853–863. https://doi.org/10.1176/appi.ajp.2018.17090978.

Koob, G. F. (2017). The dark side of addiction: The Horsley Gantt to Joseph Brady connection. *The Journal of Nervous and Mental Disease, 205*(4), 270–272. https://doi.org/10.1097/NMD.0000000000000551.

Krieger, M. S., Goedel, W. C., Buxton, J. A., Lysyshyn, M., Bernstein, E., Sherman, S. G., Rich, J. D., Hadland, S. E., Green, T. C., & Marshall, B. D. L. (2018). Use of rapid fentanyl test strips among young adults who use drugs. *International Journal of Drug Policy, 61*, 52–58. https://doi.org/10.1016/j.drugpo.2018.09.009. Epub 2018 Oct 18.

Kwako, L. E., Momenan, R., Litten, R. Z., Koob, G. F., & Goldman, D. (2016). Addictions neuroclinical assessment: A neuroscience-based framework for addictive disorders. *Biological Psychiatry, 80*(3), 179–189. https://doi.org/10.1016/j.biopsych.2015.10.024.

Larimer, M. E., Malone, D. K., Garner, M. D., Atkins, D. C., Burlingham, B., Lonczak, H. S., Tanzer, K., Ginzler, J., Clifasefi, S. L., Hobson, W. G., & Marlatt, G. A. (2009). Health care and public service use and costs before and after provision of housing for chronically homeless persons with severe alcohol problems. *JAMA, 301*(13), 1349–1357. https://doi.org/10.1001/jama.2009.414.

Liebschutz, J. M., Crooks, D., Herman, D., Anderson, B., Tsui, J., Meshesha, L. Z., Dossabhoy, S., & Stein, M. (2014). Buprenorphine treatment for hospitalized, opioid-dependent patients: A randomized clinical trial. *JAMA Internal Medicine, 174*(8), 1369–1376. https://doi.org/10.1001/jamainternmed.2014.2556.

MacArthur, G. J., Minozzi, S., Martin, N., Vickerman, P., Deren, S., Bruneau, J., Degenhardt, L., & Hickman, M. (2012). Opiate substitution treatment and HIV transmission in people who inject drugs: Systematic review and meta-analysis. *BMJ, 345*, e5945. https://doi.org/10.1136/bmj.e5945.

MacArthur, G. J., van Velzen, E., Palmateer, N., Kimber, J., Pharris, A., Hope, V., Taylor, A., Roy, K., Aspinall, E., Goldberg, D., Rhodes, T., Hedrich, D., Salminen, M., Hickman, M., & Hutchinson, S. J. (2014). Interventions to prevent HIV and hepatitis C in people who inject drugs: A review of reviews to assess evidence of effectiveness. *The International Journal on Drug Policy, 25*(1), 34–52. https://doi.org/10.1016/j.drugpo.2013.07.001.

Magill, M., & Ray, L. A. (2009). Cognitive-behavioral treatment with adult alcohol and illicit drug users: A meta-analysis of randomized controlled trials. *Journal of Studies on Alcohol and Drugs, 70*(4), 516–527.

Magill, M., Ray, L., Kiluk, B., Hoadley, A., Berstein, M., Tonigan, J. S., & Carroll, K. (2019). A meta-analysis of cognitive-behavioral therapy for alcohol and drug use disorders: Treatment efficacy by contrast condition. *Journal of Consulting and Clinical Psychology, 87*(12), 1093–1105.

Mancini, M. A., & Linhorst, D. M. (2010). Harm reduction in community mental health settings. *Journal of Social Work in Disability & Rehabilitation, 9*, 130–147.

Mancini, M. A., & Wyrick-Waugh, W. (2013). Consumer and practitioner perceptions of the harm reduction approach in a community mental health setting. *Community Mental Health Journal, 49*(1), 14–24.

Mancini, M. A., Hardiman, E. R., & Eversman, M. H. (2008a). A review of the compatibility of harm reduction and recovery-oriented best practices for dual disorders. *Best Practices in Mental Health: An International Journal, 4*(2), 99–113.

Mancini, M. A., Linhorst, D. M., Broderick, F., & Bayliff, S. (2008b). Challenges to implementing the harm reduction approach. *Journal of Social Work Practice in the Addictions, 8*(3), 380–408.

Marlatt, G. A. (1996). Harm reduction: Come as you are. *Addictive Behavior, 21*, 779–788.

Marlatt, G. A., & Gordon, J. R. (1985). *Relapse prevention: Maintenance strategies in the treatment of addictive behaviors*. New York: Guilford Press.

Mate, G. (2010). *In the realm of hungry ghosts*. Berkley: North Atlantic Books.

McHugh, R. K., Hearon, B. A., & Otto, M. W. (2010). Cognitive-behavioral therapy for substance use disorders. *Psychiatric Clinics of North America, 33*(3), 511–525. https://doi.org/10.1016/j.psc.2010.04.012.

Miller, W. R., & Rollnick, S. (2002). *Motivational interviewing: Preparing people for change* (2nd ed.). New York: Guilford Press.

Miller, W. R., & Rollnick, S. (2013). *Motivational interviewing: Preparing people for change* (3rd ed.). New York: Guilford Press.

Milloy, M. J., & Wood, E. (2009). Emerging role of supervised injecting facilities in human immunodeficiency virus prevention. *Addiction, 104*(4), 620–621. https://doi.org/10.1111/j.1360-0443.2009.02541.x.

Monti, P., Kadden, R., Rohsenow, D., Cooney, N., & Abrams, D. (2002). *Treating alcohol dependence: A coping skills training guide* (2nd ed.). New York: Guildford Press.

Mueser, K. T., Noordsy, D. L., Drake, R. E., & Fox, L. (2003). *Integrated treatment for dual disorders: A guide to effective practice*. New York: Guilford Press.

Naar, S., & Safren, S. A. (2017). *Motivational interviewing and CBT: Combining strategies for maximum effectiveness*. New York: Guilford Press.

Olsen, Y., & Sharfstein, J. M. (2014). Confronting the stigma of opioid use disorder--and its treatment. *JAMA, 311*(14), 1393–1394. https://doi.org/10.1001/jama.2014.2147.

Pinkerton, S. D. (2011). How many HIV infections are prevented by Vancouver Canada's supervised injection facility? *The International Journal on Drug Policy, 22*(3), 179–183. https://doi.org/10.1016/j.drugpo.2011.03.003.

Potier, C., Laprévote, V., Dubois-Arber, F., Cottencin, O., & Rolland, B. (2014). Supervised injection services: What has been demonstrated? A systematic literature review. *Drug and Alcohol Dependence, 145*, 48–68. https://doi.org/10.1016/j.drugalcdep.2014.10.012.

Prochaska, J. A., DiClemente, C. C., & Norcross, J. C. (1992). In search of how people change: Applications to addictive behaviour. *American Psychologist, 47*, 1102–1114.

Salyers, M. P., Stull, L., & Tsemberis, S. (2013). Assertive community treatment and recovery. In V. L. Vandiver (Ed.), *Best practices in community mental health* (pp. 103–115). Lyceum Books: Chicago.

Sharma, M., Lamba, W., Cauderella, A., Guimond, T. H., & Bayoumi, A. M. (2017). Harm reduction in hospitals. *Harm Reduction Journal, 14*(1), 32. https://doi.org/10.1186/s12954-017-0163-0.

Strathdee, S. A., Ricketts, E. P., Huettner, S., Cornelius, L., Bishai, D., Havens, J. R., Beilenson, P., Rapp, C., Lloyd, J. J., & Latkin, C. A. (2006). Facilitating entry into drug treatment among injection drug users referred from a needle exchange program: Results from a community-based behavioral intervention trial. *Drug and Alcohol Dependence, 83*, 225–232.

Substance Abuse and Mental Health Services Administration. (1999, 2012). *Center for Substance Abuse Treatment. Brief interventions and brief therapies for substance abuse.* Treatment Improvement Protocol (TIP) Series, No. 34. HHS Publication No. (SMA) 12-3952. Rockville, MD.

Substance Abuse and Mental Health Services Administration (SAMHSA). (1999). *Center for Substance Abuse Treatment. Enhancing motivation for change in substance abuse treatment.* Treatment improvement protocol (TIP) Series, No. 35. HHS Publication No. (SMA) 12-4212. Rockville, MD.

Substance Abuse and Mental Health Services Administration (SAMHSA). (2019). *Key substance use and mental health indicators in the United States: Results from the 2018 National Survey on Drug Use and Health* (HHS Publication No. PEP19-5068, NSDUH Series H-54). Rockville: Center for Behavioral Health Statistics and Quality, Substance Abuse and Mental Health Services Administration. Retrieved from https://www.samhsa.gov/data/

Tsemberis, S., Gulcur, L., & Nakae, M. (2004). Housing first, consumer choice, and harm reduction for homeless individuals with a dual diagnosis. *American Journal of Public Health, 94*(4), 651–656. https://doi.org/10.2105/ajph.94.4.651.

Tsui, J. I., Evans, J. L., Lum, P. J., Hahn, J. A., & Page, K. (2014). Association of opioid agonist therapy with lower incidence of hepatitis C virus infection in young adult injection drug users. *JAMA Internal Medicine, 174*(12), 1974–1981. https://doi.org/10.1001/jamainternmed.2014.5416.

Turner, K. M., Hutchinson, S., Vickerman, P., Hope, V., Craine, N., Palmateer, N., May, M., Taylor, A., De Angelis, D., Cameron, S., Parry, J., Lyons, M., Goldberg, D., Allen, E., & Hickman, M. (2011). The impact of needle and syringe provision and opiate substitution therapy on the incidence of hepatitis C virus in injecting drug users: Pooling of UK evidence. *Addiction, 106*(11), 1978–1988. https://doi.org/10.1111/j.1360-0443.2011.03515.x.

Watkins, K. E., Ober, A. J., Lamp, K., Lind, M., Setodji, C., Osilla, K. C., Hunter, S. B., McCullough, C. M., Becker, K., Iyiewuare, P. O., Diamant, A., Heinzerling, K., & Pincus, H. A. (2017). Collaborative care for opioid and alcohol use disorders in primary care: The SUMMIT randomized clinical trial. *JAMA Internal Medicine, 177*(10), 1480–1488. https://doi.org/10.1001/jamainternmed.2017.3947.

Wilson, D. P., Donald, B., Shattock, A. J., Wilson, D., & Fraser-Hurt, N. (2015). The cost-effectiveness of harm reduction. *The International Journal on Drug Policy, 26*(Suppl 1), S5–S11. https://doi.org/10.1016/j.drugpo.2014.11.007.

Wilson, N., Kariisa, M., Seth, P., Smith, H., 4th, & Davis, N. L. (2020). Drug and opioid-involved overdose deaths – United States, 2017–2018. *MMWR. Morbidity and Mortality Weekly Report, 69*(11), 290–297. https://doi.org/10.15585/mmwr.mm6911a4.

Wodak, A., & Cooney, A. (2004). *Effectiveness of sterile needle and syringe programming in reducing HIV/AIDS among injecting drug users.* Geneva: World Health Organization.

Wodak, A., & Maher, L. (2010). The effectiveness of harm reduction in preventing HIV among injecting drug users. *New South Wales Public Health Bull, 21*, 69–73.

Index

A

Absolutistic (all-or-nothing) thinking, 278
Act "As if" exercise, 286
Action stage, 73
Activity monitor, 284
Activity schedule, 284–286
Adjustment disorders, 242, 257, 260
Adverse childhood experiences (ACEs), 25, 97
  COPD, 197
  definition, 194
  DSM-5, 194
  health impacts, 194
  household events, 197
  HPA, 198
  interpersonal violence, 197
  longitudinal study, 197
  prevalence, 198
  toxic/traumatic, 197
Affirmations, 354
Affordable Care Act (ACA), 12, 166
Agenda-setting, 280
Agoraphobia, 257, 259, 291
Alcohol, 317, 318
Alcohol dependence (AD), 321
Alcohol use disorder (AUD), 321
Alcohol use disorder identification test
  (AUDIT), 96, 321
Alcohol, Smoking, and Substance Involvement
  Screening Test (ASSIST), 322
Ambivalence, 71
American Psychiatric Association, 248
Amyotrophic lateral sclerosis (ALS), 105
Anger management skills, 302
Antidepressants, 247
Antipsychotic medications, 145

Antisocial and borderline personality
  disorder, 158
Antisocial personality disorders (ASPD), 158
Anxiety, 86, 90, 94, 95, 97, 99, 102, 104, 105
  behavioral health disorders, 254
  behavioral health settings, 237
  behavioral/mental avoidance, 252
  diagnostic criteria, 252, 257–258
  experience, fear/nervousness, 252
  GAD-7, 254
  medical and social comorbidities, 237
  OCD, 254
  pathological, 252
  periods, 308
  physical health disorders, 254
  screening, 254
  social determinants of, 237
  social gatherings, 261
  social situations, fear, 262
  suicidal thoughts, 262
  symptoms, 254, 262
Anxiety disorders, 26, 30, 32, 158
Anxious breathing, 288
Arbitrary inference, 277
Ask Suicide-Screening Questions
  questionnaire (ASQ), 106
Assertive communication, 367–369
Assertiveness skills, 301, 302
Assessment
  areas, 88
  behavioral health, 102
  components, 87
  environmental strength, 93
  family history, 101
  interpersonal relationships, 92

© Springer Nature Switzerland AG 2021
M. A. Mancini, *Integrated Behavioral Health Practice*,
https://doi.org/10.1007/978-3-030-59659-0

Lightning Source UK Ltd.
Milton Keynes UK
UKHW050405190822
407458UK00007B/13